SECOND EDITION

Managing Oral Anticoagulation Therapy

Clinical and Operational Guidelines

Editors:

Jack E. Ansell, MD
Professor of Medicine
Vice Chairman for Clinical Affairs
Department of Medicine
Boston University School of Medicine

Lynn B. Oertel, MS, ANP, CACP
Clinical Nurse Specialist,
  Anticoagulation Management Services
Massachusetts General Hospital

Ann K. Wittkowsky, PharmD, CACP
Director, Anticoagulation Services
University of Washington Medical Center
Clinical Professor
University of Washington School
  of Pharmacy

Wolters Kluwer Health | Facts & Comparisons

The author has made every effort to ensure the accuracy of the information herein. However, appropriate information sources should be consulted, especially for new or unfamiliar procedures. It is the responsibility of every practitioner to evaluate the appropriateness of a particular opinion in the context of actual clinical situations and with due consideration to new developments. The authors, editors, and the publisher cannot be held responsible for any typographical or other errors found in this manual.

Wolters Kluwer Health
77 Westport Plaza
Suite 450
St. Louis, MO 63146-3125

Orders and Customer Service: (800) 223-0554

ISBN-10: 1-57439-210-7
ISBN-13: 978-1-57439-210-4

Printed in the United States of America

09 08 07   2 3 4

Contents

For a detailed listing of chapter contents,
please see the first page of each part.

Contributing Authors

Barbara M. Alving, MD, MACP
Deputy Director
Division of Blood Diseases and Resources
The National Heart, Lung, and Blood Institute
National Institutes of Health
Bethesda, Maryland

David R. Anderson, MD, FRCP
Professor of Medicine
Queen Elizabeth II Health Sciences Centre
Dalhousie University
Halifax, Nova Scotia, Canada

Maureen Andrew, MD*
Professor of Pediatrics
Department of Pediatrics
Hamilton Civic Hospitals Research Centre
Hamilton, Ontario, Canada
Children's Hospital at Chedoke McMaster
Hospital for Sick Children
Toronto, Ontario, Canada

Jack E. Ansell, MD
Professor of Medicine
Vice Chairman for Clinical Affairs
Department of Medicine
Boston University School of Medicine
Boston, Massachusetts

Julia H. Arnsten, MD, MPH
Assistant Professor of Medicine
Assistant Professor of Medicine and Epidemiology
Montefiore Medical Center
Albert Einstein College of Medicine
Bronx, New York

Shannon M. Bates, MDCM, FRCP(C)
Assistant Professor
Department of Medicine
McMaster University
Hamilton Civic Hospitals Research Centre
Hamilton, Ontario, Canada

Kenneth A. Bauer, MD
Associate Professor
Department of Medicine
Harvard Medical School
Boston, Massachusetts

Richard C. Becker, MD
Professor of Medicine
Director, Cardiovascular Thrombosis Research Center
University of Massachusetts Medical Center
Worcester, Massachusetts

Rebecca J. Beyth, MD
Assistant Professor of Medicine
Baylor College of Medicine
Department of Medicine
Houston Veterans Administration Medical Center
Houston, Texas

Robert D. Bona, MD
Professor of Medicine
Associate Director, Cancer Center
University of Connecticut Health Center
Farmington, Connecticut

W.G. Mimi Breukink-Engbers, MD
Public Health Physician
Managing and Medical Director
East Netherlands Anticoagulation Center ASCON
Lichtenvoorde, Netherlands

*deceased

Linda Barna Cler, MS, MT(ASCP)SH
Medical Technologist
Hematology/Coagulation
St. John's Health System
Anderson, Indiana

Janet Hiatt Dailey, PharmD
Professor, Department of Pharmacy Practice
University of Florida College of Pharmacy
Gainesville, Florida

Nichola Davis, MD
Assistant Professor of Medicine
Internal Medicine Department
Albert Einstein College of Medicine
Montefiore Medical Center
Bronx, New York

Barbara Delmore, RN, MA
Department of Medical Affairs and Nursing
New York University Medical Center
New York, New York

Jeffrey S. Ginsberg, MD, FRCP(C)
Professor of Medicine
Department of Medicine
McMaster University, faculty of Health Services
Hamilton, Ontario, Canada

Scott H. Goodnight, MD
Professor of Medicine and Pathology
Oregon Health and Science University
Portland, Oregon

Philip Hansten, PharmD
Professor of Pharmacy
School of Pharmacy
University of Washington
Seattle, Washington

Amy D. Hickey, RN, BSN, MA
Thromboembolic Research Nurse
St. Francis Hospital and Medical Center
Section of Hematology/Oncology
Department of Medicine
Hartford, Connecticut

Russell D. Hull, MBBS, MSc
Professor of Medicine
University of Calgary
Calgary, Alberta, Canada

Alan K. Jacobson, MD, FACC
Loma Linda Veterans Administration Center
Loma Linda, California

Clive Kearon, MD, MRCP(I), FRCP(C), PhD
Associate Professor of Medicine
Department of Medicine
McMaster University
Hamilton, Ontario, Canada

Michael Leaker, MD, FRCPC
Assistant Professor of Pediatrics
University of Western Ontario
London, Ontario, Canada

Katharine E. Leaning, MD
Staff Physician
Lucile Packard Children's Hospital at Stanford
Palo Alto, California

Sally Loken, MS, APRN
Primary Care Nurse Practitioner
Veterans Administration
Salt Lake City Health Care Administration
Salt Lake City, Utah

Velma Marzinotto, BScN
Clinical Research Monitor, RN
Research Institute, Hospital for Sick Children
Toronto, Ontario, Canada

Patricia Massicotte, MD, MSc, FRCPC
Director of Clinical Thrombosis Program
Department of Hematology/Oncology
The Hospital for Sick Children
Toronto, Ontario, Canada

David B. Matchar, MD
Director and Professor of Medicine
Center for Clinical Health Policy Research
Duke University Medical Center
Durham, North Carolina

William P. McCormick, JD, B.S. Pharmacy, RPh
General Counsel
CuraScript Pharmacy, Inc.
Orlando, Florida

Dennis Mungall, PharmD
Director, Virtual Education
Associate Professor of Pharmacy Practice
College of Pharmacy
Ohio State University
Columbus, Ohio

Cheryl Nadeau, RN, MS, FNP-CS, CACP
Anticoagulation Management Service
New York University Medical Center
New York, New York

Jennifer L. Wilson Norton, RPh, MBA
Director of Pharmacy and Anticoagulation Services
The Everett Clinic
Everett, Washington

Lynn B. Oertel, MS, ANP
Clinical Research, Stroke Service
Department of Neurology
Massachusetts General Hospital
Boston, Massachusetts

Gaultiero Palareti, MD
Professor in Cardiology
Head of Angiology Department
University Hospital S. Orsolo-Malpighi
Bologna, Italy

Graham F. Pineo, MD
Professor of Medicine and Oncology
University of Calgary
Department of Medicine and Oncology
Calgary, Alberta, Canada

Paul Radensky, MD, JD
Partner, Health Law Department
McDermott Will and Emery
Miami, Florida

Eileen M. Ryan, RN, MS, MPH
Risk Management Consultant (Retired)
Harwich, Massachusetts

Gregory P. Samsa, PhD
Associate Professor
Department of Biometry and Bioinformatics
Duke University Medical Center
Durham, North Carolina

Daniel E. Singer, MD
Professor of Medicine
Harvard Medical School
Boston, Massachusetts

Christine A. Sorkness, PharmD
Professor of Pharmacy and Medicine
University of Wisconsin—Madison
Director, Anticoagulation Clinics
William S. Middleton Veterans Administration Hospital
Madison, Wisconsin

Frederick Spencer, MD
Assistant Professor of Medicine
Associate Director Coronary Care and Anticoagulation
    Clinic
Medical Director, Cardiac Rehabilitation
University of Massachusetts Medical School
Worcester, Masschusetts

Orsula Voltis Thomas, PharmD, MBA
Vice President and Chief Marketing Officer
ExcelleRx, Inc.
Philadelphia, Pennsylvania

Douglas A. Triplett, MD
Vice President and Director
Department of Medical Education
Ball Memorial Hospital
Director, Midwest Hemostasis and Thrombosis
    Laboratories
Muncie, Indiana

Armando Tripodi, MD
Department of Internal Medicine
University and IRCCS Maggiore Hospital
Milano, Italy

**Gordon J. Vanscoy, PharmD, MBA, CACP, BS Pharm,
    RPh**
Assistant Dean for Managed Care and Associate
    Professor
Department of Pharmaceutical Services
University of Pittsburgh School of Pharmacy
Pittsburgh, Pennsylvania

Donna M. Wallace, RN, BS, MS
Nursing Instructor
New England Technical Institute
New Britain, Connecticut

Robert T. Weibert, PharmD
Clinical Professor
University of California San Francisco School of
    Pharmacy
San Francisco, California
Anticoagulation Clinic Director
University of California San Diego Medical Center
San Diego, California

Kari A. Wieland, PharmD, CACP
Clinical Pharmacy Specialist
Medication Use Management
Virginia Mason Medical Center
Clinical Assistant Professor
School of Pharmacy
University of Washington
Seattle, Washington

Ann K. Wittkowsky, PharmD, CACP
Director, Anticoagulation Services
University of Washington Medical Center
Clinical Professor
University of Washington School of Pharmacy
Seattle, Washington

Jeffrey I. Zwicker, MD
Clinical Fellow
Hematology–Oncology
Beth Israel Deaconess Medical Center
Boston, Massachusetts

Preface

It is with great excitement and enthusiasm that we present the publication of the second edition of *Managing Oral Anticoagulation Therapy: Clinical and Operational Guidelines*. This has been one of the most rewarding projects of our careers. The response from health care providers has been overwhelming. As educators, particularly in health care, there is no greater reward than to see the fruits of our efforts translated into improved clinical outcomes for our patients. By providing the resources and information needed to enhance the management of anticoagulation therapy, we believe health care practitioners and patients have benefited substantially.

Oral anticoagulation therapy is a growth industry. According to recent statistics, warfarin is the fifteenth most prescribed drug in the United States, and the third most prescribed cardiovascular agent. Anticoagulation management services have also flourished. Although there are no formal statistics, the Anticoagulation Forum (a national network of anticoagulation clinics) has over 1,100 clinics on its roster, and there may be well over 2,000 such programs in the United States.

Since its publication in 1997, *Managing Oral Anticoagulation Therapy* has had four supplements containing revisions and updates of approximately half of the chapters with additional chapters added as the need arose. The current text contains much more than its original publication. With the second edition, we have continued this process of revision as new studies emerge and guidelines evolve. Some chapters have been deleted, others added, and others consolidated. We have added a stronger international perspective by asking our colleagues from Europe to provide an overview of how anticoagulation therapy is managed in their countries. The manual still contains a large number of practical templates and tools useful for managing oral anticoagulation. Lastly, the chapters and pages have been renumbered in a less confusing format to help the reader locate topics of interest more readily.

Although the coumarin derivatives have been the mainstay of oral anticoagulation therapy for well over 60 years, we realize that there are other oral anticoagulants in the pipeline that may significantly impact the future of oral anticoagulation and its management. Until that time, our goal is to provide the health care provider community with the information it needs to enhance the care of patients on oral anticoagulation. We are committed to the management of oral anticoagulation in a systematic and coordinated fashion as practiced by Anticoagulation Management Services.

Jack E. Ansell
Lynn B. Oertel
Ann K. Wittkowsky

Preface from the First Edition

Few medications have had such an impact on health and illness, and such staying power, as the oral anticoagulants. Discovered over 50 years ago, little has changed in the formulation of warfarin sodium, the principal oral anticoagulant used in North America. In 1994, warfarin was the fifth most frequently prescribed cardiovascular agent and the thirteenth most frequently prescribed of all medications in the United States. However, as a narrow therapeutic index agent, warfarin requires careful management to avoid potential hemorrhagic complications associated with over-anticoagulation and potential thromboembolic complications associated with under-anticoagulation.

Over the years, investigators have concentrated on understanding the mechanism of action of oral anticoagulants, defining the appropriate indications and establishing the most appropriate intensity of therapy for specific indications. The results of these efforts have been summarized by numerous expert consensus panels. However, less emphasis has been devoted to assessing how warfarin therapy should be managed, to the consequences of substandard management practices, and to improving the clinical outcomes of patients who require warfarin therapy for the prevention or treatment of thromboembolic disease. If the consequences of therapy manifested by adverse outcomes outweigh the advantages gained by precisely determining when and how intensely to treat patients, then little has been gained in our overall efforts to improve the health and clinical outcomes of patients with thromboembolic disease. It is these issues to which this text is devoted.

The authors of this text focus on a model of anticoagulation care that is systematic, organized and coordinated: the anticoagulation management service. All aspects of development and implementation of such a model of care are addressed. A substantial portion of this text is also devoted to the actual management of patients receiving oral anticoagulants, based on an examination of available literature and on personal experience.

Most importantly, this text is written by a diverse and multidisciplinary group of health care providers, all of whom have extensive hands-on experience in the management of patients. The chapters are supplemented by numerous examples of actual policies, procedures, guidelines, algorithms, and flowsheets used in anticoagulation programs across the country. This collaborative efforts has culminated in a rich resource for clinicians.

It is our hope that this text will be used by practitioners to establish anticoagulation management services to improve the care and outcomes of their own patients treated with warfarin. Because it is in a format that allows for routine updating, this text will remain contemporary and useful for many years to come.

Jack E. Ansell
Lynn B. Oertel
Lynn K. Wittkowsky

Part 1

Establishing an Anticoagulation Management Service

Chapter 1

Historical Developments in Oral Anticoagulation

Jack E. Ansell

HISTORICAL PERSPECTIVES

The first oral anticoagulant was identified in 1939.[1,2] This event was the culmination of many years of investigation and the congruence of a number of factors. Beginning in the early 1900s, Schofield,[3] a veterinary pathologist, identified that a hemorrhagic disease of cattle was related to the consumption of spoiled sweet clover. Sweet clover had been planted years earlier in the northern United States as one of the few crops able to grow on the exhausted, overfarmed land. Occasionally, during the ensilage process, the clover spoiled and, when consumed, led to this disease. Several years later, Roderick,[4] another veterinary pathologist, identified that these cattle were deficient in prothrombin, one of the few coagulation factors known at the time.

Coincidentally, other investigators during this time were making discoveries that would be intimately linked to the future of oral anticoagulation. Henrik Dam[5] described a hemorrhagic disease in chickens fed a specially formulated diet freed of sterols, and he subsequently postulated the existence of a vitamin K, the lack of which led to the bleeding disorder.[3] Dam[6] and Almquist and Stohstad[7] subsequently isolated this vitamin, and Doisy et al[8,9] identified its structure. In 1943, Doisy and Dam shared the Nobel Prize for their work.

At approximately the same time, Armand Quick and associates[10] described the prothrombin time assay that quickly became the basis for measuring the "clotability" of blood in animals who were vitamin K–deficient and, subsequently, the basis for monitoring oral anticoagulant therapy.

In 1933, Karl Paul Link became involved in searching out the cause of this hemorrhagic disease (sweet clover disease) of cattle as the result of a chance meeting with a farmer who was irate over the death of his cattle.[1] Link, a biochemist at the University of Wisconsin, was investigating the coumarin compounds in long grasses that were responsible for the bitter taste, but sweet smell, of freshly cut hay. He was trying to produce a strain low in coumarin content. Intrigued by this hemorrhagic disease, Link eventually isolated the causative compound, dicumarol (3,3'-methyl-bis-(4-hydroxycoumarin)) in 1939.[1,11] The oxidation of coumarin to 4-hydroxycoumarin, on coupling with formaldehyde and another 4-hydroxycoumarin, resulted in the formation of dicumarol (Figure 1–1). Link immediately synthesized this compound, and in 1941 it was first used in humans as an anti-thrombotic by a group of physicians from the Mayo Clinic.[12]

Link continued to investigate the coumarin compounds throughout the 1940s and looked for related compounds with improved pharmacologic properties. One of the compounds that he synthesized, compound 42 (warfarin sodium), emerged as an ideal rodenticide in the late 1940s.[13] Its effectiveness made it the most widespread rodenticide worldwide within a few years.[1] Investigators began experimenting with warfarin during the early 1950s as a suitable anticoagulant for humans. It had much better pharmacokinetic and pharmacodynamic properties than did dicumarol. Its utility in humans, however, did not become commonplace until it was used to treat President Dwight D. Eisenhower after a heart attack in the mid-1950s.[1] Subsequently, warfarin sodium (the generic name *warfarin* is derived from the *W*isconsin *A*lumni *Re*search *F*oundation, which held the original patent on war-

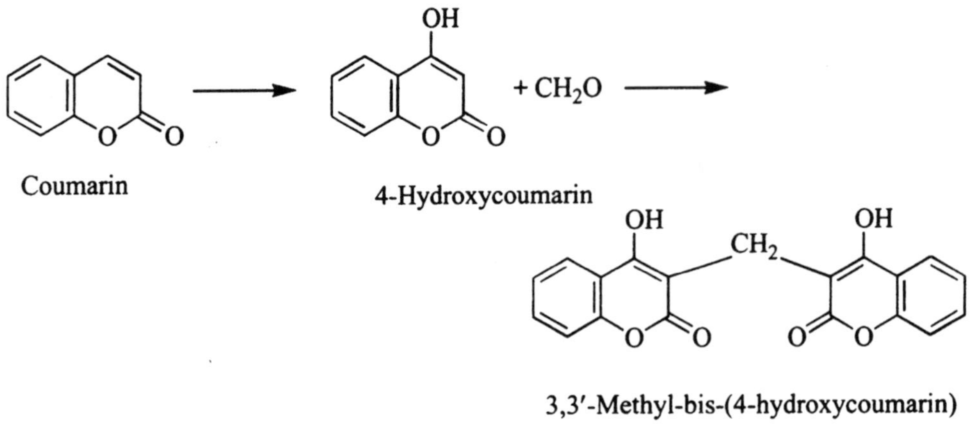

Figure 1–1 Coumarin is oxidized to 4-hydroxycoumarin and then couples, through a formaldehyde linkage, to another 4-hydroxycoumarin to form 3,3'-methyl-bis-(4-hydroxycoumarin).

farin) quickly became the major oral anticoagulant formulation used in the United States and throughout North America. Several other classes of oral anticoagulants are available and in wide use in Europe (see Chapter 29 for further discussion). Because warfarin sodium is the predominant formulation used in North America, all further discussion in this manual focuses on this particular agent.

VITAMIN K

Since the 1950s, little new has emerged regarding the development of improved orally administered anticoagulants of this class. Scientists of the last 40 years have focused on understanding the mode of action of vitamin K and the inhibitory effect of the dicumarol-type anticoagulants on vitamin K action. Although it was known at the time of discovery that vitamin K was essential for the synthesis of specific coagulation factors, not until 1974 did Stenflo et al[14] and Nelsestuen et al[15] elucidate its mechanism of action. They described the critical posttranslational modification mediated by vitamin K converting specific N-terminal glutamic acid residues in precursor prothrombin molecules to γ-carboxyglutamic acid to create functioning prothrombin (Figure 1–2). Similar modifications occur in the other vitamin K–dependent factors (factors VII, IX, and X), as well as in the coagulation inhibitors, proteins C and S, and the noncoagulation vitamin K–dependent proteins in bone, cartilage, and other tissue.[16,17] γ-carboxylation confers the calcium-mediated ability to bind to negatively changed phospholipid surfaces, an essential requirement for normal coagulation.[15,18,19] Vitamin K serves as a cofactor for a vitamin K–dependent carboxylase, thus freeing the γ-glutamyl hydrogen and leaving the carbon atom open to carbon dioxide

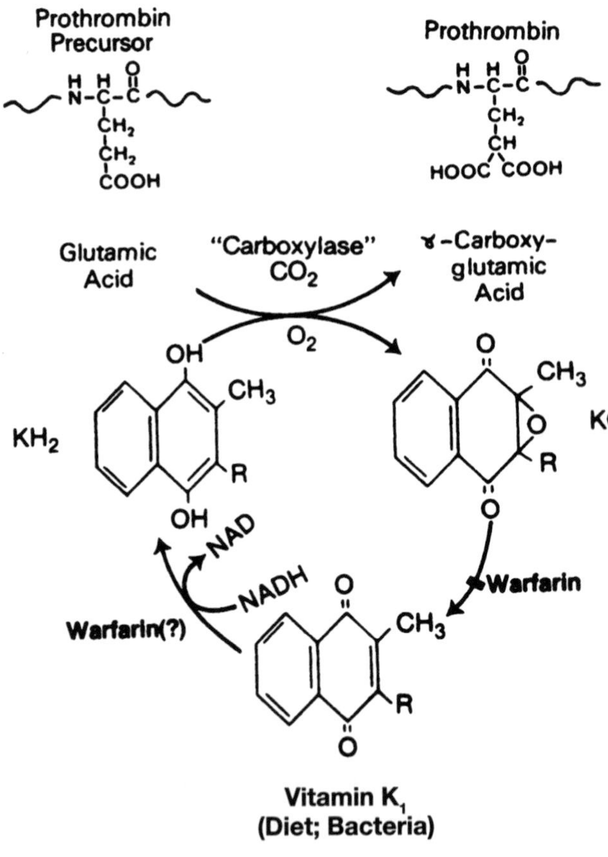

Figure 1–2 Reduced vitamin K is essential for the γ-carboxylation reaction of glutamic acid residues in precursor prothrombin or other vitamin K–dependent factors. Reduced vitamin K is oxidized in the carboxylation reaction. Vitamin KO is reduced to vitamin KH$_2$ by two enzymatic steps, the first of which is sensitive to warfarin inhibition, while the second is relatively insensitive. Source: Reprinted with permission from JE Ansell, *Archives of Internal Medicine*, Vol 153, p 587, © 1993, American Medical Association.

attack.[17] In the process, vitamin K undergoes 2,3-epoxidation and then undergoes reduction to the quinol form for recycling. This latter step is interrupted by the coumarin anticoagulants.[20-23] Orally administered anticoagulants lead to a decrease in functioning prothrombin and related factors as a result of synthesis of decarboxylated or partially carboxylated precursors.[24-27] Two reductase enzymes are involved,

the first of which is sensitive to warfarin inhibition, while the second is relatively insensitive. Thus, the defect caused by warfarin therapy can be overcome by Vitamin K_1 administration or by vitamin K_1 in the diet since this form of vitamin K bypasses the first reduction step and is not inhibited by warfarin to conversion to vitamin KH_2 at the second reduction step.

REFERENCES

1. Link KP. The discovery of dicumarol and its sequels. *Circulation.* 1959;19:97–107.

2. Campbell HA, Link KP. Studies on the hemorrhagic sweet clover disease, IV: the isolation and crystallization of the hemorrhagic agent. *J Biol Chem.* 1941;138:21–33.

3. Schofield FW. Damaged sweet clover: the cause of a new disease in cattle simulating hemorrhagic septicemia and blackleg. *J Am Vet Assoc.* 1924;64:553–575.

4. Roderick LM. Problems in the coagulation of the blood. *Am J Physiol.* 1931;96:413–425.

5. Dam H. Cholesterinstoffwechsel in Huhnereiern und Huhnchen. *Biochem Z.* 1929;215:475–492.

6. Dam H. Antihemorrhagic vitamin of the chick: occurrence and chemical nature. *Nature.* 1935;135:652–653.

7. Almquist JH, Stohstad ELR. Dietary hemorrhagic disease in chicks. *Nature.* 1935;136:31.

8. Thayer SA, MacCorquadale DW, Brinkley SB, Doisy EA. Isolation of crystalline compound with vitamin K activity. *Science.* 1938;88:243.

9. Brinkley SB, McKee RW, Thayer SA, Doisy EA. Constitution of vitamin K_2. *J Biol Chem.* 1940;133:721–729.

10. Quick AJ, Stanley-Brown M, Bancroft FW. A study of the coagulation defect in hemophilia and in jaundice. *Am J Med Sci.* 1935;190:501–511.

11. Stahmann MA, Heubner CF, Link KP. Studies on the hemorrhagic sweet clover disease, V: identification and synthesis of the hemorrhagic agent. *J Biol Chem.* 1941;138:513–527.

12. Butt HR, Allen EV, Bollman JL. A preparation from spoiled sweet clover which prolongs coagulation and prothrombin time of the blood: preliminary reports of experimental and clinical studies. *Mayo Clin Proc.* 1941;16:388–395.

13. Link KP. The anticoagulant from spoiled sweet clover hay. *Harvey Lect.* 1944;34:162–216.

14. Stenflo J, Fernlund P, Egan W, Roepstorft P. Vitamin K dependent modifications of glutamic acid residues in prothrombin. *Proc Natl Acad Sci USA.* 1974;71:2730–2733.

15. Nelsestuen GL, Zytkovicz TH, Howard JB. The mode of action of vitamin K. Identification of γ-carboxyglutamic acid as a component of prothrombin. *J Biol Chem.* 1974;249:6347–6350.

16. Lian JB, Hauschka PV, Gallop PM. Properties and biosynthesis of a vitamin K–dependent calcium binding protein in bone. *Fed Proc.* 1978;37:2615–2620.

17. Friedman PA, Przysiecki CT. Vitamin K–dependent carboxylation. *Int J Biochem.* 1987;19:1–7.

18. Nelsestuen GL. Role of gamma-carboxyglutamic acid: an unusual protein transition required for calcium-dependent binding of prothrombin to phospholipid. *J Biol Chem.* 1976;251:5648–5656.

19. Borowski M, Furie BC, Bauminger S, Furie B. Prothrombin requires two sequential metal-dependent conformational transitions to bind to phospholipid. *J Biol Chem.* 1986;261:14969–14975.

20. Whitlon DS, Sadowski JA, Suttie JW. Mechanism of coumarin action: significance of vitamin K epoxide reductase inhibition. *Biochemistry.* 1978;17:1371–1377.

21. Bell RG. Metabolism of vitamin K and prothrombin synthesis: anticoagulants and the vitamin K–epoxide cycle. *Fed Proc.* 1978;37:2599–2604.

22. Wallin R, Martin LF. Vitamin K dependent carboxylation and vitamin K metabolism in liver: effects of warfarin. *J Clin Invest.* 1985;76:1879–1884.

23. Thijssen HHW, Baars LGM. Microsomal warfarin binding and vitamin K 2,3–epoxide reductase. *Biochem Pharmacol.* 1989;38:1115–1120.

24. Friedman PA, Rosenberg RD, Hauschta PV, Fitz-James A. A spectrum of partially carboxylated prothrombins in the plasmas of coumarin-treated patients. *Biochim Biophys Acta.* 1977;494:271–276.

25. Malhotra OP, Nesheim ME, Mann KG. The kinetics of activation of normal and gamma-carboxyglutamic acid deficient prothrombins. *J Biol Chem.* 1985;260:279–287.

26. Malhotra OP. Dicoumarol-induced prothrombins containing 6, 7 and 8 gamma carboxyglutamic acid residues: isolation and characterization. *Biochem Cell Biol.* 1989;67:411–421.

27. Malhotra OP. Dicoumarol-induced 9 gamma carboxyglutamic acid prothrombin: isolation and comparison with 6, 7, 8 and 10 gamma carboxyglutamic acid isomers. *Biochem Cell Biol.* 1990;68:705–715.

Chapter 2

The Value of an Anticoagulation Management Service

Jack E. Ansell

INTRODUCTION

Why is oral anticoagulation management such an important issue? Certainly, the same degree of attention is not focused on the "management" of dosing of antibiotics, calcium channel blockers, or a wide range of other medications. What makes oral anticoagulants different? The most important factor for differentiating oral anticoagulants from other medications is the very high risk/benefit profile of these drugs compared with other medicinals. This high risk/benefit profile results from three characteristics identified below:

1. *Oral anticoagulants have a narrow therapeutic index.*
   Too much or too little medication can lead to serious consequences.
   The therapeutic response is labile and requires precise management.
   The monitoring tool (ie, prothrombin time) is an imprecise measure of responsiveness.
2. *Complications of oral anticoagulant therapy are influenced by specific patient characteristics.*
   Co-morbidities, age, diet, and other factors influence the response to therapy or the risk of complications.
3. *There are multiple points in the continuum of oral anticoagulation management subject to a breakdown in communication.*

Thus, if the therapeutic intensity is poorly maintained, if patient characteristics are not adequately accounted for, or if

communication between provider and patient or laboratory and provider is faulty, there is a high possibility for an adverse outcome such as a major hemorrhage or a thromboembolism. Further, because of this high risk/benefit ratio and issues surrounding management, many providers are reluctant to prescribe oral anticoagulation even when there is good evidence of its effectiveness.[1-3] Treating patients with warfarin for atrial fibrillation is a good example of this dilemma. A number of surveys indicate that there is widespread undertreatment with anticoagulants of patients with atrial fibrillation.[3] Surveys show that, besides knowledge of its effectiveness, fear of complications and difficulty with management are major impediments to therapy.[1,2] Clearly, any developments that would lower the risk/benefit profile and encourage the use of warfarin by physicians would be quite welcome.

Since the mid-1980s, developments have occurred that do effectively lower the risk/benefit profile. Substantial progress has been made in understanding the vagaries of the prothrombin time and standardizing reporting by use of the International Normalized Ratio.[4] A number of national consensus conferences have analyzed the literature based on levels of evidence to understand better the indications and appropriate intensity of therapy.[5] Finally, there has been a substantial increase in managing anticoagulation through a coordinated approach.[6] One might ask, however, whether such a systematic approach to managing therapy is truly better than standard models of managing patient care. And, if better, are such models cost-effective?

COORDINATED ANTICOAGULATION CARE

Most oral anticoagulation therapy in the United States is presently managed by a patient's personal physician along with all the other patients in that physician's practice. This approach might be characterized as "routine medical care." The physician might have no special system to track these patients, to make sure that they follow up with care, or to educate them about their anticoagulation. An anticoagulation management service (AMS) employs a focused and coordinated approach to managing anticoagulation. Although an AMS may vary depending on the individuals involved and the health care system or practice setting, coordinated care, in most cases, can be defined as a specialized program of patient management focused predominantly, if not exclusively, on the management of oral anticoagulation. A program is often directed by a single physician who assumes no responsibility for the primary care of the patients under management. The actual management is usually conducted by registered nurses, nurse-practitioners, pharmacists, or physician assistants. In some settings, these individuals manage a panel of patients with direction provided by different primary or referring physicians for individual patients. At a minimum, the goals of an AMS are to coordinate and optimize anticoagulation by:

- helping to determine the appropriateness of care
- managing anticoagulation dosing
- providing systematic monitoring and patient evaluation
- providing ongoing education
- communicating with other providers involved in the patient's care

This approach to managing oral anticoagulation has grown considerably during the last 10 years, but is it truly better than the routine medical care provided by physicians? Fortunately, the literature provides numerous examples and accumulating evidence that a systematic approach is better, but, unfortunately, there is little high-quality evidence based on prospective, randomized trials. In the face of this deficiency, one must rely on the literature that exists and on expert opinion as to the advantages of a specific recommendation. What support is there for a coordinated approach to the management of oral anticoagulation?

Table 2–1 summarizes those few studies available that identify the rate of complications when care is provided in a routine fashion as defined above. Although the number of studies is limited, the literature suggests that a major hemorrhagic rate of at least 6% to 7% per patient year of therapy, if not more, is expected. There is a similar rate of recurrent or de novo thromboembolism in these patients. This can be contrasted to the rates identified in a large number of retrospective or observational studies listed in Table 2–2. Even in these studies, the rate of major hemorrhage is considerably more than is reported in many large prospective studies such as the atrial fibrillation trials. These studies of coordinated care, however, more closely reflect the reality of medical practice with a variety of patients and medical conditions, whereas the atrial fibrillation trials, for example, comprise uniform, highly selected patients managed under tight oversight.

Table 2–3 summarizes those studies examining both models of management where coordinated care is measured against a control group of routine medical care within each study. These studies are mostly nonrandomized, retrospective analyses that tend to assess the care provided to patients before enrollment and after enrollment in an anticoagulation clinic, but, given this limitation, they do provide further evidence for the benefit of coordinated care. The rates for major adverse events for routine medical care are remarkably similar to those found in Table 2–1, whereas the coordinated care group is even further improved compared with the results in Table 2–2.

In a recent prospective study of routine medical care (RMC) vs AMC, Anderson et al[28] randomized 210 patients, all of whom were first stabilized by an AMS (three months) and then cared for by their private physicians or by the AMS. Although this study did show a greater time in an expanded therapeutic range for the AMS managed patients (83.6%) compared to the RMC patients (78.9%, p = 0.025), there was no significant difference in the outcomes of major hemorrhage or thromboembolism. The design of this study (the stabilization of all patients by AMS for the first three months and the possibility of a "Hawthorn" effect on the RMC group that might influence their quality of management) may have contributed to the lack of a more significant difference. Based on these reports, it appears that coordinated care offers the possibility of improved clinical outcomes and a reduction of hemorrhage or thromboembolism.

TIME IN THERAPEUTIC RANGE

Assessing the effectiveness of models of anticoagulation management by measuring the rate of major adverse events may be the ideal, but obtaining statistically valid data requires studies of large numbers of patients, which is not always possible. An alternative outcome measure is time-in-therapeutic range (TTR). A strong relationship between TTR and bleeding rates has been observed across a large number of studies with different patient populations, different target ranges, different scales for measuring intensity of anticoagulation (ie, prothrombin time [PT], PT ratio, International Normalized Ratio [INR]), and different models of dose management.[10,14,18,19] A similar relationship holds for TTR and thromboembolism rates. Table 2–4 summarizes data from studies assessing the quality of anticoagulation as reflected by TTR.

Table 2–1 Frequency of Major Hemorrhage/Thromboembolism in Patients Managed under a Usual Care Model of Management

Study	No. of Patients	No. of Patient Years	Years of Data Collection	New or Established Patients	Indications	Major Hemorrhage*	Fatal Hemorrhage*	Recurrent TE*	Definition of Major Bleed
Landefeld et al 1989[7]	565	876	1977–1983	New	Ven & Art[§]	7.4	1.1	NA	Fatal or life-threatening (surgery, angiography, irreversible damage); potentially life-threatening (≤ 3 u bleed, hypotension, hct ≤ 20).
Gitter et al 1995[8]	261	221	1987–1989	Estab	Ven & Art	8.1	0.45	8.1	≥ 2 u bleed in ≤ 7 days; life-threatening bleed.
Beyth et al 1998[9]	264	440	1986–1993	New	Ven & Art	5.0	0.68	NA	Overt bleeding that led to loss of ≥ 2 u in ≤ 7 days or life-threatening bleed
Total	1,090	1,537				6.8	0.9	8.1	

* Major and fatal hemorrhage and thromboembolism rates expressed as percent per patient year of therapy; fatal hemorrhagic events also included with major hemorrhage.
§ Ven & Art = mixed indications in the venous and arterial system.
NA = not available; TE = thromboembolism

Table 2-2 Frequency of Major Hemorrhage/Thromboembolism in Patients Managed under an Anticoagulation Management Service

Study	No. of Patients	No. of Patient Years	Years of Data Collection	New or Established Patients	Indications	Target PTR/INR	Major Hem[‡]	Fatal Hem[‡]	Recurrent TE[‡]	Definition of Major Bleed
Forfar 1982[10]	541	1,362	1970–1978	N & E	Ven & Art[§]	1.8–2.6[PTR]	4.2	0.14	NA	Significant bleed requiring medical advice (exclude bruises and epistaxis).
Errichetti et al 1984[11]	141	105	1978–1983	N & E	Ven & Art	1.3–2.0[PTR]	6.6	NA	NA	Bleed leading to hospitalization, transfusion, or discontinuing therapy.
Conte et al 1986[12]	140	153	1975–1984	N & E	Ven & Art	1.7–2.5[PTR]	2.6	NA	8.4	Bleed leading to hospitalization, discontinuing or reversal of therapy.
Petty et al 1988[13]	310	385	1977–1980	N & E	Ven & Art	NA	7.3	0.77	NA	Life-threatening bleed (GI, intracranial, subdural, or death); discontinuing therapy.
Charney et al 1988[14]	73	77	1981–1984	N & E	Ven & Art	1.5–2.5[PTR]	0	0	5.0	Bleed leading to hospitalization or discontinuing therapy.
Bussey et al 1989[15]	82	199	1977–1986	N	Ven & Art	NA	2.0	NA	3.5	Bleed leading to hospitalization, transfusion, vitamin K, or fresh frozen plasma.
Seabrook et al 1990[16]	93	158	1981–1988	N	Ven & Art	1.5–2.0[PTR]	3.8	0	2.5	Bleed leading to hospitalization, transfusion, or discontinuing therapy.
Fihn et al 1993[17]	928	1,950	NA	N	Ven & Art	1.3–1.5[PTR] 1.5–1.8[PTR]	1.7	0.2	7.5	Fatal or life-threatening bleed (CPR, surgery, angiography, irreversible damage, hypotension, Hct < 20, ≥ 3 u bleed).
van der Meer et al 1993[18]	6,814	6,085	1988	N & E	Ven & Art	2.4–5.3[INR]	3.3	0.64	NA	Fatal bleed; intracranial bleed, transfusion, or surgery; all muscle and joint bleeds.
Cannegieter et al 1995[19]	1,608	6,475	1985	N & E	Mech Valves	3.6–4.8[INR]	2.5	0.33	0.7	Fatal or bleed leading to hospitalization.
Palareti et al 1996, 1997[20–21]	2,745	2,011	1993–1995	N	Ven & Art	2.0–3.0[INR] 2.5–4.5[INR]	1.4	0.24	3.5	Fatal bleed; intracranial bleed, ocular bleed with blindness; joint, retroperitoneal bleed; surgery or angiography, > 2 gm bleed; transfusion ≥ 2 units
Total	13,475	18,960					2.8	0.39	2.6	

[‡] Major and fatal hemorrhage and thromboembolism rates expressed as percent per patient year of therapy; fatal hemorrhagic events also included with major hemorrhage.

[§] Ven & Art = mixed indications in the venous and arterial systems.

NA = not available; TE = thromboembolism; PTR = prothrombin time ratio

Table 2–3 Frequency of Hemorrhage and Thromboembolism with Routine Medical Care versus Anticoagulation Management Service

Study[†]	Type of Care	No. of Patients	Patient Years	Target PTR/INR[‡]	Major Hemorrhage[§]	Minor Hemorrhage[§]	Fatal Events[‖]	Thrombo-embolism[§]
Hamilton et al 1985[22]	RMC	49	73.25	NA*	6.8	21.0	NA*	8.0
	AMS	41	91.75		6.5	23.0		8.0
Cohen et al 1985[23]	RMC	17	NA*	1.5–2.5	9.0[#]	NA*	0	NA*
	AMS	18			6.9[#]		0	
Garabedian-Ruffalo et al 1985[24]	RMC	26	64.3	1.5–2.5	12.4	NA*	NA*	6.2
	AMS	26	41.9		2.4			0
Cortelazzo et al 1993[25]	RMC	271	677	3.0–4.5	4.7	NA*	0	6.6
	AMS	271	669	(INR)	0.1 P<.01		0	0.6 P<.01
Wilt et al 1995[26]	RMC	NA*	28	NA*	28.6	14.3	NA*	48.6
	AMS		60		0	13.7		0
Chiquette et al 1998[27]	RMC	142	102	2.0–3.0	3.9	62.8	1	11.8
	AMS	176	123	2.5–3.5 (INR)	1.6 RR = .21	26.1	0	3.3 RR = .30
Total	RMC	505+	944.8+		6.2 (4.3–26.8)			8.9 (6.2–48.6)
	AMS	532+	985.65+		1.0 (0–6.9)			1.5 (0–8.0)

* NA = Not available or not applicable.

[†] Mixed indications for anticoagulation (ie, venous and arterial disease) except the studies of Hamilton and Cortelazzo, which were for prosthetic heart valves only.

[‡] PTR = Prothrombin time ratio; INR = International Normalized Ratio.

[§] Results expressed as percent per patient year of therapy.

[‖] Fatal events expressed as individual events. Their rates are included under Major Hemorrhage.

[#] Combined major and minor hemorrhage.

Note: AMS, anticoagulation management service; RMC, routine medical care.

Source: Adapted with permission from JE Ansell and R Hughes, *American Heart Journal*, Vol 132, pp 1095–1100, © 1996, Mosby-Year Book, Inc.

TTR is a surrogate measure for adverse events and a quality measure for the management of oral anticoagulation. Another measure of quality, and thus value, of anticoagulation management is an assessment of the response of the health care provider to an out-of-range INR value or change of warfarin dose. The presumption is that a more timely follow-up to a dose change or out-of-range value is better quality care that might lead to better outcomes, although this concept has not been formally tested by measuring the outcomes of hemorrhage or thrombosis. This parameter, however, was measured in a study by Samsa et al[37] that compared the frequency of warfarin therapy for atrial fibrillation and the time in therapeutic range for three communities, only one of which had care provided by an anticoagulation management service. Besides demonstrating higher rates of treatment of atrial fibrillation and greater time in range for patients managed by the AMS, they also showed that 51% of follow-up visits

after an out-of-range INR occurred within 7 days in the AMS group compared to 34% and 32% for the two RMC groups.

COST-EFFECTIVENESS OF COORDINATED CARE

Although there is little in the literature to address the issue of the cost-effectiveness of coordinated versus routine medical care, some studies do suggest a significant benefit. The benefit is derived mainly by a reduction in adverse events and reduced utilization of hospital services. Simply taking into account the costs associated with adverse events, one can estimate the differences that are likely to be seen with RMC vs an AMS. Eckman et al[38] estimated the inpatient cost of major anticoagulant-related bleeding between $3,000 and $12,000, depending on outcome. Using $7,500 as an average

Table 2–4 Time in Therapeutic Range (a Surrogate Measure for Quality) Achieved under Different Models of Anticoagulation Management

Study	Predominant Model of Management	PTR vs INR	% Time in Therapeutic Range	% Above Range	% Below Range	Method of Determining Time in Range#	Major Dx
Garabedian-Ruffalo et al 1985[24]	RMC	PTR	64	—	—	% in range	Mixed
Gottlieb & Salem-Schatz 1994[29]	RMC	PTR	50	30	20	days in range	Mixed
Holm et al 1999[30]	RMC	INR	63	8	29	% in range	Mixed
Beyth & Landefeld 1997[31]	RMC	INR	33	16	51	—	Mixed
Horstkotte et al 1996[32]	RMC	INR	59	—	—	% in range	Valves
Sawicki, 1999[33]	RMC	INR	34	16	50	% in range	AF/Valves
Palaretti et al 1996[20]	AMS	INR	68	6	26	days in range	Mixed
Cannegieter et al 1995[19]	AMS	INR	61	8	31	days in range	Valves
Lundstrom & Ryden 1989[34]	AMS	TT	92	—	—	% in range	AF
Garabedian-Ruffalo et al 1985[24]	AMS	PTR	86	—	—	% in range	Mixed
White et al 1989[35]	AMS	PTR	75	—	—	days in range	Mixed
Ansell et al 1995[36]	AMS	PTR	68	10	22	% in range	Mixed
Conte et al 1986[12]	AMS	PTR	59	12	29	—	Mixed
Seabrook et al 1990[16]	AMS	PTR	86	7	7	% in range	Mixed

RMC = routine medical care; AMS = anticoagulation management service; PTR = prothrombin time ratio; INR = international normalized ratio; TT = thrombotest; AF = atrial fibrillation.

cost, the annual savings achieved by preventing five major events would be $37,500 for 100 patients, or $375 per patient year. Similarly, the decreased incidence of thromboembolism achieved by coordinated care is approximately five events per 100 patient year. Eckman et al[38] estimated the inpatient cost of a thromboembolism between $5,000 and $18,000, depending on outcome. Therefore, using an average cost of $11,500, the data would indicate an annual savings of $46,000 per 100 patient years, or $460 per patient year. Based on these assumptions, neither of which takes into account the long-term morbidity or costs of complications, the combined savings of coordinated care, by lowering the incidence of both major bleeding and thromboembolism, would approximate $835 per patient year. Campbell et al[39] performed an economic analysis of RMC vs AMS care based on cost estimates for the various aspects of care including the costs of adverse events that are likely to occur in each model based on reports from the literature. For a cohort of 1,000 patients with atrial fibrillation on warfarin therapy, they estimated a cost of $1.2 million for patients managed by an AMS vs $2.0 million for patients managed by RMC. Approximately 30% of the additional costs could be accounted for by the model of care, whereas the other 70% was due to an increase in adverse event rates in the RMC group. Table 2–5 summarizes those studies in which this issue has been addressed. Gray et al[40] estimated a benefit/cost ratio of 6.5, or a savings of $860 per patient year of therapy as a result of reduced hospital days per patient year. Wilt et al,[26] in their small study, found an extraordinary cost savings through a reduction in hospital or emergency department visits. Chiquette et al[27] recently reported their estimates of savings through a coordinated approach, compared with routine care, as 11 versus 41 hospital or emergency department visits for complications, which resulted in savings of $1,320 per patient year of therapy. Lee and Schommer[41] also found a reduction in hospital admissions with coordinated care but did not report the estimated dollars saved.

Taken together, these estimates provide a relatively consistent picture of cost savings that can be achieved through prevention of major bleeding and thromboembolism via coordinated anticoagulation care that approximate $1,000 per patient year. Therefore, available data indicate that not only will coordinated care reduce the incidence of adverse outcomes, but it will also save financial resources.

Table 2–5 Cost Savings Resulting from Reduced Hospital and Emergency Department Use by an Anticoagulant Management Service

Study	Cost Savings
Gray et al 1985[40]	0.48* vs 3.22* hospital days per patient year $860/patient year of therapy
Wilt et al 1995[26]	0 vs 21 hospital or emergency department visits $4,072/patient year of therapy
Chiquette et al 1998[27]	11 vs 41 hospital or emergency department visits $1,320/patient year of therapy
Lee and Schommer 1996[41]	3 vs 15 hospital admissions Dollar savings not determined

*Rates for coordinated care versus routine medical care.

REFERENCES

1. Kutner M, Nixon G, Silverstone F. Physicians' attitudes toward oral anticoagulants and antiplatelet agents for stroke prevention in elderly patients with atrial fibrillation. *Arch Intern Med*. 1991;151:1950–1953.

2. McCrory DC, Matchar DB, Samsa G, Sanders LL, Pritchett ELC. Physician attitudes about anticoagulation for nonvalvular atrial fibrillation in the elderly. *Arch Intern Med*. 1995;155:277–281.

3. Agency for Health Care Policy and Research. Life-saving treatments to prevent stroke underused. September 7, 1995. Press release.

4. Loeliger EA, Poller L, Samama M, et al. Questions and answers on prothrombin time standardization in oral anticoagulant control. *Thromb Haemost*. 1985;54:515–517.

5. Dalen JE, Hirsh J, eds. Fourth ACCP Consensus Conference on Antithrombotic Therapy. *Chest*. 1995;108(suppl):225S–522S.

6. Ansell JE, Hughes R. Evolving models of warfarin management: anticoagulation clinics, patient self-monitoring and patient self-management. *Am Heart J*. 1996;132:1095–1100.

7. Landefeld CS, Goldman L. Major bleeding in outpatients treated with warfarin: incidence and prediction by factors known at the start of outpatient therapy. *Am J Med*. 1989;87:144–152.

8. Gitter MJ, Jaeger TM, Petterson TM, Gersh BJ, Silverstein MD. Bleeding and thromboembolism during anticoagulant therapy: a population-based study in Rochester, Minnesota. *Mayo Clin Proc*. 1995;70:725–733.

9. Beyth RJ, Quinn LM, Landefeld S. Prospective evaluation of an index for predicting the risk of major bleeding in outpatients treated with warfarin. *Am J Med*. 1998;105:91–99.

10. Forfar JC. Prediction of hemorrhage during long-term oral coumarin anticoagulation by excessive prothrombin ratio. *Am Heart J*. 1982;103:445–446.

11. Errichetti AM, Holden A, Ansell J. Management of oral anticoagulant therapy: experience with an anticoagulation clinic. *Arch Intern Med*. 1984;144:1966–1968.

12. Conte RR, Kehoe WA, Nielson N, Lodhia H. Nine-year experience with a pharmacist-managed anticoagulation clinic. *Am J Hosp Pharm*. 1986;43:2460–2464.

13. Petty GW, Lennihan L, Mohr JP, et al. Complications of long-term anticoagulation. *Ann Neurol*. 1988;23:570–574.

14. Charney R, Leddomado E, Rose DN, Fuster V. Anticoagulation clinics and the monitoring of anticoagulant therapy. *Int J Cardiol*. 1988;18:197–206.

15. Bussey HI, Rospond RM, Quandt CM, Clark GM. The safety and effectiveness of long-term warfarin therapy in an anticoagulation clinic. *Pharmacotherapy*. 1989;9:214–219.

16. Seabrook GR, Karp D, Schmitt DD, Bandyk DF. An outpatient anticoagulation protocol managed by a vascular nurse-clinician. *Am J Surg*. 1990;160:501–504.

17. Fihn SD, McDonell M, Martin D, et al. Risk factors for complications of chronic anticoagulation: a multicenter study. *Ann Intern Med*. 1993;118:511–520.

18. van der Meer FJM, Rosendaal FR, Vandenbrouke JP, Briet E. Bleeding complications in oral anticoagulant therapy: an analysis of risk factors. *Arch Intern Med*. 1993;153:1557–1562.

19. Cannegieter SC, Rosendaal FR, Wintzen AR, van der Meer FJM, Vandenbroucke JP, Briet E. Optimal oral anticoagulant therapy in patients with mechanical heart valves. *N Engl J Med*. 1995;333:11–17.

20. Palareti G, Leali N, Coccheri S, et al. Bleeding complications of oral anticoagulant treatment: an inception-cohort, prospective, collaborative study (ISCOAT). *Lancet*. 1996;348:423–428.

21. Palareti G, Manotti C, D'Angelo A, et al. Thrombotic events during anticoagulant treatment: results of the inception-cohort, prospective, collaborative ISCOAT study. *Thromb Haemost*. 1997;78:1438–1443.

22. Hamilton GM, Childers RW, Silverstein MD. Does clinic management of anticoagulation improve the outcome of prosthetic valve patients? *Clin Res*. 1985;33:832A.

23. Cohen IA, Hutchison TA, Kirking DM, Shue ME. Evaluation of a pharmacist-managed anticoagulation clinic. *J Clin Hosp Pharm*. 1985;10:167–175.

24. Garabedian-Ruffalo SM, Gray DR, Sax MJ, Ruffalo RL. Retrospective evaluation of a pharmacist-managed warfarin anticoagulation clinic. *Am J Hosp Pharm*. 1985;42:304–308.

25. Cortelazzo S, Finazzi G, Viero P, et al. Thrombotic and hemorrhagic complications in patients with mechanical heart valve prosthesis attending an anticoagulation clinic. *Thromb Haemost.* 1993;69:316–320.

26. Wilt VM, Gums JG, Ahmed OI, Moore LM. Outcome analysis of a pharmacist-managed anticoagulation service. *Pharmacotherapy.* 1995; 15:732–739.

27. Chiquette E, Amateo MG, Bussey HI. Comparison of an anticoagulation clinic and usual medical care: anticoagulation control, patient outcomes and health care costs. *Arch Intern Med.* 1998; 158:1641–1647.

28. Anderson DR, Wilson J, Wells PS, et al. Anticoagulant clinic vs family physician based warfarin monitoring: a randomized controlled trial. *Blood.* 2000;96:846a.

29. Gottlieb LK, Salem-Schatz S. Anticoagulation in atrial fibrillation: does efficacy in clinical trials translate into effectiveness in practice? *Arch Intern Med.* 1994;154:1945–1953.

30. Holm T, Lassen JF, Husted SE, Heickendorff L. Identification and surveillance of patient on oral anticoagulant therapy in a large geographic area—use of laboratory information systems. *Thromb Haemost.* 1999;82(Suppl):858–859.

31. Beyth RJ, Landefeld CS. Prevention of major bleeding in older patients treated with warfarin: results of a randomized trial [abstract]. *J Gen Intern Med.* 1997;12:66.

32. Horstkotte D, Piper C, Wiemer M, et al. Improvement of prognosis by home prothrombin estimation in patients with life-long anticoagulant therapy [abstract]. *Eur Heart J.* 1996;17(suppl):230.

33. Sawicki PT, Working Group for the Study of Patient Self-Management of Oral Anticoagulation. A structured teaching and self-management program for patients receiving oral anticoagulation. A randomized controlled trial. *JAMA.* 1999;281:145–150.

34. Lundstrom T, Ryden L. Haemorrhagic and thromboembolic complications in patients with atrial fibrillation on anticoagulant prophylaxis. *J Intern Med.* 1989;225:137–142.

35. White RH, McCurdy A, Marensdorff H, et al. Home prothrombin time monitoring after the initiation of warfarin therapy: a randomized, prospective study. *Ann Intern Med.* 1989;1111:730–737.

36. Ansell J, Patel N, Ostrovsky D, et al. Long-term patient self-management of oral anticoagulation. *Arch Intern Med.* 1995;155:2185–2189.

37. Samsa GP, Matchar DB, Goldstein LB, et al. Quality of anticoagulation management among patients with atrial fibrillation: results from a review of medical records from two communities. *Arch Intern Med.* 2000;160:967–973.

38. Eckman MH, Levine JH, Pauker SG. Making decisions about antithrombotic therapy in heart disease. *Chest.* 1995;108(suppl):457S–470S.

39. Campbell PM, Radensky PW, Denham CR. Economic analysis of systemic anticoagulation management vs routine medical care for patients on oral warfarin therapy. *Dis Manage Clin Outcomes.* 2000; 2:1–8.

40. Gray DR, Garabedian-Ruffalo SM, Chretien SD. Cost-justification of a clinical pharmacist–managed anticoagulation clinic. *Drug Intell Clin Pharm.* 1985;19:575–580.

41. Lee YP, Schommer JC. Effect of a pharmacist-managed anticoagulation clinic on warfarin-related hospital readmissions. *Am J Health-Syst Pharm.* 1996;53:1580–1583.

Chapter 3

Guidelines for Development of an Anticoagulation Management Service

Orsula Voltis Thomas and Jack E. Ansell

INTRODUCTION

Recent literature identifies three principal barriers to greater anticoagulant use: (1) gaps in knowledge of or belief in its effectiveness, (2) concerns about its safety, and (3) concerns about the difficulty of managing patients on anticoagulation.[1–3] Great strides in reducing the first two barriers have been made by such efforts as the series of Consensus Conferences on Antithrombotic Therapy sponsored by the American College of Chest Physicians.[4] Less has been accomplished in a systematic way, however, to improve and facilitate the management of therapy for the primary health care provider. As discussed in Chapter 2, existing evidence suggests that coordinated anticoagulation therapy is more likely to achieve good clinical outcomes.[5–9] By improving the safety and effectiveness of therapy and by easing the burden on the primary health care provider, one might expect an increase in the use of anticoagulants resulting in further enhancements of patient care and cost reduction. Although numerous studies describe various components of anticoagulation management, there are currently no widely accepted clinical guidelines or standards of care.

Standards of care are those principles that "define the appropriate environment, process, and procedures necessary for quality medical care and optimal health outcomes."[10] The lack of standards for the treatment of disease and the reporting of outcomes is not unique to anticoagulation therapy. Health researchers note significant variations in the management of different disease states.[11] Although guidelines regarding indications for, and the optimal intensity of, warfarin

therapy for these indications have been published in the literature,[12,13] there are no current clinical guidelines for coordinated outpatient anticoagulation therapy.

In an effort to provide health care providers with guidelines for the development of anticoagulation management services and a coordinated approach to care, an anticoagulation guidelines task force recently developed a series of recommendations for coordinated outpatient anticoagulant therapy.[14] The goal of this effort was to provide primary and referring health care providers with a guide for the provision of safe and effective anticoagulation management in any setting. These standards provide clinicians with a means to:

- create a reproducible framework for the establishment of effective outpatient anticoagulation management services
- provide multidisciplinary health care providers with a mechanism for the assessment and monitoring of persons receiving oral anticoagulation
- enable patients to assume greater responsibility for self-care through health education about the safe use of warfarin, the physical signs and symptoms of bleeding or thromboembolism, and the importance of laboratory monitoring
- improve patient adherence to the prescribed regimen through education and empowerment
- decrease complications, hospitalizations, and emergency department utilization related to anticoagulation therapy
- increase patient satisfaction and improve quality of life for patients receiving anticoagulation therapy

- provide a structure for the evaluation of the outcomes and quality of outpatient anticoagulation management services

The guidelines are divided into three categories as outlined in Exhibit 3–1. This approach follows the operational format often used in the process of quality improvement with a focus on structure, process, and outcome.

GUIDELINES FOR ORGANIZATION AND MANAGEMENT

1. Qualifications of Personnel

> **1.1 Anticoagulation providers should meet minimum competencies and hold a license in a patient-oriented health-related field (eg, medicine, nursing, pharmacy).**

Comment: A review of the literature and current practice reveals that anticoagulation therapy is frequently undertaken by a multidisciplinary team representing medicine, nursing, and pharmacy[5–9,15–20] (eg, physicians, pharmacists, registered nurses, physician assistants, nurse-practitioners). Other aspects of patient management, such as scheduling, may be delegated to other, nonclinical personnel.

Studies describing both inpatient and outpatient anticoagulation management show that inexperience and lack of knowledge regarding the pharmokinetic and pharmacodynamic properties of warfarin lead to suboptimal anticoagulant therapy.[17,21] Although the educational requirements are not described, studies describing clinics indicate that some nonphysician anticoagulation therapy providers receive specialized training and education,[6,16,20,22] for example, through the American Society of Health-System Pharmacists and some state pharmacy societies that have developed an anticoagulation traineeship program to train pharmacists. These programs, however, do not extend to other health care providers. Outside of this formal mechanism, there are currently no recognized means of ensuring the competency of anticoagulation therapy providers. The anticoagulation guidelines task force suggests that anticoagulation providers should be required to demonstrate competence in the content areas summarized in Exhibit 3–2.

2. Supervision

> **2.1 The physician or health care provider with ultimate responsibility for therapeutic decisions should develop an agreed-upon policy and procedure for personnel supervision and oversight of those health care providers actually managing the anticoagulation therapy.**

Comment: The availability and accessibility of physicians are dependent on the clinic site. In an individual or group medical practice, physicians are often available to see anticoagulation patients if warranted, but, in other settings, physicians might not be present at the actual anticoagulation clinic site. The development of a policy describing the supervisory process for nonphysician health care providers is deemed essential to establish and clarify the roles and responsibilities of those involved in providing care.

3. Care Management and Coordination

> **3.1 Written protocols for the management of anticoagulation should be established.**

Comment: Policies and procedures serve as a clinical tool and a quality assurance mechanism to preserve the quality of

---

Exhibit 3–1
GUIDELINES FOR COORDINATED OUTPATIENT ANTICOAGULATION THERAPY MANAGEMENT

1. guidelines for organization and management
   - qualifications of personnel
   - supervision
   - care management and coordination
   - communication and documentation
   - laboratory monitoring
2. guidelines for the process of patient care
   - patient selection and assessment
   - initiation of therapy
   - maintenance and management of therapy
   - patient education
   - management and triage of therapy-related and unrelated problems
3. guidelines for the evaluation of patient outcomes
   - organizational components
   - patient outcomes

Source: Reprinted with permission from JE Ansell, ML Buttaro, and OV Thomas, Consensus Guidelines for Coordinated Outpatient Oral Anticoagulation Therapy Management. *Annals of Pharmacotherapy* 1997;31:604–615.

Exhibit 3–2
COMPETENCY REQUIREMENTS FOR ANTICOAGULATION PROVIDERS

- understanding of coagulation, antithrombotic therapy, and thrombogenesis
- understanding of pharmacokinetic and pharmacodynamic properties of warfarin and other anticoagulants used in the outpatient setting
- ability to describe the expected impact of and identify the medications, disease states, dietary, and lifestyle changes that alter anticoagulation therapy
- assessment skills to elicit the signs and symptoms of bleeding and knowledge of when to refer to a physician
- assessment skills to elicit the signs and symptoms of a thromboembolism and knowledge of when to refer to a physician
- skills to identify, triage, or manage other medical problems through the appropriate health care provider
- understanding the effects of socioeconomic, behavioral, psychological, and environmental factors on patient adherence

- ability to describe the meaning of prothrombin time (PT), International Normalized Ratio (INR), and International Sensitivity Index (ISI) value and the relationships between these values, their limitations, and reasons for variability
- ability to interpret INR and related laboratory values and adjust warfarin dose accordingly
- proper use of capillary blood-testing devices if they are used at the practice setting
- determination of optimal intensity and duration of antithrombotic therapy for individual patients
- determination of appropriate options for interrupting and/or reversing anticoagulation
- ability to communicate with patients and anticoagulation providers
- skills to authorize and coordinate follow-up with patients and other health care providers

care. These policies and procedures may address, but are not limited to, the areas summarized in Exhibit 3–3.

> **3.2 The anticoagulation provider should have a systematic process to identify patients who need to be scheduled for a blood sample and/or medical assessment, to schedule the necessary appointments, to retrieve laboratory results, and to provide patient instruction and follow-up.**

Comment: A major cause of suboptimal anticoagulant therapy is fragmented medical care.[21–23] It has been suggested that the success of clinic-managed anticoagulation therapy is related to the ability of the clinic to maintain continuity of care, regulate anticoagulation dosage, avoid complications by early identification of potential interferences with therapy, and provide regular monitoring with systematic follow-up and education. The system must be well defined, organized, and complete. The minimum components of this system are

- a patient database
- a systematic mechanism for transition between inpatient and ambulatory care and vice versa
- a mechanism for scheduling regular laboratory appointments and retrieving laboratory data
- a method of appointment scheduling and follow-up with patients
- other fail-safe mechanisms identified by the anticoagulation provider as necessary for continuity of care

4. Communication and Documentation

> **4.1 The anticoagulation provider should have policies and procedures regarding communications with the patient, primary care physician or health care providers, laboratory, and designated pharmacy(ies). Documentation of these interactions, as well as documentation of outcomes assessment, should be recorded in the database of the patient.**

Comment: Anticoagulation therapy requires interaction between a patient and the physicians and other health care providers. Communication with the referring physician (if not the one managing the anticoagulation) is essential. Lack of communication can result in poor patient outcomes. The mechanism by which patient communication occurs is up to the individual clinic (eg, face to face, telephone, postcards). Regardless of the method of communication and anticoagulation service setting, clear-cut processes for all patient and health care provider interactions should be established.

Copies of all letters sent to patients and other health care providers should be included in the patient's medical record. Documentation of other communication processes, including telephone calls and postcards, also should be included. The database of the patient should include information regarding patient demographics, indications for anticoagulant therapy, desired intensity and expected length of therapy,

Exhibit 3–3
POLICY AND PROCEDURE AREAS FOR ANTICOAGULATION MANAGEMENT

- patient assessment
- patient education
- indications for, intensity of, and planned duration of antico-agulation therapy
- systematic method for therapy initiation
- systematic method for interpretation of INR results and management of nontherapeutic laboratory values
- intervals for monitoring INR and other laboratory parameters pertinent to anticoagulation therapy (eg, complete blood count [CBC], urinalysis)

- adverse event protocol with definitions of minor and major bleeding and disease recurrence with appropriate actions
- method for dosage adjustment based on INR results; patient assessment; and evaluation of dietary, disease state, and lifestyle changes
- management of patient nonadherence to blood tests or clinic visits
- guidelines for discharge of patients from a clinic program, if applicable
- reimbursement procurement

tablet size(s) of warfarin prescribed and used, other disease states, laboratory values, dosage and medication adjustments, communications, and other information pertinent to the patient's anticoagulation care. Names; dose; route and frequency of administration; and start dates and stop dates for concomitant medications, including over-the-counter medications, also should be included. A flowchart documenting the INR and warfarin dose of the patient is a useful tool to track trends.

5. Laboratory Monitoring

> **5.1 The anticoagulation provider should use the INR to access patient anticoagulation control.**

Comment: A critical component of anticoagulation monitoring is the interpretation of the PT. In response to variations in sensitivity of thromboplastin reagents used to calculate the PT, the World Health Organization (WHO) developed the ISI, a reference standard to calibrate thromboplastin reagents and permit standardization.[23] The WHO calibration model is known as the INR. The INR is the PT ratio that would have been obtained if the WHO thromboplastin standard (ISI = 1) had been used (see Chapter 25 for a detailed discussion).

Failure to use the INR system can compromise anticoagulation control.[12] Although more valid than the PT ratio, the INR system has limitations. Anticoagulation providers should be cognizant that reagents with ISI values ≥ 1.5 and the type of equipment used for clot detection can affect INR values.

Anticoagulation providers should have knowledge of the laboratory testing sites in the region, the type of equipment used by the laboratories, and the quality of the laboratory reagents. They also should be familiar with the technology of the new methods of INR monitoring (eg, capillary whole blood testing) and related regulations if they are using such methods.

GUIDELINES FOR THE PROCESS OF PATIENT CARE

6. Patient Selection and Assessment

> **6.1 The referring physician or health care provider recommending anticoagulation therapy shall determine the appropriateness of anticoagulation therapy for a particular patient. The actual anticoagulation provider or director of the service, in order to manage the care, must agree on the appropriateness of the therapy.**

Comment: When considering the use of anticoagulants, one must weigh the risks of therapy versus the benefits. If the provider of anticoagulation management does not agree that a therapy is appropriate, he or she has the right to decline the management of the patient under consideration.

> **6.2 The anticoagulation provider should assess the patient's current medical, medication, dietary, and lifestyle history; level of understanding and literacy; health beliefs and attitudes; motivation for self-care behavior; and other environmental or behavioral barriers to learning and adherence when therapy is instituted.**

Comment: The initial assessment of the individual referred for anticoagulation therapy is an important component of care that can reveal the current beliefs and expectations of the patient about treatment, in addition to information regarding the patient's medical, social, and lifestyle history. Because the therapeutic outcomes of anticoagulation are affected by concomitant medications, co-morbid conditions, and variations in diet, this assessment is an integral part of the care process.

7. Initiation of Therapy

> **7.1 A patient-specific INR range, based on the medical literature and other patient-specific information, should be established.**

Comment: Establishing a targeted INR range entails careful assessment of the indication for therapy, as well as patient-specific risks and benefits. Guidelines in the peer-reviewed literature should be used to aid clinicians in selecting the appropriate intensity of therapy.

Therapy should not be initiated with a loading dose as once recommended. It has been shown to be associated with a high risk of early hemorrhage and a false sense of full anticoagulation in early treatment.[12,13] Initiation of therapy is recommended using an average or sometimes slightly higher (eg, 5–10-mg) maintenance dose unless there are reasons to initiate therapy at an even lower dose (eg, elderly or malnourished patients, those with liver diseases).[12,13,24–26]

> **7.2 The anticoagulation provider should base dosage adjustments on INR and other pertinent laboratory results, individual assessment, patient-specific response, and guidelines approved by the anticoagulation service as part of its policies and procedures.**

Comment: There is no single, standard pharmacokinetic model to predict the optimal maintenance anticoagulant dose or to perform dosage adjustments. Various equations and computer-assisted models have been developed to assist clinicians in dosage titration.[12,27] The role of such models in actual clinician practice needs further study.

Warfarin dosage adjustments should be limited to 5%–20% of total weekly (or total daily) dose because a nonlinear relationship exists between warfarin dose and pharmacodynamic response. Anticoagulation clinics use different methods for dose titration. Some clinics might instruct patients to skip doses or to take extra doses and/or alter the patient's therapeutic regimen. The anticoagulation provider should decide the method of dosage titration most appropriate for each patient. Ideally, this dosage adjustment should be verbally communicated to the patient. In extenuating circumstances, a written (postcard) intervention might be necessary.

Dosage regimens should be kept as simple as possible, with the fewest number of different-strength tablets as possible. Some clinicians advocate the use of a single-strength tablet to simplify the regimen for all patients and use fractions or multiples of the same tablet to achieve individualized dosing. The anticoagulation provider should do as much as possible to aid patient understanding and adherence (eg, written instructions, pillboxes, calendar cards.

> **7.3 Initial monitoring should occur every week or more frequently following initiation of therapy or hospital discharge, depending on the stability of the patient. After the patient's anticoagulation has been stabilized, follow-up evaluation should occur at least every four weeks.**

Comment: Initiation of anticoagulation therapy will require frequent blood sampling and dosage adjustments until the patient is adequately anticoagulated and INR results are stable. Once the INR has been stabilized, monitoring intervals can be extended to every two weeks and eventually to every four weeks. Stability with respect to other medical illnesses, medication use, diet, and lifestyle must be evaluated when establishing this interval. Because patients are most likely to experience hemorrhagic complications during the first several months of therapy, more frequent monitoring might be required throughout this period.

After the target INR of the patient has been reached and stabilized, many clinics have a four-week follow-up as a maximum time interval. The most recent American Heart Association medical/scientific statement regarding oral anticoagulant therapy currently recommends a PT test for patients who are hemodynamically stable every 4 weeks.[13] The maximum time interval reported in the literature for patients stabilized on anticoagulation therapy, however, might be as long as every 12 weeks.[28] Until more definitive information is available, the maximum recommended time interval for follow-up remains at 4 weeks.[13]

8. Maintenance and Management of Therapy

> **8.1 The anticoagulation provider should have a systematic process for follow-up evaluations focused on patient assessment for potential side effects of therapy; recurrent disease; hemorrhagic complications; drug-drug/drug-disease state, and drug-food interactions; lifestyle changes; review of laboratory results; adherence issues; and patient education.**

Comment: The positive outcomes associated with anticoagulation clinic care suggest that the frequency of follow-up is an important variable affecting outcomes. Follow-up evaluations should include assessment for changes in medications, health status, diet, and patient adherence. The patient also should be assessed for signs and symptoms of hemorrhagic complications and thromboembolism.

8.2   The anticoagulation provider should have a policy in the interval for follow-up blood testing after a dosage adjustment has been made. The determination should consider the magnitude of the nontherapeutic INR and dosage change, as well as other variables influencing patient responsiveness and stability.

Comment: Because it takes at least three days for the effect of a change in dose to be reflected in the INR, the minimum time to schedule a PT test is approximately three days after therapy has been adjusted. The maximum time should be no longer than two weeks.

8.3   Anticoagulation providers should develop guidelines regarding management of anticipated changes in anticoagulant response that result from a change in patient status, medication use, diet, or other factors.

Comment: Patients often function under the misconception that all health care providers involved in their care are aware of what the others are doing at all times. They also might assume that a diagnostic procedure or other variable is not of consequence. To help avert this type of problem, patients should be advised to contact the anticoagulation provider regarding all pending or scheduled dental, medical, or surgical appointments. The anticoagulation provider can adjust the dose appropriately or maintain the dose but reassess the PT/INR response at a shorter interval than might have occurred otherwise. All patients might also be instructed to notify the anticoagulation management service of any changes in medication, diet, or disease-state status.

9.   Patient Education

9.1   The anticoagulation provider should have a policy and procedure pertaining to the desired goals and objectives of its educational program. Patient education should be individualized according to the initial assessment, based on the patient's level of understanding; be accompanied by written information as a reinforcement; and be reviewed on a regular basis.

Comment: Well-designed educational programs have been shown to increase adherence and improve outcomes.[29,30] Anticoagulation management services provide patient education as part of their usual care. Researchers evaluating the results of anticoagulation programs conclude that the achievement of therapeutic end points, including improved stability of anticoagulation and low incidence of bleeding, are associated with continuous patient education.[6,7,15,21] Education should be targeted to meet the patient learning objectives summarized in Exhibit 3–4.

Exhibit 3–4
PATIENT LEARNING OBJECTIVES

- State the reason that the patient is taking warfarin and how it relates to clot formation.
- Recite the name of the drug (generic and trade).
- Discuss how the drug works (eg, interferes with clotting) and the problems of too much or too little anticoagulation.
- Explain the need for blood tests and the target INR appropriate for the patient's treatment.
- Recite the importance of adherence, close monitoring, regular appointments, and good follow-up.
- Describe the common signs of bleeding.
- Outline precautionary measures to decrease trauma and bleeding.

- Identify diet, drug, and alcohol usage that might cause problems with therapy.
- Female patient: Explain the importance of not becoming pregnant and the need for birth control measures (or abstinence).
- Report with accuracy and honesty changes in lifestyle, diet, medications, alcohol intake, or disease process.
- Identify the importance of informing the health care provider when dental, surgical, or invasive procedures and hospitalization are scheduled or occur unexpectedly.
- State what to do in case of an emergency.
- Identify the specific tablet or tablets, by color and markings, that the patient is taking.

The amount of information presented to the patient beginning anticoagulation therapy can be overwhelming. Research has shown that, on average, 40% of patients forget the information given to them.[31] Written information reinforces oral information, helps patients remember important facts about therapy, and enhances knowledge about their disease. Patient education materials are commonly used by anticoagulation providers. Because therapy is often long term and patient and disease characteristics are not static, periodic reassessment should be part of the educational program of the anticoagulation provider. Each component of the educational process, including assessment, educational plan, and follow-up, should be documented in the database of the patient.

10. Management and Triage of Therapy-Related and Unrelated Problems

> **10.1 Anticoagulation providers should have a policy and procedure for the management of major and minor bleeding episodes, signs and symptoms of thromboembolism, other potential anticoagulation side effects, or other medical problems not related to anticoagulation therapy. This should include the use of vitamin K or fresh-frozen plasma to correct an excessively prolonged INR or to treat serious hemorrhage.**

Comment: Because complications do not absolutely correlate with the INR, careful patient assessment, in addition to interpretation of laboratory values, is necessary. Patients must be taught to self-monitor and report immediately all signs and symptoms of possible bleeding or thrombosis to the anticoagulation management service.

A patient whose therapy is managed at the office of his or her primary health care provider should have any problems triaged by a licensed health care provider. The patient should be seen by the appropriate provider within a timely period based on the urgency of the bleeding. The referring provider should be contacted regarding the nature of the episode.

An excessively prolonged INR (>5.0) is associated with an increased risk of bleeding.[22,24,32–34] When such values are observed, the patient should be contacted by the anticoagulation management service and assessed by the appropriate health care provider. Depending on the degree of elevation of the INR and whether or not bleeding is present, the appropriate interventions should be undertaken to correct the excessive degree of anticoagulation. Besides altering the dose of warfarin, this might involve the administration of vitamin K

and/or fresh-frozen plasma. The anticoagulation management service should have established guidelines for the use of such therapy based on opinions published in the literature or on other criteria.[12]

When elevated INR values are associated with serious bleeding, immediate medical attention is required. In addition to receiving vitamin K, patients might require administration of fresh-frozen plasma and hospitalization. Anticoagulation providers should facilitate and coordinate the provision of emergency services when necessary.

> **10.2 Anticoagulation providers should have a policy and procedure for the management of anticoagulation when the patient requires an invasive procedure.**

Comment: When considering changes in a patient's current anticoagulation therapy regimen because of a scheduled medical, dental, or surgical procedure, the anticoagulation provider must carefully weigh the risk of excessive or uncontrolled bleeding against the potential for recurrent thromboembolism. Both patient-specific variables and the type of procedure (eg, major surgery, dental procedure) should be evaluated to determine the optimal treatment plan. Current practice options include close monitoring, discontinuation of anticoagulation therapy three to five days prior to the procedure, initiation of a lower anticoagulation dosage, short-term substitution of intravenous heparin therapy, and the utilization of tranexamic mouthwash.

> **10.3 Anticoagulation providers should have a policy and procedure for the management of patients who are nonadherent with therapy, appointments, or other aspects of anticoagulation treatment. This policy should include guidelines for termination of anticoagulation management by the anticoagulation service.**

Comment: Anticoagulation requires a combination of provider and patient responsibility. Some patients who require anticoagulation therapy lack the personal and social resources to comply safely with their prescribed anticoagulation therapy regimen. To protect anticoagulation providers against liability, policies and procedures regarding management of nonadherent patients must be in place. To protect both the provider and the patient, guidelines for termination of patients from the anticoagulation management service also must be present.

GUIDELINES FOR THE EVALUATION OF PATIENT OUTCOMES

11. Organizational Components

> **11.1** The anticoagulation provider should perform a program evaluation of organizational components on an annual basis or more often as deemed necessary. Anticoagulation providers should analyze the contribution of various processes to patient outcomes.

Outcome: The evaluation of organizational components should include a systematic review of all factors contributing to outcomes—systems efficiency, care processes, laboratory monitoring, and patient education. Process indicators can be used to gauge the efficiency of these components. Failure to address this evaluation can lead to a type III error—the evaluation of a program that has not been adequately implemented.[35] The purpose of this evaluation is to ensure that the outlined processes are being implemented as intended.

12. Patient Outcomes

> **12.1** The anticoagulation provider should perform an outcomes evaluation on an annual basis or more often as deemed necessary. This outcome assessment should include, as a minimum, information pertaining to degree of therapeutic effectiveness as determined by the INR, hemorrhagic complication rates, thromboembolism rates, and other complications resulting from anticoagulant therapy.

Comment: Outcomes are the ultimate objectives of a health or therapeutic intervention as related to patients, anticoagulation providers, and payers. For patients, outcomes include not only improved health but improved self-care skills and improved quality of life.[36] For payers, outcomes include decreased medical care utilization and cost-effectiveness.

Each anticoagulation provider should review the frequency of untoward events in the facility annually or more often as deemed necessary. These events should include all deaths, minor and major bleeding episodes, recurrent thromboembolism, and patient health care system utilization secondary to anticoagulation problems (eg, emergency room visits, hospital admissions). Because the frequency of complications corresponds to the variability of the INR over time,[33,37] an intermediate outcome should include the percentage of time each patient spends within the targeted therapeutic range. Anticoagulation providers should perform continuous quality assurance monitoring that targets the maintenance of therapeutic INR.

Periodic surveys regarding quality of life issues, as well as patient and referring health care provider satisfaction with services, should be included in the anticoagulation provider's outcomes evaluation. Future program planning and quality improvement strategies should be based on the results of the organizational, clinical, and patient-specific evaluation components.

CONCLUSION

These clinical guidelines provide a framework for health care providers on the facets of anticoagulation therapy needed to provide quality care. The impact of these guidelines will depend on their implementation and the perceived value of their utility. The development of clinical guidelines is a first step in providing a system or process to ensure positive outcomes for patients on oral anticoagulation therapy. Issues regarding implementation of guidelines, education of anticoagulation providers, certification of anticoagulation providers and/or clinic sites, and standardization of outcomes evaluation also must be addressed.

REFERENCES

1. Agency for Health Care Policy and Research. Life-saving treatments to prevent stroke underused. September 7, 1995. Press release.

2. Kutner M, Nixon G, Silverstone F. Physicians' attitudes toward oral anticoagulants and antiplatelet agents for stroke prevention in elderly patients with atrial fibrillation. *Arch Intern Med.* 1991;151:1950–1953.

3. McCrory DC, Matchar DM, Samsa G, Sanders LL, Pritchett ELC. Physician attitudes about anticoagulation for nonvalvular atrial fibrillation in the elderly. *Arch Intern Med.* 1995;155:277–281.

4. Dalen JE, Hirsh J. Fourth ACCP Consensus Conference on Antithrombotic Therapy. *Chest.* 1995;108(suppl):225S–522S.

5. Cohen IA, Hutchison TA, Kirking DM, Shue ME. Evaluation of a pharmacist-managed anticoagulation clinic. *J Clin Hosp Pharm.* 1985;10:167–175.

6. Garabedian-Ruffalo SM, Gray DR, Sax MJ, Ruffalo RL. Retrospective evaluation of a pharmacist-managed warfarin anticoagulation clinic. *Am J Hosp Pharm.* 1985;42:304–308.

7. Cortelazzo S, Finazzi G, Viero P, et al. Thrombotic and hemorrhagic complications in patients with mechanical heart valve prostheses attending an anticoagulation clinic. *Thromb Haemost.* 1993;69:316–320.

8. Wilt VM, Gums JG, Ahmed OI, Moore LM. Outcome analysis of a pharmacist-managed anticoagulation service. *Pharmacotherapy.* 1995;15:732–739.

9. Bussey HI, Chiquette E, Amato MG. Anticoagulation clinic care versus routine medical care: a review and interim report. *J Thromb Thrombolysis.* 1996;2:315–319.

10. Clark CM, Kinney ED. Standard for the care of diabetes: origins, uses and implications for third-party payment. *Diabetes Care.* 1992; 15(suppl 1):10–14.

11. Clinton JJ, McCormick K, Besteman J. Enhancing clinical practice: the role of practice guidelines. *Am Psychologist.* 1994;49:30–34.

12. Hirsh J, Dalen JE, Deykin D, Poller L, Bussey H. Oral anticoagulants: mechanism of action, clinical effectiveness and optimal therapeutic range. *Chest.* 1995;108(suppl):231S–246S.

13. Hirsh J, Fuster V. AHA Medical/Scientific statement, special report: guide to anticoagulation therapy part 2: oral anticoagulants. *Circulation.* 1994;89:1469–1480.

14. Ansell JE, Buttaro ML, Thomas OV. Consensus guidelines for coordinated outpatient oral anticoagulation therapy management. *Ann Pharmacother.* 1997;31:604–615.

15. Errichetti AM, Holden A, Ansell JE. Management of oral anticoagulant therapy: experience with an anticoagulation clinic. *Arch Intern Med.* 1984;144:1966–1968.

16. Conte RR, Kehoe WA, Nielson N, Lodhia H. Nine-year experience with a pharmacist-managed anticoagulation clinic. *Am J Hosp Pharm.* 1986;43:2460–2464.

17. Bussey HI, Rospond RM, Quandt CM, Clark GM. The safety and effectiveness of long-term warfarin therapy in an anticoagulation clinic. *Pharmacotherapy.* 1989;9:214–219.

18. Kornblit P, Senderoff J, Davis-Ericksen M, Zenk J. Anticoagulation therapy: patient management and evaluation of an outpatient clinic. *Nurse Practitioner.* 1990;15(8):21–32.

19. Seabrook GR, Karp D, Schmitt DD, Bandyk DF. An outpatient anticoagulation protocol managed by a vascular nurse-clinician. *Am J Surg.* 1990;160:501–504.

20. Gassmann A, Goldman S, Hager D, et al. Results with nurse-directed outpatient anticoagulant therapy. *J Cardiol Med.* 1981;6:565–569.

21. Ellis FE, Stephens MA, Sharp GB. Evaluation of a pharmacy-managed warfarin-monitoring service to coordinate inpatient and outpatient therapy. *Am J Hosp Pharm.* 1992;49:387–394.

22. van der Meer FJM, Rosendaal FR, Vandenbrouke JP, Briet E. Bleeding complications in oral anticoagulant therapy: an analysis of risk factors. *Arch Intern Med.* 1993;153:1557–1562.

23. American Society of Health-System Pharmacists. ASHP Report: ASHP therapeutic position statement on the use of the International Normalized Radio system to monitor oral anticoagulant therapy. *Am J Health-Syst Pharm.* 1995;52:529–531.

24. Fihn SD, McDonell M, Martin D, et al. Risk factors for complications of chronic anticoagulation: a multicenter study. *Ann Intern Med.* 1993;118:511–520.

25. Landefeld CS, Beyth RJ. Anticoagulation-related bleeding: clinical epidemiology, prediction, and prevention. *Am J Med.* 1993;95:315–326.

26. Landefeld CS, Anderson PA. Guideline-based consultation to prevent anticoagulant-related bleeding: a randomized, controlled trial in a teaching hospital. *Ann Intern Med.* 1992;116:829–837.

27. Porter RS, Sawyer WT. Warfarin. In: Evans WE, Schentag JJ, Jusko WJ, eds. *Applied Pharmacokinetics: Principles of Therapeutic Drug Monitoring.* 3rd ed. Vancouver, Wash: Applied Therapeutics Inc; 1992:31–46.

28. Howard MR, Milligan DW. Frequency of attendance at anticoagulant clinics. *Acta Haematol.* 1986;76:78–80.

29. Green LW, Kreuter MW. Applications of PRECEDE-PROCEED in community settings and applications in health-care settings. In: *Health Promotion Planning: An Educational and Environmental Approach.* 2nd ed. Mountain View, Calif: Mayfield Publishing Co; 1991:261–307, 390–427.

30. Morisky DE, Levine DM, Green LW, Shapiro S, Russell RP, Smith CR. Five-year blood pressure control and mortality following health education for hypertensive patients. *Am J Public Health.* 1983;73:153–162.

31. Prochaska J, DeClementi C. Toward a comprehensive model of change. In: Miller WR, Heather N, eds. *Treating Addictive Behaviors: Process of Change.* New York: Plenum Press; 1986:3–27.

32. Landefeld CS, Rosenblatt MW, Goldman L. Bleeding in outpatients treated with warfarin: relation to the prothrombin time and important remediable lesions. *Am J Med.* 1989;87:153–159.

33. Cannegieter SC, Rosendaal FR, Wintzen AR, van der Meer FJM, Vandenbroucke JP, Briet E. Optimal oral anticoagulant therapy in patients with mechanical heart valves. *N Engl J Med.* 1995;333:11–17.

34. European Atrial Fibrillation Trial Study Group. Secondary prevention in non-rheumatic atrial fibrillation after transient ischemic attack or minor stroke. *Lancet.* 1993;342:1255–1262.

35. Basch CF, Sliepcevich EM, Gold RS, Duncan DF, Kolbe LJ. Avoiding type III errors in health education program evaluations: a case study. *Health Educ Q.* 1985;12:315–331.

36. Task Force To Revise the National Standards. National standards for diabetes self-management education programs. *Diabetes Care.* 1995;18(suppl 1):94–96.

37. Albers GW. Atrial fibrillation and stroke: three new studies, three remaining questions. *Arch Intern Med.* 1994;154:1443–1448.

Chapter 4

Personnel Needs and Division of Labor

Lynn B. Oertel

INTRODUCTION

Health care professionals involved in the management of anticoagulant therapy are keenly aware of increasing demands on their time. With the growing numbers of patients on therapy and with expanding clinical indications, optimal efficacy and optimal safety are primary concerns, followed closely by efficiency and cost-effectiveness of care. A creative, multidisciplinary approach to staffing and organization will often lead to successful and productive patient management. As health care costs climb, a critical look at traditional methods of patient care delivery is appropriate. The anticoagulation management service (AMS) that incorporates a multidisciplinary team utilizing nonphysician providers is an approach that can provide the opportunity for collaboration among physicians, nurses, pharmacists, and administrative assistants and result in cost savings without sacrificing high quality of care.

GETTING STARTED

In developing a program, the purpose, goals, scope of services, and target patient population should be identified. Careful consideration should be given to defining the goals and scope of service, as these factors will determine staffing needs and daily management activities. The details of how an AMS organizes its daily operations will vary from one setting to the next; however, commonalities in the general structure and overall purpose will remain. Many of the key elements in the organizational makeup and clinic functions are depicted in Figure 4–1.

Reimbursement for services from third-party payers for AMSs without face-to-face encounters is not well established. Therefore, support from hospitals, clinic administration, or other professional departments often must be considered and the costs justified. Efforts focused on a specific population (eg, cardiology or vascular patients) can help to promote the success of the larger group or institution through development of a collaborative network between referring physicians and the organization. By documenting such benefits, a positive track record of the anticoagulation management service can be established. This track record will promote continued expansion of the AMS beyond the initial focus as patients are recruited from other departments. Thus, costly duplication efforts for attaining similar goals in other anticoagulated groups are minimized.

The following are additional financial considerations:

- operating budget (What are the projected revenues and expenses?)
- dedicated office space
- personnel salaries
- office supplies
- computer and software needs
- capital expenditures (Is there a need for a facsimile machine, copier, or additional telephone lines?)

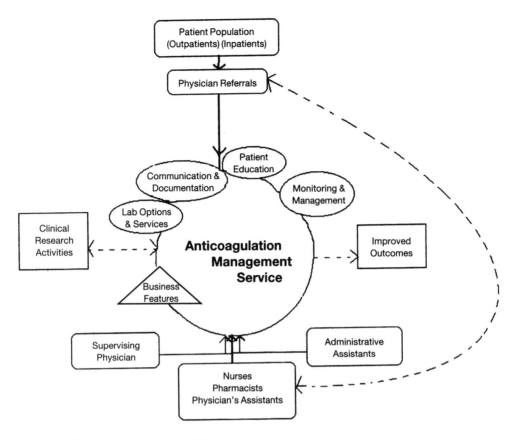

Figure 4–1 Organization and functions of an anticoagulation management service

For a more in-depth discussion on financial or business considerations, the reader is referred to Chapter 15, Developing a Business Plan for an Anticoagulation Clinic.

Evolving evidence indicates that an AMS can lead to financial savings through improved patient outcomes and such evidence can help in justifying the development of a service.[1–9] Alternatively, a retrospective data review obtained from one's own clinical setting that demonstrates less than ideal patient outcomes can be a powerful catalyst to support a new service. These data would also provide a benchmark on which to evaluate the impact of change and future performance.

Once gals and a patient population have been identified, the next step is to define specific policies and procedures. These guidelines will provide the framework on which the service operates. The following are key topics to include in a policy and procedure manual for an AMS:

- purpose and goals
- scope of services (Who is the intended population?)
- staffing: roles and responsibilities, medical consultation
- referring mechanism (How will new clients be obtained?
- educational curriculum content and methods

- anticoagulant therapy management (Will a dosing algorithm be implemented? Define the clinical guidelines for dose adjustment and prothrombin time [PT] scheduling.)
- patient tracking methods (What mechanisms are in place for patient follow-up?)
- data management tools (How will data be stored and retrieved for quality control?
- communication procedures for patient and referring practitioners
- safety procedures (Include clinical actions in response to supra- or sub-therapeutic International Normalized Ratios [INRs] or patient report of symptoms, after-hours coverage, etc.)
- evaluation methods: measures to assess quality of care and INR performance
- identification of personnel and additional resources

Ansell and colleagues[10] were the first to identify guidelines for developing policies and procedures to ensure safe and effective anticoagulation therapy management. A discussion on standards of care relative to anticoagulation management is also found in Chapter 3. However, as cautioned by D. Moniz,[11] "practitioners should develop protocols that are based on a minimum safe level and not the maximum level aimed at ideal care." This cautionary statement will help avoid problems with potential malpractice suits. Practitioners should keep in mind that once a protocol or standard is adopted by an AMS, it must be followed to minimize exposure to risk. Protocols and standards must be realistic for the individual practice and updated on a regular basis to keep consistent with research and practice trends.

Appendix 4A provides additional examples of policies and procedures developed at various AMSs.

PREDICTING AND PLANNING STAFFING PATTERNS

Questions frequently asked by those who are just beginning to establish an AMS are "How large of a staff do I need?" "What type of professional degrees should I seek?" and "What about nonprofessional support staff?" The projected numbers of patients and the scope of services will determine the labor needs specific to each practice setting. Large group practices might find it necessary to evaluate and redesign the daily work responsibilities of several workers across professional disciplines in order to maximize efficiency and optimize patient care. Conversely, smaller practices or single practitioners might need to place more emphasis on the daily work flow within the practice in order to find ways to achieve greater efficiency. Tasks need to be defined and delegated. What types of skills or expertise exist among current staff? If critical skills, such as computer skills, are deficient, then part of the overall plan should be to assist staff in acquiring those necessary skills.

Responses to the 1997 Winter Survey conducted by the Anticoagulation Forum of its membership yield descriptive data that may help to provide solutions to staffing questions. Exhibit 4–1 summarizes some of the survey's findings. The results of this survey suggest that most AMSs involve a physician at some level of participation (many are in medical director roles), whereas nurses and pharmacists have the majority of the day-to-day management responsibilities.

The staffing pattern within each AMS ideally should maximize each individual's clinical background and area of expertise. Staffing patterns currently observed in AMSs across the United States vary somewhat, depending upon the geographical location of the program and scope of services. Occasionally, some services have incorporated a primary care component into their care delivery systems. Some may offer an additional in-hospital consultation service for patient care. However, despite varying clinical makeups, the vast majority of AMSs utilize a medical director who generally is not responsible for the primary management of patients' anticoagulation therapy but who oversees the clinic from an administrative and consultative point of view. In other cases, the AMS personnel do not have a single individual providing oversight and medical backup but report and consult to a number of providers who refer patients to their service.

Anticipating staffing needs and patterns of work is difficult in the beginning as patient panels expand. Additionally, predicting personnel needs is complex due to the various clinical practice settings, resources, and experience available. A plan to incorporate flexibility among staff should be implemented to provide coverage for unexpected sick time, planned vacations, and unavoidable absences. A mechanism for training new staff is also needed, and cross-training provides a contingency mechanism for crisis control. Encouraging flexibility and creativity in positions, such as job sharing, may offer additional benefits to staff scheduling and, at the same time, promote continuity in quality patient care.

Table 4–1 provides information for planning future staffing needs based upon continued expansion of anticoagulation services. Extrapolating clinical experiences and consulting with other experts provided guidance for predicting the amount of effort required for INR management alone. The time required to perform daily AMS functions is difficult to estimate but must be accounted for in some fashion. The estimates used in this table are based upon the following assumptions:

- For ease in computing, it is assumed that, on average, patients obtain twice-monthly blood tests. This accounts for new patients needing weekly prothrombin time tests and for other patients with unstable, nontherapeutic responses who require more frequent testing.
- The model includes time required for making patient contact via telephone and/or postcard or letter preparation.

This model does *not*, however, include a time factor to account for the following essential tasks:

- an in-depth patient education session or introduction to the AMS and operations
- response to telephone calls from patients and other health care professionals regarding patient care issues
- assisting patients with brief interruptions in their anticoagulant therapy and conferring with medical professionals to make appropriate plans
- retrieval of INR values (Some AMSs may choose to perform point-of-care testing to determine INR values on site, whereas other services may choose to retrieve INR results from various clinical laboratories.)
- conducting measures of quality assurance performance (Parameters of quality assurance are imperative in order to evaluate current practice and are needed to guide

Exhibit 4–1
ANTICOAGULATION FORUM, 1997 WINTER SURVEY

- Number of surveys mailed/returned: 619/205 (33%)
- Number of individual programs responding: 161
- Number of patients managed/mean number per program: 59,000/366 per program
- Type of care provided:
  - Anticoagulation only: 62%
  - Anticoagulation plus primary care: 23%
  - Anticoagulation plus other care: 15%
- Location of programs:
  - Hospital outpatient clinics: 37%
  - Veterans Affairs medical centers: 24%
  - Private offices (group practices): 16%
  - Managed care organizations: 9%
  - Other: 5%
- Types of health care providers who participate in care, calculated by number of programs with type of providers ÷ total number of programs:
  - Physicians: 160 (99%)
  - Nurses: 74 (46%)
  - Nurse practitioners: 25 (16%)
  - Pharmacists (PharmD): 94 (58%)
  - Pharmacists (RPh): 32 (20%)
  - Physician assistants: 5 (3%)
  - Health assistants: 22 (14%)
  - Other: 43 (25%)
- Types of health care providers by effort or % full-time equivalent (FTE), based on total programs ÷ 161:
  - Physicians: 15%
  - Nurses: 30%
  - Nurse practitioners: 8%
  - Pharmacists (PharmD): 34%
  - Pharmacists (RPh): 6%
  - Physician assistants: 1%
  - Health assistants: 6%
  - Other: 15%

Source: Data from 1997 Winter Survey, Anticoagulation Forum, presented at the 4th National Anticoagulation Forum Conference, San Antonio, Texas, May 15–17, 1997.

Table 4–1 Estimates of Effort To Manage International Normalized Ratio (INR) Results Alone

| Clinic Size | Predicted Number of INRs | | | Hours/Day | % FTE |
	Per Month	Per Week	Per Day		
100	200	50	10	2	.25
200	400	100	25	5	.625
300	600	150	30	6	.75
400	800	200	40	8	1.0

Note: Estimates include decision making regarding dose adjustments and future prothrombin time (PT) scheduling, patient contact to inform of dose and PT date, additional patient assessments when indicated to assess INR response and health status, documentation of patient contact, etc.
% FTE = percent full-time equivalent.

future practice. Parameters may include time spent in therapeutic range (TTR), complication rates to therapy, frequency of INR testing, patient satisfaction, etc.)

Cataloguing the above tasks allows the clinician to document time devoted to various aspects of the anticoagulation management service. Referring to Table 4–1, one can conclude that one the patient population grows to 200 patients, over half of a clinician's time is relegated to INR management alone. The remaining time is insufficient to undertake other tasks essential to supporting a quality anticoagulation management service. Additionally, as the patient panel expands, considerations must be made to offer patient access 5 days a week as well as after-hours, weekend, and holiday coverage for emergency consultation. Once the service approaches 300 patients, adding part-time clerical assistance is warranted. As the service grows beyond 400, additional professional staff are necessary to assist with dose management, patient education, and clinical assessments. Some very efficient programs manage well with one full-time-equivalent licensed professional and one full-time-equivalent clerical individual for as many as 600 to 700 patients, but these are clearly the exceptions.

FACTORS AFFECTING STAFFING PATTERNS

The extent of person-to-person encounters after the initial orientation and educational phase varies among programs and will affect staffing needs. Several large clinics with years of experience utilize a telephone or mail system for successful patient management beyond the initial patient contact. In this model, administrative assistants perform vital tasks such as retrieving INR results, triaging telephone calls, scheduling initial patient appointments, tracking down tardy patients, and mailing postcards. By allocating these types of time-consuming tasks to nonmedical staff, licensed professionals can devote their expertise to areas where it is absolutely critical.

Another key factors in determining labor needs is the methodology used to measure INR results: Will fingerstick devices be used by staff personnel? Will a laboratory associated with the clinic be used for INR monitoring? Will the clinic utilize an off-site, independent laboratory, more conveniently located to patients, that will necessitate retrieval of results by clinic personnel? Each of these methods offers unique benefits to patient care, incurs varied costs for implementation, and requires different time commitments of personnel.

Until recently, very few sites utilized a computerized system for data storage or patient management, and even fewer incorporated a computerized dosing algorithm. That is now changing as the development and availability of patient management systems, information systems, clinical pathways, and other technology provide additional tools for anticoagulation therapy. (Details of commercially available software programs are described in Chapter 9, Software Applications in Anticoagulation Management.) Each of these has an impact on staffing needs. Such organizational tools are useful to ambulatory care clinics, community-based office practices, independent practitioner practices, and even in the inpatient setting where positive effects on anticoagulation management and utilization of resources have been noted.

PERSONNEL ROLES AND RESPONSIBILITIES

Once the overall clinic structure is defined, the next task is to provide a description of roles and corresponding responsibilities needed to achieve the goals of the work plan and organizational structure. Staff should demonstrate advanced knowledge of anticoagulants, including indications; develop an expertise in management strategies when evaluating INR responses; facilitate brief interruptions in therapy, when necessary, across various disciplines; be able to identify risk factors for untoward side effects; and perform effective education of patients. For further discussion of these roles and responsibilities, see Chapters 5 and 6.

Interest is growing for health care professionals to seek and obtain credentialing status specific to anticoagulation therapy. Such a credential provides the health care professional with the distinction of possessing advanced knowledge and skill relative to anticoagulation therapy and related disease processes. The National Certification Board for Anticoagulation Providers sponsors the only multidisciplinary certification process for health care providers in the United States.[12] The Certified Anticoagulation Care Provider credential is earned after submitting evidence of clinical practice expertise and achieving a passing score on a comprehensive examination. Chapter 7 discusses this credentialing process in further detail. Additional types of training and competency programs are available; however, most are restricted to pharmacists. For example, the National Association of Boards of Pharmacy has developed several disease state management credentialing examinations, including anticoagulation therapy. There are many reasons for professionals to seek credentialing, including recognition among peers, employers, and patients; employment advancements; or personal satisfaction. Additionally, future changes to third-party reimbursement structures and Medicaid payments may require a credentialed provider.

Nonprofessional personnel perform critical roles in the day-to-day function of an anticoagulation service. Written procedures to prioritize and accomplish tasks within designated time frames are helpful. Utilization of administrative assistants or secretaries allows for an increase in productivity and the management of an ever-expanding patient population.

A thumbnail list of daily tasks encountered by most AMSs includes:

- scheduling patient appointments for initial educational session
- providing in-depth patient teaching sessions
- retrieving INR results from an outside laboratory or from venipuncture or fingerstick tests within the clinic
- interpreting INR results for dose adjustments, if necessary, and scheduling future blood tests
- communicating with patients to inform them of test results and next blood test appointments
- tracking and identifying tardy patients
- serving as resource for referring physicians and patients
- facilitating continuity of care for patients during brief interruptions to therapy (eg, travel, hospitalization)
- performing quality control analyses

The AMS patient population is dynamic. Patients will continually be discharged from the service for various reasons, including completion of planned duration of therapy, death, complication to therapy, geographical relocation, and changes in health care coverage. Likewise, new patients will continually be added to the panel. The scope of service significantly affects staffing requirements and must be carefully evaluated and documented to make the best projections for staffing needs.

CONCLUSION

High-quality patient care is the overall primary goal of anticoagulation therapy, and individuals have a right to expect that the care provided by anticoagulation clinic staff surpasses traditional care. It is important not to lose sight of this focus. Knowledgeable staff associated with anticoagulation clinics are uniquely positioned to collaborate and offer high-quality, cost-effective care in contrast to traditional environments that are not anticoagulation focused.

REFERENCES

1. Cortelazzo S, Finazzi G, Viero P, et al. Thrombotic and hemorrhagic complications in patients with mechanical heart valve prosthesis attending an anticoagulation clinic. *Thromb Haemost.* 1993;69: 316–320.

2. Fihn SD, McDonell MB, Vermes D, et al. A computerized intervention to improve timing of outpatient follow-up: a multicenter randomized trial in patients treated with warfarin. *J Gen Intern Med.* 1994;9: 131–139.

3. Landefeld CS, Anderson PA. Guideline-based consultation to prevent anticoagulant-related bleeding: a randomized, controlled trial in a teaching hospital. *Ann Intern Med.* 1992;116:829–837.

4. Poller L, Wright D, Rowlands M. Prospective comparative study of computer programs used for management of warfarin. *J Clin Pathol.* 1993;46:299–303.

5. Skordis CM, Whitehead S. Computerised management of an oral anticoagulant clinic. *Aust NZ J Med.* 1992;22:496–497.

6. van de Besselaar AM, van der Meer FJM, Gerrits-Drabbe CW. Therapeutic control of oral anticoagulant treatment in the Netherlands. *Am J Clin Pathol.* 1988;90:685–690.

7. Garabedian-Ruffalo SM, Gray DR, Sax MJ, et al. Retrospective evaluation of a pharmacist-managed warfarin anticoagulation clinic. *Am J Hosp Pharm.* 1985;42:304–308.

8. Wilt VM, Gums JG, Ahmed OI, et al. Pharmacy operated anticoagulation service: improved outcomes in patients on warfarin. *Pharmacother.* 1995;15:732–779.

9. Chiquette E, Amato MG, Bussey HI. Comparison of an anticoagulation clinic and usual medical care: anticoagulation control, patient outcomes, and health care costs. *Arch Intern Med.* 1998;158: 1641–1647.

10. Ansell JE, Buttaro ML, Voltis TO, et al. Consensus guidelines for coordinated outpatient oral anticoagulation therapy management. *Ann Pharmacother.* 1997;31:604–615.

11. Moniz DM. The legal danger of written protocols and standards of practice. *Nurse Practit.* 1992;17(9):58–60.

12. Oertel LB. A national certification program for anticoagulation therapy providers. In: Becker RD, Alpert JS, Eds. *Cardiovascular Medicine: Practice and Management.* London: Arnold: 2001; 755–764.

Policies and Procedures Examples (Clinic Policies, Mission Statements, Scope of Service, Quality Improvement Report)

MULTIDISCIPLINARY WARFARIN CLINIC POLICY

POLICY

Referral to the clinic will be by written consultation. Ambulatory outpatients who are receiving primary/subspecialty care at this hospital and who are not being followed by hospital-based home care are eligible for enrollment in the clinic. The indication for anticoagulation, desired International Normalized Ratio range, and the duration of treatment need to be provided. When warfarin is initiated as an inpatient, written referral needs to be made prior to discharge and patient education about warfarin therapy completed by the inpatient nursing service. In addition, the following criteria must be met:

- Patients must have demonstrated capability for self-administration of medication or have a caretaker who can supervise the medication.
- Patients must have a telephone or reliable 24-hour-a-day, seven-day-a-week telephone contact established.
- Patients must be compliant and not abusing alcohol. Patients may be discharged from the clinic if they are abusing alcohol, are poorly compliant with their medication, or for failing to maintain communication or get prothrombin checks as requested.
- Patients need to have a primary care provider who is identifiable in the provider and group fields.

RESPONSIBILITY

This is a multidisciplinary clinic with shared responsibility by the primary care subspecialty medicine service, nursing service, and pharmacy service. The clinic will be staffed by registered nurses, registered pharmacists, and physician consultants. The roles of the providers are as follows:

- Designated registered nurses will be provided from the nursing service who will be credentialed to manage warfarin prothrombin times, dosage adjustment, quality assurance/improvement, and triage for anticoagulation or other medical problems.
- A designated registered pharmacist will be provided from the pharmacy service who will perform the above duties and provide drug information.
- A designated physician consultant will be provided from the primary care subspecialty medicine service for consultation and also for involvement in patient education and quality assurance/improvement activities.

PROCEDURES

Service will be provided for patients on warfarin or dicumarol only. The functions of the clinic are as follows:

- patient education to include information about drug dosage forms, prothrombin time testing, drug interactions, food interactions, disease interactions, alcohol interactions, lifestyle changes, and the need for careful follow-up and watching for complications
- dosage adjustment within established protocol guidelines
- triage for complications of anticoagulation or other clinical problems, and appropriate tests, consultation, and referrals made for any problems encountered
- maintenance of effective quality assurance/improvement program

REFERENCE

Fourth ACCP Consensus Conference on Antithrombotic Therapy. *Chest.* 1995;108(suppl):231S–245S.

Courtesy of Coumadin Clinic, Veterans Affairs Medical Center, Albuquerque, New Mexico.

ANTICOAGULATION MANAGEMENT SERVICE POLICY AND PROCEDURES

PURPOSE

The primary purpose of the Anticoagulation Management Service (AMS) is to manage the warfarin therapy of patients of _____ Hospital in order to maximize the efficacy, safety, and cost-effectiveness of therapy.

ROLE AND SCOPE

The Pharmacy Department's scope of service is to provide patient care by assisting the hospital staff in the management of patients enrolled in the AMS.

RESPONSIBILITY

The AMS is the responsibility of the Pharmacy Department and functions under the guidance of the AMS medical director. Within the Pharmacy Department, under the supervision of the clinical manager, the AMS is coordinated by a staff pharmacist, who has received specialized training in oral anticoagulation therapy management.

PROCEDURES

1. The AMS is located in _____, and hours of service are _____. Alternate appointments can be scheduled if necessary. Consultation and assistance are available Monday through Friday by voice mail or service pager.
2. The AMS will monitor any patient appropriately receiving oral anticoagulation, upon written request for consultation from a hospital physician, who has some aspect of medical care provided at the hospital. Consultation requests may be phoned or left at the AMS office.
3. Laboratory studies will be performed primarily by the _____ Laboratory. Prothrombin time results are obtained using MLA 1000 methodology and Dad Innovin reagent. Alternatively, laboratory studies may be conducted at outlying facilities for patient convenience. Prothrombin time results will be expressed exclusively as the International Normalized Ratio (INR). Results will be communicated to the AMS by the specific laboratory or visiting nurse.
4. The AMS pharmacist will interpret the INR according to the current recommendations regarding degree of anticoagulation based on the medical condition.
5. The AMS pharmacist will modify the patient's warfarin dosage regimen, if warranted, according to established protocol and communicate such modification to the patient within 24 hours.

6. The medical director of the AMS will be consulted immediately via telephone or in person regarding a patient's warfarin therapy when necessary.
7. For each AMS encounter, information will be recorded on an AMS flowsheet and subsequently entered into a computerized database. An updated patient report will be generated following each scheduled laboratory appointment and signed by the pharmacist. The reports (see **Warfarin Patient Tracking Report**) will be submitted to the patient's physician, via interdepartmental mail, for review within 24 hours of each AMS encounter. (There may be circumstances that prohibit a physician from receiving a report within the optimal 24-hour time frame; however, patients will be notified promptly of their laboratory results.) The reports will then be incorporated into the patient's chart by the Medical Records Department.
8. Patients will be seen by the AMS pharmacist on _____ from ____ AM to ____ PM, when they are scheduled for laboratory studies at the AMS clinic, to personally evaluate each patient for compliance with, and/or complications to, therapy. Personal consults can be scheduled at alternate times whenever necessary.
9. Patients presenting with severe bruising, active bleeding episodes, or excessively prolonged INRs will have their warfarin therapy managed according to AMS guidelines (see **Managing Excessive Prolongation of the International Normalized Ratio in the Outpatient Setting**). The AMS medical director or the patient's primary care physician also will be notified immediately to obtain specific interventional instructions.
10. The AMS pharmacist's competency and quality of work will be assessed through case presentations with the clinical manager of the Pharmacy Department or designee. A formal review will be conducted biannually by the clinical manager of the Pharmacy Department and the AMS medical director.
11. The physician, whose signature appears below, authorizes the pharmacist listed below, or designee, to make warfarin dose changes when medically appropriate. Authorization is limited to monitoring and dosage adjustment (including renewal of warfarin prescriptions to retail pharmacies), per established protocol for patients who are enrolled in the AMS.

Authorization as described above will be granted for a period of one year. A review of the protocol will be conducted yearly. Review of the pharmacist's performance will be conducted intermittently on an ongoing basis. Changes in the protocol, authorized prescribers, or pharmacists involved in the service will be communicated and documented via a resubmitted protocol or an addendum approved by the physicians and pharmacists involved with the AMS.

continues

Anticoagulation Management Service continued

_____   _____   _____   _____
Medical Director   Date   Clinical Manager,   Date
                                                             Department of Pharmacy

_____   _____
Pharmacist, Anticoagulation   Date
Management Service

The above-named pharmacist is hereby credentialed by the Department of Pharmacy to manage the AMS.

Courtesy of Boston University Medical Center Anticoagulation Clinic, Boston, Massachusetts.

ANTICOAGULATION SERVICE POLICIES AND PROCEDURES

PURPOSE

The purpose of the Anticoagulation Service is to complement the care provided by the physician, physician assistant, or nurse practitioner. The Anticoagulation Service is designed to provide intensive patient teaching and monitoring of oral anticoagulation therapy to maximize benefits while minimizing bleeding and thromboembolic events.

POLICY

It is the policy of the Anticoagulation Service to accept referrals to manage the anticoagulation of all patients on warfarin therapy who are under the continuing care of a physician, physician assistant, or nurse practitioner in the Physician Office Center. Anticoagulation clinic patients must continue to receive medical follow-up by a primary care provider in the clinic or be seen by the referring specialist at a minimum of every six months. The pharmacist in the Anticoagulation Service is responsible for monitoring the patient's International Normalized Ratio (INR), questioning the patient about any complaints of bleeding or thromboembolic events on a regular basis (at least every six weeks), and adjusting the warfarin dose as necessary to achieve a therapeutic level of anticoagulation as defined by the most current American College of Chest Physician guidelines. The anticoagulation clinic pharmacist will provide patient education, screen and monitor for the addition or subtraction of any interacting medications, and renew warfarin prescriptions. The physician preceptor or the patient's primary care provider should be consulted as necessary.

HOURS OF OPERATION AND PATIENT VISITS

The clinic will be staffed Monday through Friday from 8:30 AM until 5:30 PM except for clinic holidays. Patients will be scheduled to have blood drawn at the clinic when possible to coincide with provider visits. When needed, patients will be scheduled to have blood drawn at a local laboratory with results called in to the clinic or obtained electronically the same day. When home health nurses are involved with patient care, the nurse will obtain the INR at specified times and call the results in to the clinic.

PATIENT INCLUSION

All individuals who are prescribed warfarin at a target INR range and for an indication consistent with the most current published recommendations of the American College of Chest Physicians are eligible for enrollment into the Anticoagulation Service.

PATIENT REFERRAL

Physicians, physician assistants, or nurse practitioners may contact the anticoagulation clinic pharmacist Monday through Friday 8:30 AM–5:30 PM at pager #0631 to refer a patient. To facilitate patient education, the anticoagulation clinic pharmacist should be notified as early as possible when a patient is initiated on warfarin. If a patient is discharged and the anticoagulation clinic pharmacist was not available, the physician, physician assistant, or nurse practitioner must provide care to

continues

the patient until the pharmacist has been appropriately notified. A voice mail message to the pharmacist will not be considered an appropriate referral.

PHARMACIST RESPONSIBILITIES

1. Conduct an initial interview with the patient/caregiver. This meeting can be in the hospital or in the clinic. The purpose of this interview is to:
   - Obtain medical problem/medication history (may be obtained from the medical record).
   - Assess educational needs and supply warfarin booklet. This step is the beginning of the educational process, which may be completed over a period of several visits, and routinely reinforced. This booklet is reviewed in detail with patients.
   - Determine logistics of laboratory evaluations and home health needs.
   - Determine communication needs and provide patient/caregiver with telephone numbers for anticoagulation clinic pharmacist.
2. Maintain a schedule of all patient visits and upcoming laboratory values. Since many patients have their INR obtained at outside facilities, it is the responsibility of the pharmacist to follow up with patients who do not have their INR drawn at the planned time.
3. Evaluate each INR value for appropriateness for the patient's indication. Patients should be asked about medication, dietary, alcohol, or health status changes that may impact on the INR value. Compliance issues also should be addressed.
4. Assess for bleeding and thromboembolic complications, Discuss any concerns, including changes in health status with the primary care provider or the attending physician on duty in the clinic. Arrange appropriate follow-up appointments or tests as needed.
5. Make adjustments in warfarin dosage as needed based on the above information. Adjustments may be of a temporary nature if the suspected cause of the fluctuation is transient, or an actual dosage change may be made. In general, most dosage adjustments should not exceed 15 percent of the total weekly dosage, unless the patient is in the initial stages of anticoagulation and the appropriate dosage has not been determined.
6. Determine when next INR should be obtained. This interval depends on the stability of the INR and other patient changes. This interval may be several days up to six weeks. The number of days or weeks the patient has been on a specific dose and the stability of the INR during that time period should be used as a guide to determine when the INR value should be obtained (eg, patient has been on same warfarin dose for 13 days with two INR values in the targeted INR range, continue dosage and obtain next INR in two weeks).
7. Instruct the patient/caregiver about dosage adjustments and determine when the next INR is to be obtained. Inform home health of any changes and arrange follow-up INR for appropriate patients.
8. Document each patient contact in the medical record and in the anticoagulation clinic database. All notes regarding patient contact will be distributed to an attending physician for review and a signature.
9. Provide instruction to physicians and patients regarding planned interruption of therapy for procedures. Coordinate the plan of care with all involved.
10. Periodically review the patient's history to determine if warfarin therapy needs to continue. Discuss possible discontinuation of therapy with the patient's provider. Changes in medical status or complications that may warrant discontinuation of therapy also should be discussed with the patient's provider.
11. Serve as preceptor for pharmacy residents and Doctor of Pharmacy students. Provide ongoing education to physicians, physician assistants, nurse practitioners, and nursing personnel on anticoagulation issues.
12. Provide educational lectures for groups at this facility and outside facilities on matters regarding anticoagulation and antithrombotic therapy.
13. Participate in ongoing research activities related to anticoagulation.
14. Conduct periodic productivity and outcomes reviews.

DISCHARGING PATIENTS FROM THE ANTICOAGULATION SERVICE

In certain circumstances, patients may be discharged from the anticoagulation service and referred to the primary care provider or a local medical doctor for management. These include:

1. The patient with chronic alcohol abuse whose level of anticoagulation remains unacceptable despite the pharmacists' best efforts.
2. The patient who is chronically noncompliant with getting INR values obtained.
3. The patient who fails to have at least an annual follow-up with the warfarin prescriber.

Courtesy of University of West Virginia, Morgantown, West Virginia.

ANTICOAGULATION PROGRAM POLICIES AND PROCEDURES

The anticoagulation program is a service directed by a physician and staffed by registered nurses and pharmacists with specific knowledge in anticoagulation therapy. Oral anticoagulant care is managed under the supervision of physicians in the Department of Internal Medicine.

I. Purpose
  A. To manage oral anticoagulant therapy (warfarin) by evaluating the prothrombin time (PT) and/or the International Normalized Ratio (INR) and instructing patients or family of appropriate dosage of warfarin.
  B. To assess patients for possible complications related to anticoagulant therapy.
  C. To provide comprehensive and ongoing education to patients and/or family members about anticoagulant therapy with specific attention to signs and symptoms to report.

II. Policy
  A. Evaluation of patients
    1. Initial evaluation of patients will occur after consult is called to the anticoagulation program by a physician from the Department of Internal Medicine.
    2. Consults are preferably made prior to the inpatient's discharge so as to allow adequate time for chart review and patient education.
    3. Patient chart will be reviewed, and the following information will be obtained for clinic chart:
      a. past medical/surgical history
      b. hospital course
      c. medications
      d. allergies
      e. anticoagulation therapy received and date of initiation
      f. primary physician
      g. patient telephone number, address, and emergency contact
    4. Patient will be seen by a member of the anticoagulation program (RN, PharmD, RPh) who will review the following:
      a. clinic policy and procedure
      b. comprehensive patient education according to guidelines established for patient education
    5. Patients will sign anticoagulation program contract, which will outline their responsibilities as participants in the program.
  B. Target PT/INR range
    1. Target PT/INR ranges will be determined by the physician according to individual patient indication and need. Changes in these therapeutic ranges will be made as indicated by the primary or clinic physician.
  C. Expected duration of therapy
    1. Expected length of anticoagulant therapy will be determined by primary or clinic physician and will be made on an individual basis, depending on indication. When therapy has reached the expected discontinuation date, the primary physician will evaluate the need for continuation of warfarin and the decision will be documented in the patient's chart.
  D. Frequency of PT/INR testing*
    1. When anticoagulation therapy has been initiated or when a patient has been recently discharged after hospitalization, the PT/INR will be checked one or two times weekly until stable.
    2. When the PT/INR and dose of warfarin remain stable for two testing days, the PT/INR will be checked weekly.
    3. When the PT/INR and dose of warfarin remain stable for two weeks, the PT/INR will be checked every two weeks.
    4. When the PT/INR and dose of warfarin remain stable for four weeks, the PT/INR will be checked in one month.
    5. All patients must have their PT/INR checked at least monthly.
    6. After a change in dose is made, all patients are required to have their PT/INR checked at least weekly until stable.
    Note: These are only general monitoring guidelines applied to patients. Frequency of PT/INR will depend on individual patient condition and overall treatment plan.

III. Eligibility Criteria
  A. Patients must be able to attend clinic appointments.
  B. If patients are not able to meet this requirement, the final decision to accept the patient will be made by the program director. The patient will be classified as a "phone patient."
  C. Patients must agree to come in for appropriate comprehensive follow-up visits with a physician in the Department of Internal Medicine.
  D. The patients or family members should have the capacity to understand the patient's condition and implications of anticoagulant therapy.
  E. Patients must be willing to be active participants in their health maintenance.
  F. Patients must be able to travel to and from clinic appointments.
  G. Patients must be accessible by telephone.
  H. Patients must have a documented need for anticoagulant therapy.

IV. Clinic Visits
  A. Clinic hours: Tuesday mornings, 8:30 AM–12:00 noon
                    Friday afternoons, 1:00 PM–4:30 PM
  B. Clinic visits are by appointment only. If patients are unable to keep an appointment, they are to notify the office and reschedule.

continues

Anticoagulation Program continued

C. Patients will have PT/INR checked by fingerstick with the Coumatrak machine.

D. Patients will then be seen by the nurse or pharmacist and the following will be assessed:
   1. signs/symptoms of bleeding episodes (gingival bleeding, epistaxis, ecchymoses, hematuria, melena, blood per rectum, etc.)
   2. signs/symptoms of a thrombotic event (shortness of breath, pain/swelling of extremity, numbness, tingling, headache, etc.)
   3. significant changes in diet
   4. any changes in concomitant drug therapy (including over-the-counter medications and intermittent antibiotic therapy)
   5. compliance with anticoagulant therapy
   6. signs/symptoms of intolerance of drug (nausea/vomiting/diarrhea, rash, skin necrosis, etc.)

E. Based on these assessments and the PT/INR, dosage changes in anticoagulant therapy will be made if necessary and patients will be counseled on these changes.

F. Dosage changes are to be supervised by the clinic physician as evidenced by co-signature beside the documented change.

G. Patient education will be reinforced.

H. Patients will be instructed on when to return for clinic appointments.

I. Patients will be referred to the physician on site for any of the following:
   1. signs/symptoms of thrombosis
   2. signs/symptoms of serious bleeding episodes
   3. significant adverse drug reactions
   4. significantly subtherapeutic or elevated PT
   5. any other acute problem related or unrelated to anticoagulant therapy

J. Prescription for anticoagulant therapy may be renewed by telephone by the nurse or pharmacist, with documentation in the patient's chart, which is to be signed by the primary physician.

V. Phone Patients

A. Clinic hours: Tuesday afternoons, 1:00 PM–4:30 PM
                  Friday afternoons, 1:00 PM–4:30 PM

B. Patients who are unable to attend clinic because of immobility, proximity, or patient condition may have their PT/INR drawn by a laboratory other than the clinic and are classified as phone patients.

C. Phone patients are accepted into the program only at the discretion and approval of the program director.

D. Patients must have access to transportation in the case of suspected anticoagulation complications that might require medical attention.

E. Anticoagulation clinical personnel will make arrangements for blood draws for the homebound patient. Patients who are not homebound may have their blood drawn at a local hospital or laboratory in their area.

F. A clinic chart will be kept on these patients as well as a PT laboratory check file. The file will include the patient's name, telephone number, name of laboratory, laboratory telephone number, and date that next PT is to be drawn. This card will be filed under the date of the month that the blood is to be drawn plus one day. This allows the laboratory one working day to process the blood. The PT laboratory check file will be reviewed daily.

G. Anticoagulation members will obtain results from the laboratory used by the patient.

H. The patient will then receive instructions by telephone from the nurse or pharmacist during clinic hours.

I. Patients will be interviewed for complications (see Clinic Visits section).

J. Patients will be required to call the office for instructions if they do not receive a telephone call within 48 hours after a blood test.

K. Patients are still required to be followed by their primary physician or a physician within the Department of Internal Medicine. If a patient is to take a three- to six-month course of therapy, the patient is to see his or her physician in the middle of therapy and at completion of therapy. If the patient is on long-term therapy, he or she is to see the primary physician every six months.

VI. Documentation

A. Anticoagulant therapy will be documented on the monitoring flowsheet.

B. Assessments of patients during clinic visits will also be documented in the progress notes.

C. Prescription renewals and scheduled laboratory draws will be documented.

D. Letters will be forwarded to the primary physician if requested, stating the PT, ratio, INR, and dosage change.

These policies and procedures were developed and mutually agreed upon by the following:

_____	_____
Program director	Date
_____	_____
Registered nurse	Date
_____	_____
Pharmacist	Date

Courtesy of Division of Internal Medicine, Anticoagulation Program, Thomas Jefferson University Hospital, Philadelphia, Pennsylvania.

ANTICOAGULATION CLINIC—MISSION STATEMENT AND POLICIES

I. MISSION STATEMENT

The mission of the Anticoagulation (AC) Clinic is to provide safe, effective management of anticoagulation therapy for ambulatory patients of the Greater Baltimore Metropolitan area. These services are provided to all persons regardless of race, color, religion, national origin, or disability. Payment for services is an objective, but not a precondition for treating any patient.

To effect its mission, the AC Clinic is authorized to:

1. Operate a clinic providing quality pharmaceutical care and services consistent with identified community needs and fiscal feasibility in accordance with the mission of University Health Center (UHC).
2. Manage resources in an efficient and effective manner.
3. Determine the appropriate dose and duration of anticoagulation therapy for each patient based on the documented indication(s) and the current literature.
4. Stabilize and maintain therapeutic anticoagulation through skillful dosage adjustment as necessary for each patient.
5. Avoid drug-induced toxicity by careful, consistent assessment of each patient.
6. Provide timely and appropriate intervention in the event of a bleeding episode.
7. Assess each patient's knowledge regarding anticoagulation therapy and provide patient instruction that maximizes the benefit and minimizes the risk of therapy.
8. Accept referrals for hospitalized patients who will be discharged on anticoagulation therapy.
9. Include the patient in therapeutic decisions.

II. POLICY ON INITIAL VISITS TO THE ANTICOAGULATION CLINIC

All new patients referred to the anticoagulation clinic will be comprehensively evaluated with regard to the indication, benefits, risks, and goals of anticoagulation therapy. All patients will be given appropriate and thorough instruction in the safe and effective use of warfarin.

Procedure

1. Patients referred to the UHC AC Clinic will be given a specific appointment to be seen. At the appointed time, patients will report to the UHC reception desk for check-in. Patients who arrive 30 minutes late for an appointment will be rescheduled for the next available appointment.
2. Following check-in, patients with a lab request slip will proceed to the lab for fingerstick and/or venopuncture. Using the Biotrak® portable Prothrombintime (PT) monitor, the laboratory technician will measure the patient's protime. The laboratory technician will record the patient's PT and INR directly on the lab slip and the Protime Log

Form. The lab slip will be returned to the patient. Patients will then return to the patient waiting area. Patients will be seen by a clinician within 30 minutes of the appointment time, unless an urgent medical or other need requires that the patient be seen earlier.

3. The clinician will gather a complete medical history and accurately record baseline data. Baseline information will be recorded on the Anticoagulation Clinic Patient Registration and Data Form (see Appendix 8A) and the Anticoagulation Monitoring Flowsheet (see Appendix 8B). These two forms will not be placed in the patient's UHC medical record, but will be retained in a patient-specific folder systematically stored in the AC Clinic filing cabinet in the UHC Clinic.
4. The clinician will perform a brief physical exam and obtain laboratory studies (as needed) to detect evidence of bleeding or thromboembolic events. At a minimum, the assessment will include:
   - Measurement of BP (sitting and supine), HR, Temp., Ht, Wt
   - Inspection of the skin and nails for bruising, injuries, or wounds
   - Auscultation of the chest (heart and lung sounds)
   - Brief neurological exam
   - Hematocrit (baseline level, obtained within the past 14 days)
5. The clinician will provide patient education. Both oral and written information will be provided and will include:
   - Benefit(s) of therapy
   - Risks of therapy
   - Risks of therapy during pregnancy (if female of childbearing age)
   - Goal of therapy, including INR range and anticipated duration
   - Drug-drug and drug-food interactions
   - Signs and symptoms of bleeding; emergency instructions
   - Pamphlets:
     – A Patient Guide: Using Coumadin® at Home (by DuPont Pharma)
     – Guide to the UHC Anticoagulation Clinic
     – Warfarin and Pregnancy (if female of childbearing age)
   - Audio and video patient instruction (when appropriate)
6. When appropriate, patients will be referred to the primary physician or a specialist if physical or laboratory findings suggest a major bleeding episode or thromboembolic event.
7. On Anticoagulation Service Referral Form (see Appendix 8A), the clinician will record the patient's pertinent medical history, objective findings, an assessment regarding the patient's anticoagulation therapy, and a plan for action. The note will be recorded in a standardized format. The original copy of the note will be placed in the patient's UHC medical record. A copy of the note will be retained in

continues

the patient's AC Clinic folder. If requested, a copy of the note is forwarded to the referring physician or other concerned parties (with the patient's permission). The laboratory results, the previous and new warfarin dose, and RTC date will be recorded on the Anticoagulation Monitoring Flowsheet (see Appendix 8B).

8. All patients will be encouraged to ask questions. The therapeutic plan will be explained to the patient. The patient will be asked to repeat important instructions to improve retention and ensure comprehension.

9. After reviewing the master appointment calendar for available appointments, the clinician will determine when the patient should return to the clinic for follow-up monitoring. Intervals between visits are determined by the stability of the patient, in terms of both anticoagulation and general health. In general, return visits are scheduled every 7 to 14 days until a stable, therapeutic response is achieved. Once stabilized, the interval between visits will generally be four to five weeks, but in no case longer than six weeks. The clinician will record the patient's follow-up appointment (date and time) in the master appointment calendar.

10. The patient will be given an Anticoagulation Service Patient Instruction Form (see Appendix 31A) that documents the results of his or her blood test, the new dose of warfarin to be taken, any special instructions, and the next appointment date and time. The patient will be given a completed laboratory slip(s) that can to be used at the next clinic visit.

III. POLICY ON FOLLOW-UP VISITS TO THE ANTICOAGULATION CLINIC

All patients followed by the anticoagulation clinic will be closely monitored for thromboembolic events, bleeding complications, and medication adherence. Warfarin therapy will be expertly managed with the goal of maintaining the patient within an appropriate range of anticoagulation based on the literature and patient-specific considerations.

Procedure

1. Upon arrival at the UHC, patients will report to the reception desk for check-in.

2. With a lab slip(s), the patient will proceed to the lab for fingerstick and/or venopuncture. Using the Biotrak® portable PT monitor, the laboratory technician will measure the patient's protime. The laboratory technician will record the results of the PT and INR test on the lab slip and the Protime/INR Log Form. The lab slip will be returned to the patient. The patient will then return to the patient waiting area. Each patient will be seen by the clinician within 30 minutes of the appointed time, unless an urgent medical or other need requires that the patient be seen earlier.

3. The clinician will gather an abbreviated patient history and will ask the patient specifically about symptoms suggestive of major or minor bleeding and thromboembolic events. If the INR is not within the patient's goal range, the clinician will question the patient to explore the etiology. The patient will be specifically asked about changes in medications and diet; changes will be recorded on the Anticoagulation Clinic Patient Registration and Data Form (see Appendix 8A).

4. The clinician will perform a brief physical exam and obtain laboratory studies (as needed) to detect evidence of bleeding or thromboembolic event. At a minimum, the assessment will include:
   - Measurement of BP (sitting and supine), HR, Wt
   - Inspection of the skin and nails for bruising, injuries, or wounds
   - Auscultation of the chest (heart and lung sounds)
   - Brief neurological exam

5. When appropriate, patients will be referred to the primary physician or a specialist if physical or laboratory findings suggest a major bleeding episode or thromboembolic event.

6. The clinician will provide patient education. Both oral and written information will be provided to reinforce topics previously discussed and to address specific patient problems or questions.

7. On the Anticoagulation Clinic History Sheet (see Appendix 8A), the clinician will record a brief patient history, objective findings, an assessment regarding the patient's anticoagulation therapy, and a plan for action. The note will be placed in the patient's UHC medical record. If requested, a copy of the note will be forwarded to the referring physician or other concerned parties (with the patient's permission). The laboratory results, the previous and new warfarin dose, and RTC date will be recorded on the Anticoagulation Monitoring Flowsheet (see Appendix 8B).

8. All patients will be encouraged to ask questions. The therapeutic plan will be explained to the patient. The patient will be asked to repeat important instructions to improve retention and ensure comprehension.

9. The patient will be given the Anticoagulation Service Patient Instruction Form (see Appendix 31A) that documents the results of his or her blood test, the new dose of warfarin to be taken, any special instructions, and the next appointment date.

IV. POLICY ON DISCHARGING PATIENTS FROM CLINIC

After consultation with the referring physician, the patient will be discharged from the clinic when the anticipated duration of therapy has been completed or when the risks of therapy outweigh potential benefits. In an effort to maximize clinic resources, a patient also may be discharged from the clinic if he or she repeatedly fails to adhere to clinician recommendations.

continues

Anticoagulation Clinic—Mission Statement and Policies continued

Procedure

1. After the patient has completed the originally anticipated duration of anticoagulation therapy without experiencing a (recurrent) thromboembolic event, the referring physician will be contacted. The referring physician will be informed of the patient's status and a recommendation for discontinuation or continuation of therapy will be explained. If the clinician and the referring physician concur, the patient will be instructed to stop taking warfarin and any potential risks will be explained (eg, thromboembolic events). Emergency instructions will be reemphasized. The plan and instructions will be recorded on the Anticoagulation Clinic History Sheet (see Appendix 8A).

2. If the patient's medical condition changes, such as to place the patient at greater risk of bleeding complications *or* new data are reported in the literature that alters the clinician's original recommendation to use warfarin, the referring physician will be contacted. The clinician will explain his or her new recommendations in light of the change in the patient's health or literature data. If the clinician and the referring physician concur, the patient will be discharged from the clinic (as above). If the referring physician does not concur with the recommendation to discontinue therapy, the clinician may discharge the patient to be followed thereafter by the referring physician (or other provider) but only after informing the patient and the referring physician *in writing*.

3. If the patient repeatedly fails to keep clinic appointments, have laboratory tests done, or take warfarin as prescribed, the patient may be discharged from the clinic at the discretion of the clinician. Patients who are physically or verbally abusive to staff or students, who place other patients at risk of injury, or who intentionally deceive the clinician(s) may be discharged from the clinic at the discretion of the clinician. In some cases, the clinician may ask the patient to enter into a patient-provider contract. The contract will specify the behaviors that are expected of both parties and the consequences if the contract is broken. If the clinician decides to discharge the patient from the clinic, the referring physician and the patient will be informed of the decision *in writing*. All reasonable efforts will be made to guarantee the patient's access to follow-up care. The decision to discharge the patient will be reconsidered if extenuating reasons for the patient's behavior are identified.

Courtesy of University of Maryland, School of Pharmacy, Baltimore, Maryland.

Anticoagulation Service Quality Improvement Report

Patient Demographics		1st Quarter	2nd Quarter	3rd Quarter	4th Quarter
Number of patients monitored on Warfarin					
Indication for anticoagulation	Atrial fibrillation				
	Valve				
	DVT/PE				
	Other				
New starts					
Discontinued therapy					
Number of patients on Warfarin with fatal outcomes					

Clinical Outcomes	1st Quarter	2nd Quarter	3rd Quarter	4th Quarter
Number of Protimes Monitored				
INR > 4.5				
INR < 1.8				
INR between 1.8 and 4.5				

continues

continued

Summary of Severe Complications

Complication	Benchmark	1st Quarter			2nd Quarter			3rd Quarter			4th Quarter		
		#	# of prevent-ables	1st qtr total	#	# of prevent-ables	2nd qtr total	#	# of prevent-ables	3rd qtr total	#	# of prevent-ables	4th qtr total
Major hemorrhagic events	2.4–3.0% 2.7/100 yr												
Thrombotic events	3.3%/ pt yr												
Fatal events	0.6%/yr 0.64/100 pt yr												

Reversal of Anticoagulation

Reversal of Anticoagulation	1st Quarter	2nd Quarter	3rd Quarter	4th Quarter
Number of hospital admissions ONLY for reversal of anticoagulation				
Number of patients receiving oral vitamin K				
Related to drug-drug interactions				
Related to discontinuation of another drug that interacts with Coumadin				

Observations and action taken:

Recommendations:

Report submitted by:

Courtesy of Kaiser Permanente Hawaii, Department of Pharmacy, Honolulu, Hawaii.

Anticoagulation Clinic Protocol: Clinical Pharmacists

The scope of practice for clinical pharmacists includes initiating orders for selective drug therapies and diagnostic tests according to established protocols.

Clinical pharmacists are the responsible providers for the anticoagulation clinic. The following procedure is authorized:

- Review the clinical record including indications for the anticoagulant, prothrombin times, and medications.
- Prescribe anticoagulants (renew orders, adjust dosage, etc.) without co-signature for patients in the anticoagulation clinic. They may also renew maintenance prescriptions for anticoagulation clinic patients with the exception of controlled substances.
- Provide patient instruction regarding the safe and appropriate use of the anticoagulation therapy.
- Utilize medical staff guidelines when prescribing anticoagulants. Criteria for protimes as defined in the medical staff guidelines will be utilized.
- Clinical concerns will be addressed to the primary care provider.

Pharmacist_____

Recommend Approval: _____
                     Chief, Pharmacy Service

                     _____
                     Chief, Clinical Service

                     _____
                     Chief of Staff

Approved/Disapproved: _____   _____
                      Director   Date

Courtesy of Anticoagulation Clinic, Royal C Johnson Memorial Hospital/Veterans Affairs, Sioux Falls, South Dakota.

Statement of Scope of Practice of Clinical Pharmacist

A statement of category I, full scope of practice, activity, or procedure may be conducted according to a preestablished protocol in accordance with all stipulations for the following individuals:

Clinical pharmacy scope of practice includes, but is not limited to, the following:

- initiating orders for selective drug therapies and diagnostic tests according to established protocols
- developing, ordering, and adjusting individualized patient dosing regimens with the consent of responsible physicians
- conducting and coordinating clinical drug investigations and research under Food and Drug Administration guidelines and regulations and approved by the local Research and Development Committee
- serving as clinical managers of drug and drug-related programs in clinics and wards in conjunction with the chief of the specific clinical service
- identifying and recommending corrective actions for drug-induced problems in association with the clinical staff
- implementing protocols approved by the Pharmacy and Therapeutics Committee in the use of nonformulary drugs and restricted drugs

_____   _____
Signature (Pharmacist)   Signature (Pharmacist)

Recommend Approval: _____
                                        Chief, Pharmacy Service

                                        _____
                                        Chief, Clinical Service

                                        _____
                                        Chief of Staff

Approved/Disapproved: _____   _____
                                        Director   Date

Courtesy of Anticoagulation Clinic, Royal C Johnson Memorial Hospital/Veterans Affairs, Sioux Falls, South Dakota.

Proficiency Skills Checklist for Point-of-Care Devices

Name _____   Date _____

Certifier's Name _____

	Yes	No
1. Explain procedure to patient.		
2. Assemble materials:		
– Protime monitor		
– Adapter plug		
– Control cartridge		
– Gauze, alcohol, Band-Aid, gloves		
3. Calibrate machine properly using control cartridges:		
– Insert control cartridge No. 1.		
– Push button at command, "Apply drop of blood."		
– Record results, range, International Normalized Ratio on daily log.		
– Repeat above using control No. 2.		
4. Perform test accurately:		
– Wear gloves and clean skin on fingertip with alcohol, then dry with gauze.		
– Insert reagent cartridge in monitor.		
– At command, "Apply drop of blood," perform needlestick with autolet and milk finger to obtain a large hanging drop of blood.		
– Place blood drop on center hole in cartridge, and maintain finger there for 2–3 additional seconds after monitor reads, "Measurement in progress."		
– Apply gauze to fingertip, and instruct patient to apply pressure.		
– Apply Band-Aid to fingertip.		
5. Record patient result on appropriate daily log.		
6. Discard cartridge, fingerstick lancets, and gauze in appropriate container.		

Courtesy of Anticoagulation Clinic, University of Virginia Medical Center, Charlottesville, Virginia.

Management of No-Shows

I. The patient is responsible for rescheduling all missed appointments.

II. The first time a patient misses a scheduled appointment:
   A. The patient will be notified by telephone.
   B. Another appointment will be scheduled.
   C. A note will be written in the progress notes of the patient's chart stating that the appointment was missed.

III. The second time a patient misses a scheduled appointment:
   A. The patient will be notified by telephone.
   B. Another appointment will be scheduled.
   C. A letter will be sent to the patient.
   D. A copy of above letter will be placed in the correspondence section of the patient's chart.
   E. A note will be written in the progress notes of the patient's chart stating that the appointment was missed.

IV. The third time a patient misses a scheduled appointment:
   A. The patient will be notified by telephone.
   B. Another appointment will be scheduled. The urgency and importance of this will be stressed.
   C. The program director will be notified.
   D. A letter co-signed by the program director will be sent to the patient's primary physician.
   E. A copy of above letter will be placed in the correspondence section of the patient's chart.
   F. A letter will be sent to the patient.
   G. A copy of above letter will be placed in the correspondence section of the patient's chart.
   H. A note will be written in the progress notes of the patient's chart stating that the appointment was missed, and that the program director and the primary physician were notified.

V. The fourth time a patient misses a scheduled appointment:
   A. The patient will be notified by telephone. The patient will be told that a letter will be sent by certified mail. If the patient fails to respond after letter sent, then patient will be terminated from the anticoagulation program.
   B. A letter signed by the program director outlining alternative forms of care will be sent via certified mail.
   C. A copy of above letter will be placed in the correspondence section of the patient's chart.
   D. A note will be written in the progress notes of the patient's chart stating that the appointment was missed, and that a letter was sent via certified mail.

VI. If the patient has not contacted the office within 10 working days:
   A. The program director will be notified.
   B. A letter will be sent to the patient's primary physician stating that the patient has been terminated from the anticoagulation program.
   C. A termination note will be written in the progress notes of the patient's chart.

Courtesy of Division of Internal Medicine, Anticoagulation Program, Thomas Jefferson University Hospital, Philadelphia, Pennsylvania.

Warfarin Patient Tracking Report

Next Visit _____   Medical No. _____

Social Security No._____

Name_____

Birth Date _____   Day Telephone _____

Sex _____ Age _____   Night Telephone _____

Other Contact _____   Contact Telephone _____

MEDICAL INFORMATION

Medical Site_____

Primary Physician _____   Telephone_____

Referring Physician _____   Telephone_____

Diagnosis_____

Recommendation _____

Other Medications _____

Complications _____

Current Dose_____

PROGRAM STATUS AND TARGET VALUES

Health Status		Low	High
Start Date _____			
Education Date _____	Seconds:	0.0	0.0
Ending Date_____	INR:	2.00	3.00
Reason for Termination _____	PT Ratio:	0.00	0.00

LABORATORY VALUES

Date	Current Dose	Laboratory Values				New Dose	Notified By	Return Date
		Control	Seconds	INR	PT			

Key: INR, International Normalized Ratio; PT, prothrombin time.

Managing Excessive Prolongation of the International Normalized Ratio in the Outpatient Setting

INR	Recommendation
4–6	Omit one or more doses of warfarin; consider reduced dose.
6–10	Hold warfarin until INR is therapeutic, then reinstitute at a reduced dose.
10–20	Consider vitamin K, 0.5–2.0 mg*; check INR in 12–24 hours and repeat vitamin K if necessary; reinstitute warfarin at a reduced dose.
>20	Consider vitamin K, 1.0–5.0 mg*; close observation and consider fresh-frozen plasma depending on degree of INR elevation and specific patient risks for bleeding; reinstitute warfarin at lower dose when INR becomes therapeutic.

Note: Serious bleeding requires the use of fresh-frozen plasma to replace missing factors and parenteral vitamin K*; factor concentrates may be considered in life-threatening or intracranial hemorrhage.

*Because of the potential for hypersensitivity reaction or anaphylaxis to intervenous vitamin K, it should be given slowly (not >1 mg/min); alternatively, it can be given by the subcutaneous route or orally, but response might be delayed if absorption is impaired. Vitamin K can lead to a brief period of relative warfarin resistance and difficulty in reestablishing a therapeutic range; higher doses of warfarin may be needed, but frequent monitoring is imperative.

Courtesy of Boston University Medical Center Anticoagulation Clinic, Boston, Massachusetts.

PROTOCOL FOR ROLE OF NURSES IN THE MONITORING AND EDUCATION OF PATIENTS

POLICY

The anticoagulation clinic is a service directed by a physician knowledgeable in anticoagulant therapy. It is staffed by two nurse-practitioners (NPs) and a registered nurse (RN) with specific knowledge in anticoagulation therapy and with job-specific training as defined in this protocol. The nurses manage patients' oral anticoagulant care in collaboration with the physician.

PURPOSE

- To manage oral anticoagulant therapy by evaluating the prothrombin time (PT) and advising patients/family of the proper dose of anticoagulant medicine.
- To assess patients for possible complications of or problems with oral anticoagulant therapy.
- To educate patient and family about the use of anticoagulants so that therapy will be successful and complications will be prevented.
- To provide inservice education regarding anticoagulation therapy.

GENERAL INFORMATION

The anticoagulation clinic specializes in the care of patients receiving oral anticoagulants to prevent blood clots. Patients are referred by physicians from the inpatient and outpatient areas of the hospital as well as the community. All patients are determined to be able to care for themselves or have appropriate caregivers such as parents, other family members, home health, or nursing home providers. Ideally, inpatients will be scheduled for their initial visit one to three days after discharge. The initial referral is per telephone by the physician. The physician documents written orders on a consultation form that includes indication for anticoagulation therapy, expected duration, current anticoagulation dosage, desired therapeutic International Normalized Ratio (INR), and the name of the primary care physician responsible for the medical management of the patient's care.

THERAPEUTIC ADJUSTMENTS

The therapeutic goal of warfarin therapy is to maintain the patient's prothrombin time between 1.3 and 2.5 times the normal control values as expressed in INR units; however, this increases the potential for adverse bleeding episodes rather than the degree of therapeutic response and therefore must be established for each patient and thereafter maintained through the expected duration of therapy.

Patients presenting with PT values outside the therapeutic range, previously maintained in good control, will be questioned in an attempt to identify precipitating factors that, if controlled, would obviate dose adjustment. If no responsible factor can be identified, warfarin will be adjusted in accordance with past dose-response data and kinetic parameters, and a return visit will be scheduled for no later than two weeks.

If the most recent PT is shorter than the therapeutic range, poor compliance may be the cause. Other variants commonly implicated in decreased response to be considered are drug-drug interactions, dietary alterations, increased alcohol intake, fever, and gastrointestinal illness.

If the most recent PT is no longer than desired, patients will fall into two categories: (1) those without evidence of excessive hypocoagulability who require a downward adjustment in dose and careful monitoring to regain therapeutic control and (2) those with actual or suspected signs of a bleeding episode whose dose should be downward adjusted and referred to an ambulatory care clinic staff physician for evaluation.

Only in extreme cases should warfarin dose be completely discontinued and/or vitamin K be administered because of the inherent problems in reestablishing therapeutic hypocoagulability. If a major bleed should occur precluding further therapy, whole blood or fresh-frozen plasma, followed by vitamin K administration in some cases, will normally return clotting factors to normal levels.

DOSE MANAGEMENT OF WARFARIN

Each patient's therapeutic range is categorized by the physician according to the diagnosis.

Deviations from these ranges will be made on an individual basis by the anticoagulation clinic physician and/or the referring physician as required by past history, current condition, risk factors, or other problems.

Diagnoses and Therapeutic Ranges

Diagnoses	INR Range
1. DVT (uncomplicated)	2.0–3.0
2. DVT (complicated)	2.5–3.5
3. PE (uncomplicated)	2.0–3.0
4. PE (complicated)	2.5–3.5
5. Chronic venous disease	2.0–3.0
6. Atrial fibrillation TIA/CVA	2.0–3.0
7. Prosthetic valve (mechanical) TIA/CVA	3.0–4.5
8. Prosthetic valve (biologic) TIA/CVA	2.0–3.0
9. Cardiomyopathy TIA/CVA	2.0–3.0
10. Left ventricular thrombus TIA/CVA	2.0–3.0
11. Peripheral arterial disease graft	2.0–3.0
12. Acute myocardial infarction	2.0–3.0
13. Coronary artery stent	2.0–3.0
14. TIA	2.0–3.0
15. CVA	2.0–3.0
16. Orthopaedic fracture or joint replacement	1.5–2.0
17. Oncology patients per protocol	Varies
18. Any of above with recurrent thrombo-embolism on anticoagulant	Shift up 0.5–1.0 INR unit

Key: CVA, cardiovascular accident; DVT, deep venous thrombosis; PE, pulmonary embolus; TIA, transient ischemic attack.

continues

Protocol for Role of Nurses continued

If bleeding risk is high, therapy should be aimed at the low end of the INR range.

The following table provides specific schedules for doses from 5 mg/week to 145 mg/week:

Dosage Schedule

	Sunday	Monday	Tuesday	Wednesday	Thursday	Friday	Saturday
5	0	2.5	0	0	2.5	0	0
7.5	0	2.5	0	2.5	0	2.5	0
10	2.5	0	2.5	0	2.5	0	2.5
12.5	2.5	0	2.5	2.5	0	2.5	2.5
15	0	2.5	2.5	2.5	2.5	2.5	2.5
17.5	2.5	2.5	2.5	2.5	2.5	2.5	2.5
20	5	2.5	2.5	2.5	2.5	2.5	2.5
22.5	2.5	5	2.5	2.5	5	2.5	2.5
25	2.5	5	2.5	5	2.5	5	2.5
27.5	5	2.5	5	2.5	5	2.5	5
30	5	2.5	5	5	2.5	5	5
32.5	2.5	5	5	5	5	5	5
35	5	5	5	5	5	5	5
37.5	7.5	5	5	5	5	5	5
40	5	7.5	5	5	7.5	5	5
42.5	5	7.5	5	7.5	5	7.5	5
45	7.5	5	7.5	5	7.5	5	7.5
47.5	7.5	5	7.5	7.5	5	7.5	7.5
50	5	7.5	7.5	7.5	7.5	7.5	7.5
52.5	7.5	7.5	7.5	7.5	7.5	7.5	7.5
55	10	7.5	7.5	7.5	7.5	7.5	7.5
60	7.5	10	7.5	10	7.5	10	7.5
65	5	10	10	10	10	10	10
70	10	10	10	10	10	10	10
75	15	10	10	10	10	10	10
80	10	15	10	10	15	10	10
85	10	15	10	15	10	15	10
90	15	10	15	10	15	10	15
95	15	10	15	15	10	15	15
100	10	15	15	15	15	15	15
105	15	15	15	15	15	15	15
110	20	15	15	15	15	15	15
115	15	20	15	15	20	15	15
120	15	20	15	20	15	20	15
125	20	15	20	15	20	15	20
130	20	15	20	20	15	20	20
135	15	20	20	20	20	20	20
140	20	20	20	20	20	20	20
145	25	20	20	20	20	20	20

continues

Protocol for Role of Nurses continued

DETERMINATION OF NEXT PT BLOOD TEST

1. The PT should be checked one or two times weekly when anticoagulation therapy has been initiated or when a patient has recently been discharged after hospitalization.
2. Once No. 1 is achieved, the PT should be checked at least weekly until the PT remains therapeutic at the same dose of anticoagulant medicine for at least one more measurement, unless otherwise indicated by a change in patient's condition and/or overall treatment program.
3. Once No. 2 is achieved, the PT should be checked approximately every 2 weeks until the PT remains therapeutic at the same dose of anticoagulant medicine for at least one more measurement, unless otherwise indicated by a change in the patient's condition and/or overall treatment program.
4. Once No. 3 is achieved, the PT should be checked approximately every 3 weeks until the PT remains therapeutic at the same dose of anticoagulant medicine for at least one more measurement, unless otherwise indicated by a change in the patient's condition and/or overall treatment program.
5. Once No. 4 is achieved, the PT should be checked approximately every 4 weeks if the PT level remains therapeutic at the same dose of anticoagulant medicine, unless otherwise indicated by a change in the patient's condition and/or overall treatment program.
6. Very stable patients (ie, those who will be anticoagulated for life) can be scheduled at longer intervals (up to 12 weeks) at the discretion of the RN. When indicated, the RN will collaborate with the NP or the physician.

PROTOCOL

1. *Visits:* By appointment only (excluding emergency visits). If unable to keep an appointment, the patient and/or significant other is responsible for calling the anticoagulation clinic and rescheduling the appointment.
2. *Laboratory testing:* Performed by an in-house or outside laboratory, according to physician request or the specific requirements of the patient, as long as an approved testing and reporting mechanism is in place.
3. *Frequency of blood testing:* Initially, PT checked once or twice weekly. As the PT and the dose of anticoagulant stabilizes, the test will be done weekly, every two weeks, every three weeks, then monthly. All patients must have their PT checked at least monthly except in rare circumstances (eg, those who are proven to be very stable).
4. *Initial visit:* After blood testing, new patients meet with the nurse for the initial patient education, which lasts approximately one hour.
5. *Pharmacy consultation:* The nurse consults with the pharmacist for current sources of information, regarding potential drug-drug, drug-food, and drug-disease interactions.

6. *Patient progress:* Assessed at least once every six months by a physician to determine the need for continued anticoagulation therapy. Clinic staff will ensure that this reassessment is performed in collaboration with a physician.

PATIENT EDUCATION

1. *Indication:* Discuss specific indication for anticoagulants (ie, valve replacement, deep venous thrombosis, pulmonary embolus, atrial fibrillation, transient ischemic attack).
2. *Action of drug:* Discuss action of anticoagulant medicine and its interference with the clotting mechanism of the blood to prevent blood clots from forming but not so much as to cause bleeding.
3. *Administration:* Discuss the administration of anticoagulants.
   - Know the strength (number of milligrams) of the prescribed anticoagulant medicine tablet.
   - Take the anticoagulant medicine once each day at the same time, usually in the early evening.
4. *Monitoring progress:* Explain how the anticoagulant medicine is monitored. The PT is the blood test used to evaluate how long it takes for the blood to clot. If the blood clots too quickly, the patient needs to take more anticoagulant because the risk of developing a blood clot is greater. If the blood takes too long to clot, the patient needs to take a smaller amount of anticoagulant because risk of a bleeding problem is greater. The PT should be measured approximately 12 hours after warfarin ingestion. Thus, evening dosing should be followed by morning testing.
5. *Signs of bleeding:* Instruct the patient regarding potential signs of bleeding problems.
   - Nosebleeds
   - Bleeding gums
   - Coughing up blood
   - Easy bruising
   - Blood in urine and/or bowel movements
   - Abnormal or excessive vaginal bleeding
   - Cuts that do not stop bleeding
6. *Medication interactions:* Discuss medication interactions.
   - Many medications can potentiate anticoagulants, whereas others can inhibit the action of anticoagulants.
   - Inform the staff of any new medications or changes in current medications.
   - Strictly avoid any products that contain aspirin. The risk of bleeding greatly increases when aspirin and anticoagulants are taken together.
   - Avoid multivitamins that contain vitamin K. Vitamin K counteracts anticoagulants.
7. *Diet:* Discuss dietary influences.
   - Fish and leafy green vegetables may be eaten as long as their intake remains consistent from week to week.

continues

Protocol for Role of Nurses continued

- Any major diet changes (eg, weight reduction or decreased appetite and food intake) should be reported as these changes can influence the action of anticoagulants.
8. *Alcohol restriction:* Discuss the effect of alcohol with anticoagulants.
    - Both alcohol and anticoagulant medicine are metabolized (broken down) in the liver. An excessive amount of alcohol can cause the anticoagulant medicine to work differently.
    - Avoid alcohol or keep to a minimum.
9. *Safety precautions:* Discuss safety precautions.
    - Because anticoagulants interfere with the blood's clotting ability, any injury can be more serious.
    - Avoid situations that might lead to injury (eg, sharp instruments, contact sports, certain occupations).
    - Do not walk barefoot outdoors.
    - Shave with an electric razor.
    - Use extreme care with sharp knives, tools, garden equipment, and broken glass.
    - Use an ID card, medallion, or bracelet to show that you are on anticoagulation therapy.

REVISITS

Return patients who have PTs drawn in another site should call the nurse after blood testing if they have any questions or problems or need further patient education. Patients who have PTs done will discuss results and dosage schedule with the nurse whenever possible.

1. The nurse will try to discuss PT results on the day of the test. This can be accomplished in person, over the telephone, or by postcard if the patient's PT is stable and no change is indicated. The following issues should be reviewed when discussing PTs and warfarin regimen:
    - current dose
    - any bleeding problems
    - medication changes/diet changes/alcohol use/life changes
    - dosage changes
    - next scheduled testing date/appointment
2. It is important to supply patients with telephone numbers to reach staff during clinic hours, evenings, weekends, and in case of emergency. Advise the patient to contact the staff regarding:
    - problems/questions with anticoagulant medicine
    - medication changes
    - upcoming dental work or surgical procedures
    - prescription refill

MANAGEMENT OF MISSED APPOINTMENTS

1. The patient is responsible for rescheduling all missed appointments.

2. When the patient does not keep an appointment and is a no-show, the following steps will be taken in an attempt to reach the patient:
    - The RN will call the patient's home.
    - If unable to contact by phone, the RN will send an appointment slip to the patient to reschedule the missed appointment.
    - No-shows will be documented on the progress note and the flowsheet in the notebook.
3. If the patient is a no-show three times, he or she will be referred to the medical director of the anticoagulation clinic by the nurse in the following manner:
    - The patient will be notified by telephone.
    - The medical director will be notified.
    - Documentation of the no-shows will be made on the progress sheet.
    - The primary physician will be notified by telephone and a copy of the progress sheet will be sent to the physician.
    - If a new appointment is made, it will be sent by certified mail.

DOCUMENTATION

1. Record on the progress note or anticoagulation summary (outpatient) sheet:
    - subjective complaints regarding bleeding, medication changes, and problems
    - PT results
    - Old warfarin dose and new dose
    - Date of next blood test/appointment
    - Aspects of patient education
    - Physician name and consulting physician who are copied
2. Copy of progress note sent to referring physician, which includes the medical information listed in No. 1.
3. Appointments and/or testing dates missed.
4. Testing location (clinic laboratory, outside laboratory, or other).

ANTICOAGULATION NURSE DUTIES

Clinic Duties

1. Manages all patient interactions as appropriate.
    - Informs patients of PT results and gives follow-up appointment.
    - Recognizes patient problems and refers any concerns regarding medication regimen, bleeding, or other adverse physical conditions to physician.
    - Telephone interactions are conducted in the following manner:
        - Identify self with first and last names, title, and name of clinic.

continues

Protocol for Role of Nurses continued

- Identify patient/responsible caregiver by first and last names.
- Ask if the patient is having any problems, specifically bleeding; if yes, refer call as in No. 1 (second entry).
- Encourage patient to adhere to plan of care as established by RN and physician.
- Give PT results and follow-up appointment to RN and physician.

2. Appropriately assists/directs patients arriving in the clinic.
3. Takes vital signs as needed and refers patient to medical clinic when indicated.
4. Performs prothrombin blood tests and records appropriately.

Clerical Duties

1. Prepares a list of pending PTs and no-shows daily.
2. Accurately records and coordinates new referrals and discharge status of current inpatients.
3. Obtains all PT results (pending first) from the clinic, outside laboratories, and hospitals for daily review and records appropriately.

4. Schedules all clinic PT appointments/arrivals, home PTs, and outside laboratory PT draws daily.
5. Checks no-show list, and calls patients to remind them of missed appointments.
6. Registers new patient referrals appropriately.
7. Completes and sends patient status reports to referring physicians.
8. Obtains medical records when requested.
9. Sends progress notes to medical records.
10. Mails patient education material to patients.

Setup and/or Maintenance

1. Checks control accuracy on near-patient testing device and records daily.
2. Keeps patient care area for PT testing clean, neat, and well stocked.
3. Cleans and properly disposes of blood-testing equipment.
4. Keeps statistics for the clinic.
5. Prepares new patient education.

Courtesy of Anticoagulation Clinic, University of Virginia Medical Center, Charlottesville, Virginia.

Chapter 5

Nursing Issues

Lynn B. Oertel

The practice of nursing is based on health promotion, disease prevention, and patient/family education and counseling. It incorporates both science and art. As Katims describes, "the art of nursing is considered that part of nursing that is not grounded in scientifically-derived or theoretical knowledge. It is, instead, the expressive, creative, and intuitive application of formal knowledge."[1] These qualities provide nurses with vital skills to effectively manage and monitor patients' anticoagulation therapy in a vast variety of practice settings.

Nurses strive to assist patients and their families in achieving a better level of wellness. They provide care to patients along the various points of the illness-wellness continuum. How lifelong prescribed therapies, such as oral anticoagulation, can affect a patient's perception of this illness-wellness continuum is but one example of the unique challenges nurses face during care delivery. The impact that therapy has on each patient must be considered in developing overall nursing goals and plans. Other variables such as concurrent medical diagnoses, medications, and dietary changes also must be evaluated throughout the course of therapy to achieve optimal outcomes.

Nurses have developed specialized roles in the care delivery of many anticoagulation management services (AMSs) across the country.[2,3] Brosnan[4] describes how multidisciplinary involvement within a medical center helped develop an anticoagulation pathway that improved service to patients and, at the same time, clarified and strengthened the nurse's role. Advanced-practice nurses in primary care practices have also effectively implemented protocols for anticoagula-

tion management services.[5,6] In such ways, nurses employ their expertise to make improvements in the care delivery systems in which they work. Clinical decisions regarding anticoagulation must include specific knowledge about patients' current health status as well as their response to therapy.

Depending upon the practice setting, nurse roles differ according to individual state practice acts. Therefore, it is imperative for nurses to review their respective state's nurse practice act. State nurse practice acts "set licensure requirements for the profession of nursing, define the scope of practice and authorize boards to enforce the laws regulating nursing practice."[7] As defined by Eskreis,[8] "the traditional standard for nurses is that degree of skill, care and diligence exercised by members of the nursing profession, practicing in the same or a similar locality." A significant phrase of this statement is "in the same or similar locality." Practitioners should take care to individualize protocols and standards to address their specific needs and scope of patient services within their locale.

Nurse practice laws also address the issue of delegating tasks. Since many AMSs employ various unlicensed personnel, this is a noteworthy issue. State boards may use different definitions of "delegation" as it applies to nursing practice. Therefore, delegating nursing activity by a licensed nurse to an unlicensed person requires careful consideration. Does the unlicensed person have a job description that permits performance of specific delegated acts? Does the employer have policies and procedures permitting this person to carry out specific delegated acts? Decisions about what nursing activities can be safety delegated are also within the scope of the individual nurse's judgment. The Massachusetts Board of Registration lists five questions to aid with the decision-making process for delegating specific nursing activities to an unlicensed assistant. These five questions are:[9]

1. Is the activity within the nurse's (RN/LPN) scope of practice to perform?
2. Based on the nurse's assessment, are the activities to be performed ones that require nursing assessment and judgment during implementation?
3. Is there an unlicensed assistive personnel available who is able to perform the activity safely?
4. Is the nurse able to provide appropriate supervision of the unlicensed assistive personnel during implementation/performance of the activity?
5. Are there any other considerations that would prohibit delegation by a reasonable and prudent nurse?

The response to each of the above questions determines the next step and whether or not the activity can be legally delegated.

On occasion, nurse roles may be further modified by institutional guidelines for practice, including clinical decision-making algorithms.[10] In some instances, practice standards address the "ideal" versus the "realistic" standard that can be met at all times and in all settings. The danger of writing protocols and standards that describe the "ideal" situation is that this practice also exposes the practitioner to unnecessary legal risk.[11] Using legal case studies, Eskreis[8] summarizes common mistakes nurses have made and highlights actions that might avoid a repeat occurrence. Failure to follow established protocols and failure to provide sufficient monitoring are described in some of these examples.

Guidelines or protocols are enacted for the purposes of standardization, cost-effectiveness, and improved patient outcomes and require a careful review process. Algorithms help support and guide practice for selected populations with specific needs. Further, policies and procedures should be routinely reviewed and revised to meet the changing needs of the patient population and clinical practice trends. The legal department for medical centers or private practices may "approve" such guidelines after endorsements are obtained from appropriate department heads and practice committees. Documentation of the roles and responsibilities of various staff members employed within an AMS will facilitate safe and effective care. Examples of nurse roles specific to an anticoagulation management service appear in Appendix 5A.

By virtue of their training and education, advanced-practice nurses bring a set of special skills to their function as primary health care providers. Nurse practitioners (NPs) continue to expand their power and influence on health care delivery in our country. Reimbursement mechanisms for services provided are improving at the state as well as the federal level, an important observation for the future of AMSs and their ability to generate revenue. Nurse practitioners are often the principal providers of primary care in rural, urban, and long-term care facilities, and they may initiate and manage oral anticoagulant therapy for their patients. Mahoney[12] describes the caring, listening, supporting, and empowering qualities that NPs possess as unique qualities that are highly valued by the patients they serve. Additionally, prescriptive authority has allowed NPs greater autonomy in their respective practices. Some form of prescriptive authority for NPs (may/may not require some degree of physician collaboration or may/may not include controlled substances) is law in all 50 states, including Washington, D.C. Additionally, 43 states now allow NPs the authority to receive and/or dispense drug samples.[13] These regulatory changes have greatly increased the autonomy of NPs as they continue to provide high-quality, comprehensive, and cost-effective patient care.

Collaboration among physicians, pharmacists, and nurses is vital to the successful delivery of care for anticoagulant therapy. Frequently, boundaries between these disciplines merge and many responsibilities are shared. Nevertheless, the primary goal to optimize therapy remains consistent. The continuing changes in the health care delivery system, along with issues pertaining to reimbursement and cost-effectiveness, will ultimately dictate further changes. The role of nurses, however, will remain instrumental in formulating specific interventions needed to achieve the most effective anticoagulation therapy for their patients.

REFERENCES

1. Katims I. Nursing as aesthetic experience and the notion of practice. *Scholarly Inquiry for Nursing Practice*. 1993;7:269–282.

2. Errichetti AM, Holden A, Ansell JE. Management of oral anticoagulant therapy: experience with an anticoagulation clinic. *Arch Intern Med*. 1984;44:1966–1968.

3. Oertel LB, Lake ME. Workshop: data management for a 2000-patient anticoagulation clinic. *J Thromb Thrombolysis*. 1996;2:305–307.

4. Brosnan J. A patient-focused pathway for ambulatory anticoagulation care. *J Nurs Care Qual*. Dec. 1996; 11(2):41–53.

5. Becker DM, DeMong LK, Kaplan P, et al. Anticoagulant therapy and primary care internal medicine: a nurse practitioner model for combined clinical service. *J Gen Intern Med*. 1994;9:525–527.

6. Kornblit P, Senderoff J, Davis-Ericksen M, Zenk J. Anticoagulation therapy: patient management and evaluation of an outpatient clinic. *Nurse Practitioner*. 1990;15:21–32.

7. Crawford L. Regulation of registered nurses. *Reflections on Nursing Leadership*. 2001;28–29, 34.

8. Eskreis TR. Seven common legal pitfalls in nursing. *AJN*. 1998;98(4):34–41.

9. Massachusetts Board of Registration in Nursing. *Nursing Board News*. 1997;3(2):1,6.

10. Gawlinski A. Practice protocols: development and use. *Crit Care Nurs Clin N Am*. 1995;7(1):17–23.

11. Moniz DM. The legal danger of written protocols and standards of practice. *Nurse Pract*. 1992;17(9):58–60.

12. Mahoney DR. Marketing health care programs to older adults: strategies for success. *Geriatr Nurs*. 1994;15:10–15.

13. Pearson LJ. Annual legislative update: how each state stands on legislative issues affecting advance nursing practice. *Nurse Pract*. 2000;25(1):16–28.

Sample Nurse Role Description Associated with Anticoagulation Services

POSITION DESCRIPTION FOR REGISTERED NURSE IN A SPECIALTY CENTER
(INCLUDES ANTICOAGULATION EDUCATION REQUIREMENTS)

Title: Registered Nurse RN
Department: Specialty Center
Reports to: Clinical Coordinator

Date: _____

Signatures:

_____

Department Director

_____

Human Resources

POSITION SUMMARY

Under the direction of the Nurse Clinical Coordinator, the Specialty Center RN assists the specialty provider in the delivery of patient care in the office setting.

Demonstrates professional, customer-focused, service-oriented manner, displays and promotes respect, care, and dignity for all internal and external customers; facilitates a team-oriented attitude, striving continuously for service excellence.

ESSENTIAL FUNCTIONS AND PRIMARY RESPONSIBILITIES

1. Assists visiting physicians with provision of health care in the office.
2. Provides appropriate health care patient education and follows protocols related to specific clinics.
3. Prepares and maintains patient chart for office visit and exam room.
4. Triages phone calls and refers to appropriate providers.
5. Provides direct patient care and administers medications within the scope of the Maine Nurse Practice Act.
6. Maintains work areas and equipment in clean, safe condition; follows fire, safety, and infection control policies and procedures.
7. Gathers data related to performance improvement, goals, and objectives.

The above statements are intended to describe the general level of work being performed by people assigned to this job. They do not necessarily include all responsibilities and duties usually associated with the job title.

QUALIFICATIONS/COMPETENCIES:

LICENSES, REQUIRED:
Registered Nurse—State of Maine

STAFFING EDUCATION REQUIREMENTS FOR ANTICOAGULATION SPECIALTY CLINIC

Registered Nurses employed by the Specialty Center will be involved in the Anticoagulation Clinic. In order to provide safe and effective care for those patients who are enrolled in the Anticoagulation Clinic, the following competency requirements for Anticoagulation Providers are needed to maintain continuity of care within the Protocols set for this clinic:

- Understanding of coagulation, antithrombotic therapy, and thrombogenesis.
- Understanding of pharmacokinetic and pharmacodynamic properties of warfarin and other anticoagulants used in the outpatient setting.
- Ability to describe the expected impact of and identify medications, disease states, and dietary and lifestyle changes that alter anticoagulation therapy.
- Assessment skills to identify the signs and symptoms of bleeding and knowledge of when to refer to the primary physician.
- Understanding of hypercoagulable states.
- Understanding of hemostasis and normal coagulation.
- Skills to identify and triage other medical problems and refer to Primary Physician.
- Understanding of the effects of socioeconomic, behavioral, psychological, and environmental factors on patient adherence.
- Ability to describe the relationship between the PT, ISI value, and INR. Ability to discuss limitations and reasons for variability.
- Ability to interpret INR and related lab values and adjust warfarin dose according to the protocol.
- Understanding of age-specific growth and development and how this may impact therapy.
- Understanding of the protocol for the Anticoagulation Clinic, Education Guidelines, and No Show/Noncompliant Policy.

The Specialty Center Clinic RN will be evaluated on a quarterly basis when first employed in the Specialty Center, then on a yearly basis. The nurse will also be expected to maintain ongoing education in this field through workshops, articles, etc. related to anticoagulation therapy. The Nurse Coordinator will conduct chart audits every 6 months to ensure that the nurses maintain protocol parameters.

Courtesy of Maine General Medical Center, Augusta, Maine.

NURSE CLINIC ANTICOAGULATION PROGRAM
Protocol for the Role of Nurses in the Monitoring and Education of Patients

POLICY

The Nurse Clinic Anticoagulation Program is a physician directed, nurse managed service. It is staffed by Nurse Clinic Registered Nurses with specific knowledge in anticoagulation therapy. Oral anticoagulation care is managed under the direction of physicians in the departments of Internal Medicine and Family Practice.

PURPOSE

- To manage oral anticoagulation therapy by evaluating the International Normalized Ratios (INR) and instructing patients or family of appropriate dosage of warfarin.
- To access patients for possible complications related to anticoagulation therapy.
- To provide comprehensive and ongoing education to patients and/or family members about anticoagulation therapy with specific attention to signs and symptoms to report.

GENERAL INFORMATION

The Nurse Clinic Anticoagulation Program specializes in the care of patients receiving oral anticoagulants to prevent blood clots. Patients are referred by physicians from the departments of Internal Medicine and Family Practice. All patients are determined to be able to care for themselves or have appropriate caregivers such as parents, other family members, home health, or nursing home providers. Ideally, inpatients will be scheduled for their initial visit one to three days after discharge. The physician completes a written refusal using the Nurse Clinic Anticoagulation Program Referral which includes: indication for anticoagulation therapy, desired INR, expected duration, date therapy began, most recent INR/date, current anticoagulation dosage, date next INR due, special anticoagulation risks, and the name of the primary care physician responsible for the medical management of the patient's care.

PROTOCOL

1. Nurse Clinic Visits: Follow-up visits by appointment. If unable to keep an appointment, the patient and/or significant other is responsible for calling the Nurse Clinic and rescheduling the appointment.
2. Initial Visit: New patients meet with the nurse for initial patient education, which lasts approximately one hour.
3. INR Monitoring: Nurse will check patients' INRs via fingerstick using the *ProTime Microcoagulation System*.
4. Frequency of INR Testing: Initially, INR checked once or twice weekly. As the INR and dose of anticoagulant stabilizes, the test will be done weekly, every two weeks, then monthly. All patients must have their INR checked at least monthly except in rare circumstances (eg, those who are proven to be very stable).
5. Patient Progress: Nurse Clinic Anticoagulation Program Physician Renewal Orders will be completed at least once every six months by a physician to verify need for continued anticoagulation therapy. Nurse Clinic staff will ensure that this reassessment is performed in collaboration with a physician.

Courtesy of Dartmouth-Hitchcock Nurse Clinic, Nashua, New Hampshire.

Chapter 6

Pharmacy Issues

Robert T. Weibert

INTRODUCTION

Anticoagulation as a Pharmacy Issue

Oral anticoagulation therapy involves careful drug dosing to a specific laboratory end point. Anticoagulant therapy has complex pharmacology, complex pharmacokinetics, and a relatively narrow margin of safety. In one sense, all aspects of anticoagulation therapy are pharmacy issues. Pharmacists receive specific training in pharmacology, pharmacokinetics, drug products, drug interactions, and other drug therapy issues, all of which constitute important assets of anticoagulation management programs.

Pharmacists and Anticoagulation Management

Inpatient Services

Patients on long-term anticoagulant therapy are likely to encounter pharmacists in a variety of practice settings. Pharmacy practitioners in hospital settings often monitor anticoagulant therapy and provide dosing advice for patients on heparin and warfarin during the initiation of oral anticoagulant therapy. Patients on long-term anticoagulant therapy might be hospitalized for related or unrelated problems, and their anticoagulant therapy is often interrupted or changed.

Careful follow-up and coordination are needed when patients are discharged.

Home Care

Patients are frequently discharged from the inpatient hospital setting to home care follow-up. Often, they are not physically able to travel to a hospital, clinic, or office for prothrombin time (PT) testing and receive care by home care nursing services. Patients might have complex intravenous therapy provided by home-infusion pharmacists, who can assist in the close follow-up of anticoagulation therapy during the critical early days of treatment.

Outpatient Prescriptions

Almost all outpatient pharmacies dispense warfarin prescriptions to patients. Ensuring an accurate and continuing supply of medication is essential to the success of anticoagulation therapy. However, this process can easily be overlooked and can increase the risk of critical errors.

Anticoagulation Management Specialists

Pharmacists have practiced as specialists in the management of anticoagulation therapy in both inpatient and clinic or office settings for more than 25 years.

PRACTICAL PHARMACY ISSUES: AVOIDING MISTAKES

Three of the most important factors in determining the response to warfarin anticoagulant therapy are key issues in pharmacy practice: (1) dose prescribed, (2) dose dispensed, and (3) dose taken.

Dose Prescribed

Prescribing Errors

Prescribing errors are a potential source for dosing errors. An anticoagulation management service focuses on the determination of the correct warfarin dose for each patient. Warfarin is available under the trade name Coumadin in seven color-coded tablet strengths. Some anticoagulation practices have limited the tablets to one strength, usually 5-mg warfarin tablets, and make dose adjustments in 1/2-tablet increments or different doses on different days of the week. Because the dose of warfarin changes frequently in some patients, adherence to one tablet strength or fractions thereof can avoid the likelihood of patients having multiple-strength tablets at home and mistakenly taking the wrong tablet. Many practitioners, however, also use all of the available tablet sizes for increased flexibility in dosage adjustment and prescribe the most convenient tablet size for patients. This practice may work best for patients who are relatively stable.

Written prescriptions for warfarin should be carefully reviewed to avoid potential errors. When warfarin prescriptions are written, fractions should be used to denote 1/2-mg tablet sizes in order to avoid any possible confusion from decimal place errors. Prescriptions should be double-checked to avoid inadvertent changes in tablet strength.

When switching to a new tablet size, it is critical to review the new instructions with the patient. Both the milligram dosage and the number of tablets required for the dose should be emphasized. Patients should repeat the new directions to reduce the chance for errors. Patients must be warned not to take both the old tablets and the new tablets if tablets of a different strength had been prescribed earlier. Indicating that the prescription is a new tablet size can help alert the dispensing pharmacist and reduce the potential for mistakes.

Refills

Prescription refills allow patients to keep an adequate warfarin supply and encourage patient compliance. Patients who have proved to be reliable and are on indefinite anticoagulant therapy can be given multiple refills to reduce unnecessary telephone calls for refill authorizations. Most pharmacists will refill prescriptions for up to one year. When patients do not have refills and encounter obstacles in obtaining prescription renewals, they may go without warfarin for days or reduce their warfarin dose to stretch their tablet supply until they obtain a refill. Occasionally, the supply of warfarin must be limited for patients who have problems with compliance or who otherwise would not have follow-up testing performed.

Additional factors can influence patients as to when they obtain prescription refills. Many patients are limited by rules from governmental or insurance drug plans. Some patients have prescription drug coverage limited to a set number of prescriptions a month. In some states, for example, Medicaid programs might limit patients to a total of six prescriptions per month. Because of reduced co-payments, patients might use mail-order prescription services and need to plan further in advance for their renewals. Finally, insurance plans often will not refill prescriptions for a three-month period until the previous prescription is used. If the patient's dosage has been increased over the prescription directions, refills might be denied until the directions have been clarified or a new prescription is issued.

Dosing Change Instructions

The warfarin dose is often changed from the dose on the prescription label. Dose changes sometimes involve an increase or decrease of 1/2 tablet per day on one to three days per week. Some patients have two or more tablet strengths and alternate or combine tablets during the week. A pillbox is a valuable tool for patients with dosing schedules that vary during the week.

Generic Warfarin Products

In the 1980s, generic warfarin products were believed to have caused significant changes in anticoagulant control.[1] Because of their limited use, these early generic warfarin products were no longer manufactured. In the late 1990s, three generic warfarin products were marketed and a controversy developed as to the therapeutic equivalence of these products relative to the original brand warfarin product (Coumadin®) then manufactured by Dupont Pharmaceuticals.[2] The Food and Drug Administration then issued comments that drugs labeled as bioequivalent were in fact therapeutically equivalent.[3] Currently, there are four marketed warfarin products manufactured by Apothecon Inc., Barr Laboratories, Bristol-Myers Squibb Pharmaceuticals (Coumadin®), and Taro Pharmaceuticals.

A multicenter, single-blind, randomized crossover study demonstrated that Apothecon warfarin and Dupont warfarin (Coumadin®) provided equivalent anticoagulation in patients with atrial fibrillation.[4] A smaller study of Barr and Dupont warfarin found comparable anticoagulant activity.[5] A cohort study did not observe apparent differences following a switch from brand to generic warfarin.[6] In contrast to sporadic case reports of possible differences in anticoagulant control associated with generic products, the data available from controlled trials have not demonstrated any clinically important difference. However, pharmacists should be encouraged to dispense a consistent warfarin product and not to switch between different generic warfarin products.

Write It Down

New dosage instructions should be written for patients to take home. An example of a dosing sheet from an anticoagulation clinic is shown in Exhibit 6–1. Again, patients should be instructed both as to the number of tablets to take and the milligram dosage. Copies of outdated written instructions are possible sources of dosing errors, however, and old dose instructions should be discarded when new directions are given.

Dose Dispensed

Dispensing errors are potential sources of dosing errors. Patients should recognize the color of their tablets and know to ask questions of their pharmacist and anticoagulation clinician to resolve any unexpected changes before starting new tablets of a different color. Patients should be asked if they still have a supply of their tablets from the previous prescription. If any tablets remain, patients should clearly explain what they plan to do with those tablets. The following case is an example of a significant dispensing error:

A patient anticoagulated for an aortic valve replacement with warfarin, 2 mg daily, was hospitalized for acute congestive heart failure. On discharge, he received a prescription for warfarin 2-mg No. 10 tablets. He returned to his anticoagulation clinic with the new vial without using the new tablets. The vial contained white 10-mg tablets dispensed in error because the quantity was 10 tablets. Despite the problem of a language barrier, this patient correctly refused to take the tablets because they were a different color.

This case illustrates several problems, including the increased chance for mistakes when a patient is discharged from the hospital with a new prescription and a dispensing error stemming from a simple misreading of a prescription.

To reduce the risks of anticoagulant therapy, pharmacists should review key safety questions with patients when dispensing warfarin prescriptions. (See Exhibit 6–2.)

Dose Taken

Inadequate or confusing directions can lead to patient dosing errors, but they can occur despite good directions and instruction. Following are several examples of dosing errors.

Dosing for Symptoms and Failing First Follow-Up

A patient was discharged following hospitalization for a deep venous thrombosis. He was on warfarin, 5 mg daily. Two weeks later, he presented with excessive anticoagulation (International Normalized Ratio [INR] >6). He had failed his first clinic visit, as he did not want to leave home because of leg pain. He also understood that the warfarin prescription was for the problem of swelling and pain in his legs, and he had doubled his dosage to 10 mg daily.

Exhibit 6–1
WARFARIN DOSING INSTRUCTIONS

Patient:							
Date:							
Day	*Sunday*	*Monday*	*Tuesday*	*Wednesday*	*Thursday*	*Friday*	*Saturday*
No. of tablets							
Milligrams (mg)							
Tablet strength: _____				Tablet color: _____			
Special instructions: _____							

Courtesy of University of California San Diego Medical Center Anticoagulation Clinic, San Diego, California.

Exhibit 6–2
SEVEN KEY WARFARIN SAFETY QUESTIONS FOR PHARMACISTS

1. When was your last INR determination? What was your last INR value?
2. What is the strength and color of your warfarin tablets? Has the warfarin dose changed from the directions on your prescription?
3. Are you eating poorly or have you made an intentional change in your diet?
4. Have you started or stopped any other medications?
5. Have you been acutely sick or noticed a change in any chronic illness?
6. Have you developed any bleeding or changes in the color of your urine or stools?
7. Are you planning to have any surgery, dental surgery, or other invasive procedures or have you had any injury or a hard fall?

Confusion between Brand and Generic Drug Names

A patient had been started on anticoagulation with a prescription from a chain-store pharmacy labeled "Coumadin 5 mg." He was then hospitalized with increasing chest pain for a percutaneous transcoronary angioplasty. On discharge, he received a prescription from the hospital pharmacy labeled "warfarin 5 mg." Despite their identical appearance, he took both tablets and presented to the anticoagulation clinic with an INR >10, which was successfully reversed.

Avoiding Foods with Vitamin K

One week later, the same patient mentioned above returned to the clinic, again with an INR >10, but he had been taking the correct warfarin dose of 5 mg daily. Because of repeated warnings from several health care professionals during his hospitalization about the dangers of foods with vitamin K, he had eliminated all foods containing vitamin K. The result was a vitamin K deficiency.

Confusion about New Directions

A patient instructed to withhold a dose or to take an extra dose for one or two days as a one-time change might continue to follow the new dosing instructions on a weekly basis. Alternatively, a patient instructed to change the dosage on a weekly basis might change it for only the first week and then return to the previous dosing schedule. The patient should accurately repeat the new dosing instructions to reduce the chance of a mistake.

Confusion about New Tablets

When a patient is given a prescription for a different strength of warfarin tablets, there are several possibilities for errors. Both the prescriber and dispensing pharmacist should carefully review the new regimen to avoid having the patient make a dangerous dosing mistake. Common dosing errors include following old directions when taking new higher-strength tablets or taking both the new and old tablets.

Look-Alike Tablets

A patient anticoagulated for atrial fibrillation had excellent control while her medications were being managed by her daughter. Upon her return from a trip without her daughter, her INR was >10. She was found to have confused her green 2½-mg warfarin tablets with her green 20-mg isosorbide tablets and had been taking warfarin three times daily.

Other Practical Issues

Ensuring Follow-Up

The basis for safety in oral anticoagulation is frequent monitoring during times of change or risk. Pharmacists should be encouraged to verify when follow-up testing is scheduled. This verification of appointments is particularly important when a patient is receiving a new prescription at hospital discharge. Pharmacists should also verify that monitoring is scheduled when there is a large change in the warfarin dosage ($\geq 20\%$).

Patient Compliance

Long-term patient compliance is the basis for successful anticoagulation therapy. Pharmacies with computerized prescription records can screen for poor compliance and can be a source of information about patterns of medication compliance. Patient information booklets and instruction sheets are useful tools for most patients. Patients also should use pillboxes, which are particularly helpful for patients on alternating schedules with varying doses of warfarin on different days of the week.

Drug Costs/Indigent Patient Programs

Bristol-Myers Squibb Patient Assistance Foundation will provide temporary assistance to patients with a financial hardship who have no private prescription drug insurance and are not eligible for prescription drug coverage through Medicaid or other governmental programs. Patient eligibility is based on income, liquid assets, and prescription drug coverage. Prescribers can contact the foundation at 800-736-0003. Qualified patients may receive two three-month supplies of Coumadin® through the prescriber. Requalification is needed for additional supplies. Other pharmaceutical manufacturers have medication assistance programs that may be important for other drugs.[7]

Instructions for Dose Changes

Simpler dose regimens are preferred and patients can often be changed to a higher or lower tablet strength with less complicated directions. For example, a patient taking 5 mg daily Sunday, Tuesday, Thursday, and Saturday alternating with 2.5 mg Monday, Wednesday, and Friday (27.5 mg per week) should be changed to 4 mg once daily (28 mg per week). Simplified dosing regimens are preferred by patients and may reduce confusion and errors.[8]

Patient Self-Testing

The availability of reliable, portable prothrombin time coagulometers has led to the expansion of patient self-testing (PST). The advantages are that the ease of testing can lead to more frequent and timely testing. In some settings patient self-dosing using a defined protocol has been added to self-testing. The British Society on Haematology has proposed recommendations for patients undertaking self-management of oral anticoagulation.[9] Pharmacists may be involved in PST in providing equipment and supplies or as clinicians in anticoagulant management services.

Drug Interactions

Drug interactions are an important factor in causing both subtherapeutic and excessive anticoagulation. Patients should be encouraged to use a single pharmacy for all of their prescription services because interacting drugs are often prescribed by multiple prescribers. Pharmacy computerized drug-interaction screening of patient profiles can help to identify when interacting drugs are added. Anticoagulation services should encourage pharmacists to call when an interacting drug has been prescribed. Clinicians should ask patients to "brown bag" their medications and carefully review all current drugs at an anticoagulation clinic visit. Patients should be specifically reminded to include nonprescription products. Self-use of nonprescription nonsteroidal anti-inflammatory agents, H-2 blockers, and vitamin K–containing multiple vitamins may result in significant drug interactions.

PHARMACISTS AND ANTICOAGULATION SERVICES

Pharmacist-Managed Anticoagulation Clinics

The involvement of pharmacists in managing anticoagulation clinics has increased during the past 25 years.

Veterans Affairs Medical Centers and Clinics

Multidisciplinary anticoagulation clinics are in place in many Veterans Affairs (VA) medical centers and clinics. Many of these sites include pharmacists as providers.

Managed Care Programs

Some managed care organizations have implemented pharmacist-managed anticoagulation clinics. The Southern California Kaiser Permanente has such anticoagulation clinics that follow more than 14,000 patients, and Hawaii Kaiser Permanente also has regionwide pharmacist-managed anticoagulation clinics. FHP Health Care has implemented pharmacist-managed anticoagulation clinics for many patients in its Arizona region.

Published Reports

Several early reports describe clinical pharmacists participating in the management of anticoagulated patients.[10-14] A report from a VA clinic compares results for 78 anticoagulation clinic patients with results for 17 patients managed in other clinics.[15] Although anticoagulant therapeutic control for the two groups was not different, for the patients cared for in the anticoagulation clinic, there were fewer combined hemorrhagic and thromboembolic complications per treatment year (6.9% versus 9.0%). At the Medical College of Virginia, 16 patients managed by clinical pharmacists had improved anticoagulant control with 80% therapeutic PTs versus 56% therapeutic PTs in 16 patients managed by physicians.

A study at the Long Beach VA Medical Center (LBVAMC)[16] retrospectively compared 26 pharmacist-managed patients (62 patient years) to the center's prior experience (64 patient years).[17] The authors report a reduction in the percentage of patients requiring hospitalization (4% clinic versus 39% preclinic); improved anticoagulation control (85.6% therapeutic PTs clinic versus 64.2% therapeutic PTs preclinic); and fewer hospitalizations for hemorrhage (1 clinic versus 8 preclinic) or thromboembolism (0 clinic versus 4 preclinic). A follow-up report retrospectively compares these same 26 patients with 26 randomly selected control anticoagulated patients followed in other LBVAMC clinics (79 patient years), as well as with the preclinic experience.[18] Again, there was improved anticoagulant control with 84.5% therapeutic PTs in the clinic group compared with 69.2% therapeutic PTs in the preclinic group and 67% in the random control group. The interval between PT measurements was similar for all groups. The combined preclinic and control groups had 462 hospital days for hemorrhage, excessive anticoagulation, or thromboembolic complications during 143.3 patient years (3.2 hospital days/patient year). At a cost of $271.40 per medical bed at LBVAMC, the hospitalization cost was $874 per patient year. The anticoagulation clinic had 3 hospital days for 62 patient years, or 0.048 hospital day per patient year. The cost savings in hospitalizations was $860.88 per patient, for a total of $211,776 for the 246 patients on anticoagulants at LBVAMC at that time. The authors did a simplified cost-benefit analysis with a salary of $32,300 for a clinical pharmacist (1985), which resulted in an overall savings of $179,465 and a benefit:cost ratio of 6.55.

Early studies followed small numbers of patients over relatively short periods of time. Conte et al report a nine-year experience with a pharmacist-managed anticoagulation clinic.[19] It treated 140 patients for 153 patient years. Anticoagulation control was described as a PT ratio of 1.5 to 2.5 times control. Of 1,060 PTs, 28.5% were subtherapeutic; 59.2%, therapeutic; and 12.4%, excessive. The incidence of major hemorrhage was 2.6% per patient year; minor hemorrhage, 58% per patient year; and thromboembolism, 8.5% per patient year.

A study to evaluate safety, effectiveness, and stability of anticoagulation therapy reports results from 82 patients followed for 199 patient years over a 9-year period.[20,21] There were 4 major hemorrhages (2.0% per patient year); 31 minor hemorrhages (15.5% per patient year); and 7 thromboembolic complications (3.5% per patient year). The report excludes patients followed for less than 7 months in order to exclude events that occurred early during treatment, which is known to be a high-risk period.

A study at the University of Florida compared 68 pharmacist-managed patients (60 patient years) in a coordinated management program with 44 physician-managed patients (28 patient years) in a random fashion during a 5-year period.[22] The anticoagulation clinic reduced major hemorrhage (0 versus 5 events) and thromboembolism (0 versus 10 events). The control group was 20 times more likely to experience an adverse event. The control group's risk of major hemorrhage was 17.9% per patient year. Unscheduled clinic visits, emergency department visits, and hospitalizations were avoided in the clinic patients. Hospital and emergency charges for control patients were $119,000, or $4,250 per patient. The potential cost avoidance was estimated to be $4,073 per patient year.

At the University of California San Diego Medical Center, the clinical outcomes of 293 patients (212 patient years) followed in a pharmacist-managed anticoagulation clinic from 1977 through 1983 were compared with patients (192 patient years) followed in general medical clinics from 1970 through 1977 (unpublished observations). There was a 58% reduction in major hemorrhage (9.4% per patient year clinic versus 22.4% per patient year preclinic) and a 71% reduction in thrombosis (4.7% per patient year clinic versus 16% per patient year preclinic). Using an estimated cost of $17,000 per major hemorrhage and $15,000 per thrombotic event, there was a cost savings of $622,000 for patients followed in the anticoagulation clinic. Anticoagulation control was substantially improved. Using a therapeutic range of a PT ratio of 1.5 to 2.5 times control, patients in the anticoagulation clinic had 4,012 PTs with 24.6% subtherapeutic, 72.5% therapeutic, and 2.9% excessive. Patients in the medical clinics had 3,663 PTs with 23.4% subtherapeutic, 63.3% therapeutic, and 13.1% excessive. From 1990 through 1994, patients followed in the anticoagulation clinic by point-of-care testing had an annual incidence of major hemorrhage of 2.3% and an annual incidence of thrombosis of 2%.

Experience from pharmacist-managed anticoagulation clinics in a managed care organization also has been described.[23] FHP in Arizona established anticoagulation clinics in 1992 and used point-of-care testing. In 1995, approximately 17% of the anticoagulated patients in the Arizona region were managed in an anticoagulation clinic. Data from 6 months in 1995 showed a dramatic reduction of warfarin-related hospitalizations in patients managed in the anticoagulation clinic (425 patients) compared with routine medical management (2,328 patients). Clinic patients had 2 hospitalizations (0.5%) for 16 days. Nonclinic patients had 75 hospitalizations (3.2%) for 407 days. The six-month cost savings from avoiding hospitalization and decreased physician time was $134,370, or $368 per patient. The estimated annual cost benefit by enrolling all patients in the Arizona region in anticoagulation clinics is $1,984,000.

Other Practice Sites

Pharmacists have coordinated inpatient and outpatient anticoagulation services.[24] An evaluation of coordinated care showed improved PT stability at hospital discharge, referral to the anticoagulation clinic, and the number of therapeutic PTs at the initial follow-up clinic visit. Pharmacists also participate in multidisciplinary anticoagulation clinics.[25]

Pharmaceutical Care

The concept of providing complete pharmaceutical care and focusing on patient outcomes has led to greater interest by pharmacists in managing anticoagulant therapy. Pharmacists in increasing numbers are practicing in the area of anticoagulation, including community practice settings.[26,27]

Prescriptive Authority

Many states authorize prescriptive authority for pharmacists practicing under protocols. A 1993 survey of clinical pharmacy services found that 59% of anticoagulation clinics authorized pharmacist prescribing.[28]

Reimbursement

Reimbursement continues to be a challenging issue for all anticoagulation practices. A business plan for a pharmacist anticoagulation clinic showed that, at a charge of $33 per visit, an anticoagulation clinic became profitable at 300 visits per month.[29]

Pharmacists with established drug-therapy management protocols have been limited to billing anticoagulation management visits "incident-to" a physician, which is limited reimbursement. Ongoing efforts of a coalition of pharmacy organizations have proposed the Medicare Pharmacist Services Coverage Act to amend the Social Security Act to allow pharmacists to bill Medicare for providing high-level patient care services.

Emergency Identification

All patients should carry a wallet card that identifies that they are taking warfarin. Many patients will choose to wear a Medic Alert bracelet stating that they take warfarin. In the event of traumatic injury, it is critical that emergency personnel know that warfarin anticoagulation may aggravate bleeding and that emergency reversal of anticoagulation should be considered.

ASHP Foundation Anticoagulation Traineeships

A formal anticoagulation therapy training program has been developed through the American Society of Health-System Pharmacists (ASHP) Research and Education Foundation. The ASHP Anticoagulation Service Traineeship (AST) is a one-week training program for pharmacists developing an anticoagulation practice. More than 280 pharmacists have participated in traineeships during the past 16 years.[30] Currently, there are seven AST sites that train 32 pharmacists annually to establish anticoagulation services.

CONCLUSION

Warfarin therapy requires detailed micromanagement and a sound understanding of complex pharmacologic, pharmacokinetic, and laboratory monitoring issues. Outcomes are greatly influenced by patient compliance and behavior. There is substantial benefit from maintaining therapeutic control, but there is high risk if patients are poorly controlled. Pharmacists have successfully contributed to the care of anticoagulated patients for more than 25 years. The management of patients on long-term anticoagulant therapy is an important area for participation by clinical pharmacists in order to ensure optimal pharmaceutical care for this group of patients.

REFERENCES

1. Richton-Hewett S, Foster E, Apstein CA. Medical and economic consequences of a blinded oral anticoagulant brand change at a municipal hospital. *Arch Intern Med.* 1988;148:806–808.

2. DeCara JM, Croze S, Falk RH. Generic warfarin: a cost-effective alternative to brand-name drug or a clinical wild card? *Chest.* 1998;113:261–263.

3. FDA comments on activities in states concerning narrow-therapeutic-index drugs. *Am J Health Syst Pharm.* 1998;55:686–687.

4. Weibert RT, Yeager BF, Wittkowsky AK, et al. A randomized, crossover comparison of warfarin products in the treatment of atrial fibrillation. *Ann Pharmacotherap.* 2000;34:981–988.

5. Handler J, Nguyen T, Rush S, Pham NT. A blinded, randomized, crossover study comparing the efficacy and safety of generic warfarin sodium to Coumadin®. *Prev Cardiol.* 1998;4:13–20.

6. Swenson CN, Fundak G. Observational cohort study of switching warfarin sodium products in a managed care organization. *Am J Health Syst Pharm.* 2000;57:452–455.

7. Chisholm MA, DiPiro JT. Pharmaceutical manufacturer assistance programs. *Arch Intern Med.* 2002;162:780–784.

8. Wong W, Norton JW, Wittkowsky AK. Influence of warfarin regimen type on clinical and monitoring outcomes in stable patients in an anticoagulation management service. *Pharmacotherapy.* 1999;19:1385–1391.

9. Fitzmaurice DA, Machin SF on behalf of The British Society on Haematology Task Force for Haemostasis and Thrombosis. *BMJ.* 2001;323:985–988.

10. Davis FB, Sczupak CA. Outpatient oral anticoagulation. Guidelines for long-term management. *Postgrad Med.* 1979;66:100–109.

11. Reinders TP, Steinke WE. Pharmacist management of anticoagulant therapy in ambulant patients. *Am J Hosp Pharm.* 1979;36:645–648.

12. Wiser TH, Mintzer DL. Oral anticoagulation therapy managed by pharmacy clinicians: a description with selected patient outcomes. *US Pharmacist.* 1980;12:23–30.

13. Nappi JM. Measuring the effectiveness of an anticoagulation clinic by a pharmacist. *Wis Pharmacist.* 1980;164–168.

14. McKenney JM, Witherspoon JM. The impact of outpatient hospital pharmacists on patients receiving antihypertensive and anticoagulant therapy. *Hosp Pharm.* 1985;20:406–415.

15. Gray D, Schultz H, Chretien SD. Development of an anticoagulation clinic. *QRB*. 1983;1:6–10.

16. Cohen IA, Hutchison TA, Kirking DM, Shue ME. Evaluation of a pharmacist-managed anticoagulation clinic. *J Clin Hosp Pharm*. 1985;10:167–175.

17. Garabedian-Ruffalo SM, Gray DR, Sax MJ, Ruffalo RL. Retrospective evaluation of a pharmacist-managed warfarin anticoagulation clinic. *Am J Hosp Pharm*. 1985;42:304–308.

18. Gray DR, Garabedian-Ruffalo SM, Chretien SD. Cost-justification of a clinical pharmacist–managed anticoagulation clinic. *Drug Intell Clin Pharm*. 1985;19:575–580.

19. Conte RR, Kehoe WA, Nielson N, Lodhia H. Nine-year experience with a pharmacist-managed anticoagulation clinic. *Am J Hosp Pharm*. 1986;43:2460–2464.

20. Rospond RM, Quandt CM, Clark GM, Bussey HI. Evaluation of factors associated with stability of anticoagulation therapy. *Pharmacotherapy*. 1989;9:207–213.

21. Bussey HI, Rospond RM, Quandt CM, Clark GM. The safety and effectiveness of long-term warfarin therapy in an anticoagulation clinic. *Pharmacotherapy*. 1989;9:214–219.

22. Wilt VM, Gums JG, Ahmed OI, Moore LM. Outcome analysis of a pharmacist-managed anticoagulation service. *Pharmacotherapy*. 1995;15:732–739.

23. Grier D, Ehsani FS, Mackin MG, et al. Pharmacist-managed anticoagulation clinics improve service and satisfaction. *FHP J Clin Res*. 1996;5:13–20.

24. Ellis RF, Stephens MA, Sharp GB. Evaluation of a pharmacy-managed warfarin-monitoring service to coordinate inpatient and outpatient therapy. *Am J Hosp Pharm*. 1992;49:387–394.

25. Krokosky NJ, Vanscoy GJ. Running an anticoagulation clinic. *Am J Nurs*. 1989;89:304.

26. Mason JD, Colley CA. Effectiveness of an ambulatory care clinical pharmacist: a controlled trial. *Ann Pharmacother*. 1993;27:555–559.

27. McCurdy M. Oral anticoagulation monitoring in a community pharmacy. *Am Pharm*. 1993;NS22(10):61–72.

28. Raehl CL, Bond CA, Pitterle ME. Ambulatory pharmacy services affiliated with acute care hospitals. *Pharmacotherapy*. 1993;13:618–625.

29. Wilson-Norton JL, Gibson DL. Establishing an outpatient anticoagulation clinic in a community hospital. *Am J Health-Syst Pharm*. 1996;53:1151–1157.

30. Wittkowsky AK. Pharmacists and stroke prevention. *Am J Health-Syst Pharm*. 1996;53:100.

Chapter 7

Guidelines for Anticoagulation Provider Certification

Gordon J. Vanscoy and Sally Loken

The use of anticoagulation therapy has increased dramatically in recent years. It has been estimated that proper anticoagulation may save $600 million annually and decrease the risk of stroke associated with atrial fibrillation by 50%.[1] These statistics imply that many more patients will receive anticoagulation therapy in the future. Three principal barriers to better anticoagulant usage have been identified in the literature. Two of them, gaps in knowledge or belief in the effectiveness of anticoagulant therapy and concerns regarding its safety, have been addressed by the Consensus Conferences on Antithrombotic Therapy, sponsored by the American College of Chest Physicians (ACCP).[2] The third barrier is concern about the difficulty of managing patients on anticoagulant therapy.[3] Changes in the health care delivery system have shifted patient management from acute, inpatient care to outpatient or ambulatory clinic settings. Patient care in anticoagulation clinics is frequently provided through a coordinated, multidisciplinary approach. Optimal management of anticoagulation therapy requires care expertise combined with sound knowledge of the pharmacology of antithrombotic therapy.[4]

RATIONALE FOR THE CERTIFICATION OF ANTICOAGULATION PROVIDERS

Reasons supporting a standardized certification program to validate competency in the provision of anticoagulation

therapy include (1) an expanded body of literature regarding anticoagulation and its management, (2) the move toward outpatient management of therapy, (3) the existence of numerous health care professionals with varying degrees of responsibility for patient care, (4) the uncoordinated provision of anticoagulation services, and (5) a need for demonstrated competency. Recognition of this need has resulted in anticoagulation management traineeship programs for pharmacists. Examples of such programs include those offered by the University of Illinois at Chicago College of Pharmacy and the American Society of Health System Pharmacists Research and Education Foundation. In addition, inservice programs, workshops, and college-sponsored courses are becoming more common with the increased recognition of the need for well-educated anticoagulation providers. The University of Southern Indiana recognized this need and developed a popular Internet-accessible continuing education program on anticoagulation therapy management.

Gourley and colleagues identify the existence of a systematic, structured program of education and experience as the differentiating feature between a certificate program and certification. The value of a certification program lies in its ability to enable the certified practitioner to provide better and more comprehensive patient care.[5]

DEVELOPMENT OF A NATIONAL CERTIFICATION PROGRAM

Certification has been defined as "a voluntary process by which a practitioner's training, experience, and knowledge are identified as meeting or surpassing a defined standard

Members of the National Certification Board for Anticoagulation Providers are Richard C. Becker, MD; Stuart Haines, PharmD; Sally Loken, APRN; Mary Lynn McPherson, PharmD; Geno J. Merli, MD; Lynn B. Oertel, MS, ANP; William Rock, PharmD; Gordon J. Vanscoy, PharmD, MBA; and Thomas Wiser, PharmD.

beyond that required for licensure."[5(p796)] Understanding that a rigorous, national program of education and certification would ensure provision of proper anticoagulation and enhance patient care, the Anticoagulation Provider Certification Working Group (APCWG) was formed in 1996. The name was changed in 1998 to the National Certification Board for Anticoagulation Providers (NCBAP).

The members of NCBAP are a multidisciplinary group representing medical, nursing, and pharmacy practitioners. They have created a reproducible, educational framework of competencies for all clinicians involved with anticoagulation therapy. The goals of the NCBAP are (1) to develop the objectives and process required for anticoagulation therapy providers to achieve the necessary competencies and (2) to develop a framework for a national certification process that validates achievement of anticoagulation therapy provider competencies. Exhibit 7–1 lists process steps that laid the foundation for the framework.[4]

This framework is based upon critical elements of certificate programs as outlined by the American Association of Colleges of Pharmacy (AACP) and the American Council on Pharmaceutical Education (ACPE). These critical elements[6] are

1. competency-based outcome objectives
2. input from practitioners in development

Exhibit 7–1
APCWG PROCESS STEPS

1. Assessment of the need for credentialing
2. Differentiation of levels of anticoagulation mastery
   – *Generalist*: a health care professional responsible for occasional management of anticoagulation therapy
   – *Provider*: a health care professional whose primary responsibility is the provision of coordinated care to anticoagulated patients
   – *Master*: an anticoagulation provider with either more extensive knowledge of anticoagulation therapy or broad administrative experience
3. Identification of key elements of a quality certification program
4. Assessment of published anticoagulation provider competencies
5. Understanding of the elements of a successful regional credentialing program
6. Proposal of core anticoagulation domains of knowledge and associated competencies
7. Incorporation of review and feedback into such domains and competencies

Source: Adapted with permission from GJ Vanscoy and W Rock, Workshop: Credentialing of Anticoagulation Providers: A Proposed Model, *Journal of Thrombosis and Thrombolysis*, Vol 5, pp S53–S61, © 1998.

3. measurable outcomes
4. didactic and experiential components
5. current and reliable content
6. accessible program with self-paced characteristics
7. rigorous program
8. appropriate length and cost
9. evaluations related to objectives
10. regular quality review

Experience gained through the development of a credentialing process at the Pittsburgh Veterans Affairs Medical Center in 1990 was included in this framework. Also, previously established certification programs were reviewed, such as the Certified Diabetes Educator program.[7] The NCBAP combined critical elements of such certificate programs with the goals identified by Ansell and colleagues as necessary for coordinated outpatient anticoagulation therapy management to develop core competencies and knowledge domains.[3] The initial draft of the proposed knowledge domains was published in early 1998.[4]

Throughout 1997 and early 1998, core competencies and knowledge domains were identified and further refined. Experiential requirement and examination questions were developed. Constructive criticism on the certification process was elicited from attendees at the May 1997 National Anticoagulation Forum Conference in San Antonio and the December 1997 Anticoagulation Pharmacists Invitational Conference held in Atlanta prior to the American Society of Health System Pharmacists Midyear Meeting.

Five knowledge domains forming the educational curriculum were identified: (1) applied physiology and pathophysiology of thromboembolic disorders, (2) patient assessment and management, (3) patient education, (4) applied pharmacology of antithrombotic agents, and (5) operational (administrative) procedures. See Appendix 7A for details relative to the domains, and associated competency statements for Certified Anticoagulation Care Providers.

During 1998 and early 1999, the NCBAP conducted extensive pilot testing to validate the bank of test items that had been developed. Both expert and generalist anticoagulation providers were included in the validation process. Keeping in mind the clinical importance of diligent patient assessment and management, the Board made a deliberate decision to weight the examination's content accordingly. The examination is designed to measure one's knowledge and skills related to antithrombotic and anticoagulation therapy management; however, emphasis is placed on patient assessment, management, and education—the foundation for optimizing patient care. Thus, 50% of the test items are derived from the second domain, patient assessment and management. The domain on patient education was deemed second in importance; therefore, 20% of the test items were developed using this domain's content. The remainder of the examination's content is equally divided among the remaining three domains with 10% of test items derived from each. The examination is composed of 150 multiple-choice items, and a minimum score of 80% is required to pass.

The first certification examination was offered in May 1999 in conjunction with the Fifth National Anticoagulation Forum's Conference in Vancouver, British Columbia. Since then, the examination has been offered in five different geographical sites across the United States. As of December 2000, nearly 90 practitioners, representing 30 states in the United States, had successfully completed the certification process and earned the Certified Anticoagulation Care Provider (CACP) credential. Approximately 83% of the candidates who were eligible to sit for the examination achieved a passing score on the examination.

MISSION AND COMPETENCIES

The mission of the NCBAP is "to develop, maintain and protect the Certified Anticoagulation Care Provider (CACP) credential and the certification process."[8] The NCBAP endorses voluntary certification of anticoagulation providers who meet education and patient-care experiential requirements. The purpose of the certification process is to meet a societal need to protect public health and well-being by

1. providing an accepted assessment of current knowledge, skills, and competencies necessary for individuals providing direct anticoagulation education and therapeutic management
2. promoting individual professional growth and development in the practice of anticoagulation therapy
3. nationally recognizing and validating anticoagulation providers who fulfill certification requirements

A CACP is defined as a health care professional who has met patient-care experiential requirements and demonstrates achievement of advanced knowledge and skills by passing a comprehensive examination. This prescribed set of knowledge and skills is routinely drawn upon in the course of managing and educating patients receiving antithrombotic therapies. These competencies include

1. a working knowledge of the normal physiological processes of homeostasis and thrombosis, and the etiology, risk factors, and clinical manifestations of pathologic thrombus formation
2. knowledge of the pharmacological properties of antithrombotic drugs
3. knowledge, skills, and ability necessary to manage and monitor patients receiving antithrombotic therapies. This includes assessment of efficacy and potential toxicity, achievement of therapeutic goals, and evaluation of patient-related variables that affect therapy management

4. provision of patient education regarding antithrombotic therapy in a coordinated program that includes individualized patient assessment, formulation of an educational plan with specific goals and objectives, implementation of an educational plan, assessment and evaluation of patient knowledge and skills pertaining to anticoagulation therapy, and documentation of all patient encounters
5. demonstration of an understanding of the issues, requirements, and processes involved in developing a coordinated anticoagulation clinic or service

CERTIFICATION PROCESS

The certification process is designed for practitioners whose primary roles as anticoagulation providers include systematic, organized, and ongoing therapeutic management and education. The process requires practitioners to submit substantial evidence of their clinical practice experience as well as to achieve a passing score on a comprehensive examination. Therefore, documentation is required describing one's clinical experience in the form of 75 anticoagulation-centered patient encounters. The encounters describe 25 separate patients along with two follow-up encounters per patient. See Appendix 7A for examples of the Patient Encounter Documentation Forms A and B.

To begin the application process, an application packet is requested through the Anticoagulation Forum's office. A copy of the "Candidate Handbook for the Certified Anticoagulation Care Provider (CACP) Examination" and current edition of the Knowledge Domains is provided to the candidate. Future examination dates and respective locations and application deadlines are also included in this handbook. The entire application packet consists of a demographic/registration form, a narrative description of the candidate's current anticoagulation practice in 250 words or less, photocopies of the candidate's professional license and photo identification. a disclosure statement with signature, 75 patient encounters, and a $300 application fee. The application is submitted and reviewed by a NCBAP Board member who determines eligibility to sit for a certification examination. This review process provides an opportunity to verify employment and discuss any questionable anticoagulation practices with the candidate should the need arise. Candidates are notified by mail of their examination results.

CLINICAL ATTITUDES TOWARD THE CREDENTIALING PROCESS

In March 2000, a three-page, self-administered questionnaire was developed for the purpose of obtaining feedback from all anticoagulation providers who have pursued the CACP credential regardless of performance on the examination. The survey was developed for the purposes of learning which parts of the certification process were most valuable to candidates, measuring the impact the credential has had in their practices, and assisting in further development of the certification process to adequately meet the needs of anticoagulation providers.

Of the 63 surveys distributed by mail, 78% (49) were returned. Eighty-eight percent (43) of the respondents achieved a passing score on the examination. Three of the six candidates who did not pass the examination during the first attempt planned to retake the examination in the near future. Sixty-five percent (28) of those who passed the examination intend to recertify in five years. Ninety-six percent (47) of respondents said that they would recommend the certification process to a colleague.

The majority of the respondents were pharmacists, but a variety of professions were represented (see Table 7–1). Survey results indicated that all respondents who practiced in Veterans' Administration Medical Centers, community hospitals, and physician offices passed the certification examination. The survey also evaluated the relationship between anticoagulation experience and examination pass rate. Sixty-two and one-half percent (5) of candidates with less than three years of experience passed in comparison to 93% (38) of candidates possessing three or more years of experience in managing anticoagulation.

A number of reasons were noted when participants were asked to indicate why they pursued the CACP credential, as illustrated in Table 7–2. In addition to these responses, 20% (10) practitioners believed that the CACP credential would result in quicker professional advancement or promotion, and 22% (11) received a salary increase or some other tangible recognition as a result of the CACP credential. Only one respondent indicated that preparing for the examination did not help to improve his or her antithrombotic skill or knowledge. The majority of respondents indicated that Domain II (patient management and assessment) was the most relevant to their practice. The survey also provided an opportunity to list suggestions to improve the credentialing process. Areas identified for improvement included eliminating confusing wording on some of the examination questions, decreasing the amount of documentation required in the application packet, and increasing awareness of the CACP credential.

Table 7–1 Professions Represented in Questionnaire

Profession	% (N)
Pharmacist	71 (35)
Nurse	16 (8)
Nurse practitioner	10 (5)
Physician's assistant	2 (1)

Table 7–2 Reasons for Pursuing CACP Credential*

Reasons	N
Improve clinical skills	22
Mandated by employer	6
Increase marketability/patient referrals	23
Validation/self-confidence	37
Other	5

*Multiple selections made by respondents

THE FUTURE

The future of this anticoagulation certification process is exciting, expanding, and challenging. The NCBAP is committed to sponsoring three or four examination opportunities each year at different locations around the country. Many examinations are planned in conjunction with regional or national conferences such as the Anticoagulation Forum's national conference and the American Society of Health Systems Pharmacists Midyear Meeting.

Many aspects of the NCBAP need involvement from new CACPs, including subcommittee work, test item development, and board member appointments as tenures expire for existing members. In addition, other opportunities are being explored, such as developing a Web site.

It is the goal of the NCBAP, and indeed of any clinical certification process, to provide better patient care through better-prepared care providers. The board plans to address the challenging demands of anticoagulation certification and strives to optimize the care of patients receiving anticoagulation therapy.

REFERENCES

1. Agency for Health Care Policy and Research. *Life-saving treatments to prevent stroke underused.* Washington, DC: Agency for Health Care Policy and Research; September 6, 1995. Press release.

2. Dalen JE, Hirsh J. Sixth ACCP Consensus Conference on Antithrombotic Therapy. *Chest.* 2001; 119 (suppl):1S–370S.

3. Ansell JE, Buttaro ML, Thomas OV, et al. Consensus guidelines for coordinated outpatient oral anticoagulation therapy management. *Ann Pharmacother.* 1997;31:604–615.

4. Vanscoy GJ, Rock W. Workshop: credentialing of anticoagulation providers: a proposed model. *J Thromb Thrombolysis.* 1998;5: S53–S61.

5. Gourley DR, Fitzgerald WL, Davis RL. Competency, board certification, credentialing, and specialization: who benefits? *Am J Managed Care.* 1997;3:795–801.

6. AACP/ACPE Conference on Certificate Programs. Proceedings of an invitational conference sponsored by the American Association of Colleges of Pharmacy and the American Council on Pharmaceutical Education, May 16, 1989, Washington, DC.

7. Oertel LB. Anticoagulation services: quality improvement direction— pursuing a certification process. *J Thromb Thrombolysis.* 1999;7: 153–156.

8. National Certification Board for Anticoagulation Providers. *Candidate handbook for certified anticoagulation care provider (CACP) examination.* 1999.

Provider Certification Tools

COMPETENCY STATEMENTS FOR CERTIFIED ANTICOAGULATION CARE PROVIDERS

Knowledge Domain	Goal
I. Applied Physiology and Pathophysiology of Thromboembolic Disorders	The Anticoagulation Therapy Provider must have a working knowledge regarding the normal physiological processes of hemostasis and thrombosis. In addition, the Certified Anticoagulation Care Provider must be knowledgeable regarding the etiology, risk factors, and clinical manifestations of pathologic thrombus formation.
II. Patient Assessment and Management	The Certified Anticoagulation Care Provider must possess the knowledge, skills, and competencies to manage and monitor patients on anticoagulant therapy. This includes the ability to assess the efficacy and toxicity of the prescribed antithrombotic treatment, determine if the therapeutic goals have been achieved, and identify patient-related variables that affect therapy.
III. Patient Education	The Certified Anticoagulation Care Provider must provide patient education that is tailored to the patient's specific needs to promote safety, enhance adherence, and ultimately positively affect clinical outcomes. Anticoagulation Providers must perform a baseline educational assessment, develop an educational plan, and document the educational endeavors in the patient's medical records. Documentation of ongoing assessment of patients' educational needs must be demonstrated.
IV. Applied Pharmacology of Antithrombotic Agents	The Certified Anticoagulation Care Provider must possess and maintain an in-depth knowledge regarding the pharmacological properties of antithrombotic drugs.
V. Operational (Administrative) Procedures	The Certified Anticoagulation Care Provider must possess the knowledge, skills, and competencies necessary to assist in management of an anticoagulation service. This will include (1) evaluating the need for anticoagulation services, (2) determining personnel requirements, (3) developing a proposal for an anticoagulation clinic, (4) effectively communicating among the provider, the patient, and other members of the health care team, (5) documenting patient care activities, (6) performing quality assurance and risk management activities, (7) maintaining appropriate laboratory services and complying with federal regulations governing these services, and (8) seeking compensation for anticoagulation therapy services.

Courtesy of Anticoagulation Provider Certification Working Group, Pittsburgh, Pennsylvania.

Patient Encounter Documentation Forms A and B

FORM A—PATIENT ENCOUNTER DOCUMENTATION—*Complete for 25 patients*

Provider Name	Date of Encounter	No. ___ of 25

Patient Information   clinical setting: ☐ Outpatient ☐ Inpatient

Age: | Initials: | Gender ☐ M ☐ F   ☐ Initial visit ☐ Follow-up

Any missed appointments? ☐ No ☐ Yes, Explain:

Indication for Anticoagulation
- ☐ DVT/PE prophylaxis
- ☐ DVT/PE treatment
- ☐ Mitral stenosis
- ☐ Heart valve replacement
- ☐ Stroke
- ☐ TIA

Intended INR Target Range:
- ☐ Recurrent DVT/PE
- ☐ Systemic/Peripheral emboli
- Location:_____
- Type:_____
- ☐ Atrial fibrillation
- ☐ CHF/cardiomyopathy
- ☐ Coagulopathy
- ☐ Other:_____

Date tx began: | Planned duration: ☐ 3 mo. ☐ 6 mo. ☐ 1 yr. ☐ long-term ☐ Other:_____ | Anticipated stop date:

Antithrombotic agent name: _____   strength:_____

Has the product source changed since last follow-up? ☐ No ☐ Yes, manufacturer:_____

List risk factors:
_____
_____
_____
_____
_____

List co-morbid medical conditions:
_____
_____
_____
_____
_____
_____

List all Rx and OTC medications and other supplements. *Identify those with potential for interaction with patient's antithrombotic therapy with an (*):*
_____
_____
_____
_____
_____
_____
_____
_____
_____

Subjective Information: (check 1 box below)
☐ Patient reports NO complaints, problems, or concerns.
☐ Patient reports complaints, problems, or concerns (e.g., symptoms of hemorrhagic or thromboembolic phenomenon, psychosocial issues, alcohol or diet, compliance issues, etc.) Describe:

Objective Information:

INR:	aPTT:	Other:

Current dose regimen of antithrombotic agent:

Use page 2 to provide additional details of the patient encounter. Patient assessment and plan should be documented as well as details of compliance, education, and management.

continues

Patient Encounter Documentation Forms continued

Assessment (compliance, INR value, therapeutic response, and complications):
Is INR therapeutic? ☐ Yes ☐ No

Plan (educational interventions, dosage changes, follow-up appointments, etc.):

_____   _____
Applicant's Signature   Date

Source: Copyright © 2001, Sally Loken.

continues

Patient Encounter Documentation Forms continued

FORM B—FOLLOW-UP PATIENT ENCOUNTERS—*Complete twice for each patient*

Provider Name	**Date of Encounter**	**No. ___ of 25**

Patient Information: Initials: clinical setting: ☐ outpatient ☐ inpatient

Any missed appointments? ☐ No ☐ Yes, Explain:

Indication for Rx remained the same?   ☐ Yes ☐ No Provide details/description for any "no" responses:
Target INR range remained the same?   ☐ Yes ☐ No
Antithrombotic agent remained the same?☐ Yes ☐ No
Has product source remained the same? ☐ Yes ☐ No

Any new medication (Rx or OTC)?   ☐ Yes ☐ No Provide details/description for any "yes" responses:
Any change in medical status?   ☐ Yes ☐ No

Objective Information:
INR:	aPTT:	Other:

Current dose regimen of antithrombotic agent:

Subjective Information: (check 1 box below)
☐ Patient reports NO complaints, problems, or concerns.
☐ Patient reports complaints, problems, or concerns (e.g., symptoms of hemorrhagic or
   thromboembolic phenomenon, psychosocial issues, alcohol or diet, compliance issues, etc.)
   Describe:

Assessment (compliance, INR value, therapeutic response, and complications, etc.)
in therapeutic range: ☐ Yes ☐ No

_____
_____
_____
_____

Plan (education interventions, dosage adjustments, follow-up appointments, etc.)

_____
_____
_____
_____
_____

_____   _____
Applicant's Signature   Date

Chapter 8

Information Management and Monitoring the International Normalized Ratio

Lynn B. Oertel

INTRODUCTION

Many activities routinely performed by members of an anticoagulation management service (AMS) require detailed documentation. The ability to standardize the information collection process ensures accurate and complete information. Data collection tools help to record patient data in an organized manner and allow access and retrieval of pertinent information in a timely fashion. This chapter provides an overview of commonly used forms and assessment tools that have proved helpful in the anticoagulation management setting; emphasis will be placed on International Normalized Ratio (INR) data collection and monitoring.

DATA COLLECTION AND MANAGEMENT

Many programs utilize a referral form to collect vital information directly from the patient's referring physician. This form provides details regarding the patient's indication for treatment, target therapeutic range, and expected duration of therapy. In some settings this tool has a secondary use, as a physician's order for the clinic to continue management of the patient's warfarin therapy. Following the initial visit, additional forms are used to collect critical demographic information, assess and document the patient's understanding of the disease process and treatment plan, assess the patient's learning style and develop an educational plan, and assess psychosocial factors that may impact the course of therapy.

Accurate and organized documentation of International Normalized Ratios (INRs) and corresponding doses are paramount to the success of an AMS. Records of when and by whom patients are contacted must also be maintained. Examples of data collection tools in use at a variety of anticoagulation clinics across the country can be found in Appendix 8A.

Many programs rely on paper forms for documentation that usually remain within the confines of the AMS, sometimes creating problems for access by other health care professionals. Medical record departments in most institutions have specific criteria for forms that may or may not be included in the patient's medical record, thus further impacting the access of information. To address this issue, some AMSs have created annual or biannual progress summaries to place in the medical record or to send to the referring physician. Ultimately, the AMS has the primary responsibility for maintaining and preserving accurate patient information and developing accurate recordkeeping systems.

The Significance of Quality Data Collection

In an era of managed care, great emphasis is placed on collecting and tracking data on targeted diseases. The shift toward evidence-based care requires that an AMS monitor and measure the quality of its performance.[1,2] In fact, the

National Committee for Quality Assurance (NCQA) uses atrial fibrillation and stroke prevention through effective anticoagulation as one measure for reporting quality care for managed care organizations.[3]

Some AMSs use computer software programs dedicated to their needs, while others may not. However, even rudimentary reviews of noncomputerized clinical data can set the initial stage for performance parameters. For example, a dedicated log of chronological entries pertaining to bleeding complications along with anecdotal notes relative to each patient may provide an opportunity for subsequent case review. Creating a forum (monthly staff meetings, for example) to review such cases may yield information that leads to a change in practice and improvement of patient care.

Benefits of Computerized Databases

The inefficiencies of paper recordkeeping have stimulated many AMSs to seek alternatives leading to a computerized patient database. In some set-tings, electronic databases have provided the means to electronically transfer INR values from a laboratory or point-of-care device directly into patients' anticoagulation data files. This diminishes the likelihood of entry errors as well as a delay in time involved with paper or telephone reporting systems.

The majority of AMSs operate with some degree of computerized assistance, commonly administrative applications for scheduling or billing purposes along with the more traditional paper files for anticoagulation management. A computerized database provides the opportunity to make accurate observations on response to treatment and determine whether other factors, such as co-morbid conditions, concomitant medications, or lifestyle factors, are significant. A computerized database can be further queried to provide information pertaining to patient INR performance and outcomes. Trends may be identified that indicate positive improvements or areas that require more intensive focus.

Computerization also helps to avoid adverse patient outcomes by facilitating automated interventions when specific criteria are met. For example, computer-generated lists identifying patients who are late for a scheduled blood test could allow the AMS to generate a friendly reminder to promote patient adherence. The ability to identify patients at higher risk for complications (eg, high number of concomitant medications, aspirin or nonsteroidal use, recent hospitalization or invasive procedure) allows clinicians to target interventions specific to this defined at-risk group and facilitates case management of such patients. Management strategies focused on patients with poor anticoagulant control or those with highly variable responses to warfarin therapy can also be implemented and evaluated.

Independent and institutional computerized software systems designed specifically for anticoagulation therapy clinics have been developed. Some of these systems interface with existing hospital information systems, thus providing access to all facets of patients' data. Computer systems also facilitate documentation of patient contact and communication, whether by mail, by telephone, or in person. For more on computer applications in anticoagulation, see Chapter 9.

Electronic databases provide a powerful source of patient information; however, integrity and accuracy of the data must be guaranteed from the start. Protecting and guaranteeing patient confidentiality are prime concerns, and protecting data from corruption or loss is another aspect of security. A plan to produce a backup copy of all data on a daily basis is critical. Clinicians should seek the expertise and resources of the information technology department to address the aforementioned issues.

The introduction of Web-based computer applications offers providers the additional benefit of no longer requiring a dedicated workstation to host the application and store accumulated data. Web-based technology allows easy access from virtually any location for both patients and their providers. The introduction of Web-based software systems and patient self-testing instruments has the potential to catapult patient participation and direct involvement with their care to a new level.

MONITORING THE INR

Patients requiring frequent assessment of their anticoagulation status are fortunate because nearly all laboratories now report an INR whenever a prothrombin time (PT) test is requested (see Chapter 25 for a detailed discussion of the INR). The use of the INR system has rectified many of the inconsistencies previously reported with the PT and has allowed results from different laboratories across cities, states, and even countries to have a standard point of reference.[4-7] Because many AMSs use laboratories throughout a wide geographic region, interpretation and subsequent patient management are more accurate and precise with use of the INR.

Recording and storing INR results can create a logistical challenge as anticoagulation data quickly accumulate. Flowsheets, an important part of the recordkeeping process, allow clinicians the opportunity to review anticoagulation histories and dose responses of their patients. Examples of flowsheets for INR recordkeeping appear in Appendix 8B. Drawing conclusions from a single, isolated INR could be misleading and inaccurate.

The results of venous PTs drawn in an office or hospital setting are generally available within hours of being received. This allows adequate time to contact the patient and adjust the warfarin dose. Even programs serving large geographical areas, where patients go to multiple laboratories, retrieve INR results by telephone if the scheduled date is known ahead of time. Waiting for INR results to be reported to the AMS via routine mail is insufficient and can lead to less effective control and potential jeopardy because of the longer time involved for notification. Use of point-of-care devices simplifies the entire reporting process as an INR can be performed at the time of patient interaction. This methodology represents another option for providing quality patient care in the office setting as well as at home. In the meantime, AMSs should consider procedures that allow laboratories to communicate dangerously high results to the appropriate person on call whenever the clinic is closed. Clinic personnel should become familiar with all clinical laboratory resources in the region they serve in order to recommend conveniently located facilities and to be aware of the quality of the testing and reagents used.

Measures of INR Performance

Anticoagulation management services may be required to justify their value to health care plans or institutions. To collect and analyze data for determining patient outcomes requires intense effort and statistical support. The ability to analyze INR data is less cumbersome and provides an initial summary of the clinic's ability to achieve and maintain therapeutic control. One measure of quality anticoagulation management that has a strong relationship between bleeding and thromboembolic rates is time-in-therapeutic-range (TTR). INR values as a measure of quality performance are further discussed by Ansell and colleagues.[8] They are as follows:

1. Percentage of INR tests in range: a simple calculation of number of tests in assigned range divided by total number tests performed in same period
2. Time in therapeutic range (TTR): a time-weighted INR distribution using a linear interpolation between sequential INR tests to assign a portion of time at a given INR level (also known as the Rosendaal method)[9]
3. Cross section of the files: an assessment of the percentage of patients in range at a point in time calculated by

selecting a random date and using the closest INR from every patient in a preselected group to determine percentage in range; generally need large sample to provide accurate estimate
4. Equidivision method: assumes the change between two consecutive INR measurements occurs halfway between tests[10]

As summarized by Ansell et al,[8] comparison of TTR values from clinical trials is difficult due to the different methods used and methods of data collection. The TTR values for a series of studies using different methods of anticoagulation management ranges from 34% to 92%. Taking into consideration the many variables that impact warfarin therapy as well as the inconsistent methods of analysis, a reasonable and realistic benchmark for TTR is approximately 70%. Clinics can use this figure as a benchmark to guide improvements in anticoagulation management.

CONCLUSION

The efforts to collect, collate, and store patient information, although challenging, must be done in order to create a comprehensive database and are an important function of the AMS. An organized database facilitates access to patient information, which in turn, can be analyzed to make assessments of patient performance parameters. These criteria, once defined, can be measured over time to create a means to evaluate the management system and effect of subsequent improvements. The data, whether stored on paper forms or electronic formats, may be used to provide measures of quality care for patients. The integration of computerized applications has many benefits and should be pursued whenever possible. Some means to specifically assess INR performance should be incorporated, as this is an important measure of quality performance of the AMS.

REFERENCES

1. Enns SM. Measuring practice performance. *Clinician Rev.* 2000;10(5): 132–138.
2. Henry LA. Why you should be collecting your own performance data. *Fam Pract Manage.* 1996;3(5):52–59.
3. National Committee for Quality Assurance. The State of Managed Care Quality, 1997; Washington, D.C.
4. Hirsh J, Poller L. The International Normalized Ratio. *Arch Intern Med.* 1994;154:282–288.
5. Kaatz SS, White RH, Hill J, et al. Accuracy of laboratory and portable monitor International Normalized Ratio determinations. *Arch Intern Med.* 1995;155:1861–1867.
6. Bussey HI, Force RW, Bianco TM, et al. Reliance on prothrombin time ratios causes significant errors in anticoagulant therapy. *Arch Intern Med.* 1992;152:278–282.
7. Hirsh J, Dalen JE, Anderson DR, et al. Oral anticoagulants: mechanism of action, clinical effectiveness, and optimal therapeutic range. *Chest.* 2001;119(suppl):8S–21S.
8. Ansell J, Hirsch J, Dalen J, et al. Managing oral anticoagulant therapy. *Chest.* 2001;119(suppl):22S–38S.
9. Rosendaal FR, Cannegieter SC, van der Meer FJM, et al. A method to determine the optimal intensity of oral anticoagulant therapy. *Thromb Haemost.* 1993;39:236–239.
10. Duxbury BMCD. Therapeutic control of anticoagulant treatment. *BMJ.* 1982;284:702–704.

Data Collection Tools

(Referral Forms, Initial Information Documentation Forms, and Ongoing Assessment Forms)

Anticoagulation Consultant Form

MEDICAL RECORD	CONSULTATION SHEET	
To: Anticoagulation Consultant	Request from:	Date of request:

Please educate this patient regarding warfarin therapy.

Currently this patient is an: _____ outpatient/_____ inpatient with an expected discharge date of _____

Indication for warfarin therapy: _____ AF_____ DVT _____Mechanical heart valve _____ Other_____

Duration of therapy: _____ lifelong _____ months until _____

Goal range for INR: _____

Physician who will follow patient for warfarin therapy:_____

Doctor's signature	Approved	Place of consultation	☐ Routine	☐ Today
		☐ Bedside ☐ On call	☐ 72 Hours	☐ Emergency

CONSULTATION REPORT

Signature and title			Date
Identification No.	Organization	Register No.	Ward No.

Patient's Identification

Key: AF, atrial fibrillation; DVT, deep venous thrombosis.

Anticoagulation Patient Referral

Patient name: _____

Appointment date: _____ Time:_____

To be completed by staff nurse:

   Visiting nurse referral: ☐ Yes   ☐ No

   If yes, agency name _____ Telephone _____

To be completed by physician/nurse-practitioner/physician assistant:

   Is patient currently on Coumadin (warfarin)? ☐ Yes   ☐ No

     If yes, date Coumadin (warfarin) started _____.

     If no, date Anticoagulant Therapy Unit to initiate _____.

Referring/attending physician _____

Physician who will be following patient _____

Office location _____ Office telephone _____ Page No. _____

Indication(s) for anticoagulant therapy_____

Requested duration of treatment _____

Requested therapeutic range   Please circle range below: _____

     A.   INR 2.0–3.0: Low intensity (eg, AF, CVA, TIAs, DVT prophylaxis, acute DVT)

     B.   INR 2.5–3.5: Standard intensity (eg, mechanical heart valves, recurrent thrombosis/emboli)

     C.   Other: Please contact Anticoagulation Unit

Signature of referring physician _____ Referral date _____

Key: AF, atrial fibrillation; CVA, cerebrovascular accident; DVT, deep venous thrombosis; TIA, transient ischemic attacks.

Courtesy of Anticoagulant Therapy Unit, Massachusetts General Hospital, Boston, Massachusetts.

Anticoagulation Service
Ambulatory Referral Form

Patient name _____

Medical record No. _____ Date of birth_____

Address _____

_____

Telephone _____ Alternate telephone _____

Referring physician _____ Primary physician _____

Diagnosis_____

_____

How long has patient been on warfarin? _____

Previous PT results:

	Date	PT	Dose
1.			
2.			
3.			
4.			

Other medications _____

_____

_____

_____

_____

Visiting nurse/home/laboratory/hospital_____

Agency telephone _____

Date of next PT _____

Called in by _____ Date called _____

Floor/clinic _____ Extension beeper _____

Anticoagulation Service Referral Form

Referral Process:

1. **Physician:** Complete this referral form. Please print legibly and completely fill in all requested information about the patient. Call _____ to schedule an appointment.

2. **Ward Clerk or Secretary:** Fax the front side of this form to ____(insert address)___. Photocopy the reverse side of this form for the patient. Forward the original form to the Anticoagulation Clinic, __(insert address)__.

3. **For patient:** Give a copy of the instructions on the reverse side of this form to the patient at the time of discharge. Tell the patient to report (on the scheduled day and time) to ____(insert address)____. Tell the patient to bring all medications (including non-prescription medicines) to the first appointment. **Please inform the patient he/she has an appointment with _____(name)_____** .

Questions?? _____(insert name(s) and phone numbers of clinic personnel)_____ .

Patient's Name: _____ MR#: _____ Date:_____

HPI: Diagnosis and indication for anticoagulation therapy. Indicate pertinent physical findings and special studies results (ie, US, MUGA, Venogram, VQ Scan).

PMHx:
- ❏ Heart Failure
- ❏ Peptic Ulcer Dz
- ❏ Arthritis
- ❏ IVDA/Alcohol Abuse

- ❏ Hypertension
- ❏ GI Bleeds
- ❏ Hx of falls
- ❏ Cognitive Impairment

- ❏ Diabetes Mellitus
- ❏ Seizure Disorder
- ❏ Cancer (Type: _____)
- ❏ Pregnant (Due _____)

Other PMHx:

Social History: ❏ Lives alone ❏ Smoker ❏ Vegetarian

Date Anticoagulation Therapy Initiated: _____ Initial dose: _____ Dose at discharge: _____

Most Recent Lab Data: INR: _____ Date: _____ PTT: _____ Date: _____ Hct: _____ Date: _____

Anticoagulation Prescription: ❏ Warfarin ❏ Heparin ❏ Ticlopidine ❏ Enoxaparin

   Anticipated Duration: ❏ Life ❏ 3 months ❏ 6 months ❏ Other (specify) _____

   Goal: ❏ INR = 2.0–3.0 ❏ INR = 2.5–3.5 ❏ PTT = _____ (specify) ❏ Other _____ (specify)

Current Medications (drug name, dose, directions):

May the patient take low-dose aspirin (81–325 mg) if indicated? ❏ Yes ❏ No

Do you want a report regarding the patient's anticoagulation status to you periodically? ❏ Yes ❏ No

Physician Signature: _____ Print Name: _____ Beeper #: _____

Primary Care Physician (if different): _____

Key: Dz, disease; GI, gastrointestinal; Hct, hematocrit; HPI, history of present illness; Hx, history; IVDA, intravenous drug abuse; MUGA, multiple gated angiography; PMHx, past medical history; PTT, partial thromboplastin time; US, ultrasound; VQ, ventilation-perfusion scan.

Courtesy of University of Maryland School of Pharmacy, Baltimore, Maryland.

Oral Anticoagulation Patient Information

Patient _____ Clinic No. _____

Telephone: Home _____ Work _____ Other _____

Physician _____

Diagnosis (reason for anticoagulation) _____

Other relevant diagnosis _____

_____

Medications _____

_____

Duration of therapy _____ Months _____ Yrs. _____ Indefinitely_____

Goal _____

Call physician if protime less than _____ seconds or greater than _____ seconds.

Courtesy of Jacksonville Coumadin Clinic, Mayo Clinic, Jacksonville, Florida.

Anticoagulation Clinic Information Sheet

1.   Patient name_____

2.   History number _____

3.   Referring physician _____

4.   Primary physician _____

5.   Reason for anticoagulation _____

     _____

6.   Current prothrombin time/INR_____

7.   Desired INR range _____

8.   Present warfarin dose_____

9.   Physician to send result form _____ Yes ____ No ____

10. Any significant medications_____

11. Anticoagulation Clinic appointment date_____

12. Other_____

Courtesy of Anticoagulation Clinic, University of Virginia Medical Center, Charlottesville, Virginia.

Initial Information Data Sheet

Appointment date _____   Patient name _____

Time _____   Hospital No. _____

Anticoagulation clinic No. _____   Address _____

Referring physician _____   _____

Physician telephone _____   Telephone: Home _____

Warfarin begun on_____   Work_____

Tablet size _____   Emergency name _____

Dose _____   Relationship _____

Emergency telephone _____

Indication for anticoagulation_____

_____

Anticipated length of therapy_____

_____

Other medications _____

_____

Other diagnoses _____

_____

Laboratory location _____

_____

Other information_____

_____

_____

_____

Courtesy of Anticoagulant Therapy Unit, Massachusetts General Hospital, Boston, Massachusetts.

Patient History Data Sheet

Name _____ Date of birth _____ Medical record No. _____

Indication for warfarin therapy _____

Desired INR _____ Physician _____ Initial visit _____

Expected duration of anticoagulation _____

Address _____   Contact _____

_____   Relationship _____

Telephone (home) _____ (work) _____   Telephone (home) _____ (work) _____

Referred by _____   Primary physician _____

Specialist(s) and dentist _____

Problem list:

1. _____   5. _____

2. _____   6. _____

3. _____   7. _____

4. _____   8. _____

Medications:

1. _____   6. _____

2. _____   7. _____

3. _____   8. _____

4. _____   9. _____

5. _____   10. _____

Alcohol use _____ Tobacco use _____

Hospitalizations _____

_____

_____

Complications _____

_____

_____

_____

Courtesy of Anticoagulation Clinic, University of Virginia Medical Center, Charlottesville, Virginia.

Anticoagulation Initial Assessment

Patient name _____

Date of admission _____

Chief complaint _____

Past medical history _____

_____

_____

_____

_____

_____

Past surgical history _____

_____

_____

_____

_____

Allergies_____

Hospitalization course _____

_____

_____

_____

_____

_____

_____

_____

_____

Medications _____

_____

_____

_____

_____

_____

_____

Signature_____

continues

Anticoagulation Initial Assessment continued

Education_____

_____

_____

_____

_____

Progress note _____

_____

_____

Date	PT	INR	Dose of Warfarin
_____	_____	_____	_____
_____	_____	_____	_____
_____	_____	_____	_____
_____	_____	_____	_____
_____	_____	_____	_____
_____	_____	_____	_____
_____	_____	_____	_____
_____	_____	_____	_____
_____	_____	_____	_____
_____	_____	_____	_____
_____	_____	_____	_____

Patient's telephone: Home _____ Work _____

Emergency contact telephone_____

Patient's primary physician _____

Signature_____

Courtesy of Division of Internal Medicine, Anticoagulation Program, Thomas Jefferson University Hospital, Philadelphia, Pennsylvania.

Anticoagulation Clinic Patient Registration and Data Form

Date: _____

Patient: _____ _____ ____ History #: _____
                    Last   First   MI

DOB: ___ / ___ / ___   Sex: M F

Address: _____ Tel #: _____

   City:_____ Zip: _____

Primary Care Physician: _____ Tel #: _____

Secondary Physician: _____ Tel #: _____

Clinical Information:

Indication:_____

Drug: ❑ Warfarin   ❑ Ticlopidine   ❑ Enoxaparin   ❑ Heparin

Significant Medical History: _____

_____

_____

Allergies: _____
(include type of reaction)

Medication	Dose	Start	Stop

Courtesy of University of Maryland, School of Pharmacy, Baltimore, Maryland.

Documenting Initial Anticoagulation Unit Interview

Patient name: _____

Address: _____

GENERAL INFORMATION

Diagnosis: _____

Primary care provider: _____ Telephone: _____

Mg. size warfarin: _____ Current dose: _____

Other medications: _____

Other diagnoses: _____

_____

PATIENT TEACHING

Understands the following: _____

Need for warfarin   ☐

Interaction of other drugs; acetylsalicylic acid ☐   alcohol ☐ _____

Others   ☐   _____

Signs and symptoms of elevated prothrombin time   ☐   _____

Bleeding precaution   ☐

Postcard system   ☐

Where to call in an emergency   ☐   _____

NURSING ASSESSMENT

Patient's perception of illness: _____

Social situation:

Lives alone   ☐   Visiting nurse   ☐

Lives with family   ☐   Significant other   ☐

Compliance with program: _____

_____

_____

_____

Courtesy of Anticoagulation Therapy Unit, Massachusetts General Hospital, Boston, Massachusetts.

Patient Enrollment/Assessment Form

Patient _____ Room No. _____ MR No. _____ Patient No. _____

Date of birth ___/___/___ Gender   M   F   Home telephone _____ Work telephone _____

Address _____ Significant other_____

Weight _____ Height _____ Significant other telephone _____

Insurance 1. _____ 2._____

ANTICOAGULATION: Diagnosis _____/_____/_____/_____

Date of admission ___/___/___   Provider _____ Specialist _____

Date discharge ___/___/___   Start warfarin _____ Start heparin _____ D/C heparin _____

MEDICAL Hx/RISK FACTORS: (Circle and date)

HBP _____ Diabetes _____ CHF _____ MI _____ CAD _____ Hx CVA _____ Hx TIA_____

Hx adm thrombus/emboli _____ Other _____

Reason for admission _____

MEDICATIONS: Allergies/Intolerance _____

PTA
_____   _____   _____

_____   _____   _____

Hospital
_____   _____   _____

_____   _____   _____

Discharge
_____   _____   _____

_____   _____   _____

BLEEDING Hx/RISK FACTORS: (circle) None

Falls	ETOH	Female	PID	Hosp. adm for bleed (date)_____
Rectal bleed	Oral bleed	Vaginal bleed	Upper GI bleed	Guaiac + – ___/___/___ ND
Lower GI bleed	Hct < 30%	Urinary bleed	Hx stroke	Renal insufficiency
Recent MI	HTN	Seizure	> 65 years old	Other_____

Description_____

DIET Hx: Vitamin K intake _____ Consistent   Y   N   ETOH _____

continues

Patient Enrollment/Assessment Form continued

BASELINE LABS:

Date _____ BIL _____ GOT/GPT _____ Scr/BUN _____ Plt _____ Alb _____ BP _____

Date _____ BIL _____ GOT/GPT _____ Scr/BUN _____ Plt _____ Alb _____ BP _____

Date	Dose	INR	PT	APTT	Hct	Date	Dose	INR	PT	APTT	Hct

OTHER LABS: Guaiac: +   – U/A: _____ Other: _____

DIAGNOSTIC: (Echo, ultrasound, V/Q, etc.): _____

Echo: _____ EF: _____% LA size: _____mm (Circle if yes): MS   MR   AS   AR   Other _____

US/Other _____

PATIENT CONSULTATION

Previous anticoagulation Hx: None   Yes   Preexisting knowledge of AC: None   Yes

Checklist: Discussed the following with (patient name)_____

__ Provided information materials on ACS and warfarin (dosing calendar, ID card, video tape)

__ General information, ACS: diagnosis, expectations of therapy, and patient obligations

__ Diet (Vitamin K consistency/ETOH use/GI illness)

__ OTC medication use and avoidance of NSAIDs and ASA

__ Prescription of drug use and obligation to inform ACS of new prescriptions/changes

__ Risk of bleeding, major and minor, and precautions (shaving/dentist visits/minor cuts, etc.)

__ Importance of contacting ACS if patient becomes ill

__ Compliance and what to do if miss a dose

__ Discussed the risks and benefits of AC (provided specific information sheet for diagnosis, if available)

__ Patient comprehends all of the above information and is ready for AC outpatient therapy.

continues

Patient Enrollment/Assessment Form continued

Assessment

Risk: 1. Thrombosis/embolism: high   moderate   low   other _____

       2. Bleed (major)—estimated risk/year _____

INR range   2–3   2.5–3.5   other _____

Duration AC   3 months   6 months   life   other _____

Current dose: _____   Recommended dose: _____

Tablet strength: _____   Next INR: _____/_____/_____

Comments _____

_____

_____

_____

_____

_____

_____

_____

_____

_____

_____

_____

_____

_____

_____

_____

_____

_____

ACS consultant _____ Date _____

Key: AC, anticoagulation; ACS, anticoagulation service; adm, admission; alb, albumin; APTT, activated partial thromboplastin time; AR, aortic regurgitation; AS, aortic stenosis; ASA, acetylsalicylic acid; BIL, bilirubin; BP, blood pressure; BUN, blood urea nitrogen; CAD, coronary artery disease; CHF, congestive heart failure; CVA, cardiovascular accident; D/C, discontinue; Echo, echocardiogram; EF, ejection fraction; ETOH, alcohol; GI, gastrointestinal; GOT, glutamic-oxaloacetic transaminase; GPT, glutamate pyruvate transaminase; HBP, high blood pressure; Hct, hematocrit; HTN, hypertension; Hx, history; ID, identification; INR, International Normalized Ratio; LA, left atrial; labs, laboratory tests; MI, myocardial infarction; MR, mitral regurgitation; MS, mitral stenosis; NSAID, nonsteroidal anti-inflammatory drug; OTC, over the counter; PID, pelvic inflammatory disease; Plt, platelets; PT, prothrombin time; PTA, prior to admission; Scr, screen; TIA, transient ischemic attack; US, ultrasound; V/Q ventilation/perfusion.

Courtesy of Anticoagulation Services of Rochester, Wilson Medical Center, Rochester, New York.

Anticoagulation Record

Name _____ Age _____ Date of birth _____ Today's date_____

Race _____ Religion _____ Education _____

Address _____

_____ Method of transportation _____

Mail _____ Internist _____

_____

Telephone _____ Alternate telephone _____ Referral source _____

Occupation _____ Primary language _____

Hours of work _____ Emergency contact person _____ Telephone_____

FAMILY HISTORY

__ Cancer	_ Epilepsy	_ Obesity
__ Tuberculosis	_ Gout	_ Bleeding
__ Diabetes	_ Heart disease	_ Migraine
__ Endocrine	_ Hypertension	_ Psychosis
__ Anemia	_ Kidney disease	_ Alcohol
__ Jaundice	_ Allergies	

SOCIAL HISTORY

Residence _____

_____

Social and economic status_____

_____

Day's activities (summary of duties) _____

_____

Diet—type and adequacy _____

_____

Habits:

__ Smoking

__ Alcohol

__ Drugs

Family status

_____

_____

continues

Anticoagulation Record continued

Other _____

_____

Medications (name, dose, frequency) _____

_____

_____

_____

_____

_____

_____

_____

_____

_____

_____

_____

SIGNIFICANT PAST MEDICAL HISTORY

Height _____

Weight _____

__ Infections

   __ Rheumatic fever

   __ Tuberculosis

__ Arthritis

__ Neurological conditions

   __ Head trauma

   __ Epilepsy

   __ Cerebrovascular disease

   __ Other _____

__ Respiratory

__ Cardiovascular

   __ Coronary disease

   __ Myocardial infarction

   __ Angina

   __ Arrhythmia

   __ Other _____

   __ Valvular disease

   __ Hypertension

continues

Anticoagulation Record continued

__ Cardiomyopathy

  __ Congenital defect

  __ Congestive heart failure

  __ Phlebitis

  __ Varicosities

__ Gastrointestinal problems

  __ Ulcer

  __ Hemorrhoids

  __ Liver disease

__ Genitourinary tract

  __ Renal disease

  __ Hematuria

  __ Other _____

__ Menstrual and pregnancy history _____

_____

__ Endocrine—Diabetes

  __ Thyroid

  __ Other _____

__ Hematology

  __ Bleeding

  __ Anemia

__ Allergies _____

_____

Indication for anticoagulation_____

_____

Date initiated _____   Estimated length of therapy _____

Identified risks _____

Patient's understanding of health status _____

_____

Problems identified by patient _____

_____

_____

_____

continues

Anticoagulation Record continued

ANTICOAGULATION TEACHING CHECKLIST

Topic	Date of Initial Instruction and Initials for Accountability	Reinforced	Comments	Initials
1. Assessment of patient knowledge				
2. Anatomy and physiology pertinent to anticoagulation				
3. Explanation of warfarin with other medications				
4. Need for regular blood tests				
5. Use of warfarin with other medications				
6. Symptoms to report				
7. Pregnancy				
8. Missed pills				
9. Time of day to take pills				
10. Alcohol use				
11. Emergency department				
12. ID card and guidelines				
13. Calendar				
14. Call back/contact system				
15. Activities of daily living				
16. Travel				

Signature_____ Date _____

PROBLEM LIST	HISTORY COMMENT
_____	_____
_____	_____
_____	_____
_____	_____

Courtesy of Framingham Heart Center, Framingham, Massachusetts.

Anticoagulation Surveillance Form

Patient name _____ Warfarin dose _____ mg/week _____

Indication _____ Daily regimen _____

Duration of treatment _____

1. Bleeding:

☐ Epistaxis   ☐ Black/tarry stools
☐ Gingival bleeding   ☐ Abnormal bruising
☐ Hematuria   ☐ No bleeding complications
☐ Hemoptysis   ☐ Other

2. Symptoms of recurring primary event (check any that apply):

☐ Chest pain   ☐ Dyspnea
☐ Palpitations   ☐ Headache
☐ Dizziness   ☐ Edema
☐ Confusion   ☐ Slurred speech
☐ Weakness   ☐ Vision changes
☐ Tender/swollen/red extremities
☐ Other_____

3. Medication changes: ___Yes ___No

4. Vitamin K intake: ___consistent

5. Missed doses (within past week): ___Yes ___No

6. INR results: _____ Dosage adjustments: _____

7. Reviewed dose with patient _____ Provided written instructions_____

Comments:

_____

_____

_____

_____

_____

_____

_____
Pharmacist signature   Date

Warfarin Patient Tracking Report

Next Visit _____ Medical No. _____

Social Security No. _____

Name _____

Birth Date _____ Day Telephone _____

Sex _____ Age _____ Night Telephone _____

Other Contact _____ Contact Telephone _____

MEDICAL INFORMATION

Medical Site _____

Primary Physician _____ Telephone _____

Referring Physician _____ Telephone _____

Diagnosis _____

Recommendation _____

Other Medications _____

Complications _____

Current Dose _____

PROGRAM STATUS AND TARGET VALUES

	Health Status		Low	High
Start Date _____				
Education Date _____	Seconds:		0.0	0.0
Ending Date _____	INR:		2.00	3.00
Reason for Termination _____	PT Ratio:		0.00	0.00

LABORATORY VALUES

Date	Current Dose	Laboratory Values				New Dose	Notified By	Return Date
		Control	Seconds	INR	PT			

Key: INR, International Normalized Ratio; PT, prothrombin time.

Courtesy of Boston University Medical Center Anticoagulation Clinic, Boston, Massachusetts.

Patient Encounter and Monitoring Form

To _____   Date _____

Patient _____   Medical record No. _____

Date of service _____

Dosage _____

INR   (____)
         (Protime)

Target INR: ☐ 2.0–3.0   ☐   2.5–3.5   ☐   _____

Previous INR summary:

Date	INR	Dose	Comment
_____	_____	_____	_____
_____	_____	_____	_____
_____	_____	_____	_____

PATIENT ASSESSMENT:

	Yes	No	Comment
Bleeding	☐	☐	_____
Shortness of breath/chest pain	☐	☐	_____
Neurologic symptoms	☐	☐	_____
Diet	☐	☐	_____
Medications	☐	☐	_____
Illness	☐	☐	_____
Hospital/Emergency department	☐	☐	_____
Compliance	☐	☐	_____

Suggest: ☐ No change in dosage regimen; continue
            ☐ New regimen_____

Next evaluation _____

Anticoagulation Services (signature) _____

Primary care physician (initials)_____

Courtesy of Anticoagulation Services of Rochester, Wilson Medical Center, Rochester, New York.

SOAP Format Record Sheet

ANTICOAGULATION CLINIC

Date _____ Telephone_____

Problem _____

SUBJECTIVE

Warfarin dose_____

Warfarin compliance: yes ___ no ___ explain _____

Bleeding symptoms: no ___ yes ___ explain _____

Medication changes: no ___ yes ___ explain _____

Dietary changes: no ___ yes ___ explain _____

Alcohol: no ___ yes ___ explain _____

Other _____

OBJECTIVE

PT _____ INR _____ Converts to INR _____

Other _____

_____

ASSESSMENT

PT/INR _____ >/< within _____ desired therapeutic range of_____

per Dr_____

copy to Dr_____

PLAN

Return to clinic_____

Guide written: Yes   or   No

_____

_____

_____

_____

Anticoagulation Clinic History Sheet

❑ New patient (if female, childbearing age? ❑ Yes ❑ No)   ❑ Follow-up   ❑ Telephone Contact Age:

	Since last anticoagulation clinic visit, has the patient experienced:

Indication:

Drug (name/strength):   Dose:

Goal INR: Duration of Tx: ❑ life   ❑ 3 mo   ❑ 6 mo   ❑ Other

Significant PMHx:

S:

Yes*	No	
❑	❑	Unusual bruising or bleeding
❑	❑	Nosebleeds
❑	❑	Blood in urine or change in color
❑	❑	Blood in stool or change in color
❑	❑	Change in medications
❑	❑	Change in diet
		(⇑ ⇓ intake of vitamin K rich foods)
❑	❑	Alcohol intake
❑	❑	Acute illness in past 10 days (eg, fever, sore thoat, diarrhea)
❑	❑	Change in overall health (eg, worsening CHF, renal failure)
❑	❑	Missed doses (per patient)
❑	❑	Falls or injuries
❑	❑	TE Event (eg, TIA, stroke, DVT, PE)
❑	❑	Hospitalization/ER Visit

*If yes, see note for detailed description

O: BP: /   HR: Wt: lbs

LABS PT _____ sec   INR _____   Hct _____

Platelet _____   WBC _____   ANC _____

A: ❶ Anticoagulation:

P: ❶ Dose:

❷ RTC   /   /   at   PM with preclinic ❑ PT/INR ❑ CBC w/differential ❑ Hct/Hgb

❸ Patient Education:

Rx(s) written: ❑ medical assistance

Signature(s):

Key: A, assessment; ANC, absolute neutrophil count; BP, blood pressure; CBC, complete blood count; CHF, congestive heart failure; DVT, deep venous thrombosis; ER, emergency room; Hct, hematocrit; Hgb, hemoglobin; HR, heart rate; O, objective; P, plan; PE, pulmonary embolism; PMHx, past medical history; PT, prothrombin time; RTC, return to clinic; S, subjective; TE, thromboembolic event; TIA, transient ischemic attack; WBC, white blood count.

Courtesy of University of Maryland, School of Pharmacy, Baltimore, Maryland.

Coumadin Therapy Record

Name _____

MR # _____

Date _____

Tablets on hand: ____ Coumadin ____ mg ____ mg   Warfarin ____ mg ____ mg

Since your last INR, have you:

- Missed any doses of Coumadin? ____ no ____ yes
- Changed from brand Coumadin to generic? ____ no ____ yes
- Started, stopped, or made changes taking medications, including prescription and OTC, especially: antibiotics, antidepressants, anti-inflammatory, cholesterol-lowering, heart, thyroid, birth control pills, estrogen, laxatives, aspirin or non-aspirin products, creams or ointments containing aspirin (i.e., Ben Gay)? ____ no ____ yes
- Started, stopped, or made changes taking any vitamins or herbal supplements? ____ no ____ yes
- Increased or decreased the amount of alcohol you use? ____ no ____ yes
- Changed your diet, including nutritional supplements? ____ no ____ yes
- Changed your exercise habits? ____ no ____ yes
- Changed employment? ____ no ____ yes
  (____ ST disability ____ LT disability ____ unemployed ____ retired)
- Had bleeding from:
  ____ Gums   ____ Nose   ____ Rectum   ____ None
  ____ Blood in urine   ____ Black stools   ____ Unexplained bruising
  ____ Prolonged bleeding from cuts ____ Increased menstrual flow or vaginal bleeding
- Been in the hospital? ____ no ____ yes
- Had a fever or illness, such as vomiting, diarrhea, infection, pain, or swelling? ____ no ____ yes
- Noticed numbness or tingling in your arms or legs? ____ no ____ yes
- Noticed any visual changes or loss of vision in either eye? ____ no ____ yes
- Noticed dizziness or fainting? ____ no ____ yes
- Chest pain, trouble breathing, or coughing up blood? ____ no ____ yes
- Had a fall or injury? ____ no ____ yes
- Become pregnant or planning a pregnancy? ____ no ____ yes ____ NA
- Been scheduled for any upcoming medical, surgical, or dental procedures? ____ no ____ yes
- Made plans to travel in the near future? ____ no ____ yes

Fingerstick INR: _____   Finger incised: R/L 1 2 3 4 5

Comments _____
_____
_____
_____

Signature _____ Date _____

Courtesy of Dartmouth-Hitchcock Nurse Clinic, Nashua, New Hampshire.

INR Flowsheet Tools

Warfarin Therapy Flowsheet

Indication:						Date therapy initiated:				
Duration of therapy: _____ indefinite /_____ months until (date) _____						INR goal:				
Physician signature: _____						Date:				

Graph	Date:									
I N R	—5.0— —4.5— —4.0— —3.5— —3.0— —2.5— —2.0— —1.5— —1.0—									
Current dose (mg)										
INR										
New dose (mg)										
Follow-up INR date										
Education (see key)										
Comments: (eg, outside laboratory used, compliance, etc.)										
RN signature/initials										
To be completed by physician/provider if complications or nontherapeutic INR occur:										
Food interaction (y/n)										
Drug interaction (y/n)										
Bleeding (y/n)										
Thrombi/emboli (y/n)										
Physician/provider Signature/initials										

	Education Key: A = dose change; B = diet; C = alcohol use; D = over-the-counter drugs; E = warfarin basics; F = other.	
	Signature/Initials	

Courtesy of Prime Care Clinic, Veterans Affairs Medical Center, Dayton, Ohio.

Anticoagulation Monitoring Flowsheet

Patient: _____ Tel #: _____

Indication: _____

Goal INR: _____ Anticipated duration of Tx: _____ (D.C. date:_____)

Date	PT (sec)	INR	Current Dose	New Dose	Other Labs and Comments	RTC

Key: D.C., discontinue; RTC, return to clinic; Tx, treatment.

Courtesy of University of Maryland, School of Pharmacy, Baltimore, Maryland.

Anticoagulation Monitoring Sheet

Patient name		MR No.		Date of birth	
Telephone (home)		Laboratory			
Telephone (work)		Home draw laboratory			
Telephone (relative)		Visiting nurse service			
Diagnosis		Pharmacy			
Physician		Tablet size			
INR range		Duration		Discharge date	

Date	Current Dose	Control	PT	PT Ratio	INR	New Dose	Next Appt	Initials	Comments

Courtesy of Division of Internal Medicine, Anticoagulation Program, Thomas Jefferson University Hospital, Philadelphia, Pennsylvania.

Anticoagulation Flowsheet

DOB_____ Reason for anticoagulation_____ Valve type _____

Telephone #_____ Physician/Clinic_____

INR goal range_____

Date	PT	INR	Dose	Comments
				Dose Verified Missed Doses Med Changes
				Diet Changes S/S Bleeding/Clotting
				INR Therapeutic Dose Change
				Comments:
				Dose Verified Missed Doses Med Changes
				Diet Changes S/S Bleeding/Clotting
				INR Therapeutic Dose Change
				Comments:
				Dose Verified Missed Doses Med Changes
				Diet Changes S/S Bleeding/Clotting
				INR Therapeutic Dose Change
				Comments:
				Dose Verified Missed Doses Med Changes
				Diet Changes S/S Bleeding/Clotting
				INR Therapeutic Dose Change
				Comments:
				Dose Verified Missed Doses Med Changes
				Diet Changes S/S Bleeding/Clotting
				INR Therapeutic Dose Change
				Comments:
				Dose Verified Missed Doses Med Changes
				Diet Changes S/S Bleeding/Clotting
				INR Therapeutic Dose Change
				Comments:

Key: S/S, signs and symptoms.

Courtesy of Red Primary Care Team, Veterans Affairs Medical Center, Salt Lake City, Utah.

Anticoagulation Clinic

Patient Name _____ ID No. _____

Address _____ Date of Birth _____

Telephone _____

Reason for Anticoagulation _____

INR Goal _____ Duration of Therapy_____

Date	Current Warfarin Dose	Control PT	Patient PT	INR	New Warfarin Dose	Next Appt	Seen by	Comments

Courtesy of Anticoagulation Clinic, Royal C Johnson Memorial Hospital/Veterans Affairs, Sioux Falls, South Dakota.

Progress of Anticoagulation

Indications _____ Name _____

Desired INR _____ Medical record number _____

Duration _____ Strength of warfarin _____ q _____

	Date										
	Protime										
INR Coumatrak											
Coagamate											
Other											
Warfarin dose 17.5											
15.0											
12.5											
10.0											
7.5											
5.0											
4.0											
3.75											
3.0											
2.5											
2.0											
1.25											
0											
Visit/No-Show Telephone											
Return in Weeks											

Comments:_____

_____

_____

_____

_____

_____

_____

_____

_____

_____

_____

Courtesy of Anticoagulation Clinic, University of Virginia Medical Center, Charlottesville, Virginia.

Anticoagulation Center Patient INR Record

Patient name _____ Sex _____ Date of birth/age _____

Patient address _____ Social Security number _____ Telephone _____

Reason for anticoagulation _____ Duration of anticoagulation _____

Referring physician _____ Clinic entry date _____ Target INR range _____

Date	Dose	Mg/week	Changes	2.0	3.0

continues

Anticoagulation Center Patient INR Record continued

Past Medical History

Condition	Diagnosis/Treatment Date	Active Treatment (Y/N)

Medication History

Name	Strength	Dosage	Start/Stop Date

Miscellaneous

	Y	N	Explain/Quantify
Drug allergies			
Tobacco use			
Alcohol use			
Previous warfarin use			
History of bleeding			

Courtesy of Lutheran General Health System Anticoagulation Center, Niles, Illinois.

INR Flowsheet

Name _____ Birth date _____ Medical record _____ Telephone _____

Risks _____ Physician _____ Location _____

Indication _____ INR Target _____ Tablet _____

Prescription _____

Date	Day	INR	PT	Lab	Dose	Last	New	Assessment/Comments
								☐ Bleed ☐ SOB ☐ CP ☐ Neuro ☐ Med ☐ Illness ☐ Hosp/ED ☐ Compl ☐ Diet Next:
								☐ Bleed ☐ SOB ☐ CP ☐ Neuro ☐ Med ☐ Illness ☐ Hosp/ED ☐ Compl ☐ Diet Next:
								☐ Bleed ☐ SOB ☐ CP ☐ Neuro ☐ Med ☐ Illness ☐ Hosp/ED ☐ Compl ☐ Diet Next:
								☐ Bleed ☐ SOB ☐ CP ☐ Neuro ☐ Med ☐ Illness ☐ Hosp/ED ☐ Compl ☐ Diet Next:
								☐ Bleed ☐ SOB ☐ CP ☐ Neuro ☐ Med ☐ Illness ☐ Hosp/ED ☐ Compl ☐ Diet Next:
								☐ Bleed ☐ SOB ☐ CP ☐ Neuro ☐ Med ☐ Illness ☐ Hosp/ED ☐ Compl ☐ Diet Next:
								☐ Bleed ☐ SOB ☐ CP ☐ Neuro ☐ Med ☐ Illness ☐ Hosp/ED ☐ Compl ☐ Diet Next:
								☐ Bleed ☐ SOB ☐ CP ☐ Neuro ☐ Med ☐ Illness ☐ Hosp/ED ☐ Compl ☐ Diet Next:
								☐ Bleed ☐ SOB ☐ CP ☐ Neuro ☐ Med ☐ Illness ☐ Hosp/ED ☐ Compl ☐ Diet Next:
								☐ Bleed ☐ SOB ☐ CP ☐ Neuro ☐ Med ☐ Illness ☐ Hosp/ED ☐ Compl ☐ Diet Next:
								☐ Bleed ☐ SOB ☐ CP ☐ Neuro ☐ Med ☐ Illness ☐ Hosp/ED ☐ Compl ☐ Diet Next:
								☐ Bleed ☐ SOB ☐ CP ☐ Neuro ☐ Med ☐ Illness ☐ Hosp/ED ☐ Compl ☐ Diet Next:
								☐ Bleed ☐ SOB ☐ CP ☐ Neuro ☐ Med ☐ Illness ☐ Hosp/ED ☐ Compl ☐ Diet Next:

Key: Bleed, bleeding symptoms; Compl, compliance; CP, chest pain; Hosp/ED, hospitalization/emergency department visit; INR, International Normalized Ratio; Lab, laboratory; Med, medication change; Neuro, neurological symptoms; PT, prothrombin time; SOB, shortness of breath.

Courtesy of Anticoagulation Services of Rochester, Wilson Medical Center, Rochester, New York.

Anticoagulation Therapy Flowsheet

Concurrent Medications: _____	Name
_____	Account No.
_____	Cardiologist
_____	Insurance
_____	Special Instructions _____
_____	_____

Indications for warfarin _____   Internist _____

Length of therapy _____

Telephone _____   Therapeutic range _____

						Daily Dosage of Warfarin Tablets										
Date	BP	PT	INR	Hct	UA	M	T	W	T	F	S	S	Bleeding and/or Bruising	Next Appt	Notes (—med changes —ETOH intake)	Acct Initials

Codes: + = Positive   +/N = Positive—refer to notes
         − = Negative

Accountability Signatures _____   _____

Full Name and Title _____   _____

Key: Acct, accountability; Appt, appointment; BP, blood pressure; ETOH, alcohol; Hct, hematocrit; INR, International Normalized Ratio; Med, medication; PT, prothrombin time; UA, urinalysis.

Courtesy of Framingham Heart Center, Framingham, Massachusetts.

Anticoagulation Summary for Outpatient

Diagnosis _____

_____

_____

_____

_____

Referring   Telephone
Physician _____   _____

                       Telephone
Pharmacy _____   _____

                       Telephone
Laboratory _____   _____

                       Taken at
Warfarin tablet size_____mg _____

| Name |
| Address |
| Birthdate/Age   Sex |
| Unit Number |
| Telephone   Estimated duration of prescription |

Medication

_____

_____

_____

_____

Date	Initial Dose	PT / Control	Prescribed Dose	Comment

Courtesy of Anticoagulation Clinic, University of Massachusetts Medical Center, Worcester, Massachusetts.

Patient Data Flowsheet

Patient No. _____

Name _____

Reason for Anticoagulation			Duration of Anticoagulation			Goal INR	Medications
Date	Current Dosage	INR	New Dosage	Next Appt	Bleed Y/N	Comments	

Courtesy of Boston University Medical Center Anticoagulation Clinic, Boston, Massachusetts.

Anticoagulation Monitoring Form

Patient's name_____   PCP:_____

Medical record #_____   Rm #_____   ___no PCP assigned

Attending physician:		Date of admission:		RPh:

Diagnosis:						
Indications for anticoagulation:		___ A-fib	___ Valve replacement	___ DVT	___ PE	
		___ Other:				
Pre-admission:	Warfarin strength:	Dose:				

Other significant information:		
Age:	Gender:	
Phone number:		

Date	Warfarin Dose	INR	APTT	On I.V. Heparin?	Notes
					____D/C home on warfarin
					____D/C home, warfarin on hold
					____D/C home, warfarin discontinued
					____Patient expired
					Date of discharge:_____ Time:_____
					Follow-up with:_____ Date: _____
					Lab slip given for PT/INR on:_____
					Warfarin dose: _____ RPh: _____

Key: A-fib, atrial fibrillation; APTT, activated partial thromboplastin time; D/C, discharged; DVT, deep venous thrombosis; I.V., intravenous; PCP, primary care physician; PE, pulmonary embolism; RPh, resident physician.

Courtesy of Kaiser Permanente Hawaii, Department of Pharmacy, Honolulu, Hawaii.

Chapter 9

Software Applications in Anticoagulation Management

Lynn B. Oertel and Dennis Mungall

INTRODUCTION

The need to individualize oral anticoagulant therapy has been apparent since its initial use more than 50 years ago. This need is driven by the desire to avoid the frequent complications of too much or too little therapy. Additionally, as the number of anticoagulation management services or clinics increases, clinicians search for tools to enhance the performance of their services and the quality of patient care. Traditionally, paper flowsheets and paper records have supported clinical decision making and documented patient interactions. However, technical advances and access to computerized software have resulted in the availability of several software products that are designed to meet the needs of busy anticoagulation management services. Numerous approaches to tailor therapy to individuals have been explored and include developing algorithms that mimic physician behavior, developing equations that predict an average dose based upon patient history, and developing dynamic models to describe anticoagulant response.[1] The decision made for each patient is complex, and a multitude of factors must be considered including drug interactions, food interactions, dosage decisions, method of prothrombin time (PT) testing, educational level of the patient, concurrent disease states, compliance and motivation, and optimal time to schedule future blood tests. This chapter reviews the historical development of software systems, describes attributes of an ideal system, and supplies a brief description of several software products to aid patient management that are specific to anticoagulation therapy.

HISTORICAL OVERVIEW

The idea of using computer techniques to assist in the management of the anticoagulated patient was originally put forth by Nagashima et al[2] in 1969. They realized that it was necessary to be able to predict response accurately to prevent too much or too little anticoagulation. Using an IBM mainframe computer, they modeled the data of 30 normal volunteers and set the stage for future attempts at predicting anticoagulant response. In 1969, Sheiner[3] used a similar model to compare the capabilities of the IBM mainframe program to that of cardiologists in predicting the daily requirements of patients with pulmonary emboli. The program was superior to two of three cardiologists.

Theophanis and Smolen[4] in 1972 proposed a model for describing both single dose and multiple dose relationships between warfarin and prothrombin complex activity. In 1973, Theophanis and Barile[5] performed a retrospective study with data from recently discharged hospital patients and showed that the model described both the early and steady state pharmacologic responses to warfarin.

Sawyer and Fin[6] compared the Theophanis and Barile model with an analog model of Barr,[7] which also had required the use of an IBM 370 mainframe computer. An interesting sidelight on the Barr model was that it was used to dose warfarin for President Richard Nixon when he developed a deep venous thrombosis in 1970. The maintenance dose was chosen to achieve a PT of 2.0 (likely equivalent to an International Normalized Ratio [INR] of 3.0–4.5).

The Anticoagulant Therapy Unit (ATU) at Massachusetts General Hospital is among the largest and oldest outpatient anticoagulation clinics in the country and provides an example of a fully computerized system for patient management, including functions for computerized dosing, patient communications using an automated postcard system, detailed reports for performance, and more. This anticoagulant management service was implemented in 1969, and a computer-based information system was added in January 1973 to accommodate the growing number of patients and large volume of anticoagulation data.[8] It has a current population of 2950 patients, and to date, the system has been used to manage over 15,700 patients. The system runs on a mainframe platform in MUMPs software, which is not available commercially.

Although revisions to the software have been made over time, the basic principles involving the dosing algorithm and other patient management functions remain essentially unchanged. The computerized dosing algorithm suggests a dose and future blood test date for about 85% of the 250 to 300 daily new INR entries. However, nurses always review and approve all computer-suggested doses and blood test dates before patients are contacted. Suggestions can be overridden as nurses apply their clinical knowledge and expertise in tailoring patient management. A computer-generated postcard system has also been used for over two decades that informs patients of test results, current dose, and future blood test date.

The ATU's computerized system at Massachusetts General Hospital is vital to the growth of the clinic, and positive results are achieving by using the computerized applications. The percentage of time patients are maintained in assigned therapeutic range is about 79% in the most frequently used INR range of 2.0 to 3.0. The success of this specific computer software applied to a large patient population over a long period of time supports the helpful and critical role played by information systems and specialized software in health care delivery systems today.

A series of papers by Powers et al,[9] O'Leary and Abbrecht,[10] and Abbrecht et al[11] tested a pharmacodynamic model that included a term for protein binding and automatically downweighted early PTs. In 1982, the first desktop personal computer (PC) marketed by IBM set in motion the ability to perform tasks that previously required a mainframe computer. The work of Abbrecht and coworkers in 1982 was among the first studies to use computer-assisted dosing prospectively to manage the inpatient initiation of warfarin therapy. Although the sample size was small (N = 200), the computer-assisted group remained within the therapeutic range a greater percentage of time than the control group (83% versus 60%).

In 1984, Wilson and James[12] described an outpatient microcomputer-assisted anticoagulation system. Their approach was to quantitate the average physician response to changes in warfarin dose for a given level of anticoagulation. They developed an empirical formula and compared it with their previous manual system. They also included a systematic approach for return visits based on the degree of anticoagulation control. The computer system was virtually identical to the manual system (17.4% manual versus 14.2% computer outside an INR of 2–4).

Mungall et al[13] in 1985 described the population of pharmacokinetics in 32 adult hospitalized patients and 131 adult outpatients. This information set the stage for the development of a new approach to the modeling of response to warfarin. Svec et al[14] had suggested an approach that embedded population information directly into a predictive pharmacokinetic/pharmacodynamic model. This approach had intuitive appeal in that all decisions made by the computer program were weighted on past experience. This statistical linking of a pharmacokinetic/pharmacodynamic model with previous experience was termed *bayesian forecasting*.

A series of papers[14–21] published from 1985 to 1995 use a bayesian forecasting approach and clearly establish the stability to predict day-to-day and steady state PT response. In 1987, White et al[22] published the first and only randomized trial of computer-assisted warfarin versus standard physician dosing in hospitalized patients. This was the first PC-DOS/Windows program for managing anticoagulation. Computer-assisted dosing consistently outperformed physicians in key areas such as individual therapeutic dosing, time in therapeutic range, and shortened hospital length of stay. A second randomized trial of computer-assisted therapy versus skilled care in outpatients was performed by White and Mungall.[23] They demonstrated that the program in outpatients was comparable to someone with several years of experience in managing patients. The significance of this finding is that anticoagulation expertise could be immediately available to the novice.

In 1988, Carter et al[24] utilized the analog computer system used in 1971 to titrate President Nixon's warfarin dose. The model, functionally similar to the one used by Svec, retrospectively predicted the daily PT response for 29 patients. The best prediction was after four days of therapy. Carter and colleagues confirmed the ability of a computer model to predict response, but the system was useful only as a research tool and inferior in ease of use to modern PC-based systems.

Ryan et al[25] in 1989 described an outpatient system designed to recommend a new warfarin dose, schedule patients, supply a drug interaction database, and record bleeding events. They used an empiric guideline for changing dosage. The percentage of range increased from a baseline of 46% to 63% after six months of use.

In 1998, Casimiro and Mungall developed the first Microsoft Windows–based anticoagulation clinic program.[26] This program was unique in that it was the only anticoagulation management system that directly modeled the response to warfarin by using a pharmacodynamic model for describing the relationship between warfarin dose and INR. It had a bleeding risk assessment module, a prospective quality assessment system for evaluating the outcomes of the patient population, and a multimedia information system for clinicians and patients. Prospective evaluation of this system showed a marked improvement in percentage of patients within the therapeutic range (36% at baseline to 78% at 6 months).

Using two approaches similar to those of Ryan et al[25] and Wilson and James,[12] Poller and colleagues[27] in 1993 performed a randomized trial in 186 patients receiving long-term warfarin treatment. The two computer approaches were compared with traditional methods in the clinic. This prospective interventional study evaluated 575 dosings in these patients. Dosing by physicians resulted in 50.4% of the visits in the therapeutic range, and the computer-generated dosing ranged from 53.0% to 56.5%.

Margolis et al[28] described the development of a warfarin management program and the results of implementing this program in their clinic in 1994. The program was developed for the IBM PC and tested in 151 patients. Prior to use of the computer, 48% of the patients were within an INR of 2–3. After implementation, 44.8% were within range. The program had an empiric dosage guide and a statistical package for prospectively evaluating its database.

In 1994, Fihn et al[29] developed and tested a computer system for assisting in optimally scheduling patients. Using this method, they were able to identify patients who needed more intense follow-up and those who required less follow-up.

Since the 1990s, more reports have appeared in the literature evaluating the impact of various computer programs on dose management and INR control, cost-effectiveness, and other measures.[31–37] They and continuing studies demonstrate that computerized dosing systems can make a significant improvement in patient management. The previously mentioned studies are summarized in Table 9–1.

Traditionally, anticoagulant therapy involves a great deal of physician time to educate and monitor patients. Computerized models can optimize the decision-making process regarding dose adjustments and intervals between periodic testing. Both economically and medically, the full impact of these technological breakthroughs hardly has been realized.

The distinction between inpatients and outpatients in the management of anticoagulated patients is rapidly fading in the evolving health care environment. Continuity of care is essential, and a system that initiates therapy in the hospital and then follows anticoagulated patients in the outpatient setting will lead to the most efficient management of these patients.

CHARACTERISTICS OF AN IDEAL ANTICOAGULATION SYSTEM

There are numerous factors to consider when evaluating a computer application specific to anticoagulation management. Before choosing a system, one needs to perform an analysis of needs. Exhibit 9–1 outlines factors to be considered for this analysis.

The remainder of this chapter provides brief summaries of commercially available software products. The primary purpose is to disseminate information about such software applications—not to endorse any specific product but to furnish facts concisely in an easy-to-read format as a service to interested clinicians about the specific products described here. The following material is provided largely by the respective company or software developer; therefore, the information may not be completely objective. We encourage interested individuals to perform a careful needs assessment of their clinic, contact vendors directly for further information, and conduct a detailed software evaluation of their own. Table 9–2 lists the salient features of the software products described.

Table 9–1 Historical Review of Anticoagulation Computer Systems

Author/Year	Subjects	Type of Study	Outcome
Nagishima et al 1969[2]	30 normals	Modeling of response	Developed dynamic model
Sheiner 1969[3]	17 patients PE	Computer (MF) vs MD	Computer better than two thirds of cardiologists
Theophanis and Smolen 1972[4]; Theophanis and Barile 1973[5]	2 patients	Modeling of response	Improved the modeling
Hoffer et al 1975[8]	420 patients	Outpatient evaluation (MF)	57%–72% in range
Sawyer and Fin 1979[6]	12 patients	Computer (MF) inpatient	Predict PT response
Powers et al 1980[9]; O'Leary and Abbrecht 1981[10]; Abbrecht et al 1982[11]	20 patients/surgery	Matched control, PC-based model vs MD inpatient	Days in control = 60%; PC model = 83%, p<.05
Wilson and James 1984[12]	132 patients	Empiric computer dosing vs historical control	Computer and manual equal
Mungall et al 1985[13]	163 patients DVT/A-fib/CHF/valve	Kinetic/Modeling	Established kinetic model for warfarin, age vs clearance; 1% reduction every year after 18
Svec et al 1985[14]	45 patients DVT/PE/graft	First bayesian forecasting modeling of PT response incorporated kinetic model/dynamic model	R = 81 predicted vs observed PT
White et al 1987[22]	75 patients DVT/PE/A-fib/valve TIA	Bayesian forecasting model (PC) vs MD randomized, prospective inpatient and outpatient	Stable PT 3.7 days sooner, 85% PC vs 42% on follow-up, fewer overanticoagulations
Carter et al 1988[24]	29 patients DVT/CVA/PE/TIA	3 doses of 10 mg, analog MF computer prospective prediction of PT response after 3 days, inpatient	After 7 days, R = .88 to predict next day's PT
Ryan et al 1989[25]	400 patients/688 visits outpatient	Empiric dosage algorithm vs historical control	46% control vs 63% computer assisted
Farrow et al 1990[17]	40 patients DVT	Daily prediction of PT response in inpatients using PC bayesian forecasting	Predicted vs observed error 5%–13%
Poller et al 1993[27]	186 patients DVT/A-fib/CVA/arterial	Prospective/randomized computer (MF) vs clinician empiric dosage algorithm, outpatient	Clinician 50.4% vs computer 57% in range overall for INR, 3.0–4.5, 36% MD vs 59% computer
Margolis et al 1994[28]	151 patients	PC-based, empiric dosage algorithm, computer managed vs historical control, outpatients	48% before, 45% after in range
Fihn et al 1994[29]	620 patients DVT/PE/A-fib/stroke/valve	Evaluate computer scheduling model, outpatients	Interval of 4.4 weeks computer vs 4.1 weeks for noncomputer
Sun and Chang 1995[21]	20 patients DVT/PE/A-fib	Bayesian forecaster (PC) vs MD dosing warfarin, inpatients	MDs vs computer needed more PTs to establish stable dose (9 vs 4)

continues

Table 9–1 continued

Author/Year	Subjects	Type of Study	Outcome
Vadher et al 1997[30]	148 inpatients	Randomized, controlled trial comparing quality of anticoagulant control achieved with computerized decision support system vs traditional method	Computerized decision support system was safe and effective; improved quality of initiation and control of warfarin
Poller et al 1998[31]	285 patients discharged from hospital within 6 weeks of start of anticoagulation	Randomized, multicenter trial comparing computer-generated dosing vs traditional methods	Computer program provided better INR control than experienced medical staff
Fitzmaurice et al 1998[32]	28 patients in inner-city general practice	Prospective evaluation of INR control and costs using computerized decision support and near patient testing	Mean percentage of patients in therapeutic range was 72%; nurse-delivered anticoagulation monitoring was cost-effective
Chatellier et al 1998[33]	9 trials, including 1,336 patients from 1996 to 1997	Meta-analysis of published randomized trials to assess effectiveness of computer-assisted dose systems	Use of computer programs increased the proportion of visits where patients were treated appropriately by 29%; hemorrhages tended to be less frequent
Casimiro and Mungall 1998[26]	42 patients DVT/PE/A-fib/valve	Bayesian forecasting outpatient INR vs historical control	35% INR in range before vs 78% after

Key: A-fib, atrial fibrillation; CHF, congestive heart failure; CVA, cerebral vascular accident; DVT, deep venous thrombosis; INR, International Normalized Ratio; MD, physician; MF, mainframe; PC, personal computer; PE, pulmonary embolism; PT, prothrombin time; TIA, transient ischemic attack; tPA, tissue plasminogen activator.

Exhibit 9–1
GENERAL CONSIDERATIONS FOR SELECTING AN ANTICOAGULATION SOFTWARE PROGRAM

Basic Features

- Hardware requirements and compatibility
- Interface possible with existing applications in work environment?
- Interface capability with standard software applications such as MS Word, Excel, or other statistical packages
- For Web-based applications, Internet access and browser requirements
- Additional platforms support using lap top, personal digital assistant, or a wireless connect

Software Functionality

- User manuals provided? How detailed?
- Ease of use and speed for users, single or multiple users?
- Functions for patient follow-up or tracking?
- What type of standard form letters included? Can they be customized? Are communication needs for patients and other health care professionals met?
- What types of reporting mechanisms are included? Can they be customized to fit needs?
- Is a dosing algorithm included? Has it been validated?
- Ability and ease to export data to other applications?
- What quality performance measures are included?
- How secure and reliable is software?
- What type of safety or clinical alerts are included?
- On-line links to references or sites?

User Support

- Installation—Does user or company perform? Additional cost?
- Assistance to transfer existing database from old to new platform—can vendor help and at what fee?
- What type of technical and user training provided and for how long? On site or remote?
- What type of ongoing technical support is planned?
- What are contact methods? Is there phone/fax/Internet access to vendor? Is phone toll free? Is there a clinician (pharmacist, nurse, or physician) on staff?
- Upgrades to program provided on regular basis? Any fee?
- Technical support fees?
- Maintenance fees—what is included?
- Does product come with a 30-day, money-back guarantee?
- References—Will vendor supply references of sites using program?

Resource Considerations

- Affordability and fees
- Capital expenses for new or additional hardware
- Interface with existing hardware/software
- Technical support fees
- Upgrades
- Staff training
- Billing and reimbursement issues

SOFTWARE PRODUCT DESCRIPTIONS

ANTHEMA (ANticoagulation THErapy MAnagement), homeTAO, e-MedicalMonitor S.L.

Outpatient oral anticoagulation clinics are the cornerstone of oral anticoagulation therapy (OAT) management in several European countries. Although this organizational model is successful in delivering high-quality therapy, there is also a trend toward moving OAT management, or at least parts of it, closer to patients. Two approaches are gaining momentum:

- the decentralization of OAT testing or management to primary care practices/family physicians
- the rise of patient self-testing and self-managing models

Notwithstanding this diversification, most therapy management models continue to demand a center of reference and excellence, eg, the specialized OAT clinic. Thus, OAT clinics will often monitor patients that are followed in different clinical settings. Appropriate information and communication systems become key enabling factors at the time of implementing new models for managing OAT. These systems play a critical role when addressing the apparent contradiction between the forces of centralization and those for decentralization.

ANTHEMA, the ANticoagulation THErapy MAnagement software marketed by e-MedicalMonitor S.L. (Barcelona, Spain) allows primary care practices and family doctors to monitor patients under the general supervision of a specialized clinic. ANTHEMA also allows the provision of direct services to patients. ANTHEMA incorporates the PARMA therapeutic decision support system, which has been validated after many years of clinical investigations and use.[34] It can also support alternative therapeutic protocols.

The ANTHEMA software architecture is located on the Web, accessible through standard Web browsers without the need for local software. ANTHEMA provides Web patient management capabilities under an application service provider (ASP) agreement under which e-MedicalMonitor maintains and operates the hardware and software infrastructure. The ASP reduces the need for investment of human and technological capital.

e-MedicalMonitor has developed ANTHEMA's functionality with a number of direct services for patients. Figures 9–1 and 9–2 are examples of ANTHEMA's screens pertaining to INR management. EasyTAO is one service that allows clinics to automate the reporting of anticoagulant dose information to patients. The patient chooses a communication channel (fax, mobile phone, or e-mail) to have an automated drug prescription sent after a routine INR test. Patients may also receive daily reminders of the drug prescription and of their next appointment for a blood test. HomeTAO is a service designed for programs involving self-testing and/or self-managing under the general supervision of anticoagulation clinics or primary care practices. HomeTAO provides a

means for the self-testing patient to communicate the INR value, along with other relevant data, from home to the supervising clinic or practice through the Web, cellular phone, etc. Figure 9–3 is a view of a patient interface screen used by homeTAO patients. On the basis of this information, the OAT practitioner at the clinic/practice uses ANTHEMA to adjust the drug dosage, which once validated, is automatically reported back to the patient by the channel of choice (eg, fax, cellular phone, e-mail, etc.).

Anticoagulation Management Program (AMP), TeleHealth Systems, Inc.

The Anticoagulation Management Program (AMP) focuses primarily on patient management through a PC-based automated telephone patient follow-up system. The company has previously developed successful systems for congestive heart failure, diabetes, chronic obstructive pulmonary disease, and women's health issues. TeleHealth began business in 1993 to assist in the monitoring of various high-risk obstetrical conditions. The specific anticoagulation applications have been developed with the assistance of a

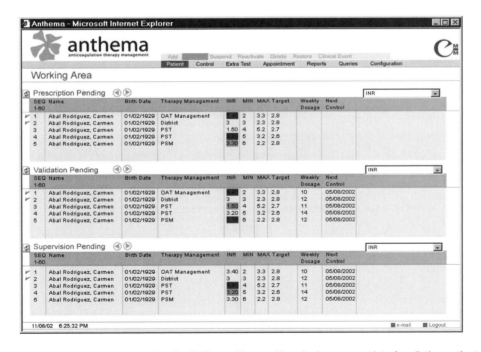

Figure 9–1 ANTHEMA working area screen. Provides the OAT practitioner with a single, compact interface listing patients for whom the drug dosage must be manually adjusted (prescription pending) or for whom the drug dosage automatically suggested by the therapeutic decision support system must be validated (validation pending). Patients are listed regardless of whether the INR determination has been performed at the clinic, primary care practice, or home. ANTHEMA also provides OAT clinics with a list of patients for whom the drug dosage adjusted by other practitioners is to be supervised (supervision pending). Courtesy of e-MedicalMonitor, D'Amunt, Spain.

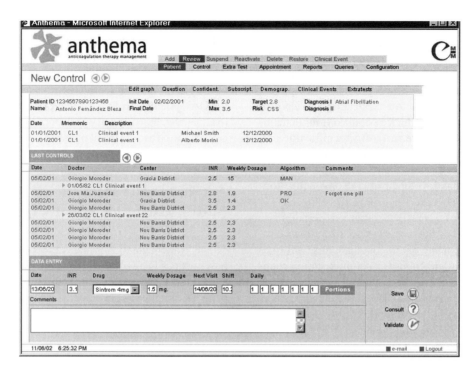

Figure 9–2 ANTHEMA's new INR determination page. The screen displays a summary of patient information (demographics, diagnostic data, lists with recent clinical events, and INR determinations, etc.) and a dosage adjustment section at the bottom. Upon entry of the INR value, the therapeutic decision support system suggests the anticoagulant drug's weekly dosage along with its weekday distribution, which can then be confirmed or overridden. Courtesy of e-MedicalMonitor, D'Amunt, Spain.

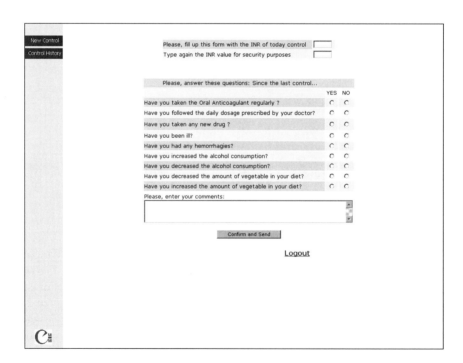

Figure 9–3 Patient screen from ANTHEMA, homeTAO. This patient interface provides a simple means through which patients enter the data associated to a specific INR. Once confirmed, the data are communicated to the OAT practitioner, who uses it as the basis for adjusting the patient drug dosage. Courtesy of e-MedicalMonitor, D'Amunt, Spain.

cardiology consultant. It is designed to begin patient follow-up as soon as warfarin therapy is prescribed. Once a patient has two consecutive in-range lab results, TeleHealth begins its "automated" follow-up to assist the health care provider in a timely collection of patient information. AMP consists of three algorithms called care tracks. The tracks are determined partly by the method of INR measurement and partly by the patient's compliance history. Patients can be moved from one care track to another as dictated by the provider. TeleHealth provides "electronic visits" to enrolled antico-agulation patients by using one of several special question algorithms to monitor individual progress. Each care track has a prescribed level of TeleHealth contacts or visits. The questions are specific to anticoagulation and can be easily answered by the patient or his or her caregiver in 3 minutes or less. A nurse or pharmacist can be paged at the end of each contact, if warranted by the patient response. This PC-based system is located at the provider's site.

Five sets of warfarin follow-up questions have been developed on the basis of patient blood test method and other patient features. Each is designed to meet the particular needs of a predetermined group of patients. These five sets are

1. *Coumadin Self-Test*—Patients respond to a group of questions about medications, food, alcohol, and symptoms. In addition, patients report their last protime result using their self-testing device.
2. *Coumadin Self-Test Inbound*—The same set of questions as above, but used only for the most compliant patient group. These patients call into TeleHealth and deposit their data on a predetermined, regular basis.
3. *Coumadin INR Inbound*—A simple question application for the group of patients who have been on Coumadin for some period of time and are self-testing. Patients enter their INR results only. Then if there is something abnormal, the protime department will call to make further inquiries.
4. *Coumadin Lab*—The same set of questions as used for the Self-Test Inbound group, except that patients are not asked for their protime results.
5. *Coumadin Lab Inbound*—The same set of questions as used for the Coumadin Lab group but for the more compliant group of patients.

Essentially, TeleHealth provides a cost-effective and timely contact method, namely "electronic visits" for larger health care providers who need to gather frequent patient information. Calls are scheduled and conducted at times that the patient expects them to be coming. Automatic requeuing of calls to handle answering machines and busy signals is built into the system. Patient response reports can be generated that provide a written copy of patient responses to the various questions. A nurse/pharmacist breakout feature is available

that allows the patient to press any key in order to page the clinician at the conclusion of the questions. A nurse/pharmacist comment section provides text files to document follow-up to a particular patient's set of responses. These might outline further instructions, observations, or an intervention. A team of well-trained nurses, pharmacists, and physicians is key to the overall management of this patient population and type of follow-up system.

The company turnkeys each system to meet individual customer needs. The services include installation and training, customer support, and periodic system enhancements. Multilingual capability is also available. Volume and growth can be accommodated by adding more phone lines and workstations. Additional uses can be added to handle other areas of concern such as compliance issues by setting up a "protime reminder call." Such calls can be designed to phone patients at 6-week intervals to remind them to visit the lab and have their blood test. Future directions for this specific application will be directed to patient self-testing and finally self-management by selected patient groups.

In summary, this system operates on the basic premise that more frequent patient contacts will yield tighter INR control and therefore will maximize the time patients spend within a designated therapeutic INR range. Patients who play a major role in their therapy and management will achieve greater success in their health care outcomes.

Clever Clog, Dr. M.A. Bradley and Mr. J.W. Bradley

This design and construction of this software program arose when the demand on a growing anticoagulation clinic's time in the United Kingdom convinced a general practitioner that the work should be delegated to a practice clinician aided by computer software.

The Development of the Clever Clog Algorithm

To create an algorithm that is individualized for each patient, a statistical analysis is performed on pairs of INRs and dose values in order to establish a dose that would provide a mean INR value equal to the target INR for that particular patient. The Clever Clog protocol assumes that previously well-controlled patients who have a result just outside the 0.5 target tolerance are still satisfactorily controlled. For a patient with a target of 2.5, a single INR result of 1.8, 1.9, 3.1, or 3.2 would not trigger a change in regular dose. Results outside 0.75 of target do trigger a change. A change will also be recommended if two consecutive results are more than 0.5 outside of target. Changes in dose are recommended when the dose are required, calculated statistically as above, drifts from the current prescribed dose.

Clinical Experience

The Clever Clog program has been in use for four years with few modifications. The program is able to produce two types of audit reports: an audit for individual patients and a summary for a group of selected patients. An example of audit results for a group of patients is provided in Figure 9–4.

CoagCare® Management System, ZyCare®, Inc.

ZyCare®'s patented applications allow remotely located patients to communicate physiologic and other data to a central server that is accessible to health care providers using a Web browser. The system can identify and prioritize patient problems and systematize the implementation of remotely managed treatment programs that include medication adjustment algorithms. ZyCare® is now testing the CoagCare® Management System for the management of anticoagulation therapy with warfarin in a clinical trial at Duke University.

CoagCare® is a browser-based system for the management of patients using home self-PT-testing devices. The patient uses the Internet to connect to the CoagCare® Web page and enter the results of each home test. CoagCare® prompts the patient to answer questions about the presence of throm-boembolic or hemorrhagic symptoms, changes in medications, or major dietary or lifestyle changes. See Figures 9–5 and 9–6 for examples of such patient communications screens. Software in the CoagCare® server analyzes the results and uses a proprietary physician-specified dosing algorithm to automatically provide appropriate small adjustments in warfarin dose as needed. Automated adjustment of self-testing frequency is based on INR and reported symptoms. Large changes in the INR require physician review and approval of the new warfarin dose before that information is communicated back to the patient. All data on the CoagCare® server is continuously accessible to the patient's health care provider, who can dynamically structure each patient's individualized treatment plan with more or less automation depending upon the needs of the patient at any given time. An automated recording of patients' receipt of information is preserved.

The CoagCare® software flags patients with markedly abnormal results or recurrent problems for quick identification of problems and physician intervention, allowing the physician to focus on patients in need of attention. CoagCare® can also automatically change the PT-testing schedule based on INR data. Indications of problems increase the frequency of scheduled PT-testing, while stable INR values in the absence of other problems decrease the frequency of testing. Figure 9–7 provides an example of a health care provider's screen used in patient management.

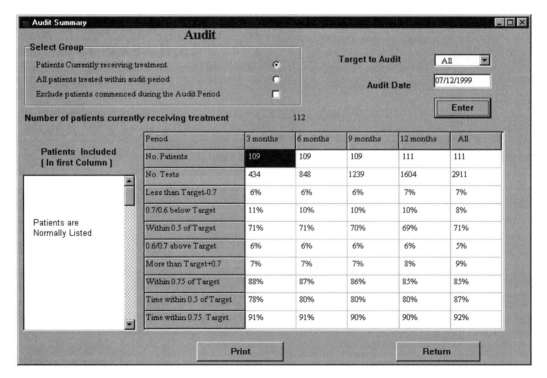

Figure 9–4 Summary of INR results from one practice using Clever Clog. This table reflects about 2 years of data. Courtesy of M.A. Bradley, England.

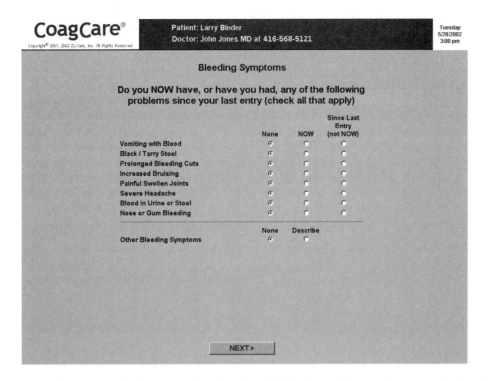

Figure 9–5 Example of a patient communication screen from CoagCare®. Patients use this screen to communicate potential symptoms to their health care provider. Courtesy of ZyCare®, Inc., Chapel Hill, North Carolina.

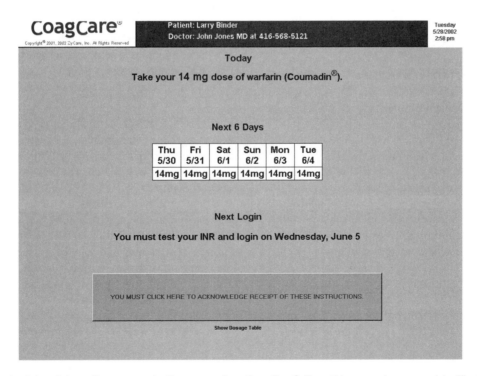

Figure 9–6 Example of dose information communication screen from CoagCare®. Once this screen is accessed, verification of this is stored. Courtesy of Zycare®, Inc., Chapel Hill, North Carolina.

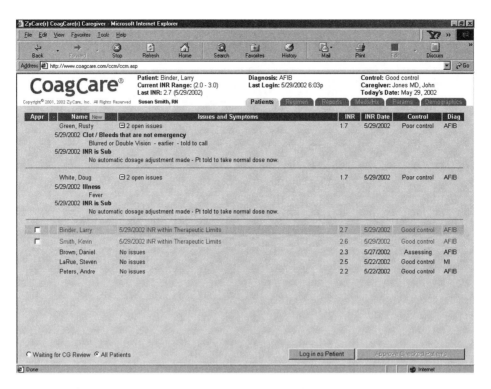

Figure 9–7 Example of a caregiver screen from CoagCare® for patient management. Courtesy of ZyCare®, Inc., Chapel Hill, North Carolina.

CoagClinic, Standing Stone, Inc.

Standing Stone's CoagClinic is designed to support the management and documentation of anticoagulation care. It is a Web-based system that is updated on a quarterly basis reflecting use.

CoagClinic is customizable by individual users and has the following options:

- Multi-office patient scheduling
- Patient follow-up listings (no more "lost" patients)
- Automated overdue visit notification
- Built-in list of ICD9 diagnosis codes and CPT billing codes
- Interactive INR guidance based upon ACCP guidelines
- User-activated, customizable dosing algorithms
- Dosing support for both warfarin and low–molecular-weight heparin
- Medication interaction notification
- Take-home visit forms for patients including customizable educational materials

- Patient INR graphs, quality control statistics, including time in therapeutic range as well as user-defined reports
- Seamless interfacing to other Windows®-based products including Word, Excel, and other reporting and data analysis tools
- Event tracking and reporting capabilities

Figure 9–8 depicts CoagClinic's main patient screen and shows all relevant information at a glance. CoagClinic tracks all visits in a flowsheet format and displays dosing schedules, low–molecular-weight heparin flags, and visit addenda as seen in Figure 9–9.

CoagClinic is offered as part of an integrated suite of disease management applications that include lipid management, diabetes, and congestive heart failure. Standing Stone offers training and support services, including a toll-free support number, e-mail support, and online help. CoagClinic can be integrated with other electronic medical records, and data can be converted to CoagClinic from other systems.

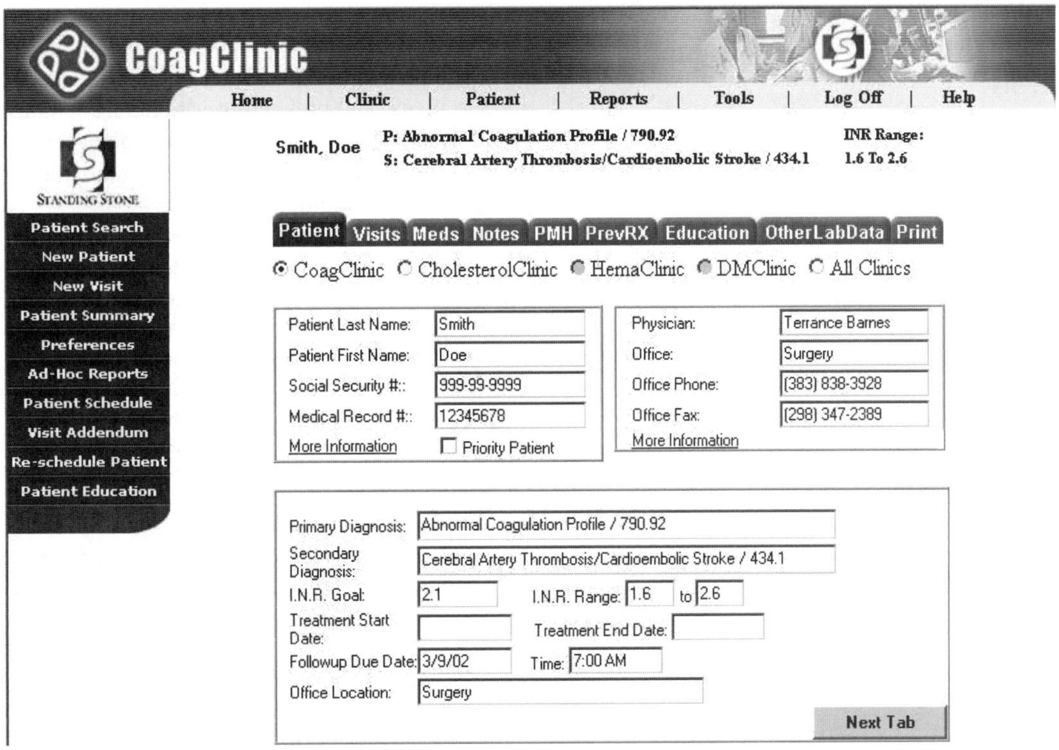

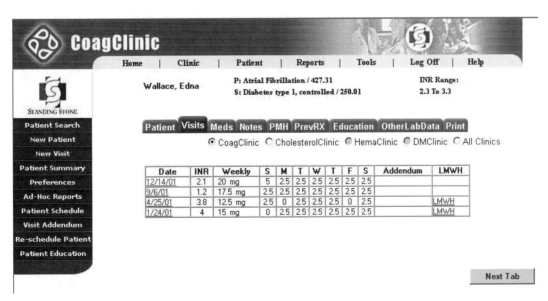

Figure 9–8 Example of CoagClinic's main patient screen shows all relevant information at a glance. Courtesy of Standing Stone, Inc., Westport, Connecticut.

Figure 9–9 CoagClinic tracks all visits in a flowsheet format and displays dose schedules, flags low–molecular-weight use, and visit addenda. Courtesy of Standing Stone, Inc., Westport, Connecticut.

CoumaCare® Patient Management System for Windows 5.1a, Bristol-Myers Squibb Pharmaceuticals

Overview

The CoumaCare® Patient Management System software is an important part of the overall CoumaCare® Process, an integrated program of specific therapy and care management strategies available from Bristol-Myers Squibb (formerly from DuPont Pharmaceuticals). This process provides a variety of resources for both new and established anticoagulation clinics, including a coumacare.com Web site.

Patient Management

In use at more than 4000 sites around the country, the CoumaCare® Patient Management System for Windows 5.1a is a computerized method of storing and retrieving information about patients who are being treated with warfarin sodium therapy. The application helps a clinic manage its warfarin patients more effectively by facilitating timely recordkeeping, automatically tracking missed appointments and lab visits, and preventing patients from simply getting "lost" to follow-up. The application also may be used to produce a wide variety of customized quality assurance and patient and clinic summary reports.

The heart of the CoumaCare® Patient Management System is the "New Patient" entry dialogue box, shown in Figure 9–10. The system assigns a unique identification number to each patient and asks the user to record a patient's name; address and phone number (including contact information for a relative or other home caregiver); anticoagulation physician, diagnosis, and any co-morbidities that may be present; and target INR range (in line with the guidelines from the 2001 *Chest* supplement).[35]

Users may specify detailed instructions concerning dosing regimens and may make extensive entries in any of several categories, including lab visits, clinic visits, and patient follow-up (Figure 9–11). They can search for and collect

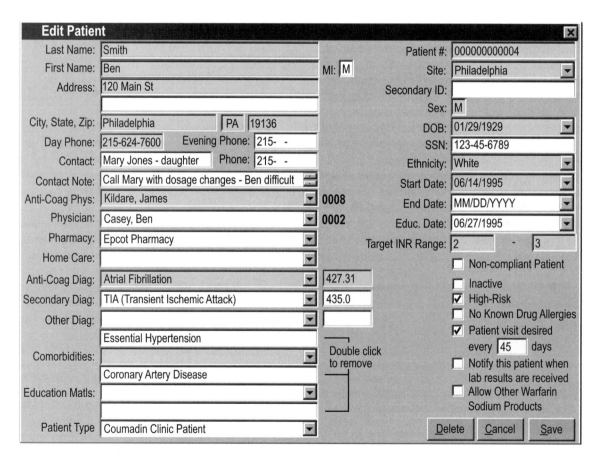

Figure 9–10 New patient entry dialogue box for CoumaCare®. Courtesy of Bristol-Myers Squibb Pharmaceuticals, Plainsboro, New Jersey. Coumadin and CoumaCare are registered trademarks of the Bristol-Myers Squibb Company. Any unlicensed use of these trademarks is expressly prohibited under the U.S. Trademark Act.

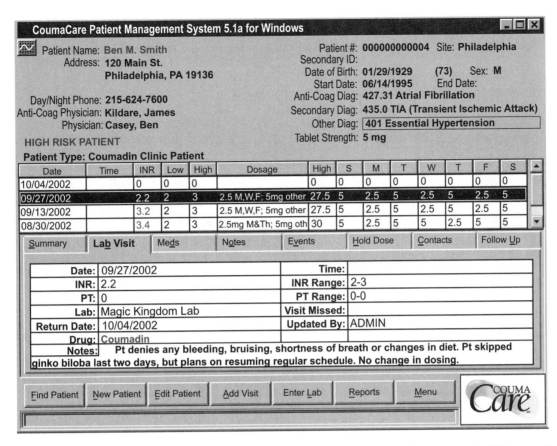

Figure 9–11 Patient management screen for CoumaCare®. Courtesy of Bristol-Myers Squibb Pharmaceuticals, Plainsboro, New Jersey. Coumadin and CoumaCare are registered trademarks of the Bristol-Myers Squibb Company. Any unlicensed use of these trademarks is expressly prohibited under the U.S. Trademark Act.

patient, physician, and therapy management data in a wide variety of ways and a wide variety of reasons: INR reviews, assessment of follow-up procedures, and tracking of high-risk patients, to name a few. The software also may be used to generate letters to patients—either customized or from a template—to remind them of missed visits.

Some of the data entry fields contained in the CoumaCare® Patient Management System software capture information being gathered for use in the Anticoagulation Consensus To Improve Outcomes Nationally (ACTION) project—a Phase IV study of anticoagulation aimed at improving patient care. Data are being collected nationwide on anticoagulation treatment practices to develop measures for quality assessment and assurance. The CoumaCare® software allows investigators ongoing access to a database used to manage patients undergoing long-term OAT. Outcomes are expected to increase knowledge on how best to manage these patients.

Dawn AC Anticoagulation Therapy Software, a Division of 4S Information Systems, Ltd

Dawn AC has been in use for 15 years and is now in its sixth version, serving over 200 anticoagulation services worldwide. Dawn AC can customize its offerings to meet the local needs in six major areas:

- Computer-aided dose change rules
- Anticoagulants used and dosing instruction format
- Test interval setting
- Letter template format and content
- Report content and format
- Patient handling, eg, home visits, clinics, transport

Several features of Dawn AC are pictured in Figures 9–12 through 9–14.

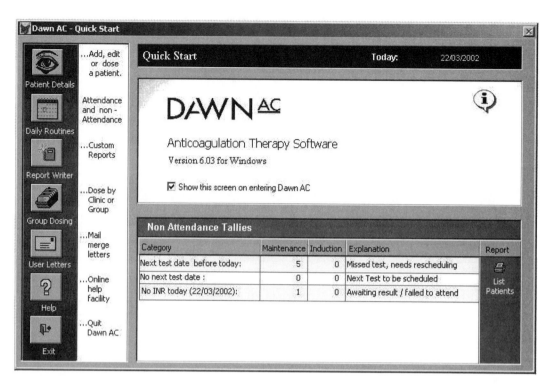

Figure 9–12 Quick Start screen from DAWN SC showing the main functions and patient non-attendance tallies. Courtesy of 4S Information Systems Ltd, Cumbria, England.

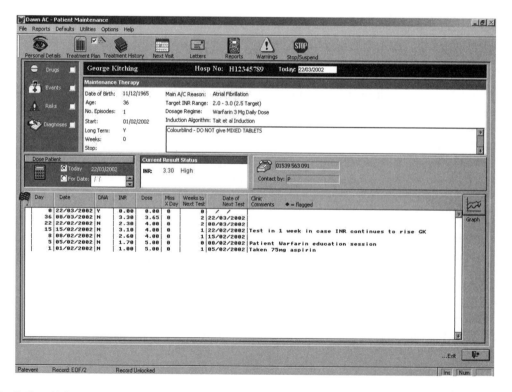

Figure 9–13 The Patient Maintenance screen from DAWN AC that provides a "whole picture" of the patient. Courtesy of 4S Information Systems Ltd, Cumbria, England.

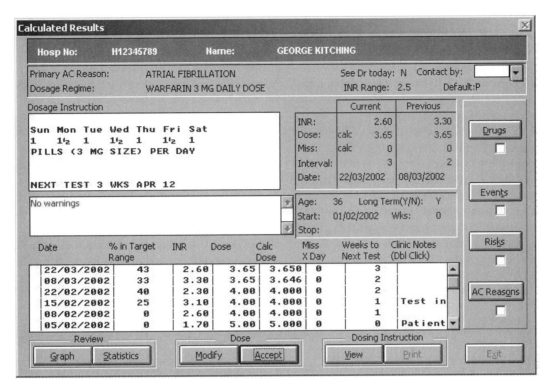

Figure 9–14 The Calculated Results screen from DAWN AC. On this screen, the clinician can accept or modify the suggested dose. Courtesy of 4S Information Systems Ltd, Cumbria, England.

Scientific studies have demonstrated the effectiveness of Dawn AC computer-aided dosing versus traditional dosing by health care professionals by demonstrating a greater time in therapeutic range for patients managed by the dosing algorithm compared to control groups.[31,35] Dawn AC is a quality management system certified to the international ISO 9000 standard and the higher United Kingdom software standard, TickIT. ISO 9000 is a general quality management standard that can be applied to any business or organization, whereas TickIT recognizes the specific nature of software development and adds further requirements to the ISO 9000.

Dawn AC can also be linked to patient administration systems and other software applications such as Microsoft Word. This facility allows users to produce highly formatted Word documents.

Dawn AC offers eight modules: three main modules and five specialist modules. The three main modules are available for maintenance or stabilized patients.

- **Dawn AC Manager.** Detailed recordkeeping of patient information allows manual setting of anticoagulant dose and the manual setting of the next test date on an individual basis. It translates the dose into a user-defined instruction for the patient, eg, pills per day. It has functions for following up patients who did not attend, for handling patients that are due to stop therapy, and for patients tested in different laboratories. It optionally has a report writer and letter definition facility.

- **Dawn AC Practitioner.** Similar in functionality to the Manager, except that the Practitioner has computer-recommended dose and next dates for handling patients on an individual basis. The operator can override the recommended decision.

- **Dawn AC Enterprise.** Indicated for large organizations with many hundred of patients managed by several staff, possibly in different locations. Sets of INR results can be progressively entered and computer recommended doses and next dates can be calculated in one operation. Enterprise allows interface with a laboratory information system.

Dawn AC offers five specialist modules:

- **Dawn AC Induction.** This offering allows patients to be initiated on oral anticoagulants over the first days of therapy. On user initiation, the software automatically transfers the patient to maintenance therapy when the patient has reached a satisfactory INR level.

- **Dawn AC Voyager.** This offering allows subsets of patient information to be taken to a remote location (in a notebook computer, eg, home visit for patient management). At the end of the remote session, data can be merged back into the central system.
- **Dawn AC Interfaces.** This offering allows Dawn AC to collect information and the INR result from a laboratory information system or other computer system.
- **Link to MS Word.** Links to Microsoft Word provides highly formatted Word documents.
- **Patient Record Book Printer.** Dose instructions may be printed directly into a record book (similar to a bank passbook) using a special printer combined with bar code reader. This provides the patient with a convenient therapy record.

Customer Services

Customer service is provided by a dedicated team and responds by telephone, email and fax. 4S staff provides classroom training on site or Microsoft NetMeeting and/or audio-visual E-Books for remote training. A benchmarking service offers clients a twice-yearly quality of care benchmarking exercise to compare treatment statistics to over 50 hospitals involving nearly 100,000 patients.

DoseResponse®, Keystone Therapeutics, Inc.

Overview

DoseResponse® is a Web-based program for managing and documenting warfarin therapy. It provides "point and click" data entry. Patient dosage instructions are fully outlined, including graphics and educational material that can be printed for the patient's home use. DoseResponse® documents the medical process for each patient encounter including the history update, progress note, and patient instructions. The automated documentation supports billing and can be formulated into a variety of administrative and quality assurance reports to help track and improve clinical outcomes.

DoseResponse® is indicated for a variety of practice settings, including physician offices, established anticoagulation clinics, and integrated delivery systems that serve from 100 to 1,000 or more patients and INRs monthly. The software (patent pending) uses SSL (abbreviation describing a security protocol developed by Netscape) to securely trans-

mit patient data, and is Health Insurance Portability and Accountability Act of 1996 compliant. Because it is Internet-based, DoseResponse® eliminates the need to install and maintain software, and supports both multiple locations and multiple users with one secure central database.

How It Works

After log on, a daily patient schedule and patient status screen comes up, helping to manage daily workflow (see Figure 9–15). The Clinician Screen provides a concise profile of the patient history including progress notes and previous dosage regimens. The Clinician Screen is prefilled with dosage and follow-up recommendations based on American College of Chest Physicians and literature-based guidelines. Figure 9–16 is an example of patient instructions including dosage, follow-up dates, and educational material.

Features

- Computerized dosing is based on published guidelines (including the American College of Chest Physicians).
- Form letters are available for missed appointments as well as for printed dosage and follow-up instructions.
- Reports include a patient history/medical record report; a patient quality assurance/graphical report; an administrative report with summary statistics such as "% Time in Range," "% INRs in Range," and "Events" for the total and segmented patient population; and other types of customized reports.
- Quality control capabilities include tracking and reporting for laboratory compliance as well as data analysis to support quality assurance and clinical outcomes assessment.
- Patient tracking includes easily viewed status of each patient (including missed appointments); changes in the patient's history including indication(s), target range, risk factors, influencing variables, and interacting medications; scheduled appointments; dosage regimens/adjustments; INR values; educational material; outcome events; and various quality assessment measures (eg, % Time in Range).

On-Line Clinical Resources

DoseResponse® provides specific clinician alerts for key clinical management issues such as serious drug interactions, oral vitamin K recommendations, excessive dosage adjustment requirements, and tablet strength changes. In addition, several links to drug information databases as well as to professional organizations are available via the Web site.

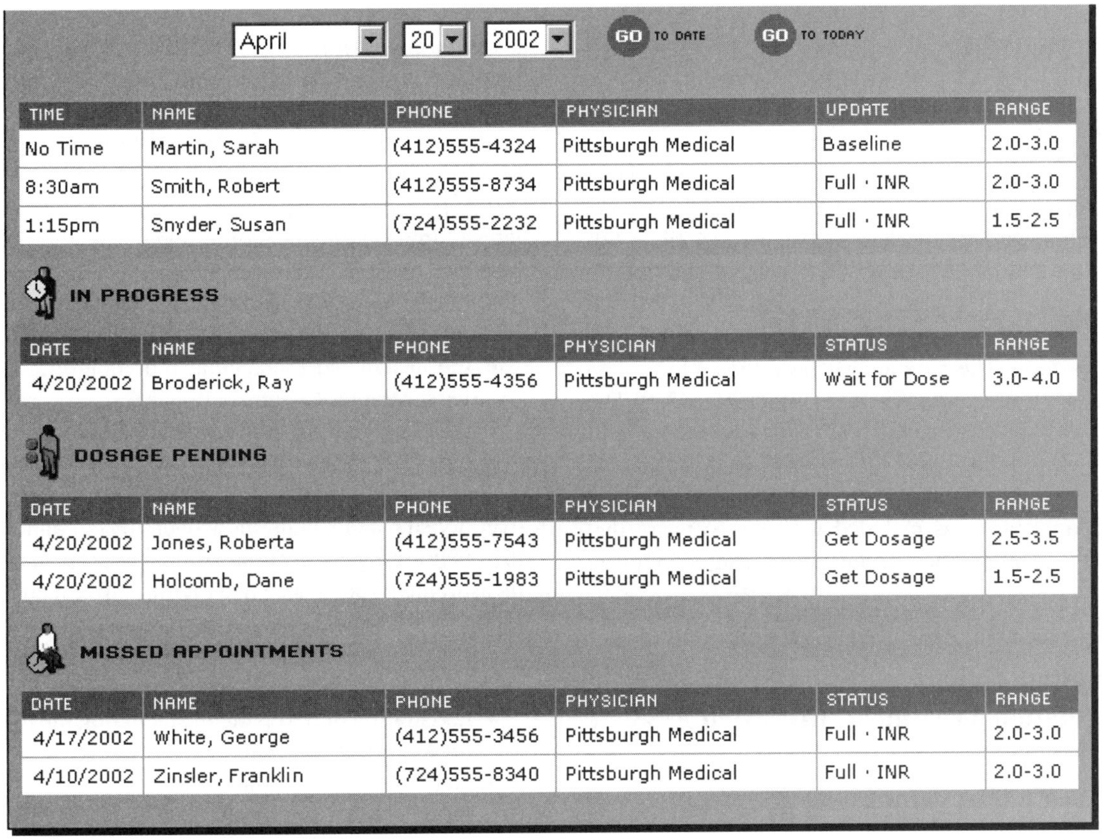

April | 20 | 2002 | GO TO DATE | GO TO TODAY

TIME	NAME	PHONE	PHYSICIAN	UPDATE	RANGE
No Time	Martin, Sarah	(412)555-4324	Pittsburgh Medical	Baseline	2.0-3.0
8:30am	Smith, Robert	(412)555-8734	Pittsburgh Medical	Full · INR	2.0-3.0
1:15pm	Snyder, Susan	(724)555-2232	Pittsburgh Medical	Full · INR	1.5-2.5

IN PROGRESS

DATE	NAME	PHONE	PHYSICIAN	STATUS	RANGE
4/20/2002	Broderick, Ray	(412)555-4356	Pittsburgh Medical	Wait for Dose	3.0-4.0

DOSAGE PENDING

DATE	NAME	PHONE	PHYSICIAN	STATUS	RANGE
4/20/2002	Jones, Roberta	(412)555-7543	Pittsburgh Medical	Get Dosage	2.5-3.5
4/20/2002	Holcomb, Dane	(724)555-1983	Pittsburgh Medical	Get Dosage	1.5-2.5

MISSED APPOINTMENTS

DATE	NAME	PHONE	PHYSICIAN	STATUS	RANGE
4/17/2002	White, George	(412)555-3456	Pittsburgh Medical	Full · INR	2.0-3.0
4/10/2002	Zinsler, Franklin	(724)555-8340	Pittsburgh Medical	Full · INR	2.0-3.0

Figure 9–15 DoseResponse® screen for daily patient schedule. Source: © 2000–2002, Keystone Therapeutics, Inc., Pittsburgh, PA.

DoseResponse™
WARFARIN DOSAGE

Issued on May 20, 2002

George White
Pittsburgh Medical

Your INR is **1.6**. Your range is 2.0 - 3.0.

Your tablet strength of warfarin (Coumadin®) is **5 mg.**

Your weekly dosage of warfarin has **changed.**

Beginning **Monday, May 20**, take your **new** dosage shown below:

START

Sun	Mon	Tue	Wed	Thur	Fri	Sat
1 tablet	1 tablet	1 tablet	1 tablet	½ tablet	1 tablet	1 tablet

Continue taking this dosage until your next INR test, scheduled for **May 27**.

PLEASE REMEMBER

Prescription medications may have a major effect on your response to warfarin. During the ... start, stop, or change the dose of a ... your INR.

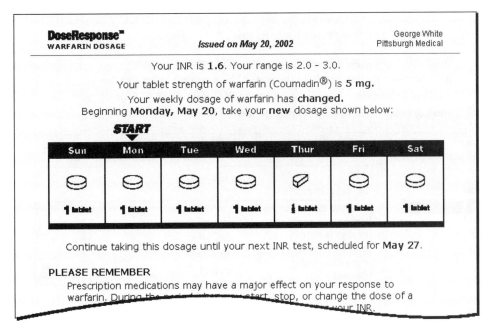

Figure 9–16 Example of patient-specific dosage printouts from DoseResponse®. Source: © 2000–2002, Keystone Therapeutics, Inc., Pittsburgh, PA.

DrugCalc, Therapeutic Technologies, Dennis Mungall, PharmD

Overview

The DrugCalc program is a bayesian forecasting system that allows the user to individualize hospital drug therapy and assists the clinician with discharge planning and clinic follow-up on an optimal dose of warfarin. (See Figure 9–17.) This same approach can be used for patients initiated on warfarin as outpatients, or to assess non–steady state response to warfarin. The program has been shown to shorten hospital stay,[23] and improve heparin therapy.[39–43] The DrugCalc program allows clinicians to manage other medications including aminoglycosides, phenytoin, theophylline, vancomycin, digoxin, lithium, etc. Additionally, a general calculation application is included with the software that allows independent creation of one's own drug monitoring programs.

Health System Organizer™ for Oral Anticoagulation Treatment, IntraMed A/S

Overview

IntraMed has developed a Web-based and scalable system for anticoagulation treatment management. The architecture is open, which allows the system to integrate with other systems, eg, laboratory hospital systems and patient administrative systems. The system was developed by Ivan Brandslund, MD, DMSx, Director and research associate professor at the Institute for Health Research, University of Southern Denmark and Vejle County Hospital.

The system has a validated, built-in algorithm that calculates a proposed medication dosage. The algorithm acts in response to three parameters:

- the difference between the two most recent INR values
- the designated therapeutic INR range for the patient versus the INR value
- a table predicting effect of dose-changes

The dosage algorithm has been validated on 500 patients over 5 years, and results show over 70% of patients in their therapeutic range at any time using an average of only 10 INR measurements per year.[44] See Figure 9–18 for an example of INR and dose history screen for a selected patient.

Software features include:

- registration of new patients, including the indication(s) for treatment
- elective or manual start of treatment
- establishment and documentation medication routines
- follow-up routines for patients who have not obtained designated INR test

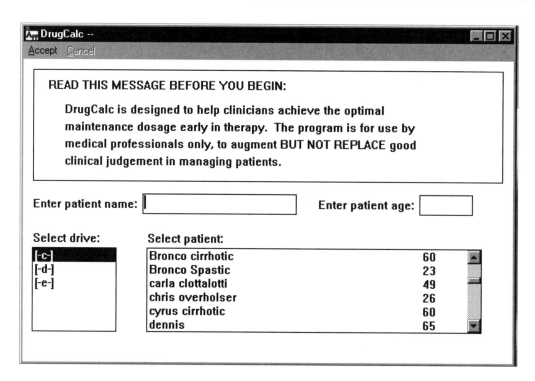

Figure 9–17 Sample entry screen for DrugCalc users. Courtesy of Therapeutic Technologies, Dayton, Ohio.

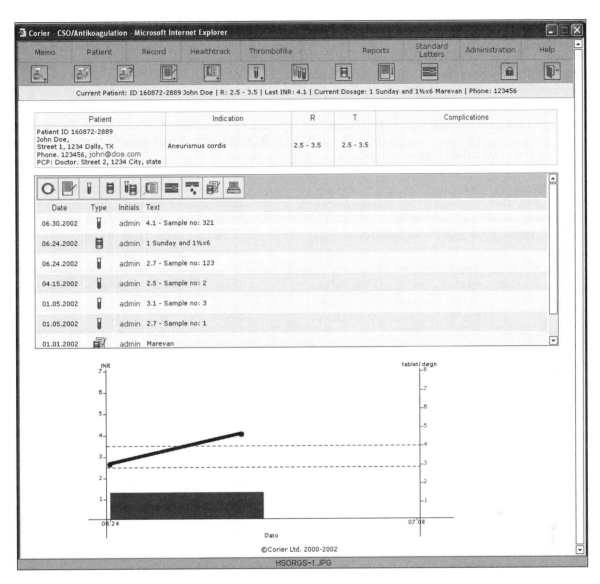

Figure 9–18 This screen shows lab results and prescribed dosage from Clinical System Organizer™ - AntiCoagulation CSO™ AC (Health System Organizer). The graph at the bottom shows INR progression and dose. On the y-axis are INR values and the solid line shows the development of the INR over time (x-axis). The y-axis on the right shows number of tablets/day. The bar shows how many tablets/day the patient received over time. Courtesy of IntraMed A/S, Denmark.

- support of local procedures for medication plans
- documentation of a health journal for patients, including test results, notes, etc.
- algorithm for diagnosis or thrombophilia
- different reports defined locally, eg, on quality aspects
- different letters automatically printed to the patient

Intelligent Dosing System™ (IDS™)

The Intelligent Dosing System™ (IDS™) is a computerized decision support system that calculates the best next dose to titrate a patient on a single drug, or combination of drugs, to achieve an optimal response. The IDS™ has an anticoagulation suite of programs for dosing both daily and weekly warfarin as well as heparin sodium. It is also able to dose insulin, immunosuppressants, multi-agent chemotherapeutic agents, and parenteral antibiotics.

Utilizing proprietary dose-response technology, the IDS™ draws a correlation between the patient's previous dose and response, the current dose and response, and a desired response to provide the next dose required to achieve the desired surrogate marker.

The IDS™ software suite contains three applications, a dose calculator (DoseRx™), a therapeutic interchange system to safely switch between agents (InterchangeRx™), and a graded simulation to practice and learn the dose and response of a new or seldom-used drug (Practice PrescribeRx™). Readily available data (previous dose-response, current dose-response, and the desired response marker) are entered into a hand-held PDA device (Palm, Win CE) or a PC and the dose required is calculated.

PARMA, Instrumentation Laboratory Spa

In the early 1980s, the Thrombosis Center of the General Hospital of Parma (Italy) developed a program for the archiving, reporting, and monitoring of anticoagulated patients (*Programma per l'Archivazione Refertazione Monitoraggio Anticoagulati*, namely PARMA), in collaboration with Ortho-Clinical Diagnostics Inc. (Milan, Italy). Currently, approximately 200 clinics use PARMA in Italy to monitor approximately 100,000 anticoagulated patients. PARMA is currently marketed by Instrumentation Laboratory Spa (Milan, Italy).

The PARMA system features a comprehensive set of patient management functions, including

- patient administrative data management
- scheduling of patient appointments

- integrated support for the coagulation analysis workflow: patient reception, blood sample labeling, preparation of laboratory work lists, online and offline laboratory data acquisition, etc.
- patient's clinical history: diagnoses, risk factors, concurrent diseases and medication, drug interactions, complications, other relevant clinical data, etc.
- built-in therapeutic decision support system for physicians
- printing of therapeutic reports for patients, including medication and dosage instructions
- analytical, therapeutic, and clinical quality control tools
- predetermined and user-defined queries and statistics over the consolidated patient database, especially useful in support of clinical studies
- data confidentiality through the use of access control lists for different user profiles

See Figures 9–19 through 9–21.

PARMA can be deployed in a variety of configurations, ranging from the one-workstation setup to a distributed configuration supporting a reception station and several clinical stations. In the latter case, the stations share a common patient database through the clinic's local area network. The PARMA system is discussed in depth by Mariani et al.[44]

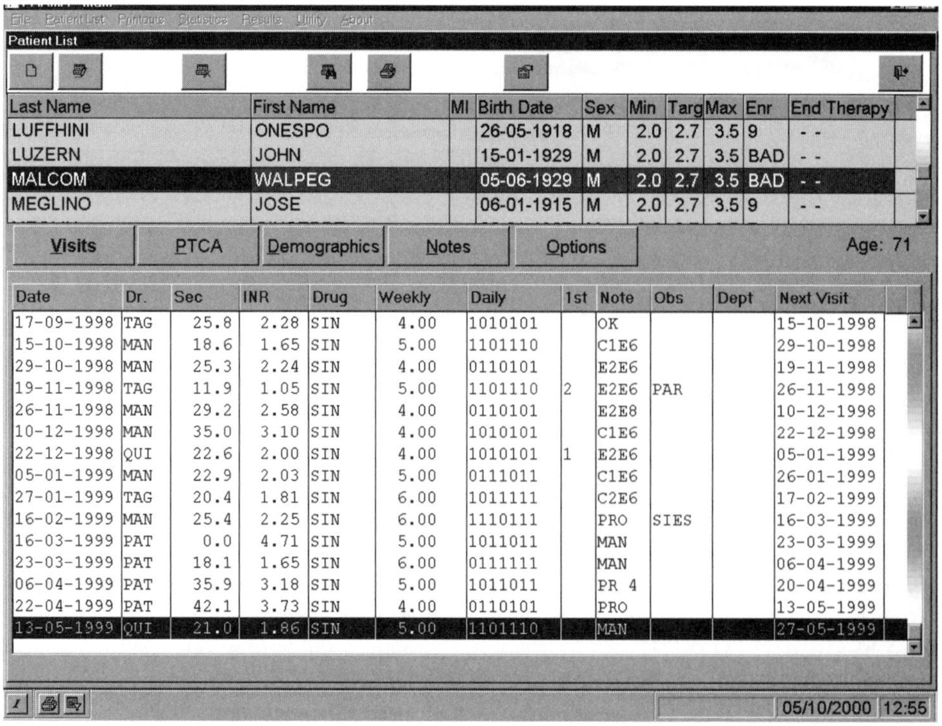

Figure 9–19 PARMA main screen, showing the clinic's patient list and, for the highlighted patient, a summary of the most recent INR controls. Courtesy of Instrumentation Laboratory Spa, Milan, Italy.

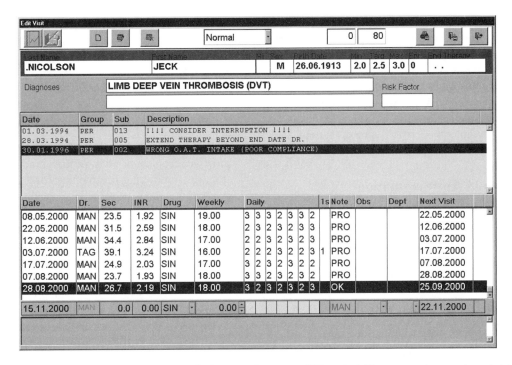

Figure 9–20 PARMA screen used to adjust the patient's therapy after a new INR control. The screen shows relevant data, including the patient's demographics, diagnoses, risk factors, past clinical events, and most recent INR controls. Once the INR value is automatically read or manually typed in, PARMA displays the dosage pattern recommendation in the bottom row, which must then be confirmed or overridden by the physician. Courtesy of Instrumentation Laboratory Spa, Milan, Italy.

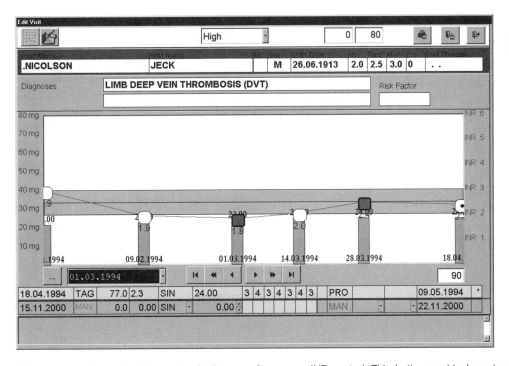

Figure 9–21 PARMA screen used to adjust the patient's therapy after a new INR control. This is the graphical version of the therapy prescription screen shown in Figure 9–20. Courtesy of Instrumentation Laboratory Spa, Milan, Italy.

PARMA employs an algorithm for dosing warfarin, acenocoumarol, and other anticoagulation therapies. Based on both logical rules and mathematical models, and under a set of conditions met in more than 90% of patient controls, PARMA suggests a dosage pattern and the date for the next control. Doctors may then confirm or override this recommendation as deemed appropriate.

The PARMA therapeutic decision support system has been validated in clinical investigations.[34,36–37,46–47]

RAID-Pro (Rapid Anticoagulation Interpretation and Dosing), HiruMed Ltd.

What is now RAID-Pro was first conceived in 1996 to provide a standardized, but flexible, computerized management system for oral anticoagulation. Initial development work was achieved primarily in the United Kingdom as a collaborative effort between HiruMed, Ltd., and Organon Teknika (UK) Ltd. but now BioMérieux (UK) Ltd. A comparative analysis was undertaken, and the Hilling-dose algorithm[48] was selected as the default dosing calculation for RAID-Pro. Clinicians worked closely with the prototype software development team, and as a result, further clinical requirements and recommendations were incorporated.

The RAID-Pro software exceeds the British Society of Haematology recommendations for minimal requirements for anticoagulation software as published in 1998.[49] The

software was influential in the formulation of the European guidelines for anticoagulant software by the European Network on Anticoagulant Treatment.

The software is divided into modules to enhance flexibility. Each module provides a discrete functionality, and all modules work together to form a comprehensive system. These modules are

1. *System Manager Module*—Defines items such as choice of anticoagulants used, primary and secondary diagnoses, interfering or noninterfering drugs, and treatment outcomes or risks. The backbone of the dosing and scheduling logic is defined in this module. The user defines a variety of tables that are used to establish the complete patient record and audit trail. The current version of the software supports 100 user-definable algorithms and induction protocols. This unique feature enables a health care professional to adapt patient therapy for factors such as diagnosis, age, and the analytical method used to determine the INR.
2. *Patient Administration Module*—Patient records are created and updated within this module. Calculated doses and appointment dates can be modified by a qualified user (via password level), and changes made to the patient file remain part of the permanent audit trail. Up to 24 previous visits can be displayed for any given patient, and archived results are readily accessible. Figure 9–22 shows a dosing screen display. The

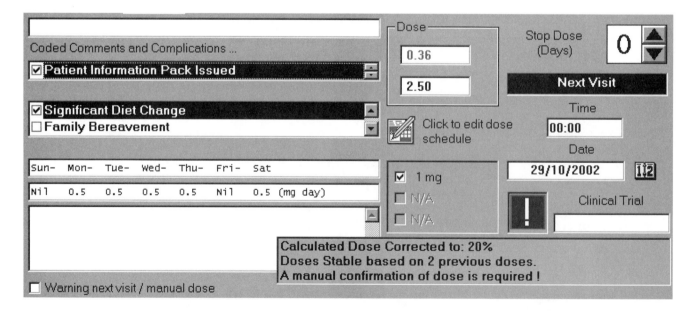

Figure 9–22 A dosing screen display for RAID-Pro. In this example, the dosing schedule is based on an average daily deliverable dose of 10.5 mg. The patient dosing instructions are user definable. The dose or date of next visit may be modified by designated users. Courtesy of RAID-Pro, HiruMed Ltd., Wiltshire, England.

software has been updated to store the additional parameters of height, weight, temperature, blood pressure, and cost center to meet requirements of billing in the US market.

3. *Database Search Module*—This is one of the most powerful modules of the system. It allows the clinician to obtain rapid statistical reports that provide useful information about the analytical or control system being used within RAID-Pro. Statistical ad hoc reports are available. The user can also specify and search on almost any field that has been entered into the patient database. Reports, letters, or export files can be generated from these searches (Figure 9–23).

4. *System Utility Module*—This module allows the user to perform various housekeeping duties and to monitor the PC system—for example, to recover from unexpected power failures or spikes.

The RAID-Pro system has several other features to add flexibility and ease of local customization. Access to the software modules can be controlled and dose authorization restricted. Audit logs are provided to track operator system activity and patient record interactions.

All of the system modules, including patient administration, system manager, induction, and the report template editor, are included in a user license. The database has, for practical purposes, an unlimited capacity. The space occupied by active patient records is reclaimed when the "episode" is closed; thus there is no requirement to purchase additional database capacity when, over time, the fixed time is exceeded. Closed episodes are transferred to an archive database that may reside on any searchable media such as a hard drive or CD-ROM. The software may be used "stand alone" or in a multiple user configuration.

The company recommends the designation of a clinical software manager, part of whose responsibility would be to initially customize the system to reflect local practice and dosing regimens. It is suggested that this individual be integrally involved with the ongoing utilizing of the RAID-Pro software within the institution or facility.

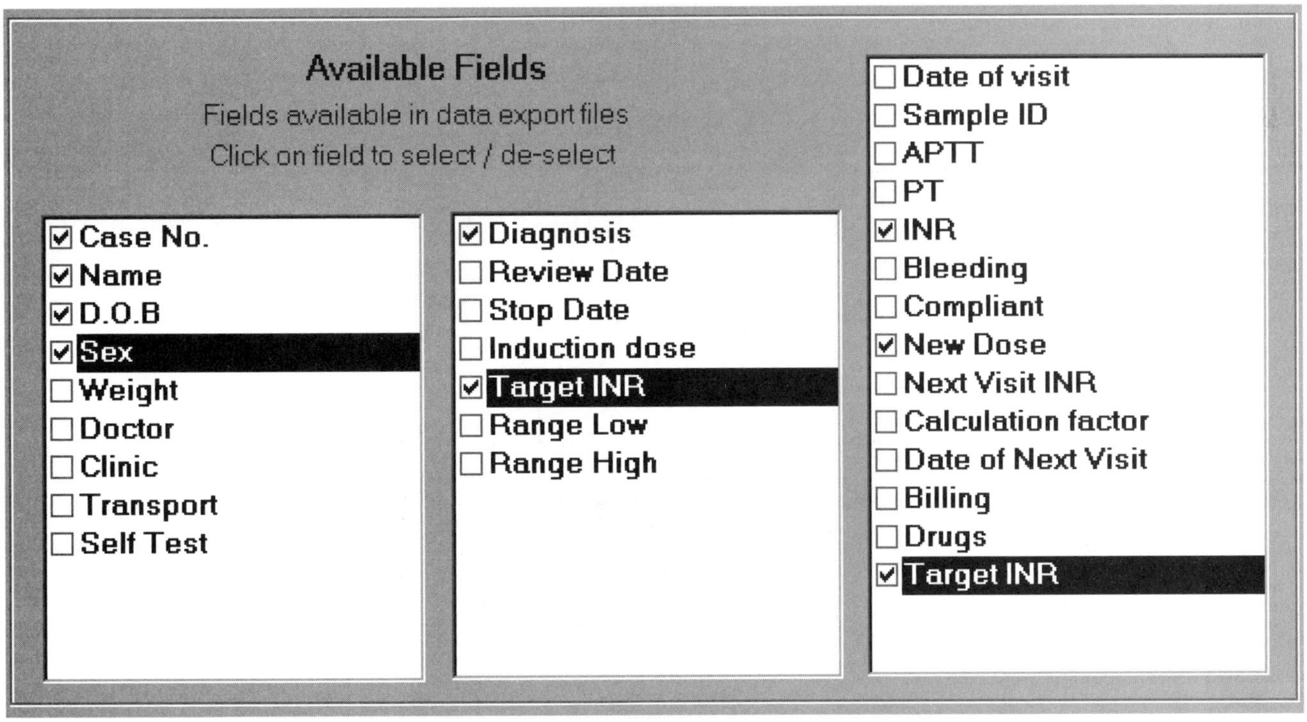

Figure 9–23 A screen display illustrating available fields to select in a user-defined database search for RAID-Pro. Courtesy of RAID-Pro, HiruMed Ltd, Wiltshire, England.

Table 9–2 At-a-Glance Reference Table of Software Products

Software Product	Vendor/Contact Information	Web Address/ E-mail	Requirements/ Interfacing Capability	Features				
				Computerized Dosing	Form Letters	Reports	Quality Assurance Capabilities	Patient Tracking
ANTHEMA (ANticoagulation THErapy Management), easyTAO, homeTAO	e-MedicalMonitor Pau Planas, CEO e-MedicalMonitorS.L. Can Malé, Lliçá d'Amunt 08186 Spain www.e-	medicalmonitor.com info@e-medicalmonitor.com	• Web-based system, requires a PC with Internet access • Supplied used an Application Service Provider (ASP) regimen. (Takes PARMA functionality to the Web)	Yes	Yes	Yes	Yes	Yes
Anticoagulation Management Program (AMP)	Telehealth Systems, Inc. Gerald H. Roesener, RPh 520 N. State Road 135, Suite M78 Greenwood, IN 46142 877-490-6161	groesener-telehealth@ worldnet.att.net www.telehlthsys.com	• NT server or stand-alone NT Workstation (This is a PC-based automated telephony patient follow-up system.)	No	No	Yes	Yes	Yes
Clever Clog	Clever Clog: Dr. M.A. Bradley Mr. J.W. Bradley 15 Rychill Ave. Brookside Chesterfield Derbyshire England 540 3PD	www.clevclog.freeserve. co.uk jwbradley@clevclog. freeserve.co.uk	• Produced for use on a typical PC with Windows 98 and is Windows 3.1 and upwards compatible • Uses less than 1Mb hard drive space • Can network a number of computers served by a central mainframe	Yes	Yes	Yes	Yes	Yes
CoagCare® Management System	ZyCare®, Inc. 3804 Sweeten Creek Road Chapel Hill, NC 27514 919-419-7228	www.zycane.com info@zycare.com	• PC with Microsoft Windows™ and Microsoft Explorer™, version 5.5 or higher with Internet access • Can work with any home Prothrombin Time monitor	Yes	Yes Web based	Yes	Yes	Yes
CoagClinic	Standing Stone, Inc. 191 Post Road West Westport, CT 06880 800-648-9877	www.standingstoneinc.com info@standingstoneinc.com	• PC with Microsoft Internet Explorer (Version 5.0 and above) and Internet access • Standalone network version also available—requires Windows 2000 server • HL7 mapping • Open architecture—ODBC access	Yes	Yes	Yes	Yes	Yes
CoumaCare® Patient Management System (v5.1a)	Bristol-Myers Squibb Pharmaceuticals P.O. Box 4500 Princeton, NJ 08543-4500 800-328-7709	www.coumacare.com	• Win 95 or 98, or Windows NT 3.51/4.x • CoumaCare® v5.1a is designed for a local area network (LAN) • Will run on Novell 3.1x and 4.x or a Windows NT 3.51 and 4.x LAN for up to seven concurrent users • CoumaCare® will not run on UNIX or Macintosh systems	No	Yes	Yes	Yes	Yes

Software Product	On Line Clinical Resources	Costs	Technical Support	Clinical Experiences	Published Reports	Future Plans and Development
ANTHEMA	No	Not available at present	Yes	Pilot test starting in 2002/Q3 Computerized dosing already validated by PARMA	No	Deployment in Italy, Spain and USA On line clinical resources via Web
Anticoagulation Management Program	No	Telehealth Suite: $25,000 single user license, additional charges as applicable	Yes On-site installation and training, annual software maintenance at a fee	Installed at one large cardiology site (2,500 patients), other sites planned, no data available yet specific to anticoagulation, but data available from other health programs (congestive heart failure, women's health)	No	Target selected patient groups such as those who self-test and self-manage
Clever Clog	Yes	Cost is currently £170 (UK Sterling) for a practice Price negotiated for larger practices	Free technical support available by e-mail during first year of use	The software has been well established in the UK for approximately 4 years. Audit of centers using Clever Clog indicates that it is effective in providing a high quality of control.	No	Future enhancements for patient self-testing and self-management protocols
CoagCare® Management System	Yes	To be determined.	Yes, for patients and care providers.	Currently have 60 patients enrolled in a clinical trial at Duke University Medical Center. The project is supported by a Small Business Innovation and Research (SBIR) grant to ZyCare® from the National Heart, Lung, and Blood Institute, a division of National Institute of Health (NIH)	Clinical trial in progress and seek additional sites	Commercial introduction of the CoagCare® System in 2003
CoagClinic	Yes	Web version is $2.00 per patient per month or can be included with point of care supplies cost. Stand-alone version is $25,000.	Telephone support 8 AM EST to 4 PM PST E-mail support Online help files Users manuals	50+ users, nearly 10,000 patients with over 50,000 visits recorded.	Yes	Quarterly upgrade cycle based on user input
CoumaCare® Patient Management System (for Windows 5.1a)	http://www.coumacare.com	No cost to customers	Live support available weekdays 8 AM–8 PM by calling 800-327-7709	In use at 4,000 sites in the US	Phase IV study ACTION® Patient registry (Anticoagulation Consortium To Improve Outcomes Nationally) in data analysis phase	

continues

Table 9–2 continued

Software Product	Vendor/Contact Information	Web Address/ E-mail	Requirements/ Interfacing Capability	Features				
				Computerized Dosing	Form Letters	Reports	Quality Assurance Capabilities	Patient Tracking
DAWN AC Anticoagulation Therapy Software v 6.03	4S Information Systems Ltd. 4 The Square, Milnthorpe, Cumbria La7 7QJ United Kingdom 011-44-15395-63091	www.4s-dawn.com sales@4s-dawn.com	• Windows 3.1 or higher • Operates on standalone workstation or on server • Modest hardware specifications • Interfacing capabilities	Yes	Yes	Yes	Yes	Yes
DoseResponse®	Keystone Therapeutics, Inc. 2736 Bingham Drive Pittsburgh, PA 15241 Mark Hudson Vice President of Sales 1-800-633-8642	www.doseresponse.com mhudson@doseresponse. com	• Operating system: any capable of running an Internet browser • Network connection: 28K+ modem, ISDN, DSL, or cable modem • Web browser: any supporting SSL and 128 bit encryption, (successfully tested with IE 5+, Netscape 4.7+, etc.) • Printer: networked or direct connection	Yes	Yes	Yes	Yes	Yes
DrugCalc	Therapeutic Technologies Dennis Mungall, PharmD	www.clinpharmacologist. bigstep.com TherTch@aol.com	• Windows 3.1 or above • Internet access for download	Yes	No	Yes	No	No
Health System Organizer™ for Oral Anticoagulation Treatment	IntraMed A/S Research and Development Manager: Jesper Leck Managing Director: Birgitte Christoffersen IntraMed A/s Naverland 31, DK-2600 Glostrup Denmark +45 70 22 62 60 **US Sales and Technical Support:** Dave F. Varnell, Director Corier Ltd. 3225 Louis Drive Plano, Texas 75023 972-618-3107	intramed@intramed.dk dfv.corier.com	• Windows 95 or higher, with Internet access using Internet Explorer 5.0 or higher • The system is developed in Java2EE browser-based technology and has user interfaces for the patient, general practitioner (GP), homecare, outpatient clinic, and other hospital departments	Yes	Yes	Yes	Yes	Yes
Intelligent Dosing System (IDS)	Jason Powers 248-321-0971	Info@RxFiles.net Jpowers@RxFiles.net	• Windows 95 or higher • Interface with hand-held PDA device and PC	Yes				
PARMA™	Instrumentation Laboratory Spa (Milan, Italy) Lourdes Nuñez, PhD, e-Medical Monitor S.L. Can Malé, Lliça d'Amunt 08186 Spain	lnunez@ilww.com	• WIN95/98 • Pentium PC 100Gig • Will run in a LAN environment	Yes	Yes	Yes	Yes	Yes
Raid-Pro™ (Rapid Anticoagulation Interpretation and Dosing)	HiruMed Ltd 1 Jubilee Estate Purton Swinton Wiltshire SN5 4EU England Tel: 01793 772786 Fax: 01793 772831	mail@hirmued.co.uk	• Windows 95/98/NT 4.0 • 486 or higher • 32 MB RAM • 20 MG free hard disk space • VGA video monitor	Yes	Yes	Yes	Yes	Yes

Software Product	On Line Clinical Resources	Costs	Technical Support	Clinical Experiences	Published Reports	Future Plans and Development
DAWN AC Anticoagulation Therapy Software v 6.03	Yes	Sliding scale for pricing is available. Some examples: DAWN AC Practitioner—starting at $758 and up depending on # of patients and other variables. DAWN AC Enterprise—starting at $2,850 and up.	Support by telephone, e-mail and fax Classroom training on site or remote can be provided Computer-based training E-books utilized	200+ sites worldwide Offers eight modules, depending on needs Currently involved in 6 clinical trials in Europe, USA, and Canada	Clinically validated, see references #31, 35 Other trials underway	Search and testing on mobile palm top versions, integrating with the Web, and integrating with other software underway
DoseResponse®	Yes	"Per patient per month" and "per INR test" pricing quotes are available by specific request	Yes, includes free transfer of data from existing CoumaCare® program	In use for almost two (2) years, can be configured to a variety of clinical settings, supports single location as well as multiple locations in both office and clinic settings that manage hundreds of patients	In progress	Immediate product development plans include the addition of monitoring programs for low molecular weight heparin and lipid management
DrugCalc	Limited	Free download from Web-site	Not available	200+ sites using DrugCalc	Modeling approach validated in several studies, see references 23, 39–42, 43	Palm version in development
Health System Organizer™ for Oral Anticoagulation Treatment	Yes	$26,000 US as a startup cost, includes server and education Price per patient per year $17 US Prices subject to change	Yes, support available in native language of user via user manuals, e-mail, phone, fax, Web-site	The system is installed in University of Southern Denmark and Vejle County Central Hospital in the outpatient clinic	Yes, see reference 43	Installation with English version in US available September 2002
Intelligent Dosing System		Not available		A precursor has 10 years clinical experience in immunosuppressant therapy	In progress	Multiple drug regimens for specific disease states
PARMA™	Common drug interactions	Not available	Yes	Installed and operating at approximately 200 sites in Italy, monitoring over 100,000 patients	See references 34, 36–37, 46–47	Improvements in several functional areas
RAID-Pro™ (Rapid Anticoagulation Interpretation and Dosing)	ACCP guidelines or British Society of Haematology guidelines as defaults	Pricing dependent on system design Not available in US	To be handled with the existing HiruMed technical support structure	Multiple installations in UK and Ireland with several sites having an active database in excess of 2,500 patients References available by contacting company	Pending	Release of version 1.0.7 and automated dosing server for Fall 2002

REFERENCES

1. Holford NHG. Clinical pharmacokinetics and pharmacodynamics of warfarin: understanding the dose-effect relationship. *Clin Pharmacokinet.* 1986;11:483–504.

2. Nagashima RA, O'Reilly RA, Levy G. Kinetics of pharmacologic effects in man: the anticoagulant action of warfarin. *Clin Pharm Ther.* 1969;10:22–35.

3. Sheiner LB. Computer-aided long-term anticoagulation therapy. *Comput Biomed Res.* 1969;2:507–518.

4. Theophanis TG, Smolen VF. Multiple-dose kinetics of pharmacologic effects of indirect anticoagulants. *J Pharm Sci.* 1972;61:980–982.

5. Theophanis TG, Barile RG. Multiple-dose kinetics of oral anticoagulants: methods of analysis and optimized dosing. *J Pharm Sci.* 1973; 62:261–266.

6. Sawyer WT, Fin AL. Digital computer-assisted warfarin therapy: comparison of two methods. *Comput Biomed Res.* 1979;12:221–231.

7. Barr W. Computer aided anticoagulation. Presented at American Society of Hospital Pharmacists Institute on Advanced Pharmacokinetics; 1975; Lexington, KY.

8. Hoffer EP, Marble KD, Yurchak PM, Barnett GO. A computer-based information system for managing patients on long term oral anticoagulants. *Comput Biomed Res.* 1975;8:573–579.

9. Powers WF, Abbrecht PH, Covell DG. Systems and microcomputer approach to anticoagulant therapy. *IEEE Trans Biomed Eng.* 1980; 27:520–522.

10. O'Leary TJ, Abbrecht PH. Predicting oral anticoagulant response using a pharmacodynamic model. *Ann Biomed Eng.* 1981;9:199–216.

11. Abbrecht PH, O'Leary TJ, Behrendt DM. Evaluation of a computer-assisted method for individualized anticoagulation: retrospective and prospective studies with a pharmacodynamic model. *Clin Pharm Ther.* 1982;32:129–136.

12. Wilson R, James AH. Computer assisted management of warfarin treatment. *Br Med J.* 1984;289:422–424.

13. Mungall DR, Ludden TM, Marshall J, Hawkins DW, Talbert RL, Crawford MH. Population pharmacokinetics of racemic warfarin in adult patients. *J Pharmacokinet Biopharm.* 1985;13:213–227.

14. Svec JM, Mungall DR, Ludden TM. Bayesian pharmacokinetic/pharmacodynamic forecasting of prothrombin response to warfarin therapy: preliminary evaluation. *Ther Drug Monit.* 1985;7:174–180.

15. Hong R, Murray W, Daschback M, Venook A, White RH, Mungall DR. Computer assisted warfarin therapy. *AAMSI Congress.* 1985;3: 310–314.

16. Lee C, Coleman R, Mungall DR. Effect of using warfarin concentration in bayesian forecasting of prothrombin time response. *Clin Pharm.* 1987;6:406–412.

17. Farrow L, Mungall DR, Raskob G, Hull R. Predicting the daily prothrombin time response to warfarin. *Ther Drug Monit.* 1990; 12:246–249.

18. Lubetsky A, Seligsohm U, Ezra D, Halkin H. The effect of the plasma levels of C and S on the prediction of warfarin maintenance dose requirements. *Clin Pharm Ther.* 1992;52:42–49.

19. Weiss P, Halkin H, Shlomo A. The negative impact of biological variation in the effect and clearance of warfarin on methods for prediction of dose requirements. *Thromb Haemost.* 1986;56: 371–375.

20. Boyle DA, Ludden TM, Carter BL, Becker A, Taylor J. Evaluation of a bayesian regression program for warfarin. *Drug Intell Clin Pharm.* 1986;20:465.

21. Sun J, Chang MW. Initialization of warfarin dosages using computer modeling. *Arch Phys Med Rehabil.* 1995;76:453–456.

22. White RH, Hong R, Venook A, Dashbach M, Murray W, Mungall DR. Initiation of warfarin therapy: comparison of physician dosing with computer assisted dosing. *J Gen Intern Med.* 1987;2:141–148.

23. White RH, Mungall DR. Outpatient management of warfarin therapy: comparison of computer predicted dosage adjustment to skilled professional care. *Ther Drug Monit.* 1991;13:46–50.

24. Carter BL, Barr W, Rock W, Taylor JW. Warfarin dosage predictions assisted by the analog computer. *Ther Drug Monit.* 1988;10:69–73.

25. Ryan PJ, Gilbert M, Rose PK. Computer control of anticoagulant dose for therapeutic management. *BMJ.* 1989;299:1207–1209.

26. Casimiro J, Mungall D. Patient oriented, technology based anticoagulation clinic. *Physicians and Computers.* 1998;2:36–39.

27. Poller L, Wright D, Rowlands M. Prospective comparative study of computer programs used for management of warfarin. *J Clin Pathol.* 1993;46:299–303.

28. Margolis A, Flores F, Kierszenbaum M, et al. Warfarin 2.0—a computer program for warfarin management: design and clinical use. *Proc Annu Symp Comput Appl Med Care.* 1994;846–850.

29. Fihn SD, McDonell MB, Vermes D, et al. A computerized intervention to improve timing of outpatient follow-up: a multicenter randomized trial in patients treated with warfarin. *J Gen Intern Med.* 1994;9:131–139.

30. Vadher B, Patterson DL, Leaning M. Evaluation of a decision support system for initiation and control of oral anticoagulation in a randomised trial. *Br Med J.* 1997;314:1252–1256.

31. Poller L, Schiach CR, MacCallum PK, et al. Multicentre randomized study of computerised anticoagulant dosage. *Lancet.* 1998; 352:1505–1509.

32. Fitzmaurice DA, Hobbs FD, Murray ET. Primary care anticoagulant clinic management using computerized decision support and near patient International Normalized Ratio (INR) testing: routine data from a practice nurse-led clinic. *Fam Pract.* 1998;15:144–146.

33. Chatellier G, Colombet I, Degoulet P. An overview of the effect of computer-assisted management of anticoagulant therapy on the quality of anticoagulation. *Int J Med Inf.* 1998;49:311–320.

34. Manotti C, Moia M, Palareti G, Pengo V, Ria L, Dettori AG. Effect of computer-aided management on the quality of treatment in anticoagulated patients: a prospective, randomized, multicenter trial of APROAT (Automated PRogram for Oral Anticoagulant Treatment). *Haematol.* 2001;86:1060–1070.

35. Ageno W, Turpie AGG. A randomized comparison of a computer-based dosing program with a manual system to monitor oral anticoagulant therapy. *Thromb Thrombolysis.* 1998;5:S69.

36. Manotti C, Guazzaloca G, et al. Prospective study on the prescription of the oral anticoagulant therapy (OAT): use of a computerized program. The APROAT Study (Automatic Prescription of Oral Anticoagulant Therapy) Part I—Stabilization Phase. *Thromb Res.* 1998;91(suppl 1):S84.

37. Manotti C, Quintavalla R, Pattacini D, Tagliaferri A, Pini M. Evaluation of a computer-assisted dosage prediction method for oral anticoagulant therapy. *Thromb Haemost.* 1997;(suppl):699.

38. Dalen JE, Hirsh J, et al. Oral anticoagulants: mechanism of action, clinical effectiveness, and optimal therapeutic range. *Chest.* 2001;119 (suppl):8S–21S.

39. Mungall DR, Raskob G, Rosenbloom D, Ludden T, Hull R. Pharmacokinetics and dynamics of heparin in patients with proximal vein thrombosis. *J Clin Pharmacol.* 1989;29:896–900.

40. Mungall DR, Floyd R. Bayesian forecasting of APTT response to continuously infused heparin with and without warfarin administration. *J Clin Pharmacol.* 1989;29:1043–1047.

41. Kershaw B, White RH, Mungall DR, Van Houten J, Brettfeld S. Computer-assisted dosing of heparin: management with a pharmacy based anticoagulation service. *Arch Intern Med.* 1994;134:1005–1011.

42. Mungall DR, Anbe D, Forrester PL, et al. A prospective randomized comparison of the accuracy of computer-assisted versus GUSTO nomogram directed heparin therapy. *Clin Pharmacol Ther.* 1994;55:591–596.

43. Mungall D, Lord M, Cason S, et al. Developing a system to improve the quality of heparin therapy in patients with acute coronary syndromes. *Am J Cardio.* 1998;82:574–579.

44. Lassen JF, Brandslund I. Antonsen S. International normalized ratio for prothrombin times in patients taking oral anticoagulants: critical difference and probability of significant change in consecutive measurements. *Clin Chem.* 1995;41(3):444–447.

45. Mariani G, Manotti C, Dettori AG. A computerized regulation of dosage in oral anticoagulant therapy. *Ricerca Clinica Laboratorio.* 1990;20:119–125.

46. Ghirarduzzi A, Ioro A, et al. Different management of oral anticoagulant therapy; a prospective cohort study. *Thromb Res.* 1998;91(suppl 1): S70.

47. Manotti C, Guazzaloca G, et al. Prospective study on the prescription of the oral anticoagulant therapy (OAT): use of a computerized program. The APROAT Study (Automatic Prescription of Oral Anticoagulant Therapy) Part 2—Stabilized Phase. *Thromb Res.* 1998;91(suppl 1):S84–85.

48. Wilson R, James AH. Computer assisted management of warfarin therapy. *Br Med J.* 1984;289:422–424.

49. Guidelines on anticoagulation, 3rd ed. *Br J Haematol.* 1998;101:374–387.

Chapter 10

Education Curriculum for Patients and Teaching Methods

Lynn B. Oertel

INTRODUCTION

The diverse clinical indications for which warfarin is prescribed encompass a broad patient population whose educational needs are varied and complex. A careful, individualized assessment of patient needs, therefore, helps in tailoring the educational process to optimize clinical outcome and to facilitate adherence. Anticoagulation management services are particularly adept at responding to the vast educational needs of patients.

Varied educational levels, literacy skills, native language, and cognitive function each play a part in patients' interpretation and integration of the knowledge provided by health care professionals. Diverse backgrounds, life experiences, and perceptions of their health status affect the ability of patients to understand their therapies. Family, employment, and society also have an important impact. It is vital to assess all of these issues if an educational program is to succeed. Health educators who make themselves aware of such issues are able to focus educational interventions properly and thus provide constructive and realistic teaching sessions.

THE EDUCATIONAL PROCESS

The goal of patient education is to provide knowledge of a disease process and its treatment in order to foster adherence to the prescribed regimen and to promote self-care. Educational needs can change over the course of therapy, particularly in patients who require lifelong anticoagulation therapy. Health care providers must educate patients on

health maintenance and disease prevention. Many indications for chronic anticoagulation are preventive in nature, and patients must be educated on the benefits of preventive regimens.

A detailed review of specific adult learning theories and their application to patient education is not included in this chapter because the theories are available from many sources.[1-4] It is important, however, to recognize the influence of these principles on health education today. Educators in anticoagulation therapy must possess advanced knowledge about drugs, monitoring, and patient management issues and safety. They should develop skills in applying principles of adult education to their teaching efforts. Educators must possess the necessary skills and characteristics that are deemed important from the patient's point of view. A list of such characteristics obtained from patient interviews is presented in Exhibit 10–1. Effective education can be provided by physicians, nurses, pharmacists, social workers, and other professionals in the health care field. The multidisciplinary approach frequently used in anticoagulation management encourages each discipline to make valuable contributions to the overall educational process.

Factors Affecting the Educational Process

Illiteracy

The educational process must be conducted in a manner and level appropriate to a patient's expectations, knowledge, and ability to comprehend. The literature indicates that 20%

Exhibit 10–1
CHARACTERISTICS OF THE EXCELLENT HEALTH EDUCATOR

- CONFIDENCE
  - selects what to teach
  - alleviates the patient's anxiety
  - provides appropriate learning environment
  - prepares appropriate teaching plan and material
- COMPETENCE
  - decides what is important to teach
  - ensures the patient's safety
  - provides individualized written instructions
  - teaches home management of special problems

- COMMUNICATION
  - gives clear directions
  - uses simple pictures or models
  - speaks the patient's language
- CARING
  - has empathy
  - recognizes patient concerns
  - provides encouragement
  - ensures adequate time
  - demonstrates sensitivity to patient's mood

Source: Reprinted with permission from SH Rankin and KD Stallings, *Patient Education—Issues, Principles, Practices*, 3rd ed, p 149, © 1996, Lippincott-Raven Publishers.

of Americans lack the necessary literacy skills to benefit from even the simplest handouts or videotaped programs.[4]

Williams et al[5] report on the proportion of patients lacking the basic literacy skills necessary to function in the health care environment. More than 40% of patients with English as their native language tested at two urban public hospitals were unable to understand the directions provided for taking medications safely, and 25% were unable to assimilate information presented to them for scheduling future appointments. The results of this study suggest that patient educational materials are too often written at a reading level higher than most patients can comprehend.

Reading comprehension levels of patients and reading materials were examined in a study by Davis et al.[6] On average, patient reading levels were far below the comprehension level required to read patient education materials in current use at the clinics involved in the study. Of the 150 pieces analyzed, only 6% were written below a ninth-grade level, whereas average patient reading comprehension was at the fifth- to sixth-grade level. There appears to be a striking discrepancy between the average reading comprehension of patients and that required for them to benefit from educational materials designed for their use that are commonly found in physician offices and hospitals.

Teaching patients who possess poor literacy skills presents unique challenges, but the guidelines listed in Exhibit 10–2 can help in restructuring existing methods and materials to improve patient education.

Cognitive, Functional, or Physical Impairments

Some patients present to the office or anticoagulation clinic with cognitive or processing impairments that impose additional challenges on the learning process. A stroke or major surgery can lead to further functional impairments that create special needs. Physical limitations can hamper pa-

tients in opening pill bottles or splitting pills for dose adjustments. Hip or knee surgery can impose limitations in mobility and access to laboratories for blood tests. The learning needs of the elderly require special consideration because many patients on anticoagulation therapy are beyond age 60. Methodologies are needed to address potential sensory deficits, intellectual abilities, and short-term memory deficits. The inclusion of a responsible family member or close friend in the educational session is important to provide support for the patient and reinforcement of information in such instances.

Patient Readiness To Learn

Patients usually begin their courses of warfarin therapy in the hospital, and this is the first opportunity for patient teaching to take place. The detail and amount of education that occurs and the amount of information that the patient retains, however, are usually insufficient. The ability for hospital nurses to plan and provide quality education pertaining to anticoagulation is hampered by shorter lengths of hospital stay and increased patient acuity. Reiley and colleagues[7] compared the predictions of nurses with patient reports of their functional status two months following discharge and found that nurses consistently underestimated the functional ability of their patients. These data have implications for community-based nurses in that an assessment of learning needs must be ongoing to fill knowledge voids or to correct misunderstandings. The time immediately following hospital discharge is a unique transition period when patients adjust to their illness and regain control over health care decisions. Anticoagulation clinics can achieve their educational goals at this time by providing in-depth education when the patient is most ready to learn.

Even during the immediate posthospitalization period, however, anxiety pertaining to recent surgery, diagnoses,

Exhibit 10–2
GUIDELINES FOR TEACHING PATIENTS WITH LOW LITERACY SKILLS

- Focus information on the core of knowledge and skills that patients need to survive and to cope with problems.
- Teach the smallest amount of information possible.
- Make the point vivid. Put important information either first or last.

- Sequence information logically, for example, step by step (1, 2, 3), chronological (a timeline), or topical (use of three or four main topics).
- Ask the patient to restate and demonstrate.
- Review.

Source: Reprinted with permission from SH Rankin and KD Stallings, *Patient Education—Issues, Principles, Practices,* 3rd ed, p 192, © 1996, Lippincott-Raven Publishers.

new medications, and other factors can overwhelm a patient's ability to integrate new information. Varied strategies or techniques might be necessary to instruct patients about warfarin therapy. Appropriately written educational materials are useful as reinforcements. With some patients, follow-up telephone calls offer providers the opportunity to assess the accuracy of their knowledge and provide the opportunity for patients to ask additional questions that have arisen. Collaboration and communication among all members of the health care team, including local pharmacists, community and home health nurses, and physicians, are particularly important in providing quality care, effecting patient adherence, and reinforcing new knowledge.

EDUCATION AND COMPLIANCE ISSUES

Rates of nonadherence to medication regimens range from 30% to 70% and can be even more problematic for preventive treatment, which requires a long duration,[8,9] or for treatment of the elderly, who take greater numbers of medications.[10,11] In the studies cited, knowledge of prescription drugs was found to be inversely related to the number of medical problems and the number of prescribed medications. Higher rates of medication errors in patients with poor knowledge of their drugs also are described by others.[12] Reports such as these emphasize the need for improving strategies for health teaching so that patients have greater knowledge of their prescribed medications.

When assessing how a warfarin regimen impacts a patient's perception of health and wellness, it is helpful to "put oneself in the patient's shoes." Health care providers should listen to what patients value most. Restriction of contact sports might be necessary for patient safety, but allowing recreational bike riding with appropriate safety gear could be a reasonable compromise. How clinicians interact with patients can significantly affect patient intentions to comply. Incorporating an assessment of lifestyle, risk factors, and current health behaviors into the educational process can improve teaching strategies. The success or failure of the teaching process is further

impacted by the patient's attitudes, beliefs, and perceptions about the treatment plan.[13]

Compliance with the therapeutic regimen pertaining to oral anticoagulation requires two specific behaviors: (1) dose taking as prescribed and (2) obtaining blood tests as scheduled. Patient self-report of pill-taking behavior might not be reliable, but results of the International Normalized Ratio can provide a reasonable measure of a patient's compliance. Nontherapeutic results might be indicative of the patient's not taking the prescribed dose, but further assessment of additional factors always should be undertaken.

One of the first studies to assess features of poor compliance specifically associated with anticoagulation therapy was undertaken by Arnsten and colleagues.[14] Significant differences were found between noncompliant patients and matched controls. The most notable independent predictors of noncompliance were younger age, absence of a regular physician, lack of knowledge regarding the reason for anticoagulation, and low confidence in warfarin's ability to prevent blood clots. Arnsten et al demonstrate how education can be directed proactively to increase the effectiveness of therapy.

CURRICULUM CONTENT

Exhibit 10–3 outlines a basic curriculum content for educating patients about warfarin therapy. The teaching session is viewed more positively when it is presented as a collaboration between patient and provider. In fact, the health care provider whom the patient perceives as attentive and caring has a positive effect on patient care in general. Schauffler et al[15] show that patients who reported that they received health education were nearly twice as likely to be satisfied with their providers. This sets the stage for developing a good relationship and communication between patient and clinician. The provider should discuss the most important items first; reinforce key information; and use a variety of media, including booklets, information sheets, and audio- or videotapes. Certainly, other aspects of therapy are important and relevant

Exhibit 10–3
BASIC CURRICULUM CONTENT FOR PATIENT EDUCATION IN ANTICOAGULANT THERAPY

- **Drug knowledge**
  - names of the drug (generic and brand)
  - action
  - indication and duration for patient
- **Safety**
  - recognition of potential side effects and appropriate action to take
  - patient identification for taking anticoagulants and/or use of Medic-Alert
  - minimization of risks for bleeding
  - limitations in daily activities
- **Dose Administration**
  - individualized dose, which might change over time
  - color-coded tablets with numeric imprint of milligrams
  - identification of best time of day for consistently taking prescribed dose
- **Factors influencing a stable response to therapy**
  - dietary Vitamin K
  - concomitant medications—prescription and over-the-counter

  - illness
  - alcohol use
  - lifestyle changes
  - health perceptions
  - motivators for adherence
- **Periodic blood testing to monitor therapeutic effect**
  - name of test—prothrombin time/International Normalized Ratio, what it measures, and how it is interpreted
  - frequency of testing
  - laboratory location and arrangements or office appointments for blood testing
- **What to report to anticoagulation clinic**
  - changes in overall medical condition
  - additions and/or deletions in medications—prescription and over-the-counter
  - missed dose or missed scheduled blood test
  - situations requiring temporary interruption in therapy
  - changes in dietary habits
  - extended travel and vacation plans
  - worrisome symptoms of bleeding or thromboembolism

for successful management, but keeping a narrow focus on such core concepts as taking the warfarin dose as prescribed daily, having blood tests when requested, and recognizing and acting on potential bleeding symptoms will help many patients. Continued follow-up by an anticoagulation management service provides the opportunity for reinforcement at the appropriate time for each patient.

HELPFUL POINTS IN PATIENT INSTRUCTION

Throughout the course of the education session, the provider should assess the patient's understanding of the medical terminology being used. For example, a common misconception among patients is that stroke and heart attack mean the same thing. The results of a 1994 Gallop poll show that fewer than 50% of the people surveyed could accurately identify the brain as the organ of insult in stroke.[16] The National Stroke Association is promoting the term *brain attack* to describe stroke and properly identify the organ affected. The term also implies that this is a medical emergency that can strike suddenly and requires immediate medical care. Misunderstanding of medical terms can have a deleterious effect on safety and compliance.

Dose instructions provided to patients must be precise to avoid misinterpretation. Hanchak et al[17] report on patient misunderstandings with the intended dosing regimen. Demo-

graphic variables, such as age, gender, race, education, or marital status, showed no relation to patients' understanding. In a study by Fletcher et al,[18] only 58% of patients could accurately recall their dose schedules for all of their medications. Therefore, ambiguity in dose instructions must be avoided. A common instruction, "Take your medicine in the evening," might not be as helpful as the phrase, "Take your medicine at 7 P.M. every day." Considering and adapting to the patient's routines at home, if necessary, are also practical. If 6 A.M. happens to be a preferable time for a patient, this information can be incorporated into dose instructions. Patients should understand that they can take a particular day's dose, if missed, later that same day, but they should not double the next day's dose if one is forgotten. If doses are missed, the anticoagulation clinic or monitoring clinician should be informed to help with continued assessments of compliance and future dosing. Lack of understanding of dose instructions can be an important factor contributing to nontherapeutic results and incorrect labeling of patients as noncompliant.

Creating an environment conducive to learning is incumbent upon the provider. A sufficient amount of time must be allocated for teaching sessions that allow for questions and special needs. Group teaching sessions are not typical in most anticoagulation clinics, but they might be an option with some patients. Group teaching has advantages, such as more effective utilization of time, and it creates a forum in which patients can learn from each other's questions and comments.

Guimon[19] describes a medication group program implemented to diminish negative attitudes associated with chronic neuroleptics that resulted in increased compliance through modifying prejudices against the chronic drug therapy. The group program had traits similar to a patient self-support group. Negative attitudes or prejudices, such as the association of warfarin with rat poison, are often described by patients taking warfarin. Patients are also fearful of potential side effects; as Lancaster et al[20] report, bleeding, even minor, was the most important factor leading to negative perceptions of health status by warfarin patients in their study. Developing and evaluating different approaches for educating patients is needed, especially because of the increasing numbers of patients who require anticoagulation therapy.

RECOMMENDATIONS FOR THE FUTURE

Future efforts should explore and validate the educational process: How effective is it? What do patients learn, and how much do they remember? How satisfied are they? An evaluation of the effectiveness of the teaching process is often lacking in current programs. Methods should be developed that assess the degree of integration and assimilation of the educational content into the patient's daily living and should be utilized to determine changes over the patient's lifetime.

Health professionals play a significant role in increasing patients' knowledge of their diseases and treatment plans. Providing health education specifically for anticoagulation therapy requires time and patience, along with continual reinforcement.

The economic incentives for promoting patient education are clear. It is logical to prevent patient misunderstanding or nonadherence with such a potentially dangerous medication as warfarin. Effective and safe use of oral anticoagulants demands that quality education be a critical component for success in achieving optimal patient care.

EXAMPLES OF EDUCATIONAL MATERIALS

A variety of methods, media, and theoretical approaches have been used to develop teaching materials to augment and reinforce content. Some institutions have supported the production of patient education videos specific to anticoagulation that are broadcast on in-hospital television stations. Appendix 10A presents a selection of educational materials, currently used in the teaching process from sites across the United States and Canada, that includes samples of work from a cross section of settings (eg, academic medical centers. Veterans Affairs medical centers, and community-based practices). The immense efforts made by individuals in these and many other health care organizations to develop high-quality educational programs and materials for their patients deserve special recognition. The intent of Appendix 10A is to provide examples of different approaches to promote the educational process, benefit patient care, and stimulate new ideas that can be incorporated at other sites. The editors feel privileged to share these materials and greatly appreciate the contributions.

In addition to patient-teaching materials, many clinicians utilize aids developed by DuPont Pharma, Wilmington, Delaware (1-800-4PHARMA). A vast selection of materials designed specifically for patient education is available courtesy of DuPont Pharma. The teaching materials are continually updated to reflect trends from current data in clinical research. One of the more popular and helpful aids is a booklet titled *Multilingual Support for Your Patients on Coumadin Therapy*. The booklet contains 30 translations (including English) of practical information about warfarin therapy for patients. An example of the Spanish translation page is in Appendix 10A. Other frequently used teaching aids from DuPont Pharma include a patient information booklet, weekly pill dispensers, and audiotapes in English and Spanish.

REFERENCES

1. Knowles M. *The Adult Learner: A Neglected Species.* Houston, TX: Gulf Publishing Co; 1973.

2. Rankin SH, Stallings KD. *Patient Education: Issues, Principles, Practices.* 3rd ed. Philadelphia: JB Lippincott Co; 1996:192.

3. Woldum KM, Ryan-Morrell V, Towson MC, et al. *Patient Education, Foundations of Practice.* Gaithersburg, MD: Aspen Publishers; 1985.

4. Redman BK. *The Process of Patient Education.* 6th ed. St. Louis, MO: CV Mosby Co; 1988.

5. Williams MV, Parker RM, Baker DW, et al. Inadequate functional health literacy among patients at two public hospitals. *JAMA.* 1995:274:1677–1682.

6. Davis TC, Crouch MA, Wills G. The gap between patient reading comprehension and the readability of patient education materials. *J Fam Pract.* 1990;31:533–538.

7. Reiley P, Iezzoni LI, Phillips R, et al. Discharge planning: comparison of patients' and nurses' perceptions of patients following hospital discharge. *Image: J Nurs Scholarship.* 1996;28:143–147.

8. Sackett DL, Snow JC. The magnitude of compliance and noncompliance. In: Haynes RB, Taylor DW, Sackett DL, eds. *Compliance in Health Care.* Baltimore, Md: Johns Hopkins University Press; 1979:11–23.

9. Marston MV. Compliance with medical regimens: a review of the literature. *Nurs Res.* 1970:19:312–323.

10. Everitt DE. Drug prescribing for the elderly. *Arch Intern Med.* 1986; 146:2393–2396.

11. Kendrick R, Bayne JRD. Compliance with prescribed medications by elderly patients. *CMA J.* 1982;127:961–962.

12. Hulka BS, Cassel JC, Jupper LL. Disparities between medications prescribed and consumed among chronic disease patients. In: Lasagna L, ed. *Patient Compliance.* Mount Kisco, NY: Futura Publishing Co; 1976.

13. Day JL. Why should patients do what we ask them to do? *Patient Educ Counseling.* 1995;26:113–118.

14. Arnsten JH, Gelfand JM, Hughes RA, et al. Determinants of compliance with anticoagulation. *J Gen Intern Med.* 1995;10:105A.

15. Schauffler HH, Rodriguez T, Milstein A. Health education and patient satisfaction. *J Fam Pract.* 1996;42:62–68.

16. National Stroke Association, 1994, 8480 East Orchard Road, Suite 1000, Englewood, CO, 80111–5015.

17. Hanchak NA, Patel MB, Berlin JA, et al. Patient misunderstanding of dosing instructions. *J Gen Intern Med.* 1996;11:325–328.

18. Fletcher SW, Fletcher RH, Thomas DC, et al. Patients' understanding of prescribed drugs. *J Community Health.* 1979;4:183–189.

19. Guimon J. The use of group programs to improve medication compliance in patients with chronic diseases. *Patient Educ Counseling.* 1995:26:189–193.

20. Lancaster TR, Singer DE, Sheehan MA, et al. The impact of long-term warfarin therapy in quality of life. *Arch Intern Med.* 1991;151: 1944–1949.

Patient Education Materials (Teaching Guides/Curriculums, Interdisciplinary Flowsheets, Contracts, Anticoagulant-Related Patient Information Sheets, Checklists, Patient Self-Tests)

ANTICOAGULATION (WARFARIN) THERAPY:
PATIENT EDUCATION AND ASSESSMENT

I.   PURPOSE: To outline policy, procedure, and responsibilities of nurses in education, assessment, documentation, and implementation of anticoagulant therapy.

II. POLICY
   A. All patients taking warfarin should be assessed for their response to the medication.
   B. All patients taking warfarin should be educated about basic information needed for safe administration of the medication.
   C. Documentation of the assessment and education will be done in accordance with hospital policy.

III. PROCEDURE
   A. Equipment/supplies needed:
      1. Warfarin therapy flowsheet
      2. Warfarin therapy patient education flowsheet
      3. Anticoagulation consultant consult form
      4. Appropriate forms to document patient progress
   B. Main steps and key points
      1. When the patient is being started on warfarin, a consult will be forwarded to the anticoagulation consultant, who will educate the patient regarding warfarin therapy. The anticoagulation consult form provides important information for the consultant and other registered nurses (RNs) who will be assessing the patient on warfarin therapy on an ongoing basis. It provides data from the physician about indication for therapy; length of treatment; International Normalized Ratio (INR) goal. The form can be started by an RN, but the physician needs to sign it. The nurse-practitioner (NP) anticoagulation consultant is available to both inpatients and outpatients.
      2. The patient will receive initial education related to anticoagulant therapy prior to initiation of warfarin therapy. It is best also to instruct a significant other. Patient education is essential to assist in medication compliance, effectiveness, and safety. If the anticoagulation consultant is not available, the RN must initiate education.
      3. The warfarin therapy patient education flowsheet will be used to document education. It will be initiated by the person starting warfarin education, the NP anticoagulation consultant or another RN. This flowsheet will be used on an ongoing basis to document warfarin therapy education.
      4. The patient will be given an educational assessment to determine ability to learn and willingness to comply with the medical regimen. If a problem with the patient's ability for self-care in regard to warfarin therapy is determined, the physician must be notified.
      5. If the patient is unable to learn the essentials of warfarin therapy management, and there is a willing and able caregiver, that person must be in-

structed. For safe administration of warfarin, the patient or caregiver must have a sufficient knowledge base about warfarin therapy.
      6. The NP anticoagulation consultant will be contacted to educate the patient that day. If the consultant is unavailable to see the patient the day therapy is initiated, the RN will give some basic/essential information regarding warfarin therapy to the patient. An appointment should be made with the NP anticoagulation consultant for a follow-up education visit.
      7. Patient and/or caregiver will be instructed on the following:
         a. Medical indication for warfarin. Patients are more compliant when they understand the importance of warfarin. Common indications include:
            (1) Atrial fibrillation (AF)
            (2) Aortic valve replacement (AVR)
            (3) Mitral valve replacement (MVR)
            (4) Pulmonary embolism (PE)
            (5) Deep venous thrombosis (DVT)
         b. Medication. Warfarin interferes with the ability to form clots. Warfarin tablets are color-coded with the dose inscribed on them.
            (1) Action of the drug
            (2) Current dose
            (3) Preferred time, 5 PM
            (4) To be taken as prescribed
         c. Adverse drug reactions. Patient should seek medical attention for the following signs and symptoms, which could indicate an elevated prothrombin time (PT)/INR or an adverse response to warfarin even when PT/INR is kept in therapeutic range:
            (1) Prolonged bleeding from a cut
            (2) Blood in urine, stool, or emesis; dark urine or tarry stool
            (3) Bleeding from gums, epistaxis, hemoptysis
            (4) Unexplained bruises, or very large bruises
            (5) Severe headaches, dizziness, or stomach pain
         d. Follow-up schedule:
            (1) Required close follow-up with blood tests (PT/INR) to assess blood clotting and whether a change in warfarin dosage will be required. It is important to keep the patient's PT/INR within a specific therapeutic range, and this necessitates frequent blood tests.
            (2) Patient should seek medical treatment for illness as soon as it occurs (eg, diarrhea, vomiting, infection, dyspnea). A change in a patient's physical condition (eg, congestive heart failure) can alter his or her response to warfarin and possibly change the PT/INR to dangerous levels.

continues

Anticoagulation (Warfarin) Therapy continued

    (3) Patient should report signs and symptoms of a thromboembolic event (ie, dizziness, visual disturbance, paresis, extremity pain or swelling, dyspnea).

  e. Dietary considerations:

    (1) Avoidance of alcohol. Chronic use of alcohol can lower the PT/INR; binge drinking can raise it. It also puts the patient at higher risk for gastrointestinal bleeding.

    (2) Consistency and limitations on foods high in vitamin K. Patient should be given a list of foods high in vitamin K. High intake of vitamin K will necessitate a higher dose of warfarin. A consistent low to moderate intake of vitamin K foods should be encouraged.

    (3) Patient needs to inform provider if his or her diet changes.

  f. Drug interactions:

    (1) Patient needs to remind all providers prescribing medications that he or she is taking warfarin. Many prescription drugs interact with warfarin, sometimes dramatically.

    (2) Patient must avoid aspirin, aspirin-containing drugs, and nonsteroidal anti-inflammatory drugs (NSAIDs) unless specifically prescribed by physician. Aspirin and NSAIDs increase the risk for bleeding while on warfarin.

    (3) Patient should not take any over-the-counter (OTC) drugs without getting approval from physician. Many OTC drugs interact with warfarin.

  g. Adjuncts to therapy:

    (1) Using a seven-day pillbox.

    (2) Wearing a Medic-Alert tag, necklace, or bracelet, indicating that the anticoagulant warfarin is being taken.

  h. Exercise:

    (1) Patient should notify provider of change in exercise patterns.

    (2) Patient should avoid activities that increase risk for trauma or injury. Electric shavers are encouraged. Fall risks need to be identified and reported. Contact sports can cause excessive bruising or bleeding into joints.

  i. Preoperative/other provider considerations. All other providers (eg, dentists, surgeons, emergency department, other clinics, local physicians) should be notified of the patient's anticoagulant therapy. Patient might have multiple providers who order medications or perform procedures affected by warfarin use.

  j. Hospital and community resources:

    (1) Videotape on using warfarin safely

    (2) Handout on patient's guide to using warfarin at home

    (3) Handout on vitamin K and warfarin therapy instructions

  k. Family responsibility:

    (1) Patient and significant other will agree on caregiver responsibilities. Caregiver's responsibilities can vary (eg, supportive, knowledgeable about diet and risks, monitoring medication compliance, administering medication, bringing patient to appointments).

    (2) If there is a visiting nurse, his or her role in warfarin therapy needs to be clarified (eg, obtaining blood specimens for PT/INR, filling pillbox). The visiting nurse must be contacted and informed of initiation of warfarin therapy, and his or her role.

8. RNs may see patients between primary care provider visits for warfarin therapy assessment. Patients are usually scheduled to come to the laboratory for a PT/INR and then report to the clinic to see an RN by appointment.

9. Some patients get their laboratory work done through a visiting nurse or an outside laboratory. In these cases:

  a. The laboratory data will be obtained by fax or telephone.

  b. Assessment will be done by telephone through conversation with the patient and/or the visiting nurse or caregiver.

    Management of a patient using an outside laboratory requires patient compliance to report for blood work on prescribed dates and availability by telephone. If there is any concern about the patient's condition, the patient should be evaluated in the clinic or emergency department.

10. Assessment of the clinic patient on warfarin therapy includes:

  a. Knowledge of the patient's:

    (1) Indication for warfarin therapy. Common indications are AF, AVR, MVR, DVT, PE, and severe cardiomyopathy.

    (2) Duration of treatment. This can vary from a few weeks to lifelong.

    (3) INR goal set by the physician. Commonly, it is 2.5–3.5 for mechanical heart valves and 2.0–3.0 for most other indications.

  b. Vital signs:

    (1) Blood pressure (BP). A very high BP might be a contraindication to continued warfarin therapy because of an increased risk of cerebrovascular accident.

    (2) Pulse. It should be noted if patient's pulse is irregular.

  c. Today's INR. The INR is a mathematical correction of the PT and is the preferred laboratory data for management of warfarin therapy. The patient's INR might or might not be within the therapeutic INR goal set by the physician.

continues

Anticoagulation (Warfarin) Therapy continued

 d. Assessment for any factors that might increase or decrease the PT/INR:

  (1) Alcohol. Chronic use of alcohol decreases the PT/INR; binge drinking increases it.

  (2) Change in vitamin K intake. A decrease in vitamin K intake will increase the PT/INR; an increase in intake will decrease the PT/INR. Increased intake of leafy green vegetables often occurs during the summer.

  (3) Changes in eating or exercise habits. Dieting or increase in physical activity can increase the PT/INR.

  (4) OTC self-medication. Many OTC medications interact with warfarin.

  (5) Prescription medication changes. Patient should be asked if he or she has been taking any new medications or had any dose changes on previous medications.

  (6) Change in health status. Infection, CHF, and diarrhea can raise the PT/INR. Patients need to be assessed for thromboembolic event.

 e. Assessment of patient for signs and symptoms of bleeding. Patient should be questioned regarding excess bleeding from cuts, bleeding gums, hematuria, dark tarry stools, bruising, and nosebleeds.

 f. Current warfarin dose. It is important to ask the patient, because the answer might differ from chart documentation or pharmacy profile.

 g. Assessment for knowledge deficits regarding warfarin therapy during patient interview. Patients frequently need review and reminders regarding important points of warfarin therapy.

 h. Report of patient assessment to physician, who will further assess patient as needed. Physician will prescribe new warfarin dose, determine follow-up time, and sign the warfarin therapy flowsheet. Documentation contains medical diagnosis and treatment, thus necessitating physician's signature.

 11. Education of the patient regarding the following:

  a. New warfarin dose. Written directions are often helpful.

  b. Follow-up appointment. Usual follow-up is in one month if the patient is on a stable dose. If the dose has had a moderate adjustment (10%–20% per week), usual follow-up is in one to two weeks. If there is a big adjustment in dose or there are other factors present that might affect the PT/INR (eg, being started on an antibiotic), the patient should be seen sooner.

  c. Instruction to the patient in any areas of warfarin therapy where knowledge deficits are identified. If the patient, during the course of anticoagulant therapy, needs more extensive review of warfarin education, a consult should be requested of the anticoagulation consultant for this purpose.

 12. Documentation of patient education and assessment:

  a. Warfarin therapy patient education flowsheet. Patient education, initial and ongoing, should be documented on this form by all who provide the teaching.

  b. Warfarin therapy flowsheet. This form provides an ongoing record of a patient's warfarin dose and response to warfarin therapy. The form should be designed to follow the patient from inpatient to outpatient status and be available to all providers through easy accessibility in the chart.

  c. Progress note, overprinted anticoagulation progress note, and prime care encounter form are used to document complete assessment and intervention.

IV. RESPONSIBILITIES

 A. RNs in prime care will assess the patient's response to anticoagulant (warfarin) therapy and document their assessments.

 B. The physician will determine and document (in accordance with hospital policy) the indication for anticoagulant therapy, the INR goal, the length of treatment, the next PT/INR check, the prescribed dose of warfarin, and any adverse drug reactions or thromboembolic events. The physician might need to do further assessment of the patient. The physician will refer the patient to the anticoagulation consultant for warfarin therapy education as needed.

 C. RNs in prime care will instruct patients and caregivers regarding prescribed warfarin dose and educate in any areas of knowledge deficit regarding warfarin therapy. RNs will document this education on designated forms.

 D. The anticoagulation consultant will respond to consults for warfarin education for both inpatients and outpatients and document on appropriate forms.

V. REFERENCES

Ansel JE, Holden A, Nozzolillo E. Oral anticoagulant therapy: practical considerations. *Nurs Pract Forum.* June 1992;3:105–112.

Dalen JE, Hirsh J. Introduction. *Chest.* October 1992;102 (suppl):303S.

Dalen JE, Hirsh J. Introduction. *Chest.* October 1995;108 (suppl):225S.

Hirsh JE, Dalen JE, Deyken K, Poller L. Oral anticoagulants: mechanism of action, clinical effectiveness, and optimal therapeutic range. *Chest.* October 1992: 102(suppl):312S–326S.

Loken S, Shioshita G. Factors that influence therapeutic anti-coagulation control. *Nurs Pract Forum.* June 1992;3:95–104.

Peric-Knowlton W. Addendum from the editor: warfarin dosage changes. *Nurs Pract Forum.* June 1992;3:113.

VI. RESCISSION

None.

NURSE'S GUIDE FOR TEACHING PATIENTS ON ANTICOAGULATION THERAPY

This guide was devised for the purpose of providing the nurse with a tool for teaching patients requiring long-term and/or short-term anticoagulation therapy. This tool includes pertinent information regarding the why and how of taking warfarin and the necessary clinical follow-up.

PURPOSE

To provide a tool for the nurse for teaching patients requiring anticoagulation therapy.

OBJECTIVE

This tool should be used only as a guide for teaching patients about the how and why of taking warfarin. The information given to the patient and the teaching to be done will be determined by the patient and his or her response to the information.

REMEMBER

Anticoagulation teaching is an ongoing process:

- Begin teaching after the nurse has assessed the patient's needs and level of understanding.
- Allow for questions and correct misunderstandings as you progress.
- Throughout the teaching sessions, continue to assess what the patient wants to know, what the patient needs to know, and how the patient interprets the explanations given.
- Be sure to document what has been taught, the patient's response, and any fears or concerns that the patient verbalizes.

TEACHING ASPECTS

1. Assessment of Patient's Knowledge

Content: To provide baseline for information giving and to assess the patient's level of understanding. The following questions can be used:
- Do you know why you're taking warfarin?
- What do you understand about the drug?
- What kinds of symptoms do you need to watch for?
- Do you have any problems with taking medication?

2. Anatomy and Physiology Pertinent to Anticoagulation

Content:

- Blood clotting, or *coagulation*, is a normal body process that keeps you from bleeding too much.
- There are many factors that both increase and decrease clot formation.

- When you develop a blood clot, or *thrombus*, your blood clots too easily or is too thick.
- For patients with atrial fibrillation: Your heart beats irregularly so that not all of the blood gets pumped with each beat. Some of it just sits around. When this happens, there is an increased risk of clot formation.

3. Explanation of Warfarin

Content: Warfarin is a drug that prevents your blood from clotting too easily. If you do, or did, have a clot, this drug will prevent it from getting any bigger or prevent any more clots from forming.

4. Need for Regular Blood Tests

Content: Before starting to take warfarin, you will have a blood test to check your prothrombin time (PT) and corresponding International Normalized Ratio (INR). From these results, the decision is made as to how much warfarin you will take. After you start, the only way to measure the level of warfarin is by testing your blood regularly and frequently. Initially, you will be coming once a week. After your medication is adjusted, the longest you will go without a blood test is four weeks.

5. Use of Warfarin with Other Medications

Content:

- Many drugs can affect how well the warfarin will or will not work.
- Don't take any medication without first checking with your physician or nurse.
- Inform the clinic whenever you start or stop a medication.
- You should be careful about any drugs (even if you've taken them before), such as aspirin (acetylsalicylic acid), sleeping pills, and headache medication.

6. Symptoms To Report

Content: Just as your blood can be too thick, it can also be too thin, which indicates that your blood level of warfarin is too high. You might be able to tell by the following symptoms and should call the clinic immediately:

- red or brown urine
- tarry black bowel movement
- increased menstrual bleeding

continues

Nurse's Guide for Teaching Patients continued

- feeling dizzy, faint, or weak
- nosebleeds
- bleeding from any place on your body
- easy bruising or black-and-blue spots
- swollen joints or large swelling from a bump

You should also call the clinic should you become ill in any way (eg, infection, virus, diarrhea).

7. Pregnancy

Content: You should not become pregnant while on warfarin because it can cause abnormalities in an unborn child. Should you discover you are pregnant, call the clinic immediately. Feel free to discuss birth control with the clinic staff.

8. Missed Pills

Content: If you forget a pill, don't double the next day's dose to make up for it. Do try and make taking the pill part of your daily routine (eg, with a particular meal, brushing your teeth).

9. Time of Day To Take Pill

Content: It is not necessary to take the pill at a special time as long as you take it at the same time every day. We recommend taking it in the evening so that, on the days your blood is checked, we will have time to change your dosage if necessary. It is not necessary to take your pill with a meal.

10. Alcohol Use

Content: Use of alcohol should be avoided because it prolongs the action of warfarin and can make your blood "thinner." If you feel that not using alcohol can be a problem, please let us know.

11. Emergency Treatment

Content: Should you need to see another physician or dentist for anything, be sure to tell the physician or dentist that you are taking warfarin.

Courtesy of Framingham Heart Center, Framingham, Massachusetts.

12. Identification Card

Content: This card has the physician's name, nurse's name, clinic telephone number, and the name of the drug on it. You should have this on your person at all times. This is so you will always have the name of the drug should you forget it, and so you can inform anyone who needs to treat you medically.

13. Medication Instructions

Content: You should receive directions for taking your warfarin each time you have your PT drawn. Based on your test results, you will be told the amount of warfarin to take each day. If you have any questions or concerns about your dose, do not hesitate to contact us.

14. Call-Back/Contact System

Content: Depending on where your blood is drawn, you might be instructed to call back for results and instructions. If you can't call back, attempts will be made to reach you or leave you a message. In case of an emergency when you cannot be reached by telephone, a telegram might be sent. If you have not received a call or telegram, continue taking your warfarin as prescribed and call the clinic for your instructions and follow-up appointment.

15. Activities of Daily Living

Content: You should be particularly careful about doing things in which you might injure yourself. For example, be careful using sharp knives; use an electric razor instead of a regular blade for shaving; and remove or protect hazards in your home, such as sharp objects that you could walk into. For those of you who are sports-minded, avoid rough contact sports.

16. Travel

Content: If you plan on being away for any length of time, let us know so arrangements can be made. You might need extra pills to take with you, or might need to have your blood checked at your travel destination. If you are going abroad, you need to discuss this in case your dosing schedule needs adjustment because of time zone differences.

ANTICOAGULANT THERAPY PATIENT TEACHING

Anticoagulant therapy patient teaching can be divided into four basic steps:

1. *Assessment.* Managing patients on anticoagulant therapy requires a planned educational intervention to deliver safe care. By establishing a written standard of care for patient teaching, accuracy and consistency in teaching content are ensured in addition to providing an assessment of teaching outcomes.
2. *Planning.* Using the **Anticoagulant Therapy Patient Teaching: Learner Objectives**, the health care provider can identify the appropriate topics, based on the assessment, for the individual patient. Some objectives might be inappropriate because of the patient's condition or prescribed regimen.
3. *Implementation.* Educational interventions are considered a treatment modality delivered on an interdisciplinary level. All health care professionals share responsibility for teaching patients about anticoagulant therapy when it is instituted. Patients on anticoagulant therapy in the ambulatory care setting can be referred by a primary physician to the Anticoagulation Clinic on a consultation sheet.
4. *Evaluation and documentation.* Health care providers are encouraged to review the teaching objectives listed on the **Interdisciplinary Patient/Family Teaching Record**. This format documents what the patient has been told and whether the objectives have been met.

Knowing what is important for a patient to learn about a disease and its management is one aspect of patient education, but knowing how to facilitate patient learning is equally important. The following information provides concrete suggestions keyed to these four steps in the educational process.

ASSESSMENT

Assessment areas relevant to the teaching-learning process are the patient's readiness, motivation, knowledge, experience with a regimen, and lifestyle.

Readiness

Patient readiness refers to the patient's capacity or ability to learn about a particular topic. It includes the patient's physical and emotional condition. Patients vary considerably on these dimensions; the health care provider must assess the patient's readiness and desire for information in order to decide whether it is appropriate to help the patient learn at this time. At times, the patient will profit more from contact with clergy or social workers to relieve emotional distress than from any patient education efforts.

Motivation

Motivation is the desire to learn. There are several dimensions to motivation, each of which needs to be considered when helping a patient learn about a disease and its management:

- Learning is most effective when the patient wants to learn something.
- Patients vary in their willingness to participate in decision making and management.
- Sources of patient motivation need to be identified.

Knowledge

There are a variety of reasons for assessing what the patient or family already knows. Listening to patients talk about their own experiences helps the provider to understand how they interpret information, as well as how they feel about their conditions. By identifying information that they understand or misunderstand, the provider can save valuable time in selecting teaching priorities. Observation of patients' psychomotor skills is an equally important strategy for assessing knowledge. What patients say and do are often very different

Experience with Regimen

The purpose of assessing a patient's experience with a regimen is to understand what problems have interfered with the regimen and what supports or strategies can minimize these problems. This assessment can also suggest ways that the regimen will need to be adapted to the patient's needs.

Lifestyle

Unless recommendations are convenient for a patient to follow, there is little chance that the patient, even if highly motivated, will follow the prescribed regimen. It is equally important to think about how the patient and family members learn best. The following questions summarize what to ask about or watch for:

- *Reading.* Does the patient spend time by reading books, magazines, or newspapers?
- *Audiovisual.* Does the patient like to watch movies or listen to tapes?
- *Conversational/verbal.* Would the patient like to talk to others who have the same condition?
- *Role playing.* Would the patient benefit from practicing how to ask questions of the physician?

continues

Anticoagulant Therapy Patient Teaching continued

- *Special learning problems.* Does the patient speak English fluently? Can the patient see and hear well?

PLANNING

Most planning for an individual patient's learning occurs informally and is likely to take little time, especially if general learning objectives already have been established. By using a general list of learning objectives or teaching areas for the patient population, the health care provider can try to identify which are appropriate for an individual patient based on the assessment. Some objectives will be inappropriate because of the patient's condition or prescribed regimen. The remaining objectives should be evaluated according to priority. It is far better to set a few realistic objectives than to generate a long list that can lead only to frustration.

IMPLEMENTATION

During the implementation phase of the teaching-learning process, the following teaching techniques can be used to achieve the learning objectives:

- offering positive reinforcement
- giving examples or asking the patient for examples
- encouraging patients' questions
- avoiding unnecessary medical jargon
- providing opportunities for practice

If a patient has a history of nonadherence, it is important to identify and deal with the reasons. One reason might be that the patient was not sure what to do. Written information should be provided, and family members should be involved if they can be a helpful resource. Another reason for nonadherence may be that the patient found the schedules too inconvenient or had difficulty with side effects and decided the benefits were not worth the costs of taking medications.

Some patients will choose not to follow recommended regimens regardless of how much the health care provider works with them. The provider has a responsibility, however, for ensuring that these patients understand what they can do to control their condition and to reduce the probability of new or further complications. It needs to be clear that patients make the ultimate choices and are responsible for the consequences.

EVALUATION AND DOCUMENTATION

Evaluation, like assessment and planning, should not be a separate step in the patient-teaching process. It occurs throughout the time the patient is being taught.

With shared teaching responsibilities throughout a health care organization, it becomes even more critical to complete the evaluation process with accurate and complete chart documentation. The Joint Commission on Accreditation of Healthcare Organizations provides standards for education and requires that patient education be interactive. Feedback from patients must be obtained to ensure the information is understood, appropriate, useful, and usable.

Courtesy of Coumadin Clinic, Veterans Affairs Medical Center, Albuquerque, New Mexico.

ANTICOAGULANT THERAPY PATIENT TEACHING: LEARNER OBJECTIVES

Learner Objective	*Content*
Following instruction, the patient will be able to:	
1. State the reason for taking anticoagulant medication.	1a. According to patient's individual condition necessitating anticoagulant therapy, explain as clearly and simply as possible the medical condition involved.
2. State the name, action, and dosage of anticoagulant medication.	2a. Ascertain that patient is able to verbalize name and dosage of anticoagulant medication. Warfarin is available in different strengths; each strength is a different color.
	2b. To avoid patient confusion and error, it is advisable for patient to use one tablet strength consistently. Patient should be able to identify tablet by strength rather than by color.
	2c. Ascertain that patient understands that anticoagulant medication acts to prolong the time for blood to form clots. Because of patient's condition (elaborate on individual situation), this is a good effect. Explain, however, that because taking this drug can cause the opposite effect (ie, bleeding), it is important that patient be monitored closely. Present in such a manner so as not to frighten patient but simply to assure patient that monitoring and patient awareness of reportable situations renders the drug safe and beneficial for specific problem.
3. State the importance of taking exact dosage prescribed at the same time each day.	3a. Explain to patient that although time of day is not important, it must be taken at the same time each day to maintain a constant blood level. (Example: If a dosage is taken in the evening and repeated the next morning, with only a 12-hour interval between, the patient could become overdosed and increase the potential for bleeding.)
4. State why dosage might be changed and why record of dosage schedule is kept.	4a. Explain to patient that monitoring will include a blood test at least every 4 weeks while on this medication. Depending on the blood test results, dosage might have to be changed. Blood tests might be required more often if results are not in therapeutic range.
	4b. Emphasize that patient must take only the dosage most recently prescribed because this dosage is based on blood test results. Explain that increasing or decreasing dosage would be dangerous. Instruct the patient never to make up a skipped dosage and emphasize the rationale behind this. Advise patient that it is better simply to note on calendar that dosage was omitted.
5. Describe two signs of observable bleeding and the action to take.	5a. Any of the following signs indicate bleeding and should be reported to an appropriate person immediately: bright red or dark or rusty brown urine, bright red or black stools, unexplained bleeding of any kind (nose, ear, vomiting blood), severe or prolonged headache or stomachache, unusual weakness or dizziness, coughing or spitting up blood, any cut that does not stop bleeding within reasonable period of time (but explain that because patient is on an anticoagulant, it can take a bit longer for a cut to stop bleeding), appearance of bruise spots on skin without apparent injury to area, abnormal or excessive menstrual flow, joint pain, or immobility.
	5b. Explain that although the above symptoms can be significant, they are not necessarily dangerous. Reporting them early can prevent more serious complications. This is an important aspect of monitoring—often, reporting bleeding symptoms early results only in a change in medication dosage. Instruct patient to apply cold to the area of bruising and to apply pressure to areas of acute bleeding. For observable bleeding (eg, black, "tarry" stools or "coffee ground" emesis), patient should go to closest hospital immediately and stop taking anticoagulant medicine.

continues

Anticoagulant Therapy Patient Teaching: Learner Objectives continued

Learner Objective	*Content*
6. State the name and normal limits of the blood test performed.	6a. Tell patient that the protime will be reported as the International Normalized Ratio (INR). To be effective in prolonging the body's ability to form blood clots, INR values should be within a therapeutic range. Recommended therapeutic ranges for INR values to follow patients on long-term anticoagulation are INR = 2.0–3.0 Primary and secondary prevention of venous thrombosis INR = 2.5–4.0 Prevention of recurrent venous thrombosis (2 or more episodes) INR = 3.0–4.5 Prevention of arterial thromboembolism, including patients with mechanical heart valves
7. State what the blood test results signify and the importance of regularly scheduled blood tests.	7a. Explain that if INR value is not within therapeutic or physician-ordered range and patient is taking the medication as instructed, the medication dosage probably will be adjusted (see 6a). 7b. To ensure that the medication is maintaining a good protime range and to ensure safety of the medication, the blood test is done at least every four weeks, or more often if indicated.
8. State that the anticoagulant can interact with other drugs, including alcohol.	8a. The action of anticoagulant medication is easily affected by the interaction of many drugs; alcohol is the most common. Depending on specific substance involved, anticoagulant action of the medication can be diminished or enhanced. Alcohol is known to do both. After any change in medication, a protime should be done to see if adjustment in warfarin dosage is needed. 8b. The patient must understand that either effect of a substance interaction can be detrimental to treatment: – Increased action of the drug can increase danger of bleeding. – Decreased action of the drug can increase potential for forming clots. 8c. Instruct patient to take only medications prescribed by physician. Depending upon the medications, they might also interact with the anticoagulant, but current blood tests reflect this interaction and dosage is adjusted accordingly. If a physician introduces a new drug, the patient's protimes will be monitored closely to ensure that effect of the new medication on the anticoagulant will be compensated by a dosage adjustment. 8d. Because aspirin itself has anticoagulant properties, it enhances the effect of an anticoagulant medication and is always contraindicated unless specifically ordered by a physician. This should be stated emphatically to the patient on anticoagulant therapy. 8e. Acetaminophen does not have the anticoagulant effect of aspirin and can be taken safely with anticoagulant agents. Advise patients to take acetaminophen instead of aspirin but not to abuse it or take it without knowledge of attending physician. 8f. Emphasize to patient to inform the physician about all other drugs he is taking, including nonprescription "over-the-counter" drugs such as Pepto-Bismol, etc. Some of these drugs may cause bleeding when taken with warfarin. 8g. Ask if patient is taking – aspirin or arthritis medicines – thyroid hormones – antibiotics – clofibrate (Atromid-S)

continues

Anticoagulant Therapy Patient Teaching: Learner Objectives continued

Learner Objective	*Content*
	– phenylbutazone (Azolid, Butazolidin)
	– disulfiram (Antabuse)
	– phenytoin (Dilantin)
	– phenobarbital
9. State the importance of carrying identification stating that patient is on anticoagulant therapy.	9a. Patients on anticoagulant medication should wear or carry some form of identification stating that they are taking an anticoagulant. Emphasize its importance in relation to possible emergencies. When cost is a consideration, expensive forms of identification, such as Medic-Alert ($15–$30) should not be promoted. Engraved discs cost much less. Minimal information— "anticoagulant"—is adequate. Identification cards can be provided, but bracelet or necklace identification should be encouraged because it is more readily noticed in an emergency situation.
	9b. Because of potential for prolonged clotting, instruct patient to inform any other care providers (eg, dentist, podiatrist, gynecologist) or if having ears pierced or donating blood that he or she is taking anticoagulant medication, and explain the reason for this precaution. Depending on specific procedures (eg, dental extraction), it is advisable for patient or care provider to contact the primary physician, who might discontinue anticoagulant therapy for a brief period before and after the procedure. In any case, a provider must be aware of the patient's medication to avoid unnecessary problems.
10. Verbalize that diet, illness, and changes in lifestyle can affect the action of anticoagulant.	10a. Because of the nature of anticoagulant medication, such factors as emotional or physical stress, changes in diet, drastic changes in lifestyle can also alter the effect of medication or alter the prothrombin time, which reinforces the need for constant monitoring as long as anticoagulant therapy is necessary. Explain this to the patient.
11. Describe the safety precautions necessary to prevent bleeding problems.	11a. Because the protime is therapeutically increased with anticoagulant medication, the danger of bleeding is present even at controlled levels. Instruct patient to avoid situations that can lead to injury:
	– Avoid use of sharp objects.
	– Avoid sports or activities that have high risk of injury.
	– Avoid vigorous nose blowing and tooth brushing.
	– Avoid use of water-jet tooth cleaners.
	– Wear shoes or slippers at all times.
	– Report pregnancy to physician immediately.
	11b. Review first-aid measures for bleeding. For all previously stated reasons, patient should be convinced of importance of ongoing follow-up while on anticoagulant therapy. Follow-up should include routine visits at least every 3-6 months to primary physician, as well as scheduled blood test (protime) at least every 4 weeks, with follow-up of test results by designated nurse or primary physician.
	11c. Provide the patient with literature to reinforce above teaching.

Physician concurrence:

_____

Signature   Date

Courtesy of Coumadin Clinic, Veterans Affairs Medical Center, Albuquerque, New Mexico.

continues

Living with Coumadin (Warfarin) Therapy Program

PROGRAM: Living with Coumadin (Warfarin) Therapy

TOPIC(S): Information for patients, family members and caregivers about Warfarin therapy

GOAL: To learn how to live with Warfarin therapy safely.

INSTRUCTOR(S):

TIME:

LEARNING OBJECTIVES (State in measurable terms)	CONTENT (Relate to objectives)	Instructional Materials	Instructional Activity/Evaluation
1. State the action of Warfarin.	1. Warfarin is used to prevent harmful blood clots from forming. It interferes with the action of vitamin K in the blood clotting process. It lowers the body's ability to make blood clots. It is a very old and common drug (> 50 yrs old), but a patient needs to have knowledge about the drug and be compliant with treatment in order to take it safely.	1. Coumadin Therapy and You. Brief Patient Guide to Coumadin Therapy. (DuPont Pharma videotape & handout)	1. Videotape—10 min., 27 secs. Discussion
2. State reason for taking Warfarin.	2. Harmful blood clots can cause a stroke ("brain attack"), a heart attack, or blood clots in the legs, lungs or other organs. For people with the heart condition of atrial fibrillation, the chance of having a stroke goes down 84% for women and 60% for men when taking Warfarin. Warfarin reduces the chance of forming harmful blood clots.	2. Wall chart—Atrial Fibrillation and Your Heart (DuPont Pharma)	2. Discussion
3. State the dose, pill color, how and when to take Warfarin.	3. All tablets are scored, color-coded, and have dose and Coumadin marked on the tablet. Generic Warfarin is dispensed from some pharmacies. Switching from Coumadin to a generic brand (or vice versa) may necessitate more frequent follow-up INR checks for a while. Warfarin can be taken with or without food, and should be taken about the same time every day. Traditionally, Warfarin is taken in the afternoon. This makes it possible to adjust the dose on the same day, when an INR is drawn in the morning.		3. Discussion

continued

continues

LEARNING OBJECTIVES (State in measurable terms)	CONTENT (Relate to objectives)	Instructional Materials	Instructional Activity/Evaluation
4. State the need for compliance with the prescribed dose.	4. Use a 7-day pillbox, so the chances of missed doses or double-dosing is minimized. Record your doses on a calendar. If you forget to take a pill or take extra or an incorrect dosage, always tell your provider/nurse at the time of an appointment. Call if you do this more than once. Do not try to catch up if you miss doses.	4. 7-day pillbox or Med-Planner; a 7-day QID pillbox. Coumadin Dosage Calendar (DuPont Pharma)	4. Discussion
5. State the need for compliance with INR checks.	5. Your dose of Warfarin is regulated by testing how quickly your blood is clotting. This blood test is called a PT (Prothrombin time) or INR (International Normalized Ratio). For most patients on Warfarin, the INR goal for therapy is 2–3. For patients who have had a mechanical heart valve surgery, the goal is usually 2.5–3.5. These blood tests need to be done fairly frequently when first starting Warfarin, but then gradually the spacing interval lengthens to every month if your INR and dose are stable. In Prime Care, you will probably see an RN for INR checks between provider appointments.		5. Discussion
6. State that there are drugs that interact with Warfarin.	6. Discuss all medicines you are taking, even OTC medicines, vitamins, or aspirin, with your provider/nurse. Avoid taking ASA or NSAIDS (name some) unless your provider specifically directs you to do so. These can increase the risk for stomach bleeding. Many prescription drugs interact with Warfarin. Discuss any questions or concerns with your provider.	6. Drug Interaction Considerations with Coumadin (DuPont Pharma chart)	6. Discussion
7. Identify the need to keep diet consistent in regard to vitamin K intake.	7. Vitamin K interferes with the action of Warfarin. If your intake varies, it will be hard to keep your INR stable. Keep your diet steady, so that intake of vitamin K will be consistent, and your INR will be more easily stabilized. Consistency and moderation are the keys. Review common foods high in vitamin K.	7. A Patient's Guide to Vitamin K; Food Habits Survey and Food Intake Survey (DuPont Pharma handouts)	7. Discussion

continues

LEARNING OBJECTIVES (State in measurable terms)	CONTENT (Relate to objectives)	Instructional Materials	Instructional Activity/Evaluation
8. State restriction on alcohol.	8. Alcohol should be avoided. Alcohol can cause an increased risk for stomach bleeding. Alcohol intake also can make your INR extremely hard to regulate, thus putting you at risk for bleeding if your INR is too high, or at risk for clots if your INR is too low.		8. Discussion
9. State the need to inform all providers of the use of Warfarin.	9. Always remind your doctor, dentist, pharmacist, or nurse that you are taking Warfarin. Since there are many drug interactions, always ask your provider if a new drug or change in a drug dose will interact with Warfarin (ie, starting antibiotics; changing Dilantin dose).		9. Discussion
10. Identify signs of bleeding.	10. The most common side effect associated with Warfarin therapy is bleeding. • Prolonged bleeding from cuts or nosebleeds; unusual bleeding from gums when brushing teeth; increased menstrual flow or vaginal bleeding • Red or dark brown urine; red or tarry black stools • Unusual bruising for unknown reasons • Pregnancy or planned pregnancy		10. Discussion
11. Recognize need to seek medical attention when illness or injury occurs.	11. Seek medical attention immediately if: • Any of the above (#10) occurs • Fever or illness develops, including vomiting, diarrhea, infection, pain, swelling, discomfort, or other unusual symptoms • Serious fall or trauma occurs (risk of internal or intracranial bleeding, bleeding into joint spaces, or large hematomas) • Frequent falls occur (the risk of bleeding may be greater than the benefit of clot prevention) • Any change in mental status or compliance (the person may need a caregiver to be involved)	11. A Patient's Guide to Preventing Falls at Home; Sample MMSE; Caregiver's Guide to Coumadin Therapy (DuPont Pharma handouts)	11. Discussion

continued

LEARNING OBJECTIVES (State in measurable terms)	CONTENT (Relate to objectives)	Instructional Materials	Instructional Activity/Evaluation
12. State the need for special safety measures.	12. There are certain precautions that are prudent: • Avoid activities with a high risk of injury (football, soccer). • Wear a Medic Alert tag. • Notify your provider if problems develop with frequent falls, or mental status change. • Contact Prime Care or provider/nurse if you have questions.	12. Prime Care and telephone triage telephone numbers 13. Post-test	12. Discussion 13. Written true-false test.

Courtesy of Prime Care Clinic, Veterans Affairs Medical Center, Dayton, Ohio.

Interdisciplinary Patient Education Flowsheet—Warfarin Therapy

Educational Assessment (Ability To Learn, Sensory/Other Limitations, Obstacles to Following Regimen)	
In the boxes below, check the appropriate status. Date of assessment _____	
Readiness to learn	___ HA = Highly anxious ___ MA = Moderate anxiety ___ A = Accepting ___ D = Denying
Ability to learn	___ A = Alert ___ UP = Unable to participate
Existing knowledge	___ C = Comprehensive ___ G = Good ___ L = Limited ___ N = None
How does the patient like to learn?	___ By being told ___ By listening ___ By reading ___ By seeing film ___ By skill
BARRIERS	
Vision	___ G = Good ___ GWA = Good with glasses ___ PWA = Poor with glasses ___ P = Poor
Hearing	___ G = Good ___ GWA = Good with hearing aid ___ PWA = Poor with hearing aid ___ P = Poor
Language	___ English ___ Other (specify)
Cultural	Specify:
Physical	___ Able ___ Limited (specify)
Religious	Specify:
Health belief	I will get better. ___ Yes ___ No ___ Uncertain I will hold my own or stay the same. ___ Yes ___ No ___ Uncertain There is no hope. ___ Yes ___ No ___ Uncertain
Motivation	I will follow the treatment plan. ___ Yes ___ No ___ Uncertain If no, explain:
What are patient's significant other's learning goals?	
EDUCATION PLAN/GOAL/NEEDS: Date met/initial	
To learn how to live with warfarin therapy safely	
Check status: Inpatient ___ Outpatient ___ Instruction given: Patient ___ Family/significant other___ For each entry include signature/title, outcome code (as listed below). 1 = Indicates understanding or performs successfully 3 = Unsuccessful 2 = Needs reinforcement or needs to repeat demonstration 4 = Not applicable	

continues

Interdisciplinary Patient Education Flowsheet continued

Persons instructed: Pt = Patient   SO = Significant other
Indicate one of the following for each expected behavioral outcome for each person instructed:
1 = Indicates understanding 2 = Needs reinforcement 3 = Unsuccessful 4 = Not applicable

Date of Instruction: *Expected Behavioral Outcome*	*Pt*	*SO*	*Pt*	*SO*	*Pt*	*SO*
1. State reason for taking warfarin.						
2. State the action of warfarin.						
3. State the dose, pill color, how and when to be taken.						
4. State the need for compliance with dose and INR checks.						
5. Identify three signs of bleeding.						
6. Recognizes need to seek medical attention when illness or injury occurs.						
7. State restriction on alcohol intake.						
8. State limitations on vitamin K foods.						
9. Name three foods high in vitamin K.						
10. State increased risk of bleeding with ASA or NSAIDs.						
11. State danger of taking OTC medications without approval.						
12. Describe use of the seven-day pillbox.						
13. Identify need to use Medic-Alert tag.						
14. State need to avoid activities with high risk of injury.						
15. State need to inform all providers of the use of warfarin.						
Resources Provided to Patient						
1. Booklet on warfarin therapy						
2. Medic-Alert tag: necklace/bracelet						
3. Seven-day pillbox						
4. Telephone number of provider for questions						

continues

Interdisciplinary Patient Education Flowsheet continued

5. Videotape on warfarin therapy viewed						
6. Audiotape on warfarin therapy given						
7. Other						
Initials of person teaching patient and/or significant other						

Is there a caregiver or visiting nurse?	*Signature Block*	*Initials*
Name		
Telephone		
Relationship		
Care given		

Key: ASA, acetylsalicylic acid; INR, International Normalized Ratio; NSAIDs, nonsteroidal anti-inflammatory drugs; OTC, over-the-counter.

Courtesy of Prime Care Clinic, Veterans Affairs Medical Center, Dayton, Ohio.

Interdisciplinary Patient/Family Teaching Record

Date	Educational Assessment of Learning Needs, Abilities, Readiness To Learn
	☐ Large group class. Unable to complete individual assessment. ☐ No major barriers to learning. If yes, check below.
	Able to read: ☐ yes ☐ no Learns best: ☐ visual ☐ hearing ☐ doing Barriers: ☐ visual ☐ hearing Readiness to learn: ☐ yes ☐ no Cultural/religious health practices: ☐ no ☐ yes Physical/cognitive limitations: ☐ no ☐ yes Emotional barriers: ☐ no ☐ yes Language barriers: ☐ no ☐ yes Desire/motivation to learn: ☐ no ☐ yes Communicates in: ☐ English ☐ Spanish ☐ sign language ☐ other If barriers are present, describe methods to overcome:
	Educational needs/plan/goals: (Cite ways to overcome obstacles to adherence, self-care approaches, participation in decision making). Instruct patient/family using anticoagulant therapy patient education manual.
	Family/significant other/caregiver present:

Teaching Date	Anticoagulant Medication	Signature/Title	Outcome (✓ one)	
			Met	Unmet
	1. Knowledge of the reason for taking anticoagulant medication			
	2. Knowledge of the name, action, and dosage of anticoagulant medication			
	3. Knowledge of the importance of taking exact dosage prescribed at the same time each day			
	4. Knowledge of why the dosage may be changed and why records of dosage schedule should be kept			
	5. Knowledge of two signs of observable bleeding and the action to take			
	6. Knowledge of the name and the normal limits of the blood test performed			

continues

Interdisciplinary Patient/Family Teaching Record continued

Teaching Date	Anticoagulant Medication	Signature/Title	Outcome (✓ one) Met	Unmet
	7. Knowledge of what the blood test results regularly signify and the importance of regularly scheduled blood tests			
	8. Knowledge that anticoagulant can interact with other drugs, including alcohol			
	9. Knowledge of the importance of carrying identification stating patient is on anticoagulant therapy			
	10. Knowledge that diet, illness, and changes in lifestyle can affect the action of anticoagulant			
	11. Knowledge of the safety precautions necessary to prevent bleeding problems			
	12. Print materials given to patient:			
	a.			
	b.			
	c.			
Signature and title of practitioner			Date	

Patient name _____

Address _____

Courtesy of Coumadin Clinic, Veterans Affairs Medical Center, Albuquerque, New Mexico.

Contract with the Patient

- I understand that, as a participant in the anticoagulation clinic, I am required to be present at all clinic appointments.

- I understand that I will call the anticoagulation program if I do not receive instructions within 48 hours after a blood test.

- I am able to travel to the clinic for my appointments.

- I am willing to follow instructions involving compliance with warfarin dosage and administration, proper diet, and notifying the clinic regarding all drugs I am taking (even over-the-counter drugs).

- I have access to a telephone and can be reached by telephone if necessary.

- I am taking a medicine that must be followed closely in order to protect me from any complications. I understand that noncompliance with any of the above can result in serious health risks and/or termination with the program.

_____

Patient signature   Date

_____

Witness signature   Date

Courtesy of Division of Internal Medicine, Anticoagulation Program, Thomas Jefferson University Hospital, Philadelphia, Pennsylvania.

Patient-Provider Agreement (Contract with Patient)

Patient Name: _____
Patient-Provider Agreement
Anticoagulation Clinic

Warfarin (Coumadin®) is a lifesaving drug. When used correctly and under close supervision, warfarin can prevent blood clots from forming in your bloodstream. Harmful blood clots can result in a stroke or damage to vital organs. If you have a stroke, you may no longer be able to walk, use your arms or hands. speak, or even think properly. If the blood clot causes severe damage to your lungs, heart, or brain, you may die. Warfarin will work only if taken in the proper dose. The best dose of warfarin is different for every person.

Warfarin is a potentially dangerous medication. When used incorrectly or without regular blood tests, warfarin can cause some serious side effects. Too much warfarin can cause you to bleed more easily. You may even bleed internally. If you lose too much blood or you bleed inside your head, you may die.

When used carefully and in the right dose, warfarin therapy can be made much safer. Working closely with you, we can determine the best dose of warfarin for you. The dose of warfarin you need may change from time to time. For these reasons, it is very important that we see you every few weeks and perform blood tests regularly.

This document is a non-binding agreement formed between _____ and _____, Pharm.D. The purpose of this agreement is to improve adherence to warfarin therapy and recommended clinic visits. To accomplish this goal, the following promises have been made:

_____ promises to keep appointments. If I cannot keep my appointment, it is my responsibility to call the clinic to reschedule. If I miss two appointments and do not call to reschedule over the next 12 months, I understand that I will be discharged from the anticoagulation clinic and will need to have someone else follow my warfarin therapy.

I, _____, Pharm.D., have explained this contract to _____. I have informed him/her of the benefits and risks of anticoagulation therapy. Unless otherwise stated in this document, I believe the patient understands this document and the responsibilities outlined in this agreement.

Signature:_____ Date: _____

I, _____, have read this document or have had its contents explained to me. I understand that I am responsible for assisting my caregivers in maintaining my health and will abide by the terms of this agreement. I have received a copy of this document. I understand that if I am unsatisfied with the care provided, I am free to seek an alternative provider. I enter into this agreement freely.

Signature:_____ Date: _____

Courtesy of University of Maryland, School of Pharmacy, Baltimore, Maryland.

Anticoagulant Warfarin Food/Drug Interactions

Warfarin is used to prevent blood clots from forming.

DO

- Take your medicine at the same time every day.
- If you notice any bleeding, contact your doctor at once.
- Before any surgery or dental work, tell your doctor or dentist you are taking warfarin.
- Your diet should have the same amount of vitamin K foods each day. Too many servings of vitamin K foods or too few servings can prevent this drug from working as it should:
  - Too much vitamin K will make your blood too thick, and you might need more warfarin.
  - Too little vitamin K will make your blood too thin, and you might need less warfarin.

The following is a list of vegetables with a high vitamin K content. You may eat up to one serving per day of any of the following:

Vegetable	Serving Size
Broccoli (raw or cooked)	1/2 cup
Brussel sprouts	5 sprouts
Cabbage (raw)	1 1/2 cups
Collard greens	1/2 cup
Cucumber peel	1 cup
Endive (raw)	2 cups chopped
Green scallion (raw)	2/3 cup
Lettuce (raw/bib/red leaf)	1 3/4 cups shredded
Mustard greens (raw)	1 1/2 cups shredded
Spinach (raw leaf)	1 1/2 cups
Turnip greens (raw)	1 1/2 cups chopped
Watercress (raw)	3 cups chopped

- Tell the health care provider who follows your warfarin therapy:
  - If you'd like to eat more of the vegetables listed. You will need to keep the number of servings and your serving sizes the same each day.
  - If there are *any* changes in your usual eating habits.

DO NOT

- Do not eat kale or parsley.
- It is advised that you avoid alcoholic drinks, such as beer, wine, and hard liquor. If you do drink alcohol, tell the health care provider who follows your warfarin therapy.
- Do not take vitamin supplements having more than 100% of the advised daily value in any one day for the following vitamins:

Advised Daily Value	
Vitamin A	5,000 IU
Vitamin D	400 IU
Vitamin E	30 IU
Vitamin K	25 mcg
Vitamin C	60 mg

- Do not use cold medicine or pain medicine containing aspirin, such as Alka-Selzer, Aspercreme, Flex-All 454 Gen, Ben-Gay.

Courtesy of Coumadin Clinic, Veterans Affairs Medical Center, Albuquerque, New Mexico.

Common Aspirin-Containing Products

You should avoid the use of aspirin and aspirin-containing products. We list for your convenience several common products containing aspirin:

Alka-Seltzer	Empirin
Anacin	Excedrin
Ascriptin	Fiorinal
Aspergum	Fizrin
Bromo-Seltzer	Midol
Bufferin	Nytol
Congespirin	Pepto-Bismol
Coricidin	Percodan
Darvon Compound	Sominex
Dristan	Vanquish

However, you should *always* read the labels of all medications before you take them. If you see these ingredients listed—aspirin, salicylate, acetylsalicylic acid, or ASA—do not take that medicine.

Aspirin-free products, such as acetaminophen, Tylenol, and Datril, can be safely used.

If you have any questions about what is in a medication, check with your doctor, nurse, or pharmacist.

Courtesy of Anticoagulation Clinic, University of Virginia Medical Center, Charlottesville, Virginia.

Taking Warfarin

DEFINITION

Warfarin is a medication that slows the blood clotting process. It is used in persons who have either recently formed a blood clot or are at risk for forming them.

SIDE EFFECTS

Some risk is involved in taking this medication because of its effect on clotting. The risk is relatively small when it is taken properly, but cooperation is required between the patient and physician/nurse. In therapeutic doses, warfarin does not cause bleeding; it only makes it harder to stop if it occurs.

MONITORING

Periodic blood tests are needed to make sure that the proper effect is achieved. Depending on the situation, testing is necessary from every week to every few weeks.

The prothrombin time (PT) is a test of the speed of clotting that is used. The goal of therapy is to slow clotting by a desired amount, as measured by the International Normalized Ratio (INR) derived from the PT. The goal is usually an INR of 2.0–3.0 (occasionally 2.5–3.5). The INR should be available from any laboratory performing PTs.

The blood should be drawn in the morning, and the physician/nurse is notified of the results. The patient on warfarin should be contacted and the warfarin dose adjusted within 24 hours (unless other arrangements have been made). This is best performed by coming to the anticoagulation clinic immediately after the blood draw for the nurse/physician visit.

If for some reason you have not been contacted soon after the blood draw, please call the clinic.

TAKING THE MEDICINE

The warfarin should be taken at the same time each day, preferably in the late afternoon or evening. It is not taken in the morning on the day of the blood test. If a dose is forgotten, omit this dose if remembered more than eight hours later. *If two or more doses are missed, notify your physician*.

It is recommended that you obtain a Medic-Alert bracelet or necklace to be worn while you are on warfarin.

NOTIFY YOUR PHYSICIAN AND THE CLINIC IF

- Excessive bleeding occurs from the nose, cuts, gums, or vagina.
- There is reddish/brown urine or stool (or black).
- There is an abundance of bruising.
- Vomiting of blood occurs.
- There is hemorrhoidal bleeding.
- Major injury occurs.
- There is a need to start a new medication or discontinue an old one.
- You intend to become pregnant.
- There are questions about the medication.
- You omitted two or more doses of warfarin.

DRUG INTERACTIONS

Many medications interact with warfarin and need to be avoided. Notify your physician if there is concern about a particular drug.

Antibiotics

Most antibiotics should be avoided.

continues

Other Medications

Avoid the following:

- aspirin-containing products (read the labels), including Aleve, Alka-Seltzer, Allerest, Anacin, Ascriptin, Bufferin, cough/cold remedies, Darvon compound, Dristan, Easprin, Ecotrin, Empirin compound, Excedrin, Fiorinal, Nytol, Pepto-Bismol, Percodan, Vanquish, Zactirin, Zorprin, and others.
- anti-inflammatory/antiarthritic medications, including Anaprox, Ansaid, Clinoril, Daypro, Dolobid, Feldene, ibuprofen (Advil, Medipren, Motrin, Nuprin, Rufen), Indocin, Lodine, Meclomen, Nalfon, Naprosyn, Orudis, Relafen, Tolectin, Voltaren, and others.

OTHER INTERACTIONS

Alcohol

Avoid more than one ounce per day.

Diet

Certain foods contain significant amounts of vitamin K, which counteracts the effects of warfarin. The main source for Vitamin K is from green leafy vegetables. No specific dietary restriction is recommended except to avoid marked changes in the diet.

Bowel Habits

Diarrhea decreases the absorption of warfarin and decreases its effect. Constipation tends to result in more absorption of the medication and increases its effect.

Be sure to notify your other physicians/dentist that you are on warfarin.

Courtesy of Jacksonville Coumadin Clinic, Mayo Clinic, Jacksonville, Florida.

Treating and Preventing Blood Clots: What You Need To Know

INTRODUCTION

Your physician has prescribed anticoagulant medicine to treat or prevent a blood clot that may be caused by your medical condition. This booklet explains how blood clots form, how they are treated and/or prevented, and how you can take care of yourself while taking anticoagulant medicine.

HOW BLOOD CLOTS FORM

When Blood Clotting Is Helpful

You have substances in your blood that make sure that your blood clots properly. These are called clotting factors.

When you are injured and bleeding, your body forms a blood clot to stop the bleeding. This also protects against infection. When the injured area is healed, your body gradually reabsorbs the clot because it is no longer needed.

When Blood Clotting Is Harmful

Certain circumstances can cause your body to develop harmful blood clots. These circumstances include long periods of inactivity, such as from paralysis; very long surgical procedures; or when parts of the body are in a cast.

Pregnancy is also a time when the body is more prone to clotting. Near the end of pregnancy, a protective mechanism develops to prevent too much blood loss at delivery. This protective mechanism can sometimes cause unnecessary blood clotting.

Blood clots in certain parts of your body can be harmful, such as in the heart, brain, lungs, arms, or legs. The blood clot blocks blood and oxygen from reaching the area beyond the blood clot. More seriously, a piece of the blood clot can break off and travel through the circulation. This can be life-threatening.

What Are the Signs of a Blood Clot?

The signs of a blood clot are:

- Sudden weakness in the arms or legs
- Severe pain, redness, or swelling in an arm or a leg
- Numbness or tingling anywhere
- Changes or loss of sight in either eye
- Sudden occurrence of slurred speech or inability to speak
- Dizziness or faintness
- Shortness of breath
- Chest pain

CONDITIONS THAT CAN CAUSE BLOOD CLOTS

A person with any of the following conditions may have blood clots or may be prone to develop blood clots.

Deep Vein Thrombosis (DVT)

A DVT is a blood clot that forms in one of the large veins in your arm or leg. This clot causes damage by blocking blood flow that leads to swelling and discomfort in part or all of the involved arm or leg. A DVT can sometimes break off and travel to the lungs, causing a pulmonary embolism.

continues

Treating and Preventing Blood Clots: What You Need To Know continued

Pulmonary Embolus (PE)

This is a blood clot in your lung. This type of clot is dangerous because it can prevent oxygen from getting through your lung and into your body. A person with this type of clot may have shortness of breath and chest pain. The seriousness of this problem depends upon clot size and exact location in the lung.

Atrial Fibrillation (Afib.)

This condition causes an abnormal beating of your heart. The heart may beat at a faster than normal rate and the pulse may be irregular. As a result, the blood is not pumped out of your heart as it should be. This can cause a blood clot to form in your heart. The blood clot can travel to other parts of the body, such as your brain or lung, and cause a stroke or pulmonary embolism.

Artificial Heart Valve

Because an artificial heart valve is made of man-made substances, the body recognizes it as foreign and attempts to protect the body against it. Blood clots may form as a result. These clots can travel also to other parts of the body and cause serious problems, such as strokes.

Hereditary Disorders

Your body makes proteins that prevent your blood from clotting when it shouldn't. These proteins are called Protein C, Protein S, and Antithrombin III.

Some people are born with a deficiency in one or more of these proteins and are at risk for developing blood clots. Other people produce substances, such as anticardiolipin antibodies, that also increase blood clotting.

Stroke or Brain Attack

A stroke occurs when a blood clot forms in one of the blood vessels in the brain. Some people who have had a stroke and those who are at a high risk for having another stroke need to take medication to prevent blood clots from forming in the brain.

TREATING AND PREVENTING BLOOD CLOTS WITH ANTICOAGULANT MEDICATIONS

Your physician has prescribed anticoagulant medicine to prevent or treat your blood clot. These medicines include warfarin (Coumadin®) and/or enoxaparin (Lovenox®). Warfarin is in a pill form and enoxaparin is taken by injection. Both of these medicines help prevent harmful clots from forming.

How Do Anticoagulant Medications Work?

Anticoagulant medications are sometimes called "blood thinners." This is not really a correct term since the blood does not become thinner; it simply takes longer for it to clot. Anticoagulant medications prolong the time that the blood takes to clot and help prevent harmful clots from developing. They do this by reducing the amount of clotting factors.

How Long Will I Have To Take Anticoagulant Medication?

The length of time you will need to take anticoagulant medicine depends on your condition. For example, people diagnosed for

continues

the first time with a deep vein thrombosis (DVT) or pulmonary embolus (PE) usually need to take enoxaparin (Lovenox®) and/or warfarin (Coumadin®) for three to six months.

In most cases, individuals with atrial fibrillation, an artificial heart valve, hereditary disorders, or recurrent blood clots will need to take warfarin (Coumadin®) for their entire lives. Of course, treatment will be different for each person.

When Can I Stop Taking Anticoagulant Medication?

You should never stop taking medication on your own. Your physician will tell you when you may stop your medicine.

INFORMATION ABOUT ANTICOAGULANT MEDICATIONS—WARFARIN (COUMADIN®)

How Should I Take My Warfarin?

The way you take warfarin may be different from how you take other medicines. For one thing, you may not take the same dose (number of tablets) every day of the week. That's because many factors (your other medications, diet, activities, and general health) can change the effect of warfarin on your blood, which in turn may cause us to change your dose.

We will closely monitor the effect of your warfarin therapy, because too much warfarin can increase chances of bleeding and too little warfarin can increase the risk of blood clots developing. The effect of warfarin on your blood is measured by a blood test, called a protime (PT) or International Normalized Ratio (INR) test.

At the beginning of warfarin therapy we will frequently check your INR to best determine your ideal dose—the dose that has just the right effect on your blood. Once we have determined your ideal dose of warfarin, we will continue to closely monitor the effect of warfarin on your blood. When we find your INR remains stable, your blood will then only have to be checked every month or so. If your condition changes, you become ill, or you change your medications or diet, then we will need to check your INR more frequently and change your warfarin dose as needed.

How Is My INR Tested?

There are two ways for your INR to be checked. One is by drawing a blood sample from your arm to be sent to a laboratory. A second way is by a fingerstick in the physician's office. The fingerstick gives an immediate result so that your warfarin dose can be adjusted right away, if necessary. While you are taking warfarin, your INR should be 1.4 to 4.0. Your exact INR goal will depend on your medical condition.

(Normal INR for a person not taking warfarin is 1.0.) If your INR is too low, you will need a higher dose of warfarin. If your INR is too high, you will need a lower dose of warfarin.

When Should I Take My Warfarin?

Take your warfarin once a day. Follow the directions on your prescription label carefully and ask your pharmacist, physician, or nurse to explain any part you do not understand.

To avoid missing a dose, get in the habit of taking your warfarin at the same time every day. Some people find it helpful to associate

continues

another activity with taking their warfarin. For example, you may get in the habit of taking warfarin when you brush your teeth or are having dinner.

Record each dose and the time you took it on a calendar. Remember, don't stop taking this medication unless your physician tells you to do so.

What Should I Do if I Forget To Take a Dose?

Take it as soon as you remember. However, if you do not remember until the next day, do not take two doses. Take only the scheduled dose. Remember to record the date of the missed dose on your calendar. Tell your doctor at your next visit, since missing a dose of warfarin may alter your blood clotting test. If you miss doses for two or more days, call your physician promptly.

What Special Instructions Should I Follow While Using This Drug?

It is important to keep appointments with your physician and the laboratory to check your response to this drug and adjust your dose if necessary. Failure to keep appointments for these tests could result in the improper control of bleeding or blood clots. You should carry a card or wear a bracelet indicating that you take warfarin so that people treating you will know this fact in case of an accident.

What Special Diet Instructions Should I Follow While Using Warfarin?

Vitamin K, a nutrient found in food, can decrease the effects of warfarin. Your warfarin dose was based on your usual daily diet;

therefore, it is important for you to eat a diet that contains the same amount of vitamin K each day. You do not need to avoid foods that contain vitamin K; however, it is important for you not to make major changes in the amount of vitamin K that you eat on a daily basis. In particular, pay close attention that you are not changing the amount of high vitamin K foods that you eat on a daily basis. The following includes those foods that are high in vitamin K:

Foods High in Vitamin K

Broccoli	Kale
Brussel Sprouts	Mustard Greens
Cabbage	Seaweed
Cauliflower	Soybeans/Soybean Oil
Collard Greens	Spinach
Endive	Tofu
Green Tea	Turnip Greens
Mustard Greens	

Remember, keep your diet consistent.

Can I Drink Alcohol While I Am Taking Warfarin?

Drinking alcohol can affect warfarin as well. Alcohol can either increase or decrease the effect of warfarin. It is not always predictable. It is best to not have more than one glass of wine, beer, or any other alcoholic drink per day; it's even better to avoid alcohol altogether.

What Side Effects Can This Drug Cause?

Although side effects from warfarin are not common, they can occur. You should watch for signs of bleeding (see Signs of Bleeding to Watch for While You Are Taking Warfarin or Enxaparin). You may also notice fatigue, fever, chills, sore throat, mouth sores, rash, or itching.

continues

If you do notice any of these symptoms, call your physician promptly.

What Precautions Should I Follow if I Am Pregnant?

Women who are breastfeeding, pregnant, or planning a pregnancy should tell their physicians before taking warfarin. You should call your physician immediately if you think you are pregnant or are planning on becoming pregnant.

Are There Any Other Precautions I Should Follow?

Before taking warfarin, tell your physician your entire medical history, especially bleeding problems (ulcer, or lengthy or heavy menstrual periods), diabetes, liver or kidney disease, high blood pressure, arthritis, seizures, and thyroid problems. Also, tell your physician if you have an infection or have had recent surgery.

Be aware of these special precautions:

- Tell your physician and pharmacist if you are allergic to aspirin or tartrazine (a yellow dye in some processed foods and medications, including certain brands of warfarin). Do not switch your brand of warfarin because it may differ in its effect on your blood.
- If you have vomiting, diarrhea, or fever for more than a few days, call your physician. These problems can change the effect of warfarin.
- In case of an accidental overdose of warfarin, call your physician, poison control center, or nearest hospital emergency department immediately.
- Do not allow anyone else to take your warfarin.

Can I Take Other Medications While I Am Taking Warfarin?

Many drugs increase or decrease the anticoagulant effect of warfarin, resulting in bleeding or clots. Tell your physician, pharmacist, or nurse what prescription and non-prescription drugs and herbal products you are taking. It is important that all physicians and dentists taking care of you know that you take warfarin so that they can avoid prescribing medications that interfere with its effect.

Do not take any nonprescription drugs or herbal products without telling your physician. Do not stop taking any current medications unless your doctor tells you to.

Nonprescription Medications

The most important nonprescription medication to avoid is aspirin. You should not take aspirin, unless your physician prescribes it, since it also decreases blood clotting and may increase your chances for bleeding. Please refer to the following partial list of non-prescription medications you should avoid while you are taking warfarin. If you have any questions, please contact your pharmacist or physician.

Vitamins

You should avoid taking vitamin supplements that contain vitamin K. Read the vitamin label or, if you have any questions, ask your pharmacist or physician.

Prescription Medications

Many prescription drugs interfere with warfarin, especially antibiotics. Tell all of your doctors that you are taking warfarin so they

continues

Treating and Preventing Blood Clots: What You Need To Know continued

will know which medications can be prescribed for you. It is also a good idea to have all of your prescriptions filled at the same pharmacy, so that your pharmacist will be able to watch for any medications that should not be taken with warfarin.

How Should I Store My Warfarin?

Keep your warfarin in the container it came in, tightly closed, and out of reach of children. Store it at room temperature and away from light.

You *may not* take these nonprescription medications:
Actron®
Advil®
Aleve®
Alka-Seltzer®
Ascriptin®
Aspirin
Bayer®
Bufferin®
Ecotrin®
Empirin®
Excedrin®
Ibuprofen®
Ketoprofen
Motrin®
Naprosyn®
Nuprin®
Orudis KT®
Pepto-Bismol®

You *may* take these nonprescription medications:
Acetaminophen
Allerest®
Benylin® Cough Syrup
Chlor-Trimeton®
Contac®
Drixoril®
Maalox®
Mylanta®
Robitussin® Cough Syrup
Sudafed®
Tylenol®
Tylenol Cold and Sinus®

Note: If you use antacids, such as Maalox® or Mylanta®, take them at least two hours before or two hours after taking your warfarin.

---

continues

INFORMATION ABOUT ANTICOAGULANT MEDICATIONS—ENOXAPARIN (LOVENOX®)

Your physician has ordered enoxaparin sodium, an anticoagulant, to prevent harmful blood clots from forming.

How Should I Take My Enoxaparin?

You will inject your enoxaparin subcutaneously (under your skin). Your physician, nurse, or pharmacist may measure the effectiveness and side effects of your treatment by physical examinations and asking questions about how you feel. The length of treatment depends on how your symptoms respond to the medication.

When Should I Give Myself Enoxaparin?

Be sure to follow your physician's instructions carefully. Give yourself only the number of enoxaparin injections your physician has prescribed for you each day. Remember:

- Take enoxaparin at the same time each day.
- If you take enoxaparin twice a day, space the injections approximately 12 hours apart. For example, inject yourself at 8 AM and 8 PM.
- For instructions on what to do if you miss a dose, call your physician immediately.
- Continue giving yourself the injections for exactly the number of days your physician has specified.

What Special Instructions Should I Follow While Using This Drug?

It is important to keep all appointments with your physician and the laboratory. You should carry a card or wear a bracelet indicating that you take anticoagulant medication so that people treating you will know this fact in case of an accident.

What Side Effects Can This Drug Cause?

Although side effects from enoxaparin are not common, they can occur. You should watch for signs of bleeding (see Signs of Bleeding To Watch for While You Are Taking Warfarin or Enoxaparin). You may also notice fever and nausea. If you experience any of these effects, call your physician immediately.

What Precautions Should I Follow if I Am Pregnant?

Women who are breastfeeding, pregnant, or planning a pregnancy should tell their physicians before taking enoxaparin. If you become pregnant while taking enoxaparin, promptly call your physician.

Are There Any Other Precautions I Should Follow?

Before taking this medication, tell your physician, pharmacist, or nurse if you know you are allergic to enoxaparin, any other drugs, or pork products. Also tell your doctor your entire medical history, especially bleeding problems (ulcer, or lengthy or heavy menstrual periods), diabetes, liver or kidney disease, high blood pressure, arthritis, seizures and thyroid problems, and if you have had recent surgery or have ever been given heparin.

Can I Take Other Medications While I Am Taking Enoxaparin?

Because certain medications may interact with enoxaparin, always tell your physician

continues

Treating and Preventing Blood Clots: What You Need To Know continued

and pharmacist what prescription and non-prescription medications you are taking, especially anticoagulants, such as warfarin (Coumadin®), phenytoin (Dilantin®), theophylline (Theo-Dur, Slo-phyllin®, Slo-bid®), and medication for high blood pressure or depression. Also tell your physician and pharmacist if you are taking aspirin, ibuprofen (Motrin®, Advil®) or other nonsteroidal anti-inflammatory drugs (NSAIDs), or cold medicines. Do not take any nonprescription medications without asking your physician or pharmacist.

How Should I Store My Enoxaparin?

Your health care provider will give you a several-day supply of prefilled syringes of enoxaparin at a time. You should store them in the refrigerator but do not let them freeze.

HOW TO GIVE YOURSELF AN INJECTION*

Enoxaparin should be injected into the layer of fat just under the skin in your abdomen. This is called a subcutaneous injection. Enoxaparin should never be injected into muscle as bleeding may occur. By gently pinching the skin between your fingers throughout the injection, the medicine enters only the fatty tissue of your abdomen and not the muscle.

Before you administer enoxaparin, look at the solution in the syringe closely. It should be clear and free of floating material. Do not use the syringe if the medication is discolored or contains particles, if a syringe leaks, or the

expiration date has passed. Use a new syringe, but show the damaged one to your health care provider.

Steps To Follow

1. Wash your hands well with soap and water. Dry your hands.
2. Sit or lie in a comfortable position so you can easily see the area of your abdomen where you will be injecting. A lounge chair, recliner, or bed propped up with pillows is ideal.

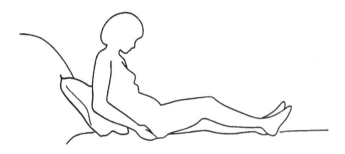

3. Select an area on the right or left side of your abdomen, at least two inches away from your belly button and out toward your sides.

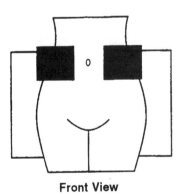

Front View

---

*Source: Reprinted with permission from Lovenox Patient Administration Guide, Rhône-Poulenc Rorer Pharmaceuticals, Inc. 1995. Collegeville, PA.

continues

Treating and Preventing Blood Clots: What You Need To Know continued

Remember:

Do not inject yourself within about two inches of your belly button or near scars or bruises. Alternate the site of injection between the left and right sides of the abdomen.

4. Clean the area you have selected for your injection with one of the alcohol swabs provided. Allow the area to dry.

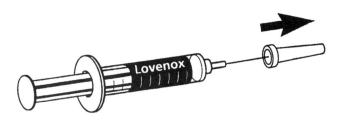

5. While the area is drying, carefully pull off the needle cap from the enoxaparin syringe and discard the cap. The syringe is prefilled and is ready to use. Do not press on the plunger before injection to expel the air bubble or medicine may be lost. To keep the needle sterile once you have removed the cap, do not set it down or touch the needle to anything.

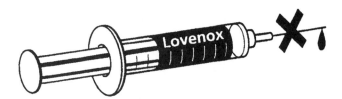

6. Hold the syringe in the hand you write with (like a pencil) and with your other hand gently pinch the clean area of your abdomen between your thumb and forefinger to make a fold in the skin. Be sure to hold the skin fold throughout the injection.

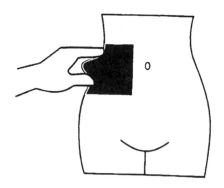

7. Vertically insert the full length of the needle (at a 90° angle) into the skin fold.

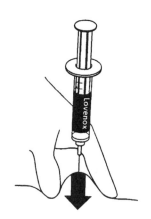

continues

Treating and Preventing Blood Clots: What You Need To Know continued

8. Press down on the plunger with your finger. This will deliver the medication into the fatty tissue of your abdomen. Be sure to hold the skin fold throughout the injection.

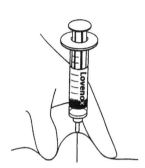

9. Remove the needle by pulling it straight out. You can now let go of the skin fold. To avoid bruising, do not rub the injection site after completion of the injection.
10. Drop the used syringe—needle first—into the sharps collector provided. Close the lid tightly and place the container out of reach of children. When the container is full, give it to your physician or home care nurse for disposal or contact your local trash service to find out if you can place it in your household trash.

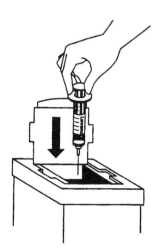

It is important to look at old injection sites for redness, pain, warmth, puffiness, discoloration of the skin, or oozing. These could be signs of infection or skin reaction.

If you do notice any of these signs listed above, contact your doctor immediately.

SIGNS OF BLEEDING TO WATCH FOR WHILE YOU ARE TAKING WARFARIN OR ENOXAPARIN

Since warfarin and enoxaparin prolong the time that blood takes to clot, it is important to watch for any signs of bleeding.

What Are the Signs of Bleeding?

Minor Bleeding

- Gums bleed while brushing teeth
- Easy bruising
- Longer periods of bleeding after minor cuts
- Prolonged menstrual bleeding
- Occasional nose bleeds

You may notice some of these types of minor bleeding while you are taking your medication. Most of the time this type of bleeding is nothing serious; however, if you are unsure whether the bleeding is significant, please call your physician. It may be necessary to decrease the dose of your medication to have your INR checked (if you are taking warfarin) to be sure.

Major Bleeding

- Blood in the urine (urine is dark red to brown in color)
- Bowel movements that are bloody, black, or tarry

continues

- Coughing up blood
- Severe headache
- Stomachache or back ache
- Bleeding into the whites of the eyes
- Very large bruises that do not heal
- Continuous or large amounts of bleeding

Call your physician right away if you notice any of these signs of major bleeding.

TAKING CARE OF YOURSELF WHILE YOU ARE TAKING WARFARIN AND/OR ENOXAPARIN

Taking anticoagulant medication should not prevent you from leading a normal, healthy lifestyle. Before making any drastic changes to your lifestyle, it is best to ask your physician for guidance.

Physical Activities

People taking anticoagulant medication can continue physical activities that are usually safe, such as walking, swimming, and gardening. These types of activities are beneficial because they help to promote good blood circulation. You should avoid body contact sports, such as football, or other activities in which injuries are more likely to occur. Discuss your current physical activities with your physician to see if you can safely continue them.

Who Should I Tell About Taking This Medication?

It is very important to tell all your physicians and your dentist that you are taking anticoagulant medication. Some treatments, such as the insertion of an intrauterine device, an injection, or pulling a tooth, can be more dangerous for people taking these medications. In such cases, let your physician or dentist know that you are taking an anticoagulant medication when making your appointment. Your physician may have to temporarily stop or change your medication before certain procedures can be done.

What Should I Tell My Physician on Regular Visits?

You should report:

- Any fall or injury
- Fever and chills that last more than one or two days
- Vomiting, nausea, and diarrhea for more than one or two days
- Severe chest pain
- Swelling of the arms or legs
- Any changes in your general health

Pregnancy

It is important to call your physician **immediately** if you think that you may be pregnant or are planning a pregnancy. Some anticoagulant medications can affect the development of the fetus during certain stages of pregnancy. Your physician can discuss with you the options for anticoagulant therapy during pregnancy.

In Case of an Emergency

If you have any signs of bleeding or clotting, it is important that you call your physician immediately. In case of an emergency, use your best judgment. If you think you need to be seen immediately, go to the nearest emergency department.

continues

Treating and Preventing Blood Clots: What You Need To Know continued

If you have any questions about your anti-coagulant medication, please call your physician.

TEST YOUR KNOWLEDGE

Please circle all of the correct answers.

1. Warfarin (Coumadin®) works to:
    a. Break down blood clots
    b. Prevent new blood clots from forming
    c. Prevent old blood clots from getting bigger
2. Enoxaparin (Lovenox®) works to:
    a. Break down blood clots
    b. Prevent new blood clots from forming
    c. Prevent old blood clots from getting bigger
3. List three signs of bleeding:
    _____
    _____
    _____
4. List three signs of a blood clot:
    _____
    _____
    _____
5. List the reason that you are taking warfarin or enoxaparin: _____
6. **True** or **False** (circle one):
    It is important to remind your dentist that you are taking warfarin.
7. Which food has a high amount of vitamin K? (circle one):
    Spinach
    Corn
    Coffee
    Milk
    Bread
8. **True** or **False** (circle one):
    It is okay to use aspirin without a prescription from your physician when you are taking warfarin or enoxaparin.

9. Eating foods that are high in vitamin K will increase or decrease (circle one) the effects of warfarin.
10. Too much warfarin can increase your chances of:
    bleeding or forming a blood clot (circle one)
11. **True** or **False** (circle one):
    Alcohol use is safe when you are taking warfarin.
12. What should you do if you notice dark urine or a red color in your urine or bowel movements?

Test Your Knowledge Answer Key

1. b and c
2. b and c
3. Bleeding gums
    Easy bruising
    Longer periods of bleeding after minor cuts
    Prolonged menstrual bleeding
    Occasional nose bleeds
    Blood in urine
    Bloody, black, tarry bowel movements
    Coughing up blood
    Severe headache
    Stomachache or back ache
    Bleeding into whites of the eyes
    Very large bruises that do not heal
    Continuous or large amounts of bleeding
4. Sudden weakness in the arms or legs
    Severe pain, redness, swelling in an arm or leg
    Numbness or tingling anywhere
    Changes or loss of sight in either eye
    Sudden occurrence of slurred speech or inability to speak
    Dizziness or faintness

continues

Treating and Preventing Blood Clots: What You Need To Know continued

Shortness of breath
Chest pain
5. Deep vein thrombosis, pulmonary embolism, atrial fibrillation, artificial heart valve, hereditary disorders, stroke or brain attack
6. True

7. Spinach
8. False
9. Decrease
10. Bleeding
11. False
12. Call your physician immediately.

NOTES:

Courtesy of Division of Internal Medicine, Anticoagulation Program, Thomas Jefferson University Hospital, Philadelphia, Pennsylvania.

Questions and Answers about Your Anticoagulant Medication

WHAT ARE ANTICOAGULANTS AND WHAT DO THEY DO?

Anticoagulants are medicines that are prescribed specifically to prevent and/or treat thrombosis. Thrombosis is the medical word for the formation of a clot inside your blood vessels. There are two types of anticoagulants:

1. *Heparin:* given by injection, usually at the beginning of treatment in the hospital.
2. *Oral anticoagulant:* taken by mouth. Warfarin sodium is most commonly prescribed.

WHY IS A CLOT DANGEROUS?

A clot may form in veins or arteries. If the clot grows, it can branch into other vessels and close them up. Rarely, it can also break into fragments—called emboli—swept along by the blood. Emboli from veins travel through the heart and lodge in lung vessels. These are called pulmonary emboli. Emboli from the heart or arteries can cause a stroke if they lodge in brain vessels or cause gangrene if they obstruct vessels in other organs or the limbs.

WHAT KIND OF MEDICATION AM I TAKING?

The medication you are taking is warfarin sodium.

HOW MUCH ANTICOAGULANT DO I NEED?

Dose

The amount of anticoagulant medication needed differs among people.

Test

To ensure that you have received the appropriate dose, your blood must be tested frequently. These tests might show that your needs for anticoagulation have changed. The test results guide your physician in modifying your dose accordingly.

WHAT IF I FORGET TO TAKE MY MEDICATION?

If, for some reason, you forget to (or cannot) take your prescribed dose at the usual time, take the dose as soon as you can or as soon as you remember. If you remember *only the next day*, carry on with your *regular dose schedule as prescribed. Do not take extra medication or double your dose to make amends.* Taking too large an amount at one time can be dangerous and cause bleeding.

If you do not take your medicine for two or three days, you should inform your physician at once. Your physician will then advise you what to do.

If you take the dose incorrectly, just continue with the proper schedule of medication.

If, for any reason, you have *not* taken your tablets as prescribed, remember to mention this to your physician at your next visit or blood test appointment, so that the results of the test will make sense and your dose schedule will not be changed needlessly.

HOW LONG DO I HAVE TO TAKE THIS MEDICATION?

The dose and the length of treatment will depend upon the illness that caused your

continues

blood to form clots. Some patients must take anticoagulant medication for the rest of their lives, but others need to take it for only three to four months.

WHAT SHOULD I BE AWARE OF?

The following are warning signs that tell your physician that your needs for the anticoagulant are changing. You must tell your physician as soon as you notice any of these signs:

- Bruises or tender swellings without obvious cause
- Severe and prolonged headaches
- Nosebleeds
- Coughing up blood
- Bleeding heavily from your gums after brushing your teeth
- Prolonged bleeding from small cuts
- Heavy bleeding at menstrual periods—such as twice the usual flow
- Swelling and tenderness or pain in your abdomen
- Vomiting red blood or material that looks like coffee grounds
- Bowel movements that are loose or contain blood or that are black and bad-smelling
- Urine that contains red blood or that is dark brown or cloudy
- Severe, prolonged back pain, without obvious cause
- If you have a fall or blow to the head, even if you do not lose consciousness or have a headache

WHAT SHOULD I TELL MY PHYSICIAN ON MY REGULAR VISITS?

You should report:

- Any fall or any injury of the head or back
- Fever and chills for more than one or two days
- Vomiting, nausea, or diarrhea for more than one or two days
- Repeated severe chest pain
- Persistent (for more than one or two days) swelling of feet and lower legs, especially if painful
- Yellow discoloration of eyes or skin or any changes to your general physical health

WHO SHOULD I TELL ABOUT TAKING THIS MEDICATION?

It is very important for you to tell your dentist or physician at the beginning of each visit that you are taking anticoagulant medication. Simple treatments, such as the insertion of an intrauterine device or even an injection, can be hazardous for patients taking anticoagulant medication. It is wise to review with the dentist or physician all of your other medications before treatment.

WHAT ABOUT PREGNANCY?

Oral anticoagulants are contraindicated for pregnant patients—meaning that you should not take this medication because it will affect the development of the fetus. If anticoagulation is required during pregnancy, heparin can be used. Heparin has no direct effect on the child or its development.

A woman who is planning to become pregnant and is on anticoagulants should tell her physician so that the physician can change her medication in time to prevent damage to the developing child.

continues

Questions and Answers continued

WHEN SHOULD I STOP TAKING MY MEDICATION?

You should not stop taking your medication on your own. Your physician will advise you when it is appropriate to do so.

WHAT ABOUT MY LIFESTYLE?

Oral anticoagulant therapy should not prevent you from leading a normal, healthy lifestyle. Before making any drastic changes to your current lifestyle (diet, alcohol consumption, exercise program) consult your physician.

Diet

Good nutrition is important for every aspect of your health, including the process of clotting. For some patients who need to eat a special diet, it is best to ask your physician to help you arrange for a visit to a dietitian for guidance. As a rule, never start on a "fad" diet or any diet radically different from your usual diet without first consulting your physician.

Alcohol

Any changes in alcohol consumption should be discussed with your physician.

Physical Activities

Patients taking anticoagulant medication can continue physical activities that are usually safe, such as walking, jogging, swimming, and gardening. These and other exercises are beneficial because they promote good blood circulation. Support stockings help in this by promoting blood flow through the veins.

Patients should avoid body contact sports and other activities in which injuries are more likely to occur. Discuss with your physician whether your current physical activities are safe enough to continue.

WHEN SHOULD I TAKE MY ANTICOAGULANTS?

It is best to take medicine at the same time every day. This establishes a routine that helps you remember your medicines and their doses.

SHOULD I EXPECT ANY SIDE EFFECTS?

Occasionally, you might experience some nausea when taking anticoagulants, as with any medicine, but this will be mild and often will pass as you become accustomed to the medicine. Rarely, some people develop a skin rash or a mild loss of hair, and they should call this to the physician's attention at the next visit.

CAN I TAKE OTHER MEDICATION?

You should not take any other medications on your own. It is best to check with your physician or pharmacist before starting to take any medicine, including such medications as cough/cold remedies, headache medicine, sleeping pills, and vitamins, because they can affect your anticoagulant therapy. This is especially important while your physician determines the best oral anticoagulant dose suited for you. Likewise, check with your physician if you stop taking any medicine because either starting or stopping medicine can easily change the way the anticoagulant acts.

continues

CONCLUSION

Anticoagulants have been prescribed for your present problem *only* and must be taken as directed. Never share this medication or any other.

KEEP YOUR MEDICATIONS AWAY FROM CHILDREN. Keep all medications out of reach of children.

KEEP YOUR MEDICATIONS IN THEIR ORIGINAL BOTTLES. There is less chance of taking the wrong medication.

NOTES:

If your physician tells you to stop taking the anticoagulant, do as directed. If there is any remaining anticoagulant, destroy it safely so that it will not be taken by mistake—by you or anyone else.

If any information in this handout worries you or if you would like to have more details, please ask your physician, but do not stop taking your medication, unless you are bleeding or otherwise ill, as described above.

Courtesy of Thrombosis Interest Group, Mississauga, Ontario.

Warfarin: Medication Information

1. Why is this medication prescribed?

   - To help prevent the formation of blood clots
   - To decrease the blood's ability to form clots.

2. How should it be used?

   - Exactly as ordered by your physician
   - Take at same time each day, with supper if possible

3. What should I do if I forget to take my warfarin?

   - Take it that day as soon as you remember.
   - If you skipped a whole day, do not take a double dose to catch up. Continue on dose as prescribed. Tell the nurse at your next protime if you missed a dose.

4. What side effects can this drug cause? Check with your physician if any of these occur:

   - Blood in urine (pink-tinged, red, or dark brown)
   - Red or black stools
   - Nosebleeds
   - Prolonged bleeding from cuts
   - Increase in menstrual flow or vaginal bleeding
   - Coughing or spitting up blood or material that looks like coffee grounds
   - Rash or hives
   - Fever or diarrhea
   - New onset of severe or continuing headache

   - All patients bruise easier while on warfarin, but massive or large areas of bruising are not considered normal and you should notify your physician

All medications have the potential for causing side effects. This usually occurs shortly after starting the medication or soon after an increase in the dose.

Other side effects might occur that usually don't require medical attention and frequently go away as your body adjusts to the medication. Call your physician, however, if any of the following side effects continue more than one or two days or are bothersome:

   - Bloated stomach or gas
   - Loss of appetite
   - Stomach cramps

5. What specific instructions should I follow while using this drug?

   - Avoid alcoholic beverages; they can react with warfarin. Contact your physician if you have questions.
   - Do not take any prescription or over-the-counter medications (including antibiotics and vitamins) without first checking with your physician.
   - Do not take aspirin unless your physician instructs differently.
   - Avoid *excessive* amounts of food that are high in vitamin K, such as leafy vegetables and broccoli. It is okay to eat normal servings each day. *No binge eating.*
   - Avoid crash diets.

continues

Warfarin: Medication Information continued

- Inform your physician immediately if you are or are planning to become pregnant.
- Please check with the physician or protime nurse before starting on any extended trip as this might influence your medication availability, scheduled protime tests, and eating habits.
- Inform other physicians and your dentist that you are taking warfarin. Before having any kind of surgery (including dental surgery) or emergency treatment, tell the physician (or dentist) that you are taking warfarin.

- Report any signs of bleeding to your physician.
- Get protimes (laboratory tests) as your physician instructs.
- If you experience severe bleeding, go to the nearest emergency department.
- When starting or stopping medicines, check with your physician.
- Initially, frequent adjustments of your warfarin dose might be necessary. If you do not hear from the protime nurse by 4 PM on the day of your laboratory test, please call for your warfarin instructions.

NOTES:

Courtesy of Indiana Heart Physicians, Beech Grove, Indiana.

Anticoagulants

This handout has been given to you because you are on an anticoagulant. It is important for you to know as much about this medication as possible. Coumadin is the trade name for warfarin sodium, which is the most commonly used anticoagulant. Anticoagulants are often called "blood-thinners" but they don't thin the blood. Warfarin decreases the clotting ability of blood and helps to prevent harmful clots from forming.

RESPONSIBILITIES

It is your responsibility to:

- Know the information in this booklet.
- Cooperate with your health care providers in managing your anticoagulation.
- Inform your health care providers of any problems that you think are related to your anticoagulation.

WARFARIN EFFECTS

- There are many different reasons to use an anticoagulant. You need to know why you are on this medication. The effect of an anticoagulant can vary greatly from person to person. Even within the same person, the effects can vary over time. That is why it is so important to have your blood level checked regularly.
- The blood test is called "prothrombin time," or PT for short. The PT is used to calculate a number called the INR (International Normalized Ratio). Your INR range is _____.

WARNING SIGNS

You must always watch for symptoms that might be problems caused by your warfarin.

- The following signs might indicate that you are bleeding:

  - Red or dark brown urine
  - Red or black, tarry bowel movements
  - A severe headache or stomachache
  - Unexplained bruising, frequent nose-bleeds, bleeding gums, or other unusual bleeding
  - Vomiting or coughing up blood
- The following symptoms should make you suspicious of a new clot:
  - New leg swelling, pain, or redness
  - New shortness of breath or other breathing difficulties
  - Sudden new visual or speech problems, numbness, tingling, difficulty using an arm or leg, or other neurologic changes worrisome for a stroke

If you experience any of these signs or symptoms, contact your physician, your warfarin care provider, or your primary care team, or come to the hospital admitting office *immediately!*

DIET

Diet can affect anticoagulants:

- Don't drastically change your eating habits.
- Maintain a *steady* diet.
- Vitamin K works against warfarin. Vitamin K is high in leafy green vegetables (broccoli, kale, collard greens, cabbage, cauliflower, spinach).

continues

Anticoagulants continued

OTHER MEDICATIONS AND ANTICOAGULANTS

- Many medications can interact with an anti-coagulant. Some increase your bleeding time (PT); others can decrease it. Please let the Anticoagulation Clinic know if your prescribed medications are:
  - Increased
  - Decreased
  - Stopped
  - New ones begun (especially *antibiotics*)
  We will check your INR as soon as possible.
- Medications you buy without a prescription can also affect anticoagulants:
  - Avoid aspirin (acetylsalicylic acid); use Tylenol instead (acetaminophen).
  - Notify your warfarin care provider if you decide to start any new vitamin or herbal product or other over-the-counter products.
  - Read the labels on nonprescription medications to be sure that aspirin-containing drugs are not included in the preparation.

HINTS YOU NEED TO KNOW

- Take your anticoagulant at the same time every day. If you miss a dose, *do not* try to catch up.
- Keep a written medication calendar—mark down the dose for each day, and cross it off when you take it. Or, use a seven-day pillbox.
- Keep a written record of your dose schedule. The dose might change often.
- Call or come to the hospital if you:
  - Have a fall or other injury
  - Have a big change in your diet
  - Have a major change in your life
  - Have anything that you think might be affecting your bleeding time

REMEMBER

- Wear a Medic-Alert identification bracelet or necklace.
- Carry a completed medical alert history card in your wallet.
- When you go to any doctors or dentists, tell them you are taking an anticoagulant. Show them your Medic-Alert card.
- Avoid alcohol. The interaction of an anti-coagulant and alcohol can be very serious.
- Guard against the risk of accidents. For example:
  - Wear shoes.
  - Wear gloves for woodworking, gardening, and similar activities.
  - Use an electric razor to shave.
- Keep your scheduled laboratory test appointment. Call if you are unable to keep your appointment.

PROBLEMS OR QUESTIONS

If you have a problem, especially any signs of bleeding, contact your warfarin care provider, your primary care team, or the hospital admitting office. Your warfarin care provider is: _____.

The telephone number is: _____.

The hospital admitting office telephone number is: _____.

Please call your warfarin care provider on the afternoon of the lab test for:
- PT results
- Next PT date

Remember: to help prevent complications, it is critical that you work closely with your warfarin care provider.

Courtesy of Red Primary Care Team, Veterans Affairs Medical Center, Salt Lake City, Utah.

Anticoagulation Clinic Patient Education Form

Date: _____

DOSAGE

- It is important for you to take the warfarin dosage prescribed. Because this dosage can change from visit to visit, we *strongly* recommend using a pillbox. When you fill the pillbox, check the pills to be sure you are using the correct:

       – Milligram dosage   – Number of tablets
       – Color   – Correct brand name

- You must take your warfarin tablets on an unchanging schedule. You should take them:
  – At the same time every day
  – Only in the prescribed amount
- If you completely forget to take a tablet, let me know at your next visit. *Do not* take another tablet to "catch up." If you forget to take a tablet at the usual time, you may take it later on the same day.
- Because many other medicines can affect the action of warfarin, you should check with me when you begin taking any other medicines. You should not take such over-the-counter drugs as aspirin or ibuprofen. You may take Tylenol.
  – Inform me if you have any illness that might require any other medication.
  – Inform other physicians or dentists that you are taking warfarin.
  – Inform me *before* making any change in current medications.
- Women: Inform me immediately if you are *pregnant or* if you are planning to become pregnant.

LIFESTYLE

- In general, you should report any lifestyle changes to me.
- Because many factors can affect the action of warfarin, it is important that you maintain a *consistent* (unchanging) lifestyle in terms of:
  – Eating habits (especially in regard to the amount of green vegetables you eat)
  – Alcohol consumption
  – Exercise
- Please check with me before starting on any extended trip as this might influence your medication availability, scheduled protime tests, and eating habits.

continues

SPECIAL CONSIDERATIONS

- Because warfarin therapy affects the clotting factors in your blood, it is important that you call me promptly if any of the following occur:
  - Bleeding—prolonged bleeding from cuts, increased menstrual flow or vaginal bleeding, nosebleeds, or bleeding of gums from brushing
  - Unusual bleeding or bruising
  - Red or dark brown urine or red or tar-black stools
  - Diarrhea, infection, or fever
  - Pain, swelling, or discomfort

IMPORTANT REMINDERS

- *Please report for all protime tests at scheduled times!* This blood test is important. We will use this test to monitor the balance of warfarin in your blood and make adjustments to your dosage to keep it at the appropriate level.
- If you have any questions regarding warfarin therapy or if you need to change an appointment time, please call me at _____ or call the clinic at _____.
- If you have an emergency after hours or on weekends, please contact the Emergency Department at _____.

Patient's signature _____

Date_____

Nurse Practitioner's signature _____

NOTES:

Courtesy of Anticoagulation Clinic, University of Virginia Medical Center, Charlottesville, Virginia.

Anticoagulation Services

Welcome! Now that you've been prescribed an anticoagulant medication (warfarin), you've become part of a very special program. The program is designed to help you and your physician during the time you will be taking this medication. We will discuss warfarin in depth with you, as well as the routine you can expect in the future. You'll also receive various information materials designed to assist you in taking the medication properly. You will play an important role in ensuring the success of your therapy. You'll probably have many questions about warfarin. This handout will answer some of those questions, but always feel free to call us with any concerns that may arise.

WHAT IS ANTICOAGULATION?

Coagulation is a term that refers to formation of blood clots, a normal body reaction if, for example, you cut yourself. Warfarin is called an anticoagulant because it works against the formation of blood clots that could be harmful to you. Although warfarin is sometimes called a "blood-thinner," it works in the liver to decrease the production of natural blood components called clotting factors. In many cases, warfarin is used as a preventive treatment to reduce the chance of forming a blood clot that could hurt you. Warfarin therapy is also used by people who have already experienced a serious blood clot.

HOW IS TREATMENT WITH WARFARIN MONITORED?

Your body's response to warfarin is monitored by a blood test, the result of which is called the International Normalized Ratio (INR). The blood test can be done by two methods:

(1) by drawing a small amount of blood from the arm and (2) by a fingerstick to obtain a drop of blood. When you begin taking warfarin, this blood test must be done frequently (once or twice weekly) to determine your body's sensitivity to the medication. As you become stabilized on warfarin (after a few weeks), the frequency of blood test monitoring will be gradually reduced. Most people taking warfarin on an ongoing basis require a blood test only once a month.

WHAT IS THE INR?

The International Normalized Ratio is the name for the blood test used to monitor your warfarin. Because the test result may normally vary from day to day, we try to maintain your INR number within a desired range (never a specific number). The goal INR range for most people is 2.0 to 3.0, although some people require a reading of 2.5 to 3.5 (or higher). We will discuss with you what your target range will be. Remember, changes in your overall health, physical activity, diet, or other medications can affect your INR reading.

WHY DOES MY WARFARIN DOSAGE CHANGE?

The effect you get from the amount of warfarin you take depends on several things, including changes in your other medications, illness, your diet, and your general lifestyle. To ensure that you continue to take the correct amount of warfarin, you should do three things:

1. Take warfarin each day, according to the directed schedule. Your warfarin calendar will help you keep track of the correct dosage.

continues

Anticoagulation Services continued

2. Have your blood test done regularly as scheduled by the anticoagulation staff.
3. Always report all changes in your other medications, health, and lifestyle to us. Call us anytime at _____.

WHEN SHOULD I COME IN FOR MY WARFARIN BLOOD TEST?

Each time you have your INR test done, the staff will tell you the next date to have your blood tested again. If you are having your blood tests done by the fingerstick method, you will be given a specific appointment time with the staff. If you are having blood drawn from your arm at the laboratory, you can have your test done (without an appointment) during normal business hours, but mornings are preferred so that we may contact you with the report the same day. A standing order for the INR test is kept in the laboratory during the entire time you take warfarin. *If you are unable to have your blood tested on the date specified by the staff, please call our office immediately.*

WHY IS IT IMPORTANT TO USE THE WARFARIN CALENDAR?

Because your warfarin dosage can change from one day to the next, we strongly encourage you to keep track of your doses in the calendar provided. *Check the calendar each day to see how much warfarin to take—don't guess.* If you get confused, just give us a call.

WHEN IS THE BEST TIME TO TAKE MY WARFARIN EACH DAY?

Warfarin is taken just *once each day.* As a general rule, we advise all patients to take warfarin at approximately the same time each day, usually about 6 PM. If you have difficulty remembering to take warfarin in the evening, please discuss this with the staff. You can take warfarin with or without food (it won't upset your stomach). You can also take warfarin at the same time as most other medications.

WHAT ABOUT MY OTHER MEDICATIONS?

Any medication (prescription or over-the-counter) can potentially affect your body's response to warfarin. *Always let us know whenever you begin a new medication or stop taking an old one.* In most cases, we are able to predict how other medications will affect your warfarin, and we will adjust your dosage accordingly. Other important points to remember:

- Never take aspirin (along with warfarin) without our knowledge. If your physician has recommended that you take one coated aspirin/Ecotrin daily, do not take more than this while you are taking warfarin. Your daily coated aspirin/Ecotrin dose should never exceed 325 mg.
- Do not take ibuprofen (Advil, Motrin, Nuprin, Medipren, Excedrin IB, Haltran, Midol 200, Pamprin-IB, Trendar, or others), naproxen (Aleve, Naprosyn, Anaprox), ketoprofen (Orudis, Actron), cimetidine (Tagamet HB), orfamotidine (Pepcid AC) while taking warfarin.
- Do not take vitamin E or vitamin C supplements without our knowledge.

WHAT CAN I TAKE SAFELY ALONG WITH WARFARIN?

- For headache or pain relief: acetaminophen (Tylenol)

continues

Anticoagulation Services continued

- For constipation: Metamucil or Milk of Magnesia
- For cold symptoms: Sudafed (to decongest), Chlor-Trimeton or Benadryl (for runny nose/sneezing/watery eyes), and Robitussin (for cough).

WHAT IF I'M SCHEDULED TO SEE ANOTHER DOCTOR OR MY DENTIST?

- Tell *all* health care providers that you are taking warfarin.
- Contact us if and when you will be seeing another physician, particularly if surgery or dental procedures are involved. We might need to adjust your warfarin dosage before your appointment. Some people (with artificial heart valves) will also need antibiotics beforehand, even for such a minor procedure as teeth cleaning.
- Call and let us know about any new medication that anyone prescribes for you before you begin taking it.

WHAT ARE WARFARIN'S SIDE EFFECTS?

Warfarin is relatively free of side effects; it will not make you drowsy, change your blood pressure, make your mouth dry, or increase your heart rate. If something feels different from normal that you think might be caused by the medication, however, please call so that we can discuss it.

MUST I CHANGE MY DIET WHILE TAKING WARFARIN?

Some foods are high in vitamin K, which can counteract the effect of warfarin. You may continue to include these foods in your diet in moderation, that is, one normal serving-size portion (3–4 oz) per day. Common foods high in vitamin K include green leafy vegetables (broccoli, brussel sprouts, cauliflower, spinach, other greens), chick peas, beef and pork liver, and green tea (served in Oriental restaurants). Most important, be consistent with what you normally eat, and notify us if you wish to go on any special diet. Likewise, you should also call us if you're ill (vomiting/diarrhea) and not eating at all, as this will affect your warfarin.

MAY I DRINK ALCOHOL WHILE TAKING WARFARIN?

Alcoholic beverages, *in moderation,* are safe while taking warfarin; this means a maximum of two drinks per day (1 beer = 1 glass of wine = 1 cocktail/shot). Excessive alcohol intake puts you at significant risk for injury and potential bleeding complications while taking warfarin. Use common sense, and be careful.

MUST I LIMIT MY DAILY ACTIVITIES WHILE TAKING WARFARIN?

Remember that because you're taking warfarin, you might have an increased risk for bleeding. Moderate exercise and activity are safe for most people taking warfarin, but always check with your physician before beginning any sports activity or situation that can put you at increased danger of injury.

WHAT IF I FORGET TO TAKE A DOSE OF WARFARIN?

Take it as soon as you remember, even up until noon of the following day (you'll also take that day's dose at the normally scheduled time). If you forget altogether or aren't sure what to do, please call us before taking the next dose.

continues

WHAT IF I EXPERIENCE SOME UNUSUAL BLEEDING?

Signs of bleeding include prolonged bleeding from cuts, nosebleeds, gum bleeding, increased vaginal bleeding, blood in the urine, red/black stools. If bleeding from the nose or skin, apply firm, direct pressure to the area until bleeding stops. If you notice blood in the urine or with a bowel movement, call us immediately. You might note a few more bruises on your skin while taking warfarin; this is not worrisome unless they become large or painful or don't go away in a reasonable time. When in doubt, please call. Bleeding may be a sign that your INR is too high.

WHAT IF I GET SICK?

Acute illness will change your body's response to warfarin. An episode of congestive heart failure, fever (over 101°F), flu, viral/bacterial infection, nausea, or vomiting (for more than 24 hours) can cause warfarin to accumulate in your body and your INR to go up dramatically. If you experience any of the above, please contact the staff so we can discuss how you're feeling. Remember also to *call us before you begin taking antibiotics for any reason*. Your warfarin dosage must be adjusted in almost all cases. If you should decide to have a flu shot, plan to have your INR tested 7–10 days later, as it also can affect your warfarin response.

Warfarin is a complex medicine that is helpful for many people with your medical history. You are the most important person in ensuring that your therapy is successful. Remember:

- Let all health care providers know that you're taking warfarin.
- Have your INR tested regularly as scheduled.
- Food, drink, illness, and other medications affect your warfarin.
- Call us at _____ with any questions you might have. We're here to help you.

NOTES:

Courtesy of Anticoagulation Services of Rochester, Wilson Medical Center, Rochester, New York.

Anticoagulation Service: Patient Instructions

1. Do not take any medications without contacting the anticoagulation service first, even those your doctor prescribes. Do not take aspirin, Anacin, Bayer, Nuprin, or Advil.

   Note: The medication you get in the hospital and will take at home is not a problem, but from then on, *call us.*

2. If you get ill, such as a cold, flu, stomach bug, *call us* and let us know.

3. Warfarin makes it easier for you to bleed. If you notice bleeding, *call us.* Watch your stools and urine each day. If the stool is black or red or if the urine is red, *call us.*

4. Do not drink more than two alcohol drinks in one day.

5. Do not change your diet without telling us.

6. Warfarin is taken *just once each day.* We like you to take it at about 6:00 PM or later.

7. Keep track of your doses in the calendar provided. Be sure and check how much warfarin you should take each day by checking the calendar first—don't guess! If you get confused, give us a call.

8. We will call you each time that you get a blood test in the late afternoon. We will tell you how much of the warfarin to take for the next several days so that you can put it right in your calendar.

9. If you miss a dose of warfarin for the whole day, call us before taking the next dose.

10. We will want to get a protime (the blood test) twice a week for the first couple of weeks. It is best to come into the health center between 8:30 AM and 11:00 AM and go to the laboratory desk. Tell them you are here for a protime and "your slip is on file."

11. We will call you the day you get out of the hospital (except Sunday) to make sure you know how much warfarin to take and when to come in for a blood test.

NOTES:

Courtesy of Anticoagulation Services of Rochester, Wilson Medical Center, Rochester, New York.

Anticoagulation Patient Information Sheet

PATIENT INFORMATION

1. Take warfarin at the same time each day.
2. Report for your blood test on the scheduled date.
3. Observe for any signs of bleeding.
4. *Avoid* aspirin products, multivitamins containing vitamin K, and ibuprofen.
5. Inform staff of any dietary changes.
6. Avoid/limit alcoholic intake.
7. Be safety conscious to avoid accidents and injury.
8. Inform anticoagulation clinic of all medicine changes.

REMEMBER

Report any of the following to your physician or nurse:

- Nosebleeds
- Bleeding from mouth or gums
- Coughing up blood
- Blood in urine and bowel movements
- Abnormal vaginal bleeding
- Easy bruising
- Cuts that will not stop bleeding

TELEPHONE NUMBERS TO KNOW

Weekdays, _____ AM–_____ PM: call _____

Evening, night, weekend: call _____

Note: Have this information sheet and your medical record number available when you call.

_____   Information given by   _____
Date   Signature

I understand this information   _____
                                Signature

Courtesy of Anticoagulation Clinic, University of Massachusetts Medical Center, Worcester, Massachusetts.

Hechos Importantes Acerca de su Terapia con Warfarin

Si se olvida de tomar una postilla un día, avísele a su médico. NO TOME OTRA PATRILLA PARA "RECUPERARSE."

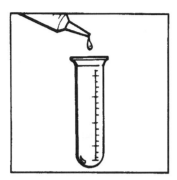

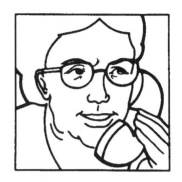

HÁGASE UNA PRUEBA DE SANGRE

Coumadin* es usado para evitar que se formen coágulos sanguineos perjudiciales. La formación de estos coágulos dañinos podría resultar en condicíones más seria. *Es importante que Ud. se someta a una prueba de sangre para determinar su tiempo de "pro-thrombin"* ("Protime").* Su Protime le permite a su médico monitorar su terapia Coumadin* y le ayuda a ajustar su dosificación. El Protime también le ayuda a saber si Ud. podria tener un riesgo de hemorragia. Esta prueba de laboratorio también se informa como "International Normalized Ratio" (Ración Internacional Normalizada) o INR.

*Protrombina

INFORME ACERCA DE CUALQUIER PROBLEMA

Llame a su médico o enfermera inmediatamente, al si tiene:

- Una fiebre o una enfermedad en desarrollo, incluyenda vómito, diarrea o infección
- Dolor, hinchazón, incomodidad, u otros sin-tomas inusuales
- Sangrado prolongado de cortaduras, y san-grado de la nariz
- Sangrado inusualmente de las encias al cepillarse los dientes
- Flujo mentrual más fuerte, o sangrado vaginal
- Orina roja o marrón (café) oscuro
- Heces rojas o de un negro similar al alquitran
- Magulladuras inusuales, por razones des-conocidas
- Embarazo o embarazo planificado

continúa

Hechos Importantes Acerca de su Terapia con Warfarin continuación

Llame a su médico inmediatamente si sufre una caida o un trauma serio.

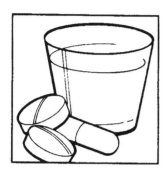

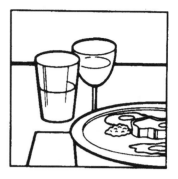

CONVERSE CON SU MÉDICO Y FARMACÉUTICO ACERCA DE CUALQUIER MEDICAMENTO NUEVO

Converse con su médico antes de comenzar a tomar, cambiar o descontinuar cualquier medicamento.

SIEMPRE CUÉTELE A SU MÉDICO, DENTISTA, FARMACÉUTICO O ENFERMERA QUE UD. ESTÁ TOMANDO COUMADIN.

TRATE DE INGERIR LA MISMA DIETA GENERAL Y EVITAR CANTIDADES EXCESIVAS DE ALCOHOL.

Source: Adapted with permission from *Multilingual Support for Your Patients on Coumadin Therapy*, © 1994, DuPont Pharma.

Checklist for Documenting Formal Instruction on Use of Warfarin

The patient has received formal instruction on the use of warfarin. Topics covered include (check all that are appropriate):

___Rationale for therapy
___How warfarin works to benefit the patient
___Potential drug interactions
___Avoidance of aspirin
___Activities
___Dietary considerations (including alcohol use)
___Laboratory monitoring (INRs)
___When to take doses
___What to do about missed doses
___Signs of overanticoagulation
___Signs of disease recurrence
___What to do in case of bleeding
___Planned length of therapy
___Dose
___Keeping log of INR results and medications

The patient has received the following materials:

___Written patient information on warfarin therapy
___Medic-Alert ID application
___Compliance aids (if appropriate)
___Appointment card
___Saw video on using warfarin safely and effectively
___Listened to audiotape on using warfarin safely and effectively

Courtesy of Lutheran General Health System Anticoagulation Center, Niles, Illinois.

What Do You Know about Warfarin (Coumadin)?

LOCATION_____   DATE_____

NAME_____

1. What is your current dose of Warfarin (Coumadin)? _____
2. I take Warfarin (Coumadin) because: _____ heart beat is not regular
                                          _____ have had blood clots in the past
                                          _____ heart valve replacement
                                          _____ other reason:

	TRUE	FALSE
3. Warfarin (Coumadin) is a helpful medication because it helps reduce clots from forming in the blood.		
4. Warfarin (Coumadin) can dissolve blood clots that have already formed.		
5. You should take your warfarin (Coumadin) at the same time every day.		
6. You should tell your health care provider about any other medicines you are taking (prescription and over-the-counter).		
7. You should ask your health care provider before you change, start, or stop taking any other medicines.		
8. You can take an extra Coumadin pill to catch up if you have forgotten a dose.		
9. Being ill may affect your PT/INR.		
10. It's okay to miss your ProTime (PT) appointment as long as you get it next month.		
11. You do not need to tell anyone else giving you medical or dental care that you are taking warfarin (Coumadin).		
12. If you have bleeding gums, nosebleeds, or bright red blood in your urine or stool, you should get your ProTime (PT) tested.		
13. Bruising can be a sign that your PT needs to be tested.		
14. Black stool or dark urine is not a sign of bleeding.		
15. Alcohol intake is always okay.		
16. It's okay to take aspirin, Advil, or Aleve without checking with your physician.		
17. Foods high in vitamin K can affect your warfarin (Coumadin) dose.		
18. Your diet does not have to be consistent while taking warfarin (Coumadin).		
19. Brussel sprouts are low in vitamin K.		
20. Absolutely no greens should be eaten while taking warfarin (Coumadin).		

continues

	TRUE	FALSE
21. Greens only need to be limited to a consistent amount while you are on warfarin (Coumadin).		
22. Fruit is high in vitamin K.		
23. All vegetables are high in vitamin K.		
24. Turnip greens, kale, and spinach are high in vitamin K.		
25. Some multivitamin supplements also contain vitamin K.		

When were you first started on Coumadin? _____

NOTES:

Courtesy of Prime Care Clinic, Veterans Affairs Medical Center, Dayton, Ohio.

Chapter 11

Quality Assurance for Anticoagulation Management Services

Christine A. Sorkness

INTRODUCTION

The purpose of an anticoagulation management service (AMS) is to increase the efficacy and safety of anticoagulation therapies through patient education, monitoring, and follow-up. In most circumstances, warfarin is the anticoagulation therapy of choice; however, heparin and low–molecular-weight heparins are increasingly prescribed alternatives for outpatients. Irrespective of the anticoagulant selected, the dual therapeutic objectives are (1) prevention of thromboembolic disease and (2) prevention of hemorrhagic complications. The following discussion provides quality assurance considerations and guidelines for an AMS in order to achieve these two important objectives.

ANTICOAGULATION MANAGEMENT SERVICE STRUCTURE

In order for an AMS to accomplish its goals effectively, an adequate administrative and personnel structure must be established. Exhibit 11–1 outlines the essential components of an AMS. First, the scope of services to be provided must be defined. These services can include patient education; initiation of anticoagulation therapies, on either an inpatient or an outpatient basis; patient monitoring; acquisition of laboratory samples; patient home visits; nursing home consultation; and anticoagulation therapy regimen adjustment. The specific days and hours of AMS operation must be established, as well as adequate physical space procured.

Mechanisms for efficient patient referral must be established, with considerations made for various patient sources (eg, inpatient consultation, hospital discharge referral, outpatient referral, and home care referral). Essential components of the referral include medical indication for anticoagulation, desired intensity and duration of anticoagulation, and relevant medical/social history that could influence anticoagulation outcomes. Adequate laboratory services must be available, with the ability to access essential anticoagulation parameters in an accurate and timely manner. A medical charting mechanism must be defined, either by utilization of institutionwide patient medical records or by dictated patient encounters transmitted to the referring physician. AMS personnel, in turn, must have access to relevant patient health information and data in order to assess the risks and benefits of anticoagulation on an ongoing basis. A quality assurance process must be defined and implemented.

A sufficient number of adequately trained and committed health professionals must be available to support the patient referral base and the scope of services provided. Each practitioner's scope of practice must be defined, with clinical privileges established and annually reapproved by the responsible institution. Exhibit 11–2 outlines the essential components in a clinical privilege statement for an AMS and its providers. It is essential that an adequate physician support system be defined if the AMS is primarily staffed by non-physician personnel (clinical pharmacists, nurse clinicians/practitioners, physician assistants) and be able to address both emergent and nonemergent patient issues.

Exhibit 11–1
ANTICOAGULATION MANAGEMENT SERVICE STRUCTURE: CHECKLIST

ADMINISTRATION	Yes	No	PERSONNEL	Yes	No
Scope of services defined	___	___	Adequate numbers to support patient base	___	___
Days/hours of operation established	___	___	Adequate training to support scope of services	___	___
Location of clinic identified	___	___	Scope of practice defined	___	___
Mechanism(s) for referral established	___	___	Clinical privileges established	___	___
Laboratory support established	___	___	Clinical privileges annually reapproved	___	___
Medical charting mechanism defined	___	___	Physician support system defined	___	___
Access to relevant patient health data/information established	___	___	Adequate visiting nurse services available	___	___
			CLIA standards met by laboratory personnel	___	___
Quality assurance process defined	___	___	Off-clinic hours personnel coverage available	___	___
			Adequate clerical personnel available	___	___

Exhibit 11–2
COMPONENTS IN A CLINICAL PRIVILEGE STATEMENT FOR AN AMS AND ITS PROVIDERS

Example 1

- Review the clinical records including indications for the anticoagulant, INRs, and medications.
- Prescribe anticoagulants (renew orders, adjust dosages, etc.) without cosignature for patients in the AMS.
- Renew maintenance medications for AMS patients, except for controlled substances.
- Utilize medical staff guidelines when prescribing anticoagulants.
- Clinical concerns will be addressed by the primary care provider.
- Provide patients with instructions regarding the safe and appropriate use of the anticoagulant therapy.

Example 2

- Initiating orders for selective drug therapies and diagnostic tests according to established protocols
- Developing, ordering, and adjusting individualized patient dosing regimens with the consent of the responsible physician
- Conducting and coordinating clinical drug investigations and research under Food and Drug Administration guidelines and regulations and approved by the local research and development committee
- Serving as clinical managers of drug and drug-related problems in clinics and wards in conjunction with the clinical staff
- Identifying and recommending corrective actions for drug-induced problems in association with the clinical staff
- Implementing protocols approved by the pharmacy and therapeutics committee in the use of nonformulary drugs and restricted drugs

If home-based patients are enrolled in the AMS, adequate visiting nurse services will be required for the acquisition of laboratory data and patient communication and supervision. All laboratory testing must be performed by clinical laboratory improvement amendments–certified personnel. Off-hours coverage (evenings, weekends, holidays) must be available. Adequate clerical personnel must be trained to maintain the necessary AMS infrastructure. Typical clerical duties include maintenance of patient referral systems, patient scheduling, medical record acquisition, communication with outside laboratories, and patient follow-up for missed appointments.

MANAGEMENT ANALYSIS

Analysis of the management of patients followed by the AMS should be included in a thorough quality assurance program. Many AMSs audit the percentage of patient encounters in which the International Normalized Ratio (INR) is either above the upper limit or below the lower limit of the designated therapeutic range. Although these statistics can be followed on an ongoing basis, it is imperative that the medical implications of these values be reviewed and that explanations for INR values outside of therapeutic range be assessed. To determine whether circumstances allow a deviation from the 100% standard, potential drug and nondrug causes of INR changes, such as laboratory or sample-handling error, drug interaction, compliance problem, dietary change, or change in medical status, must be identified.

Other management processes that can be audited on an ongoing basis include patient adherence with follow-up appointments, pharmaceutical care interventions (whether or not specifically related to anticoagulation), and the compliance of AMS practitioners with the warfarin or heparin management protocols established by the AMS.

DRUG USE EVALUATION

Applications for Anticoagulation Management Services

The Joint Commission on Accreditation of Healthcare Organizations (Joint Commission) was formed in 1951 to improve the quality of care provided to the public. Drug use evaluation (DUE) is mandatory for member institutions. The 1994 Joint Commission standards emphasize that DUE is a criteria-based, ongoing systematic process designed to maintain the appropriate and effective use of drugs.[1] DUE is a sophisticated analysis of drugs, their uses, and their contributions to various patient outcomes.[2] It can focus on a particular drug, an entire class of drugs, or the therapy of a specific condition. Anticoagulants are frequently evaluated because they meet four criteria advocated by the Joint Commission: (1) frequently prescribed, (2) known or suspected to present significant risk, (3) known or suspected to be problem prone, and (4) represent a critical component of the care provided for a specific diagnosis, condition, or procedure.[3]

Warfarin DUE criteria, titled "Criteria for Use of Warfarin in Adult Inpatients and Outpatients,"[4] serve as a starting point for application to specific AMS settings. The criteria were developed by utilizing peer-reviewed literature published in professional journals, as well as the 1992 Third ACCP (American College of Chest Physicians) Consensus Conference on Antithrombotic Therapy guidelines.[5] They address justification for use (indications for warfarin), critical (process) indicators, complications of therapy, and patient outcome measures. Each criterion consists of an element, a standard, exceptions to the element, and sources of information. The element is the minimal level of evidence needed to show that patient care is optimal. The standard defines the deviation from an element that is acceptable. If no deviation is acceptable, the standard is 100%. Exceptions to an element allow for justifiable clinical variation; they define situations that constitute probable justification for failure to meet that element.

Anticoagulant drug use in specific AMS settings can be assessed retrospectively, concurrently, or prospectively. Ret-

rospective DUEs are conducted after completion of a course of drug therapy or, in hospitalized patients, after discharge. As a consequence, follow-up action does not produce specific changes in an individual patient's drug therapy. Concurrent DUEs are conducted during the course of therapy and allow for an active intervention to correct specific problems in an individual anticoagulated patient. Prospective DUEs evaluate the anticipated drug therapy before it is initiated so that active intervention to correct problems can occur prior to drug use. DUE programs of an AMS should not be limited to or rely on any one method. Prospective and concurrent DUEs allow for impact on an individual patient; however, retrospective DUEs are often most feasible and can accommodate aggregate data analysis. In order to perform successful DUEs, especially with the retrospective method, accurate and complete medical record documentation is essential. Exhibit 11–3 outlines items for inclusion in an AMS patient encounter that are required for comprehensive DUE data collection.

Indications for Use of Warfarin

A frequently performed DUE focuses on appropriate indications of warfarin therapy in an enrolled AMS setting. Justification for the use of warfarin, as described by the DUE criteria above, are divided into two categories: (1) prophylaxis of patient at risk for thromboembolic disease and (2) treatment of pulmonary embolism or deep vein thrombosis. Table 11–1 outlines recommended criteria for use of warfarin. These criteria are largely based on those previously published[4] and modified in accordance with specific recommendations from the 1995 Fourth ACCP Consensus Conference on Antithrombotic Therapy.[6] Importantly, the justification for use of warfarin in atrial fibrillation has been updated.[7]

Medical records of enrolled AMS patients should be reviewed to determine if the use of warfarin can be justified by these criteria. Those patients who deviate from the standard require a clinical evaluation of the specific medical circumstances, an appropriate intervention (eg, discontinuation of therapy), and a follow-up assessment.

OUTCOME-BASED QUALITY ASSURANCE

A successful and relevant quality assurance program for an AMS should include an assessment of outcomes, including clinical and psychologic outcomes and resource utilization. These data are necessary for quality improvement, and they also can be used for ongoing justification of the AMS or to alter resource allocation for the AMS. Outcome analysis can be performed either retrospectively or prospectively. Ideally, independent trained abstractors should review the AMS records and use standardized, validated forms.

Exhibit 11–3
ANTICOAGULATION MANAGEMENT: PATIENT ENCOUNTER CHECKLIST

Item	Chart Documentation of Item	
Indication for anticoagulation	_____ Yes	_____ No
Target INR or activated partial thromboplastin time*	_____ Yes	_____ No
Planned duration for anticoagulation treatment	_____ Yes	_____ No
Current anticoagulant dose/regimen	_____ Yes	_____ No
Adherence assessment	_____ Yes	_____ No
Adverse events assessment	_____ Yes	_____ No
Pertinent laboratory results assessment	_____ Yes	_____ No
Potential drug interactions identified/assessed	_____ Yes	_____ No
Planned anticoagulant dose/regimen	_____ Yes	_____ No
Planned follow-up	_____ Yes	_____ No

*Dependent on specific anticoagulation therapy utilized.

Clinical Outcomes: Prevention of Thromboembolic Recurrence

Table 11–2 outlines the Warfarin Optimized Outpatient Follow-Up Study Group's criteria for classification of thromboembolic complications as either minor, serious, life-threatening, or fatal.[8] Thromboembolic rates in AMS patients should be compared with rates reported in the literature.

Clinical Outcomes: Prevention of Hemorrhagic Complications

Three published classification systems of hemorrhagic complications are outlined in Table 11–3.[8] Petty et al[9] divide hemorrhagic complications as either life-threatening or minor (all others). Landefeld et al[10,11] incorporate the elements of blood loss, hypotension, and anemia into the assessment of potentially life-threatening episodes. A bleeding severity index and algorithm for case review has been developed.[12] Fihn et al[8] recommend the most detailed scheme to classify complications as minor (no associated costs or medical consequences), serious (requiring treatment or medical evaluation), life-threatening, or fatal. Minor complications require no additional testing, referrals, or outpatient visits but are remarkable enough to report to the provider and be documented in the medical record. Conversely, serious complications require a specific treatment *or* a medical evaluation. These definitions are particularly applicable to managed care AMS organizations as a mechanism to determine cost implications or savings.

Selection of one of these hemorrhagic complication criteria is recommended to allow for comparison of audited rates with those in the medical literature. All serious, life-threatening, and fatal complications should be independently reviewed by a selected panel of knowledgeable clinicians and disagreements reconciled by discussion. If the quality assurance audit identifies that complication rates are greater than published norms, targeted interventions must be implemented.

Clinical Outcomes: Prevention of Falls

The risk for and severity of bleeding complications in elderly patients treated with warfarin is of increasing importance.[13] This is particularly relevant in the face of increasingly larger numbers of elderly patients being anticoagulated on a long-term basis for chronic atrial fibrillation. AMS settings should focus quality assurance efforts on this high-risk population. One suggested quality assurance program is directed at fall prevention as a means to reduce the chance of intracranial hemorrhage.[14] Exhibit 11–4 outlines the essential components of a comprehensive fall risk assessment, which requires a thorough medical history and an observation of a patient's gait and mobility. If this preliminary assessment identifies potential problems, a home visit for an environmental analysis is recommended. A quality assurance strategy can evaluate the success of interventions.

Table 11–1 Modified Criteria for Use of Warfarin in Adult Inpatients and Outpatients

Element	Standard 100%	Standard 0%	Exception
JUSTIFICATION FOR USE			
1. Prophylaxis of patient at risk for thromboembolic disease due to one or more of the following:	X		
a. mechanical cardiac valve prosthesis			
b. tissue cardiac valve prosthesis in patient with or without history of embolic event (not used in patient with tissue cardiac valve prosthesis in place for >3 months and no history of embolic event or documented left atrial thrombus at surgery or concurrent atrial fibrillation)			
c. AF before and after elective cardioversion (not used in patient with new onset of AF of <2 days in duration)			

d. AF in patient >65 years of age
 	
    or
 	
    AF in patient <65 years of age with any of the following risk factors: previous TIA or stroke, hypertension, CHF, diabetes, clinical coronary artery disease, mitral stenosis, prosthetic heart valves, thyrotoxicosis
			Patient who declines warfarin or is a poor candidate for anticoagulation therapy

e. valvular heart disease in patient AF, history of systemic embolism, or history of transient ischemic attack despite antiplatelet therapy			
f. anterior transmural MI or MI in patient with other risk factors (eg, AF, reduced left ventricular function, CHF, mural thrombosis, or history of thromboembolic event)			
g. dilated cardiomyopathy			
h. total hip replacement surgery or hip fracture surgery (not used in patient receiving twice-daily fixed dose low–molecular-weight heparin or adjusted dose unfractionated heparin)			
i. congenital hypercoagulable disorder (eg, antithrombin III, protein S, or protein C deficiency)			
j. acquired hypercoagulable disorder (eg, malignancy, presence of lupus anticoagulant or anticardiolipin antibody in patient with history of embolic event, or imbalance of fibrinolytic system)			
k. peripheral vascular disease in patient with history of arterial occlusion			
l. CVA in patient with probable cardiogenic embolism (not used acutely in patient with uncontrolled hypertension or evidence of hemorrhagic transformation)			
m. CVA in patient with history of noncardiogenic embolism despite antiplatelet therapy (not used acutely in patient with uncontrolled hypertension or evidence of hemorrhagic transformation)			
n. recurrent venous thromboembolic events			
o. presence of long-term indwelling central vein catheters (not used in patient receiving heparin for prophylaxis)			
2. Treatment of pulmonary embolism or deep vein thrombosis	X		Asymptomatic patient with isolated calf vein thrombosis followed up with serial noninvasive tests for 10–14 days

Key: AF, atrial fibrillation; CHF, congestive heart failure; CVA, cerebrovascular accident; MI, myocardial infarction; TIA, transient ischemic attack.

Table 11–2 Criteria for Classification of Thromboembolic Complications

| Reference | Minor | Major | | Fatal |
		Serious	Life-Threatening	
Fihn et al 1993[8]	Mild superficial thrombophlebitis	Transient ischemic attacks or suspected stroke Recurrent deep venous thrombosis Pulmonary embolism without respiratory or hemodynamic compromise	Massive pulmonary embolism Stroke with residential neurologic deficit Systemic embolism	Death

Table 11–3 Criteria for Classification of Hemorrhagic Complications

| Reference | Minor | Major | | Fatal |
		Serious	Life-Threatening (or Potentially)	
Petty et al 1988[9]	Bleeding from hip fracture Bleeding from hemorrhoid Epistaxis Hematuria Hemoptysis Intramuscular hematoma Laceration bleeding Occult blood in stool Oral bleeding Subconjunctival hemorrhage Vaginal bleeding		GI hemorrhage Hemorrhagic cerebral infarction Subdural hematoma Unspecified intracranial hemorrhage	Death
Landefeld et al 1987[10], Landefeld et al 1989[11]	Other internal bleeding not associated with blood loss: – overt or occult GI bleeding – hemoptysis – gross hematuria Symptomatic anemia ascribed to acute blood loss without an identified site of bleeding Chronic bleeding with moderate blood loss Bleeding that led to hospitalization only for observation or for therapy of a co-morbid process that was exacerbated by bleeding		Led to MI, stroke, or surgical or angiographic intervention Acute or subacute and led to 2 of 3 serious consequences: 1. Severe blood loss 2. Hypotension (>20% drop in SBP to ≤90 mm Hg) 3. Critical anemia (≥20% drop in hematocrit to ≤20%)	Death
Fihn et al 1993[8]	No associated costs or medical consequences (no additional testing, referrals, or outpatient visits) Examples: – Mild nosebleeds – Bruising – Mild hemorrhoidal bleeding – Microscopic hematuria	Specific treatment or a medical evaluation required Examples: – overt GI bleeding – occult GI bleeding if endoscopic or radiographic studies done – gross hematuria >2 days or prompting cystoscopy or intravenous urography – blood transfusion ≤2 units	Leading to cardiopulmonary arrest, surgical or angiographic intervention, or irreversible sequelae or Any 2 of the following: 1. transfusion of ≥3 units 2. hypotension (SBP <90 mm Hg) 3. critical anemia (Hct ≤0.20) 4. acute bleeding (<3 days)	Death

Key: GI, gastrointestinal; Hct, hematocrit; MI, myocardial infarction; SBP, systolic blood pressure.

Exhibit 11–4
ASSESSMENT OF FALLING RISK

- Mobility
  - walking a short distance
  - getting in and out of a chair
  - moving on and off the toilet
  - bending down and picking object off the floor
  - standing on tiptoes
  - reaching for an object on a shelf
- Medical problems
  - orthostatic hypotension
  - arrhythmias
  - vision problems
  - osteoporosis
  - musculoskeletal weakness
  - balance problems
  - foot/toe disorders
  - limitations of knee extension or stability
  - hip problems
- Gait
  - arthritis
  - orthostatic hypotension
  - intermittent claudication
  - heart failure
  - leg edema
  - neurologic abnormalities
- Contributing medications
- History of falls
  - location
  - symptoms prior to and after the fall
- time of day of fall
- activity at time of fall
- consequences of fall
- Environment
  - improper lighting
  - lack of safety railings
  - rugs or mats that move
  - unsafe stairways
  - slippery bathtubs or showers
  - deep carpets
  - toilet seats too low
  - wobbly furniture
  - pets underfoot
  - beds too high or too low
  - shelves too high
  - family supervision
- Potential interventions
  - strength training
  - flexibility training
  - correction of home hazards
  - treatment of contributing medical problems
  - osteoporosis treatments
  - gait-assistive devices with proper instruction
  - medication changes
  - home supervision
  - installation of night lights, handrails, and other assistive measures

Clinical Outcomes: Patient Education Assessment

Patient education is the foundation of improving the risk/benefit ratio of patients on long-term anticoagulation therapy. An essential component of any AMS consists of both new patient education and ongoing reinforcement. Often, a family member or caregiver must be included in the educational process. Consistent patient information, delivered in a standardized format, is recommended. Quality assurance programs must evaluate the quality of this education. Written materials must be appropriate for the patient's educational level, language, and culture, and educational effectiveness should be documented (eg, pre-test/post-test format). Minimum components of a warfarin education program are listed in Exhibit 11–5. Minimum components of a patient education and counseling program for outpatient deep vein thrombosis (DVT) treatment are outlined in Exhibit 11–6.

Exhibit 11–5
MINIMUM COMPONENTS OF A WARFARIN PATIENT EDUCATION PROGRAM

- Purpose of the warfarin therapy
- Specific instructions for the warfarin regimen and tablet identification
- Emergency contact mechanism
- Compliance requirements
- Instructions for missed warfarin doses
- Warfarin refill procedures
- Dietary recommendations
- Over-the-counter drug and alcohol restrictions
- Management of minor bleeding complications
- Management and contact procedures for major bleeding complications
- Fall and trauma prevention and management instructions
- Communication with all health care providers

Clinical Outcomes: Psychological Outcomes

The focus of any quality assurance program is continuous quality improvement. An AMS must ensure that the quality of its care meets or exceeds the expectations of both patients and referring clinicians. This can be measured with patient satisfaction and physician satisfaction surveys administered on a regular basis.[15] The results of satisfaction surveys can be used to identify areas in need of improvement and to measure the success of improvement strategies.

Clinical Outcomes: Resource Utilization

Ongoing assessment of medical resource utilization by AMS patients can be significant in some health care organizations, particularly managed care settings. Emergency department visits, unplanned clinic visits, and hospital admissions can be tracked and compared with those of non-AMS patients taking anticoagulant drugs.[16] The economic implications of these parameters are important for ongoing clinic justification and resource allocation.

CONCLUSION

The development of a detailed quality assurance program for an AMS is required for continuous quality improvement. Examples of reporting forms are provided in Exhibit 11–7. Design should be influenced by the unique characteristics of the AMS and the health care setting in which it exists, as well as by the requirements of the Joint Commission and other regulatory agencies. AMSs will continue to grow as their efforts prove successful through quality assurance strategies.

Exhibit 11–6
PATIENT EDUCATION AND COUNSELING FOR OUTPATIENT DVT TREATMENT

Discuss the topics in this checklist with patients and families:

_____ Description of DVT and its risks and complications

_____ Treatment regimen of low–molecular-weight heparin (LMWH) (dosing frequency: once-daily versus twice-daily based on the health care system's choice of LMWH and interpretation of the data to support once-daily versus twice-daily dosing), as well as potential side effects

_____ Treatment regimen with warfarin (dosing frequency, potential side effects, required monitoring of INR)

_____ Explanation of laboratory tests and subsequent warfarin dosing adjustments

_____ Demonstration of how to perform LMWH injections, site selection, and syringe disposal with observation of the patient or caregiver performing these skills

_____ Instructions specific to the health care system regarding recommended behaviors (e.g., elevation of leg, avoidance of stasis, etc.)

_____ Signs and symptoms of bleeding or worsening or progression of their thromboembolic event and how to respond

_____ Purpose and duties of the visiting nurse when necessary

_____ Phone numbers of the anticoagulation therapy service personnel or patient's physician

_____ Date and time of next appointment

Exhibit 11–7
AMS REPORTING FORMS

AMS Visits per Month (Dates: Jan. _____ to Dec. _____)

Month/Year	# of Visits	# of Patients*	Business Days**	Visits per Day	Visits per Patient
January					
February					
March					
April					
May					
June					
July					
August					
September					
October					
November					
December					
Yearly Totals					

*The number of distinct patients for the specified clinic who had one or more visits.
**The number of days on which there were one or more visits.

AMS Visit Categories (Dates: Jan. _____ to Dec. _____)

Month/Year	# Phone Visits	# Return Visits	# New Patient Visits
Yearly Totals			

continues

AMS Reporting Forms continued

AMS Resource Utilization (Dates: Jan. _____ to Dec. _____)

Month/Year	ER Visit—Warfarin Related	ER Visit—Warfarin Unrelated	Hospital Admission— Warfarin Related	Hospital Admission— Warfarin Unrelated
Yearly Totals				

AMS Monitoring Outcomes (Dates: Jan. _____ to Dec. _____)

Month/ Year	INR <2.0 # (%)	INR 2.0–4.0 # (%)	INR >4.0 # (%)	INR within Range # (%)	INR Outside Range # (%)	In Range (+/–0.2) # (%)	Outside Range (+/–0.2) # (%)
Yearly Totals							

continues

AMS Explanation for INR Outside Range (Dates: Jan. _____ to Dec. _____)

Category	# of Visits	% of Total
Change in Rx meds		
Change in OTC meds		
Change in herbal meds		
Change in medical condition/health status		
Change in dietary vitamin K intake		
Change in ETON intake		
Nonadherence/Incorrect use		
Initiation (Reinitiation) therapy		
No clear explanation		
Response to previous change in warfarin dose		
Warfarin intentionally omitted		
Totals		

REFERENCES

1. Joint Commission on Accreditation of Healthcare Organizations. *Accreditation Manual for Hospitals 1995*. Chicago, IL: Joint Commission on Accreditation of Healthcare Organizations; 1994.

2. Roseman AW, Sawyer WT. Population-based drug use evaluation. *Top Hosp Pharm Manage*. 1988;8:76–92.

3. Kubacka RT. A primer on drug utilization review. *J Am Pharm Assoc*. 1996;NS36(4):257–279.

4. Hiatt J, Wittkowsky AK. Criteria for use of warfarin in adult inpatients and outpatients. *Clin Pharm*. 1993,12:307–313.

5. Dalen JE, Hirsh J, eds. Third ACCP Consensus Conference on Antithrombotic Therapy. *Chest*. 1992;102(suppl 4).

6. Dalen JE, Hirsh J, eds. Fourth ACCP Consensus Conference on Antithrombotic Therapy. *Chest*. 1995;108(suppl 4).

7. Laupacis A, Albers G, Dalen J, et al. Antithrombotic therapy in atrial fibrillation. *Chest*. 1995;108(suppl 4):352S–359S.

8. Fihn SD, McDonell M, Martin D, et al. Risk factors for complications of chronic anticoagulation: a multicenter study. *Ann Intern Med*. 1993;118:511–520.

9. Petty GW, Lennihan L, Mohr JP, et al. Complications of long-term anticoagulation. *Ann Neurol*. 1988;23:570–574.

10. Landefeld CS, Cook EF, Flatley M, et al. Identification and preliminary validation of predictors of major bleeding in hospitalized patients starting anticoagulant therapy. *Am J Med*. 1987;82:703–713.

11. Landefeld CS, Rosenblatt MW, Goldman L. Bleeding in outpatients treated with warfarin: relation to the prothrombin time and important remediable issues. *Am J Med*. 1989;87:153–159.

12. Landefeld CS, Anderson PA, Goodnough LT, et al. The bleeding severity index: validation and comparison to other methods of classifying bleeding complications of medical therapy. *J Clin Epidemiol*. 1989;42:711–718.

13. Fihn SD, Callahan CM, Martin DC, et al. The risk for and severity of bleeding complications in elderly patients treated with warfarin. *Ann Intern Med*. 1996;124:970–979.

14. Hylek EM, Singer DE. Risk factors for intracranial hemorrhage in outpatients taking warfarin. *Ann Intern Med*. 1994;120:897–902.

15. Wilson-Norton JL, Gibson DL. Establishing an outpatient anticoagulation clinic in a community hospital. *Am J Health-Syst Pharm*. 1996; 53:1151–1157.

16. Wilt VM, Gums JG, Ahmed OI, Moore LM. Outcome analysis of a pharmacist-managed anticoagulation service. *Pharmacotherapy*. 1995;15:732–739.

Chapter 12

Reimbursement Basics for Anticoagulation Services: Coverage, Payment, and Coding

Paul Radensky

To offer high-quality anticoagulation services and achieve good outcomes in patients requiring anticoagulation, anticoagulation service providers must have revenues sufficient to cover their costs. In the health care market, revenues come from health benefit plan reimbursement. To determine whether and at what rate anticoagulation services will be paid, one must consider three issues: coverage, payment, and coding. Coverage is a threshold issue answering the question: Are anticoagulation services eligible for payment at all? This is determined by reference to the terms of the benefit plan. For public payers, like Medicare and Medicaid, coverage is determined by statute; for private payers, coverage is determined by benefit plan agreements (contract) under requirements set out by state or federal law. Depending upon the payer and the type of service (coverage category), various methods determine at what rate covered services will be paid and what, if any, copayments or coinsurance will apply. Coding addresses the mechanics—it is the language providers use to tell payers what they have done and why. (The policies under Medicare are publicly available and directed nationally by the Centers for Medicare and Medicaid Services (CMS). By contrast, the policies among private payers vary widely and also differ among the 50 state Medicaid programs. Therefore, this summary primarily presents information on Medicare policies.)

To be eligible for coverage, a service must be included under the scope of benefits of the particular health plan, and the item or service also must not otherwise be excluded from coverage. Under most benefit plans the list of covered items and services is described broadly and includes hospital, physician, clinical laboratory, skilled nursing facility, home health, and skilled nursing facility services. The scope of benefits under Medicare is set out in the Social Security Act.[1] Anticoagulation services are not listed specifically under the scope of benefits. Anticoagulation services may include physician services for evaluating a patient on therapy, obtaining blood specimens, and for administration of a low–molecular-weight heparin (LMWH); clinical laboratory services for monitoring prothrombin time (PT) levels; hospital services if the patient is evaluated and managed in a hospital setting; skilled nursing facility services if the patient is managed in that setting; and home health agency services if the patient is managed at home. Home PT monitors are covered as durable medical equipment (DME) by private payers, a separately listed item under the scope of benefits. Home anticoagulation monitors are to be covered as diagnostic services under Medicare effective July 1, 2002.[2]

Some, but not all, benefit plans will include outpatient prescription drugs, like warfarin. Medicare generally does not cover outpatient prescription drugs. Under Medicare, coverage is limited to drugs that are not usually self-administered by the patient.[3] Therefore, warfarin is not covered under Medicare because it is not included under the scope of benefits. Warfarin may be covered under certain Medicare supplement policies (ie, standard supplement policies H, I, and J).[4] An LMWH may be covered under Medicare when administered by a physician or hospital but would not be covered when self-administered by a patient.

Exclusions may apply two ways—to all beneficiaries at all times (the item or service is never covered) or only to specific beneficiaries or specific circumstances. Some items are specifically excluded (eg, hearing aids).[5] Anticoagulation services are not specifically excluded. Other items may be excluded because the payer considers the item or service to be investigational or experimental. Under these circumstances, the payer will deny coverage whenever the item or service is ordered. For example, for several years Medicare contractors denied coverage for home PT testing because the contractors believed the benefits of home testing had not yet been proved. CMS's Coverage and Analysis Group reviewed the evidence on home PT testing in 2001 and in September 2001 issued a decision memorandum summarizing the evidence on home PT monitoring and announcing that Medicare would begin covering home PT monitoring for patients with mechanical heart valves.[2]

Items and services that are generally covered also must be considered medically necessary for a specific patient at a specific time. For example, a payer may determine that it is medically necessary to order a PT test every three to four weeks, but not every three to four days. Medicare issued a national coverage decision on PT testing last fall (applies to testing other than home PT monitoring) in which it specified that PT testing usually is not required more than every two to three weeks. The policy does allow for more frequent testing, if medical necessity is shown and documented in the medical record.[6]

The payment policies that apply to covered items and services vary by the setting where the service is provided. Under Medicare, there are several prospective payment systems that define how Medicare sets the payment rate for anticoagulation services. Hospital inpatient services are paid under the per-admission, all-inclusive diagnosis-related group (DRG) rates. Medicare payment is the same, for example, for an admission to manage a patient with deep venous thrombosis whether the patient is treated with unfractionated heparin or an LMWH. The DRG payment also covers emergency department (ED) services provided by the hospital if the ED visit results in an inpatient admission, and the DRG payment covers diagnostic tests, like PT testing, performed by the hospital within 3 days before the inpatient admission.

Hospital outpatient services, such as ED visits or outpatient clinic visits, are paid under the recently initiated Hospital Outpatient Prospective Payment System (HOPPS), which provides a packaged payment for procedures performed in the hospital outpatient setting under Ambulatory Payment Classification (APC) rates. Physician services are paid under the Resource Based Relative Value Scale (RBRVS) fee schedule. PT tests are paid under the clinical laboratory fee schedule. Home health agency services are paid under the recently introduced Home Health Prospective Payment System.

Several coding systems are used to report services on claim forms. Procedures are generally reported using the American Medical Association's Current Procedural Terminology (CPT) codes. Office visits, PT tests, venipuncture, and administration of injectable drugs are all reported using CPT codes. Injectable drugs, such as LMWHs, and DME are reported using the alpha-numeric Healthcare Common Procedure Coding System (HCPCS) codes. Providers report the reason for providing services using the *International Classification of Diseases 9th Revision Clinical Modification* (ICD-9-CM) codes.

COVERAGE, PAYMENT, AND CODING FOR ORAL ANTICOAGULATION MANAGEMENT VISITS

Consider the patient who is on chronic oral anticoagulation. The patient will be seen at regular intervals and the following services may be provided: (1) PT testing, (2) specimen collection, and (3) evaluation and management. PT testing performed in the outpatient setting is covered and paid under the Clinical Laboratory Fee Schedule. The test is coded using CPT 85610: "Prothrombin time." If the test is performed in a physician office lab that has a certificate of waiver under the Clinical Laboratory Improvement Amendments, the test must be performed using a waived test device and reported using the "QW" modifier following the CPT code for the test. The 2002 Clinical Laboratory Fee Schedule payment for PT testing is $5.43 (national limitation amount). PT testing performed in an inpatient setting would be included in the rate paid to the facility for the admission. No separate payment is made for the test.

Specimen collection by venipuncture may be paid separately under HCPCS G0001 "routine venipuncture for collection of specimens" at a 2002 payment amount of $3.00 (2002 midpoint). Medicare will not pay for fingerstick sample collection. Private payers may pay for venipuncture or fingerstick sample collection under CPT 36415 "routine venipuncture or finger/heel/ear stick for collection of specimen(s)."

Evaluation and management office visit services are also covered, *but only when medically necessary* and when the services actually provided meet the intensity of services described by the CPT code for each type of service. Evaluation and management office visit service codes and payment amounts are shown in Table 12–1 for new patients and in Table 12–2 for established patients. New patients are those who have not received any face-to-face service by the physician within the past 3 years. For multispecialty groups, if the patient has been seen by a physician in the same specialty

Table 12–1 Evaluation and Management Office Visit Service Codes and 2002 Medicare Fee Schedule Payments for New Patients

Code[1]	99201	99202	99203	99204	99205
History	Problem focused	Expanded problem focused	Detailed	Comprehensive	Comprehensive
Exam	Problem focused	Expanded problem focused	Detailed	Comprehensive	Comprehensive
Medical Decision Making	Straightforward	Straightforward	Low complexity	Moderate complexity	High complexity
Problem Severity	Minor/self-limited	Low to moderate	Moderate	Moderate to high	Moderate to high
Face-to-Face Time	10 minutes	20 minutes	30 minutes	45 minutes	60 minutes
Payment (Office)[2]	$34.03	$61.54	$91.95	$130.68	$166.15

[1]2002 CPT codes copyright 2001 American Medical Association. All rights reserved.
[2]2002 Medicare Physician Fee Schedule, 66 *Fed. Reg.* 55244, November 1, 2001.

Source: Reprinted with permission of P.W. Radensky, Reimbursement for Anticoagulation Services, *Journal of Thrombosis and Thrombolysis*, Vol. 12, No. 1, pp. 73–79, © 2001, Kluwer Academic Publishers.

Table 12–2 Evaluation and Management Office Visit Service Codes and 2002 Medicare Fee Schedule Payment Amounts for Established Patients

Code[1]	99211	99212	99213	99214	99215
History	Not defined	Problem focused	Expanded problem focused	Detailed	Comprehensive
Exam	Not defined	Problem focused	Expanded problem focused	Detailed	Comprehensive
Medical Decision Making	Not defined	Straightforward	Low complexity	Moderate complexity	High complexity
Problem Severity	Minimal	Self-limited or minor	Low to moderate	Moderate to high	Moderate to high
Face-to-Face Time	5 minutes	10 minutes	15 minutes	25 minutes	40 minutes
Payment (Office)[2]	$20.27	$36.20	$50.32	$78.91	$115.84

[1]2002 CPT codes copyright 2001 American Medical Association. All rights reserved.
[2]2002 Medicare Physician Fee Schedule, 66 *Fed. Reg.* 55244, November 1, 2001.

Source: Reprinted with permission of P.W. Radensky, Reimbursement for Anticoagulation Services, *Journal of Thrombosis and Thrombolysis*, Vol. 12, No. 1, pp. 73–79, © 2001, Kluwer Academic Publishers.

within 3 years, the patient is an established patient. For the purposes of determining new versus established patients, simply performing a PT test or interpretation of an electrocardiogram is not a face-to-face service that would result in a patient's being an established patient.

Evaluation and management service codes are determined by the comprehensiveness of the history and examination and the complexity of the medical decision making required to manage the patient. The severity of the presenting problem and the time spent with the patient are also listed as guides, but the selection of appropriate evaluation and management

code is not determined by the problem severity or time.

For hospital-based anticoagulation management services, the facility would submit a claim for the technical or facility component service. This covers the room, equipment, supplies, and staff, excluding the physician's professional services. The hospital payment amounts are determined under the HOPPS under APC groups to which each CPT code is assigned. The payment amounts in the hospital outpatient setting are shown in Table 12–3. If a physician has a face-to-face encounter with the patient, the physician may also be paid a professional fee. The professional fee in the hospital

Table 12–3 Evaluation and Management Services in the Hospital Outpatient Department: Medicare 2002 Payments

Code[1] (New Patient)	99201	99202	99203	99204	99205
Hospital Payment[2]	APC 600 $44.29	APC 600 $44.29	APC 601 $48.36	APC 602 $70.25	APC 602 $70.25
Professional Fee[3]	$22.81	$45.61	$69.50	$102.81	$136.47
Code[1] (Established Patient)	99211	99212	99213	99214	99215
Hospital Payment[2]	APC 600 $44.29	APC 600 $44.29	APC 601 $48.36	APC 602 $70.25	APC 602 $70.25
Professional Fee[3]	$8.69	$23.17	$34.03	$56.11	$90.50

[1]2002 CPT codes copyright 2001 American Medical Association. All rights reserved.
[2]2002 Hospital Outcome Prospective Payment System rates effective April 1, 2002, 67 *Fed. Reg.* 9556 (March 1, 2002).
[3]2002 Medicare Physician Fee Schedule, 66 *Fed. Reg.* 55244, November 1, 2001.

Source: Reprinted with permission of P.W. Radensky, Reimbursement for Anticoagulation Services, *Journal of Thrombosis and Thrombolysis*, Vol. 12, No. 1, pp. 73–79, © 2001, Kluwer Academic Publishers.

outpatient setting is lower than the corresponding fee in the physician office setting, thus recognizing that the physician does not bear the cost of overhead and staff in the hospital setting (Table 12–3).

COVERAGE, PAYMENT, AND CODING FOR HOME PT/INR MONITORING

Effective July 1, 2002, Medicare has begun to cover home anticoagulation monitoring services provided to patients with mechanical heart valves. Medicare will provide coverage for testing up to once per week. Unlike home blood glucose monitoring, which is covered under the DME benefit, Medicare is covering home International Normalized Ratio (INR) monitoring as a diagnostic service under the RBRVS fee schedule.

The following requirements must be met for coverage of the home PT/INR monitoring benefit:

- The patient must have been anticoagulated for at least 3 months prior to use of the home INR device.
- The patient must undergo an education program on anticoagulation management and the use of the device prior to its use in the home.
- Self-testing with the device is limited to a frequency of once per week.[7]

Medicare payment for home PT/INR monitoring comprises three components: demonstration and training, ongoing monitoring through the provision of testing equipment and strips, and physician review and interpretation of test results. There are three HCPCS procedure codes used to report these services effective July 1 (see Table 12–4). The payment amounts are approximately $111 for the demonstra-

tion and training, $120 for the ongoing provision of strips and equipment per 4 tests, and $9 for physician interpretation and reporting per 4 tests. These payment amounts are considered "interim" for the remainder of 2002. Medicare is accepting comments on these payment amounts and will "finalize" the relative value units next year. Medicare will also provide payment for the demonstration and training and for the ongoing provision of equipment and test strips provided by hospital outpatient departments under the HOPPS under codes G0248 and G0249, respectively.

The demonstration and training service and the ongoing provision of equipment and strips may be provided either by physicians or by independent diagnostic testing facilities—the same type of providers who perform the technical component services of Holter monitoring, pacemaker monitoring, or free-standing diagnostic imaging services.

COVERAGE, PAYMENT, AND CODING FOR ADMINISTRATION OF LMWH

Consider next an outpatient encounter to evaluate a patient with deep venous thrombosis and to administer an LMWH. This encounter would involve the following components: (1) evaluation and management services, (2) injection of the LMWH, and (3) the LMWH drug product itself. These items and services may be provided in the physician office setting, a hospital outpatient clinic, an emergency department, or by a home health agency.

In the office setting, the evaluation and management services would be reported under CPT 99201–99205 for new patients and 99211–99215 for established patients as shown in Tables 12–1 and 12–2. For the injection of an LMWH, the physician may report CPT 90782 "Therapeutic, prophylactic or diagnostic injection (specify material injected); subcutaneous or intramuscular." The allowance under the 2002

Table 12–4 Medicare Coding for Home PT/INR Monitoring: Effective July 2002

Code	Nomenclature
G0248	Demonstration, at initial use, of home INR monitoring for patient with mechanical heart valve(s) who meets Medicare coverage criteria, under the direction of a physician. Includes demonstration, use, and care of the INR monitor; obtaining at least one blood sample; provision of instructions for reporting home INR test results; and documentation of patient ability to perform testing.
G0249	Provision of test materials and equipment for home INR monitoring to patient with mechanical heart valve(s) who meet Medicare coverage criteria. Includes provision of materials for use in the home and reporting of test results to physician; per 4 tests.
G0250	Physician review; interpretation and patient management of home INR testing for a patient with mechanical heart valve(s) who meets other coverage criteria; per 4 tests (does not require face-to-face service).

Medicare Fee Schedule for this service is $3.98. Note, however, that payment will be made under this code only if no other fee schedule service is provided on the same day. Therefore, the physician will not be paid for the injection if an evaluation and management service visit is billed on the same date. Private payer policies on payment for the injection will vary.

Under Medicare outpatient prescription drugs are generally not covered. However, drugs and biologicals that are not usually self-administered by the patient are covered when provided incident to physician services or hospital services. When administered incident to a physician's service, the payment is set at 95 percent of the national average wholesale price, as published by reference sources such as *Drug Topics Red Book* or *First Databank*. As LMWHs may be self-administered, these agents are covered only when it is medically necessary for the drug to be administered by the provider. For example, physicians may determine that a patient should have the initial injection in the office to show the patient how to self-administer and to assess for any complications with the initial injection. Many local Medicare contractors have policies covering the initial injection of LMWH. In addition, some patients may not be able to self-administer at all because of physical impairment, visual limitations, or cognitive impairment. Under those circumstances, repeat injections in the physician office setting may be medically necessary.

In the hospital outpatient setting, the facility may report the same services as the physician's office may report in the office setting. The evaluation and management services would be reported and paid at the rates shown in Table 12–3. In the hospital outpatient setting, APC 0352, to which injection code 90782 is assigned, has a payment rate of $20.87. As the injection policy limiting payment for injections to only when no other service is billed does not apply in the hospital outpatient setting, it is unclear whether payment would be made for both the injection and the evaluation and management visit. Under HOPPS, payment for drugs is generally included in the payment for the associated procedure. The LMWHs are included in the payment for the outpatient visit. Medicare has not specified its reasoning for bundling the payment for these agents. Private payers may provide separate payment for the LMWHs provided in the hospital outpatient setting if it is medically necessary to administer the drug in this setting.

In the ED setting, both the hospital and physician would report the facility and professional components services respectively. There would be an evaluation and management service, an injection, and the LMWH. Payment for the evaluation and management services is shown in Table 12–5. The injection service, if separately billed and payable, would fall under APC 0352, as above, and the LMWH would be bundled into the payment for the ED visit.

When LMWH is provided in the home health setting to homebound patients, payment for the nursing service and supplies is made under the home health prospective payment system. If the patient requires 5 or more skilled nursing visits within a 60-day encounter period (eg, to assist with the administration of the LMWH, to evaluate the leg and assess for clotting or bleeding complications, and to conduct point-of-care testing of PT for adjunctive warfarin therapy), the payment would fall under one of the home health resource groups, with payment amounts ranging from approximately $1,000 to $6,000. If the patient requires 4 or fewer visits, the payment would be on a per visit basis under what is called the "Low Utilization Payment Adjustment" (LUPA). The 2002 LUPA amount for skilled nursing visits is $99.28.

Table 12–5 Evaluation and Management Services in the Emergency Department: Medicare 2002 Payments

Code[1]	99281	99282	99283	99284	99285
History	Problem focused	Expanded problem focused	Expanded problem focused	Detailed	Comprehensive
Exam	Problem focused	Expanded problem focused	Expanded problem focused	Detailed	Comprehensive
Medical Decision Making	Straightforward	Low complexity	Moderate complexity	Moderate complexity	High complexity
Problem Severity	Self limited or minor	Low to moderate	Moderate	High	High
Facility Payment[2]	APC 610 $63.12	APC 610 $63.12	APC 611 $109.95	APC 612 $178.67	APC 612 $178.67
Physician Payment[3]	$15.93	$26.43	$59.37	$92.67	$144.80

[1]2002 CPT codes copyright 2001 American Medical Association. All rights reserved.
[3]2002 Hospital Outpatient Prospective Payment System rates effective April 1, 2002, 67 *Fed. Reg.* 9556 (March 1, 2002).
[2]2002 Medicare Physician Fee Schedule, 66 *Fed. Reg.* 55244, November 1, 2001.

Source: Reprinted with permission of P.W. Radensky, Reimbursement for Anticoagulation Services, *Journal of Thrombosis and Thrombolysis*, Vol. 12, No. 1, pp. 73–79, © 2001, Kluwer Academic Publishers.

INCIDENT-TO SERVICE RULES

Providing high-quality anticoagulation services requires a coordinated effort among many professionals. Many of the services can appropriately be provided by physician office or hospital staff and do not require face-to-face services from the physician. For example, under physician supervision, a nurse may evaluate a patient by asking about changes in medication, diet, or concurrent illnesses or occurrence of any bleeding or clotting events; by conducting a brief examination to look for signs of bleeding or clotting; drawing a specimen to run a PT test; performing a point-of-care test; informing the patient of the results; and instructing the patient on any changes in warfarin dosing.

Medicare recognizes that physicians and hospitals can provide services beyond the direct physician face-to-face encounter, and these services are covered as incident to the services of a physician, provided specific rules are followed. In the physician office setting, there are two requirements for coverage of incident-to services: (1) there must be direct personal physician supervision, and (2) the services must be furnished during a course of treatment in which the physician performs an initial service and subsequent services of a frequency that reflect his or her active participation in and management of the course of treatment.

Direct physician supervision requires that the physician be present in the office suite and immediately available to provide assistance and direction throughout the time the nonphysician is performing services. The physician need not be present in the same room, however.

To be eligible for incident-to coverage, the physician who is billing for the services must personally provide an initial service to the patient and must see the patient personally at some routine interval as medically necessary to provide adequate supervision of the patient's management. There are no specific policies on the frequency at which physicians must personally provide follow-up services.

Prior to 2002 there was a third requirement for incident-to billing: the auxiliary personnel who personally perform services, such as nurses, nonphysician anesthetists, psychologists, technicians, therapists, and other aides, were required to be employed by the physician. Beginning in 2002, an employment relationship with the physician is no longer required for incident-to services in the physician office setting: "[T]he employment relationship is irrelevant to whether a physician (or other practitioner) can effectively furnish direct supervision of the auxiliary staff."[8]

In addition to services provided by physicians or by their nonphysician staff incident to a physician's service, anticoagulation management services may be provided by nurse practitioners, physician assistants, or clinical nurse specialists—so-called advanced practice nonphysician practitioners.[9] These advanced practice nonphysician practitioners are licensed by the states under various programs to assist or act in the place of the physician. For services of a nonphysician practitioner to be covered as incident to services of a physician, the services must meet the requirements for coverage specified above: direct personal supervision during the course of treatment by the physician. When incident-to services are provided by non–advanced practice nonphysician professionals, Medicare policy limits the services to the lowest level evaluation and management visit: 99211.[10] If the services are provided by advanced practice professionals, however, there is no limitation on the intensity of evaluation and management service provided as long as the services provided are within the advanced practice professional's scope of practice under state law. Payment for services provided incident to a physician's service are paid at the full Medicare Physician Fee Schedule rate.

Advanced practice professionals also may provide services directly and not under direct physician supervision. Payment for services of advanced practice professionals performed independently (ie, not incident to a physician's service) are paid at 85 percent of the Medicare Physician Fee Schedule rate. Although physician assistants may perform evaluation and management services without direct physician supervision and their services may be billed as independent services, physician assistant services can only be billed by their employer.

Services incident to physician services may also be covered in the hospital outpatient setting.[11] These services must be provided: (1) under physician supervision, (2) by hospital personnel, and (3) on the order of a physician who sees the patient personally during the course of treatment. In the hospital setting, when services are provided on the hospital campus, the physician supervision requirement is generally assumed to be met. The hospital medical staff that supervise the services need not be in the same department as the ordering physician. Physician supervision is not assumed, however, for off-campus facilities. (A discussion of the requirements for off-campus facilities to bill as hospital outpatient departments is beyond the scope of this chapter.) Although physician supervision may be assumed for reimbursement purposes in the hospital campus setting, good medical care may require that a physician be physically close to the place where the anticoagulation management services are provided and be ready immediately to handle personally any emergency situations that arise.

As discussed above for incident-to services in the physician office setting, in the hospital outpatient setting, the hospital can bill only for services provided by its personnel or personnel the hospital provides under arrangements. A physician cannot bring his or her staff to the hospital and bill under the incident-to rules for services performed by the physician's staff. If the anticoagulation management services are provided by advanced practice professionals, these professionals may bill their professional services independent from the hospital facility fee only if the salary, benefits, and expenses of the advanced practice professionals are excluded from the hospital's cost report to Medicare and the advanced practice professionals' services are not included in the hospital's charge for the services.

As in the physician office setting, the incident-to services provided by the hospital must be during the course of care provided by a physician who initially evaluates the patient and sees the patient periodically and sufficiently often to assess the course of treatment and the patient's progress and, where necessary, to change the treatment regimen.[12] A hospital service or supply would not be considered incident to a physician's service if the attending physician merely wrote an order for the services or supplies and referred the patient to the hospital without being involved in the management of that course of treatment. The required nexus between the physician who personally sees the patients and the hospital is not defined in the regulations or policies, but it would appear that the physician referring the patient to the hospital for incident-to services should have staff privileges at the hospital.

The general framework for considering coverage, payment, and coding for incident-to services is presented above, but many questions arise from those involved in providing anticoagulation management regarding incident-to services: Who can perform these services? Who can bill for the services? How much will be paid for the services?

Two important issues should be considered to answer the question about who can provide incident-to services. First, looking at the physician, one must ask whether it is appropriate for the physician to delegate the particular service that is performed by nonphysician staff. Second, one must consider whether it is appropriate for the physician to delegate the specific service to the particular nonphysician practitioner performing the service. These issues involve state law issues about the scope of medical practice, the scope of practice of the nonphysician staff actually performing the service, and the standard of care in the community for providing these services. Physicians have greater freedom to delegate services to advanced practice professionals than to non–advanced practice professionals. Among non–advanced practice professionals, the question about whether a particular service is within the scope of practice may not be clear. Under those circumstances, the physician and the nonphysician practitioner may wish to inquire of the respective licensing authorities (medical board and board of practice for the non–advanced practice staff, if any) about the appropriateness of any physician-delegated services performed under direct physician supervision.

From a reimbursement perspective, Medicare recently clarified that any individual may serve as auxiliary personnel for incident-to service consistent with state law limitations:

> We have not further clarified who may serve as auxiliary personnel for a particular incident to service because the scope of practice of the auxiliary personnel and the supervising physician (or other practitioners) is determined by State law.... We deliberately used the term any individual so that the physician (or other practitioner), under his or her discretion and license, may use the service of

anyone ranging from another physician to a medical assistant. In addition, it is impossible to exhaustively list all incident to services and those specific auxiliary personnel who may perform each service.[12]

This would appear to allow coverage for anticoagulation clinic services provided incident to a physician's service where the face-to-face service is provided by a pharmacist or PharmD, a common practice in many anticoagulation clinic settings. It is important to understand that, under these circumstances, Medicare is not paying for pharmacy services or services provided by pharmacists. Medicare covers physician or hospital services where the staff providing the service include pharmacists or PharmDs, and all incident-to rules are met. The distinction between paying for nurse practitioner and physician assistant services but not pharmacist services is based upon Medicare law. The Medicare statute scope of benefits specifically provides coverage for nurse practitioner and physician assistant services; it does not provide coverage for pharmacy services.

In Tables 12–6 and 12–7, the incident-to coverage, payment, and coding rules and policies are summarized as understood by the application of these rules and policies on coverage and payment for anticoagulation management services. The rules, as described above, are more detailed than one easily can summarize in tabular form, however.

CONCLUSION

Proper anticoagulation can be lifesaving and can avert serious events, like strokes and pulmonary emboli. Providing high-quality anticoagulation services involves a coordinated effort among multiple professionals. The rules defining coverage, payment, and coding for these services are complex, but navigating through them properly will ensure that anticoagulation service providers receive appropriate revenues for the services provided so they may continue to offer these much-needed services.

Table 12–6 Incident-to Billing in Physician's Office Setting*

Personnel performing service	Supervision required	Reportable codes	Payment amount
Physician	None	99201–99205 (new patient); 99211–99215 (established patient)	100% MFS
Advanced practice professional (independent service)	None	99201–99205 (new patient); 99211–99215 (established patient)	85% MFS
Advanced practice professional (incident-to-service)	Direct physician supervision	99211–99215	100% MFS
Non–advanced practice professional	Direct physician supervision	99211	100% MFS

*This information is based upon Medicare rules and policies generally. However, there are no specific policies pertaining to anticoagulation management services, and coverage and payment for these services cannot be guaranteed.

Source: Reprinted with permission of P.W. Radensky, Reimbursement for Anticoagulation Services, *Journal of Thrombosis and Thrombolysis*, Vol. 12, No. 1, pp. 73–79, © 2001, Kluwer Academic Publishers.

Table 12-7 Incident-to Billing in Hospital Outpatient Setting*

Personnel performing service	Supervision required	Reportable codes	Hospital payment amount	Professional fee
Physician	None	99201–99205 (new patient); 99211–99215 (established patient)	APC 600–APC 602	100% MFS
Advanced practice professional (not included on hospital cost report)	None	99201–99205 (new patient); 99211–99215 (established patient)	APC 600–APC 602	85% MFS
Advanced practice professional (included on hospital cost report)	None	99211–99215	APC 600–APC 602	Not eligible to bill for professional fee
Non–advanced practice professional	Physician supervision (assumed on campus; not assumed off-campus)	99211	APC 600	Not eligible to bill for professional fee

*This information is based upon Medicare rules and policies generally. However, there are no specific policies pertaining to anticoagulation management services, and coverage and payment for these services cannot be guaranteed.

Source: Reprinted with permission of P.W. Radensky, Reimbursement for Anticoagulation Services, *Journal of Thrombosis and Thrombolysis*, Vol. 12, No. 1, pp. 73–79, © 2001, Kluwer Academic Publishers.

REFERENCES

1. 42 U.S.C. §1395(d) and 42 U.S.C. § 1395(k).

2. Centers for Medicare and Medicaid Services. Decision memorandum: Home prothrombin time (INR) monitor for anticoagulation management. September 18, 2001.

3. 42 U.S.C. § 1395(x)(s).

4. National Association of Insurance Commissioners. Model regulation to implement the NAIC Medicare supplement insurance minimum standards model act § 9.

5. 42 U.S.C. § 1395(y)(a)(7).

6. 66 *Fed. Reg.* 58832 (November 23, 2001).

7. Program memorandum AB-02-064 (May 2, 2002).

8. 66 *Fed. Reg.* 55268 (November 1, 2001).

9. Medicare Carrier's Manual § 2050.2.

10. Medicare Carrier's Manual § 15501G.

11. Medicare Intermediary Manual § 3112.4.

12. Medicare Carrier's Manual § 2050.1.

Chapter 13

Risk Management and Anticoagulation Therapy

Eileen M. Ryan

INTRODUCTION

This chapter introduces general concepts pertaining to risk management as it has evolved from industry to clinical risk management practiced in health care institutions today. This discussion is by no means an exhaustive review of the newly developed discipline of risk management, but it can serve as background and rationale for an understanding of the risk management process. The identification and analysis of liability risks in oral anticoagulant therapy by utilizing actual clinical situations that resulted in medical malpractice claims and suits constitute the major focus of this chapter. Based on these cases, suggestions for loss prevention and reduction are offered.

RISK MANAGEMENT: A BRIEF HISTORY

Hospital risk management programs were developed in response to the medical malpractice insurance crisis of the mid-1970s as the number of medical malpractice claims filed against physicians and hospitals dramatically escalated. There was a steady increase in claims frequency and severity (amount of indemnity paid) until 1985 when the number of claims leveled off, but the severity of claims continued to rise. Currently, insurers are again reporting a possible trend toward an increase in both frequency and indemnity.[1]

The insurance industry's initial response to its increased financial losses resulting from malpractice claims was to raise premiums to cover the losses. Because losses continued to escalate and a groundbreaking study[2] reported that roughly 1 in 126 hospital admissions resulted in patient injuries and 1 in 10 of these injuries resulted in claims, however, questions relating to the unpredictability of risk prompted many insurance companies eventually to withdraw from the market. As a result, hospitals and physicians were left uninsured. In some states, government-funded joint underwriting associations were made available for institutions and/or health care providers without the use of commercial carriers. This situation prompted the development of self-insured captives and hospital- and physician-owned insurance companies.

Many of these newly formed companies, as well as some of the commercial carriers that had remained in the market, reduced premiums to facilities that initiated risk management programs. Their actions were based on the premise that these programs would bring malpractice costs under control. Prior to the insurance crisis, the elements of claims surveillance and management, incident reporting and investigation, and equipment safety had been considered by commercial carriers to be conditions of coverage.[3] Another incentive for the development of risk management programs was their requirement in hospitals with trusts under the Medicare Conditions of Participation.[4]

Three major strategies to stem the rising tide of medical malpractice have been identified. The first is an insurance approach that merely transfers the financial risk, which can be effective in a healthy market. The second is a legislative approach through tort reform, such as placing a cap on damage awards to plaintiffs, limiting attorney fees, establishing no-fault compensation for specific types of injuries, setting requirements for expert witnesses, and shortening the statute of limitations. The third approach, and the one believed to be the most effective, is the risk management approach, which establishes systems to prevent or minimize malpractice and its subsequent liability. Orlinkoff[5] states that "the first two approaches have yet to demonstrate significant progress in reducing the frequency or severity of patient injury, reducing malpractice claims or losses or slowing the rate of acceleration of malpractice liability insurance costs."

Definitions

The concept of risk management, as developed by industry, is defined as the minimization or insurance financing of predictable losses in business. When hospitals adapted the concept, risk management was expanded to include the prediction of risk of patient injury, avoidance of exposure to predicted and other risks, and minimization of malpractice claims loss.[6] Hospital risk management is usually defined as follows:

> An organized effort to identify, assess, and reduce, where appropriate, risks to patients, visitors, staff, and hospital assets. It involves activities that are designed to (1) reduce the hospital's risk of a malpractice suit by maintaining the quality of care, (2) reduce the probability of a claim being filed after a potentially compensable event has occurred, and (3) preserve the hospital's assets once a claim has been filed.[7]

This definition implies knowledge and expertise in a variety of content areas such as financial; insurance, including claims management; legal, including liability case law; clinical; and health care organizational structures, including the evolving health care management systems. Skills in management and loss prevention techniques are essential for a functioning risk management program.

RISK MANAGEMENT PROGRAM DEVELOPMENT

Risk management programs have developed over the years into two basic models, one that focuses on safety and the other on patient injury. The latter is the more comprehensive model because it emphasizes patient care quality improvement and not merely injury reduction.[5]

Quality assessment and improvement activities overlap those of risk identification and treatment, particularly in the acquisition, analysis, and utilization of similar data for assessment, evaluation, and educational purposes. The result is a variety of organizational designs for the implementation of these functions. With some institutions, quality assurance and risk management are separate entities that report to clinical departments and legal counsel, respectively. The insurance function often reports to administration and/or finance. In other settings, either the quality assurance manager or the risk manager is the program director and the other manager has reporting responsibilities. The quality and risk management functions are integrated in some community hospitals and handled by the same individual.

Traditionally, risk management programs have focused on inpatient services and responded to the high incidence of malpractice claims resulting from events that took place in hospitals. With the shortened length of stay and the shift of care from inpatient to outpatient services, however, managers are currently developing and/or enhancing risk management programs for ambulatory services, including physicians' offices. Risk management principles underlying these programs remain the same regardless of the setting.

RISK MANAGEMENT FUNCTIONS

Those tasks considered as part of the risk management function are[4]

- controlling losses to the institution from medical malpractice
- managing claims
- reviewing contracts
- overseeing hospital safety program
- reviewing hospital policies to minimize loss exposures
- ensuring the adequacy of disaster plans
- keeping management informed of new legislation affecting operations
- identifying potential loss exposures from medical staff credentialing
- setting up risk management programs in outpatient care settings
- conducting ongoing orientation and inservice programs
- serving on hospital committees that discuss loss prevention and risk management issues
- reporting regularly to management and the board of directors on the effectiveness of the risk management program
- facilitating resolution of crisis situations in patient care areas
- managing the institution's insurance program
- complying with the standards of the Joint Commission on Accreditation of Healthcare Organizations related to risk management and safety

Risk managers approach the control of institutional loss by using a systematic process outlined below:[8]

- identification of risk
- analysis of risks identified

- treatment of risk
- evaluation of treatment strategies

Data Sources for Identification and Analysis of Risk

Risk identification at the institutional level requires the access and analysis of data relating to all actual and potential financial losses from out-of-court settlements and jury verdicts and casualty losses to the physical plant, property, staff, and visitors and/or their property. The human loss through death or disability from patient injury and the potential loss of reputation of defendants also must be calculated as real loss and taken into consideration in the risk management process.

The risk manager uses a variety of institutional data sources, including incident reports, actual and potential malpractice claims and suits, quality assessment data, patient complaints and surveys, safety and infection control data, and surveys by state licensing and accreditation bodies.

Published reports of multi-institutional studies with a focus on patient injury are valuable in determining the incidence and severity of various types of injuries and the potential loss and liability incurred by the injuries. These studies also target areas of high risk, such as drug therapy and medication errors, for detailed analysis.

MEDICATION ERRORS AND ADVERSE DRUG EVENTS

The Harvard Medical Practice Study,[9] published in 1991, reviewed randomly selected medical records of 30,195 patients hospitalized in New York state during 1989. The study identified 1,133 patients (3.7%) who suffered injuries caused by medical treatment; 27.6% of the injuries were due to negligence. The most common (19%) single type of adverse event were those resulting from drug complications. Anticoagulants, which ranked third as a drug class in the study, accounted for 11.2% of all drug-related adverse events.[10]

Actual loss through professional liability can be determined by analysis of closed claims and suits. The Physician Insurers Association of America (PIAA), a 44-member organization of physician-owned professional liability insurers, entered into a data sharing project in 1985 to collect and categorize malpractice data systematically from a variety of perspectives (eg, indemnity payments, profiles of defendants and plaintiffs, clinical specialties involved in the claims, allegations, injuries). In a 1992 study based on PIAA data,[11] of 67,650 closed claims, medication prescription (5,870 cases) gave rise to the most claims and was the most costly. Approximately one-third of the total claims in the study (21,977) were closed with indemnity payments totaling

$2.58 billion. Indemnity payments related to prescription of drugs totaled $185.53 million.

For study purposes, inpatient medication errors are categorized by the processes involved in drug therapy: ordering or prescribing, transcribing, dispensing, and administering. Prescription and administration accounted for about 81% of the errors in a study of 896 medication errors in a sample setting of slightly more than 2 million unit doses of medication.[12] Of the total errors, prescribing accounted for 323 errors; administering, 405 errors; dispensing, 110 errors; and transcribing, 58 errors.

Bates et al[13] studied 247 adverse drug events (ADEs) and 194 potential ADEs during a six-month period at three institutions and reported that 90% of the preventable ADEs occurred at the stages of ordering (56%) and administering (34%). Transcribing (6%) and dispensing errors (4%) were less frequent. The study concludes that "adverse drug events were common and often preventable."

A follow-up review of the 247 ADEs was done in order to determine errors in inpatient anticoagulant use (warfarin and heparin). Anticoagulants were responsible for 9 ADEs (4%), 4 of which were preventable. Of the 194 potential ADEs, 21 (14%) were due to anticoagulants. Together, ADEs and potential ADEs involving anticoagulants accounted for 9% of all serious drug errors in the study.[14]

Hemorrhage and thromboembolism are the major complications of drug therapy with oral anticoagulants. It has been estimated that more than a million patients at risk for thromboembolism because of prosthetic valves, atrial fibrillation, peripheral vascular disease, or cardiovascular disease are being treated with warfarin in the United States each year. The large numbers of this population and the long-term nature of the treatment increase the potential for additional risk and injury.

Landefeld and Goldman[15] studied the risk of major bleeding in 565 patients who were started on warfarin outpatient therapy at hospital discharge. Of these, 65 patients (12%) suffered episodes of major hemorrhage, and 10 (2%) of them sustained subsequent bleeding. Risk factors included

- older than age 65
- atrial fibrillation
- history of gastrointestinal bleeding
- history of stroke
- a severe co-morbid condition, such as a recent myocardial infarction, renal insufficiency, or severe anemia

A later study[16] of 928 patients receiving 1,103 courses of warfarin reported 1,332 episodes of bleeding of various severity. Age, reason for anticoagulation, use of interfering drugs, and hypertension were not associated with the risk of bleeding. A mean prothrombin time ratio (PTR) of more than 2.0 was a major indicator for risk of hemorrhage, with the highest risk during the first three months of therapy. Patients exhibiting variability in the PTR, as reflected by frequent dose adjustments, bled more frequently. The risk for thromboembolism was high when the mean PTR was less than 1.3.

The dominant risk factor in a study of 121 patients who suffered intracranial hemorrhage was a PTR greater than 2.0.[17] Age was a strong independent factor for subdural hemorrhage, and it had borderline statistical significance with intracerebral hemorrhage.

Despite the apparent conflicting reports of the antecedent patient risks of warfarin therapy, hemorrhage is a major adverse event that can be best prevented by careful monitoring of the PTR to guide dosage appropriately.

MALPRACTICE CLAIMS AND SUITS RELATED TO ORAL ANTICOAGULANTS

Adverse events involving oral anticoagulants might or might not be due to negligence; however, some of these events can result in medical malpractice claims and suits. To be successful in a malpractice suit, the plaintiff must establish

- that the health care provider owed a duty to the plaintiff/patient
- that there was a breach in that duty
- that injury occurred
- that the injury was caused by the breach (deviation of standard)

Contrary to public opinion, this is a difficult task to accomplish, and fewer than half of patients who bring suits ever receive compensation. Many claims are made, however, where there is an injury but no evidence of negligence.

A series of 10 medical malpractice claims or suits alleging failure in oral anticoagulant management is discussed below in some detail to demonstrate the complexity and multiplicity of events that resulted in the legal actions. More specifically, the focus of this review is to develop meaningful strategies for oral anticoagulant risk reduction and control based on actual case material. Legal and/or settlement outcomes are not included in the presentations.

These cases were closed between 1985 and 1994 by the self-insured captive of university-affiliated medical institutions. They involved 6 female and 4 male patients ranging in age from 6 to 74 years. Excluding the 6-year-old child, the average age was 67 and the median age was 58. The indications for warfarin therapy were prosthetic valves (4 cases), atrial fibrillation (3 cases), and pulmonary embolism and/or deep venous thrombosis (3 cases). The injuries included 7 resulting from hemorrhage and 3 from thromboembolism, which resulted in the death of 4 patients; 5 significant neurologic deficits; and 1 minor hematoma that required surgical evacuation.

Of the 7 patients who suffered injuries from bleeding, several of the antecedent risks previously cited[15] were present.

Four of the 7 patients were over age 65, 5 of the 7 had serious co-morbid conditions, and 2 had atrial fibrillation. One patient had an unidentified bleeding disorder. Correlations with the PTR were not possible because of the reporting methods.

Defendants in these claims represented a variety of medical specialties, including cardiologists, internists, and surgeons (general, vascular, urologic). In addition, 2 pharmacists and 10 institutions (8 hospitals and 2 pharmacies) were named.

Fifteen liability issues were identified for the cases:

1. no response to abnormal values
2. warfarin not reordered after invasive procedure
3. warfarin not held before invasive procedure
4. inadequate or no patient medication history
5. lack of coordination and communication
6. inadequate or no patient teaching
7. documentation problems
8. medication errors in ordering and dispensing
9. unidentified noncompliant patient
10. vitamin K not given when indicated
11. no consultation when appropriate
12. overreliance on computer-generated protocol
13. physician attitude
14. resident supervision and staffing
15. telephone assessment

Multiple issues were found in each of the 10 cases. A careful reading of these cases provides convincing evidence that most of the events might have been avoided if patients and/or families understood the goals and risks of the treatment. In addition, patients need to be empowered to question their providers when they do not understand, or are unsure of, the rationale for continuous testing and medication changes. A major role for the staff of an anticoagulation clinic is undoubtedly patient education and evaluation of patient knowledge necessary to prevent injuries and complications. The education of patients and the assessment of their knowledge constitute a major strategy to reduce liability exposure of individual providers and institutions.

CASE STUDIES

Miscommunication

Anticoagulation clinics have a major impact on the efficiency and effectiveness with which oral anticoagulation is managed. The coordination of laboratory results with drug dosage changes is performed by providers specializing in this process. Case 1 demonstrates how the lack of coordination and communication between providers resulted in the patient's death.

Case 1

A 45-year-old female undergoing chemotherapy for breast cancer was admitted with a diagnosis of pulmonary embolism and treated with heparin and warfarin for 10 days. At discharge, her prothrombin time (PT) was in the therapeutic range of 18.5/10.1 on 7.5 mg of warfarin daily. The following day, she was seen at a health center for an infected tooth and vaginal infection. She was treated with Flagyl and penicillin. Her warfarin was reduced to 5 mg because of the enhancement effect of Flagyl. The patient's PT was being monitored at the health center, but, because she was also receiving chemotherapy, she requested that her blood be drawn at the hospital when she was there for the chemotherapy. The result of the first PT done at the hospital was 11.1/10.1, and a notation was made that it be checked at the health center for the next two weeks. The abnormal PT was flagged in the record but not reported to the primary physician at the health center. The patient was not seen again until she arrived in the emergency department in cardiac arrest 13 days later. The autopsy report indicated that the cause of death was an acute thromboembolism of the right pulmonary artery and a pulmonary embolism with organizing thrombus of the left pulmonary artery. A claim was made against the primary care physician that alleged failure to monitor and manage warfarin therapy properly, which led to the patient's death.

Risk Management Issues

When more than one physician is involved in a patient's care, it is essential that it be clear to all providers and to the patient as to the individual responsible for each aspect of the care and how communication will be established and maintained. The patient must be educated regarding the use, effect, and necessity for close monitoring of the PT in order to regulate the dosage properly. It is also appropriate to tell the patient what the target therapeutic range should be. An electronic monitoring system that flags unreported laboratory results might have prevented the disastrous outcome of this case.

Medication Error

Dispensing errors in two cases resulted in a thromboembolic stroke in one patient and an intracerebral hemorrhage in the other patient.

Case 2

A 44-year-old female was maintained on anticoagulant medication for approximately seven years subsequent to replacement of her mitral valve with a Starr-Edwards valve.

She suffered a left-sided stroke one year prior to the present event as a result of a nontherapeutic level of anticoagulation. In this case, the patient's prescription was mistakenly refilled by the pharmacist with 2.5-mg warfarin tablets instead of the prescribed dosage of 5 mg. One week later, she had her PT done at a local community hospital, and the results were sent to an anticoagulation unit at a nearby medical center. When the PTR was determined to be 1.2, which was below the required 1.5-2.0, notification was sent to the patient to advise her to continue her present dosage for one week and have a repeat in another week, per institutional protocol. The patient received the notification the day before she suffered a left-sided stroke. PT on admission was 10.5/10.5. A claim was made against the pharmacist, pharmacy, and hospital.

Risk Management Issues

Case 2 involved a very–high-risk patient because of her Starr-Edwards prosthesis, which is known to be the most thrombogenic type of valve, and the fact that she had had a prior stroke. The anticoagulation clinic presumably thought this represented a transient drop in her PT and suggested continuing the same dose but repeating the PT in one week. Clinic staff were unaware of the medication error by the pharmacy. The medication administration error was the proximal cause of the nontherapeutic blood levels and resultant stroke. Electronic methods need to be developed to prevent human error in dispensing. Patients must be alerted to report any differences noted in the color, size, shape, or other aspects of their pills when their prescriptions are refilled.

Case 3

A 52-year-old female patient was placed on oral anticoagulation subsequent to aortic and mitral valve replacements. PTs were drawn weekly to biweekly. The dose and schedule of warfarin varied. At one point, the patient experienced a large hematoma and ecchymosis to her right forearm secondary to mild trauma. Her PT at that time was 37.3/11.6. Warfarin was withheld but was restarted when her PT was rechecked at 16.5/11.6. It took two months for resolution of the ecchymosis, which extended from wrist to elbow. After this episode, PTs were drawn monthly, and they remained stable. The patient telephoned her physician's office for a prescription refill, which was called in to the pharmacy by the secretary. Two weeks later, the patient reported bruising of her right arm and was instructed to stop taking the warfarin for three days and then to resume. Two days later, she presented at the emergency services with ecchymotic areas over her body, generalized headache, and vomited guaiac-positive emesis. She claimed to have stopped her warfarin as instructed. Her PT was 66/11.6, and her activated partial thromboplastin time (aPTT) was 128/33. A neurologic examination and a computerized tomography (CT) scan were negative. She was given 10 mg of vitamin K and analgesics for headache and was discharged home. The following day, the patient was admitted to the hospital with a brain stem hemorrhage secondary to warfarin-induced hypoprothrombinemia. It was ultimately determined that there was an error in the prescription refill. Instead of receiving orange-colored, 2.5-mg tablets for a daily dosage of 5 mg, the patient was given and was taking the peach-colored, 5-mg tablets for a daily dosage of 10 mg. Despite the severity of the patient's injury, the hemorrhage was totally resolved at discharge and her rehabilitation potential was for a full recovery. A claim was made against the physician, pharmacy, and secretary.

Risk Management Issues

Systems to prevent human error that can cause significant patient injury need to be developed. In retrospect, it was determined that this was a severely depressed and, at times, noncompliant patient whose PT was difficult to control. She had multiple symptoms, including headaches, for which she took four or five analgesics daily, and had had neurologic consults prior to this incident. It would appear that this type of patient would have benefited greatly from the close monitoring available through an anticoagulation clinic.

Subsequent to the incident, this patient became even more depressed and saw a psychiatrist, who placed her on medication that she took irregularly. She continued to have variability in her PTs, which created difficulty in keeping her within a therapeutic range for several years after the injury.

Physician Attitude and an Angry Patient

Patient anger directed against a physician that was not addressed prompted the claim in case 4.

Case 4

A 34-year-old male was hospitalized for anticoagulant treatment for deep venous thrombosis and a suspicion of pulmonary emboli. He was discharged on warfarin, 10 mg/day. It was unclear how or if his PTs were monitored. Ten days later, he experienced chest pain, fatigue, and breathlessness. A lung scan confirmed pulmonary emboli, and he was admitted for placement of a transjugular caval filter. He was discharged on warfarin (dosage unknown) and an analgesic for pain. The following day, he presented to triage at his health maintenance organization with incisional pain and swelling from a hematoma. His PT was 24 seconds. He was treated with analgesics and hot packs. The next day, he telephoned his primary care physician, who made an appointment to see him the following day. A consult was arranged with a general surgeon, who suggested checking the PT and reducing the warfarin if necessary. In addition, the general surgeon suggested admission if the hematoma did not resolve. A pressure dressing was applied and Tylenol given. The next day, the patient was seen by a vascular surgeon, who placed the caval filter. He had the patient admitted for evacuation of the hematoma. A claim, alleging improper treatment, was made against the general surgeon.

Risk Management Issues

This was an extremely anxious young man who had experienced a life-threatening situation. He kept a detailed diary of all medical encounters. The patient believed that he was not taken seriously by the consulting general surgeon, who had a condescending attitude and minimized his complaints (ie, prescribing Tylenol when the analgesic was ineffective). He complained that the surgeon did not answer his specific clinical questions and patted him on the shoulder, which was quite painful from the hematoma extension. The patient verbalized extreme anger with this physician to his nurse, which was not dealt with at the time. Expressions of anger by patients always should be taken seriously and reported to the risk manager or other personnel, as defined by institutional policy, so that an appropriate response can be made.

The setting for this case was a group practice where admissions, referrals, and consultations were set by policy, sometimes with resulting delays, lack of coordination, and communication lapses. The general surgeon who was covering had never seen this patient before and believed that the patient's problem belonged to the operating vascular surgeon. This attitude is one that physicians, particularly in this era of managed care, need to explore fully and to correct if they are to avoid being sued. The physician involved in this case, although respected for his clinical ability, lacked appropriate communication skills. His actions resulted in two additional suits.

Trauma

Trauma played a part in two cases of patient injury. In case 5, the parents of a six-year-old girl were given insufficient information regarding the risks of bleeding with warfarin medication. In case 6, a fatal hemorrhage might have been prevented in an elderly patient if she had been questioned regarding her medication history in the emergency room or if she had been instructed regarding the risks of trauma while taking warfarin.

Case 5

A six-year-old female had surgery for replacement of the aortic root of the ascending aorta with a Björk-Shiley valve because of an aneurysm associated with Marfan's syndrome. She was known to have a tendency for bruising and bleeding, but a coagulation workup was not done at that time. The patient was placed on warfarin and, in three days, had a PT of 15.5/12.2 on a dosage of 2 mg daily. She was discharged on the 7th postoperative day with the same dosage. Four days after discharge, she suffered a nosebleed (PT 16.5/12.7). The following day, her warfarin was increased to 3 mg/day. She subsequently had a hematology workup in an attempt to identify a specific bleeding disorder. A PT of 27.4/12.7 and an aPTT of 43.5/31.4 were reported 12 days after the increase of warfarin to 3 mg. There was some bleeding reported at the lower end of her incision two weeks later (PT, 17.2/11.4). On her next visit in 12 days, the patient's warfarin was increased to 4 mg/day (PT, 18.5/11.3) and a follow-up appointment scheduled for three months. The patient was admitted with leg weakness and paresthesia 2 days later (55 days post-hospital discharge). The history noted that she was hopping and jumping about at a party and straining while moving bowels 2 days prior to admission (PT, 21.8/12.3; aPTT, 44.4/30.1). The patient was found to have a significant, acute neurologic defect localized at the region of the first lumbar vertebra and below. Myelogram findings were consistent with extensive subdural hematoma, which was surgically evacuated. The patient developed disseminated intravascular coagulopathy treated with fresh-frozen plasma. Surgical exploration resulted in only minimal improvement in her left leg. She developed a neurogenic bladder that required long-term intermittent catheterization.

Risk Management Issues

This child presented with a difficult clinical problem. Although von Willebrand's bleeding disorder was suspected, extensive testing did not confirm this diagnosis. The bleeding disorder, however, was not implicated in the etiology of the subdural hemorrhage. Anticoagulation was difficult to control and necessitated careful and precise documentation, but there was a gap of close to a month in the documentation of the anticoagulant management. Parents of children on anticoagulant therapy need precise oral and written instructions regarding activity and prevention of trauma. No notation was made on discharge of patient/parent instruction and understanding of the risks of trauma. In a letter written by one of the physicians, the parents were warned that the child should not participate in strenuous sports or gym. Most parents probably would not interpret this child's activities, prior to her admission, as strenuous or consistent with those of gym.

Case 6

A 74-year-old female was discharged from the hospital after 12 days of treatment for congestive heart failure, atrial fibrillation, pneumonia, and flare-up of disseminated lupus erythematosus. Warfarin was prescribed in addition to multiple cardiac drugs and prednisone. Her PT on discharge was 21/10.5. Two months later, the patient was seen by a resident in emergency after she was "struck by a slow moving car." The only abnormality noted was a slight bruise over her left hip. There was no tenderness or ecchymosis. Vital signs were recorded once: blood pressure (BP), 160/80; pulse, 100; respiration, 22; temperature (T), 98.6°F. Cervical spine X-rays were negative. No past medical history was elicited. The patient was able to ambulate independently, and she was discharged without follow-up instructions. Approximately 12 hours later, she was brought asystolic to a local community hospital. The history noted "on warfarin." She was resuscitated with central but no peripheral BP. Paracentesis was negative, and hematocrit (Hct) was 21%. She was intubated and transferred back to the university hospital, where she arrived comatose with fixed dilated pupils; BP 50/palpitations; PT, 26.7/11.1. The patient's abdomen was distended without bowel signs. Hct was 18%. Exploration of the abdomen and thorax were negative for active bleeding. There was a retroperitoneal hematoma. The patient never regained consciousness and was subsequently pronounced dead. The medical examiner's autopsy report described an acute myocardial infarction, which could have been the basis for sudden acute ventricular dysrhythmia and fatal cardiac arrest precipitated by the bleeding. A claim was made alleging that the failure to obtain a history or record of warfarin medication prevented proper care and resulted in hemorrhage and death.

Risk Management Issues

Trauma patients should be routinely questioned regarding anticoagulant medication. Staff of anticoagulation clinics may need to be involved in education programs for emergency department personnel. Patients on long-term anticoagulant therapy should be encouraged to wear Medic-Alert bracelets and/or be instructed to inform caregivers of their medication history, particularly in the setting of trauma. When a history is not documented, the presumption is that it was not done. Careful documentation is always essential, even in the setting of an emergency department with multiple trauma patients who appear to require priority attention.

Invasive Procedures

Cases 7, 8, and 9 refer to patients receiving warfarin who required invasive procedures.

Case 7

A 67-year-old male, with a history of atrial fibrillation, who had been taking warfarin for 8 years was hospitalized for removal of a bladder stone. On admission, the patient stated that he was taking warfarin for "thick blood," had stopped taking it 12 days previously in anticipation of surgery, and did not know the dosage. Documentation of his history and physical examination was extremely sketchy. The stone removal by lithotripsy was unsuccessful, and plans were made to do an open procedure. The patient developed an irregular pulse, and an unsuccessful attempt was made to contact his cardiologist (who was not on the staff of that hospital). He was discharged and returned one week later for the open surgical procedure. Preoperative tests included a PT of 10.3/10.8 and an aPTT of 29.0. The preanesthesia workup noted that the patient had had chronic atrial fibrillation for 12 to 14 years, had taken no warfarin for three to four weeks, and had an irregular pulse. An electrocardiogram (ECG) showed atrial fibrillation, right bundle branch block, and changes consistent with anterior ischemia. It was noted that the patient's old chart was unavailable for comparison, but, because he had no symptoms, it could be "presumed" that the ECG changes were old ones. A cystolithotomy and transurethral prostatectomy were performed without incident, and the patient was discharged on the sixth postoperative day. He reported slight weakness in his left hand four days later and was advised to see his cardiologist. One week later, he suffered left-sided weakness, facial droop, and slurred speech, and he was admitted to the hospital. CT scan was consistent with an acute right middle cerebral artery infarct. The patient's condition gradually worsened over several days, and he subsequently expired. The patient's family claimed that the stroke could have been prevented if the warfarin had been restarted.

Risk Management Issues

It is essential that patients and/or their families be given careful, detailed instruction regarding the goals of anticoagulant therapy. It is particularly important for providers to reinforce instruction and check understanding periodically when a patient is on long-term therapy. After eight years of taking warfarin, this patient demonstrated little understanding of his medical status or treatment. If he and his family had better understood his clinical situation, this outcome might have been averted. A patient with a long history of cardiac difficulty should have a careful preoperative workup, including a cardiac consultation. It is unclear why this patient's cardiologist was never contacted, either by the surgeon or by the patient himself after he was instructed to do so. It would have been appropriate in view of his history to have a preoperative cardiac workup at the institution where the surgery was performed, particularly because the medical record noted that his past medical records were unavailable.

Physicians in non-cardiology specialties might need updating in oral anticoagulation management and the appropriateness of seeking consultation with staff members of anticoagulant clinics.

Case 8

A 73-year-old woman was admitted with carotid artery occlusion for an elective arteriography of the neck arteries via a right axillary route. She had diffuse cardiovascular disease and had undergone bilateral femoral bypass procedures. In addition, she had a history of myocardial infarction, hypertension, pulmonary embolus, and cerebral episodes. In addition to taking 5 mg of warfarin a day, the patient was on Lopressor, digoxin, and hydrochlorothiazide. On admission, the patient's PT was 21.6/12.1. Even though she had been advised to discontinue her warfarin six days prior to admission, she experienced hypertension and profuse bleeding while the arteriography was in process. A vascular surgeon was called to control the bleeding. He successfully accomplished hemostasis under adverse conditions but, in the process, ensnared the median nerve with a silk suture (which was removed during a subsequent operation). The patient developed a neuropathy along the distribution of the right upper extremity and made a claim against the vascular surgeon who had responded to the emergency situation.

Risk Management Issues

Because the PT was not allowed to return to normal, this patient was placed at greater risk for bleeding. Vitamin K supplements, if administered preoperatively, might have accelerated the return to a normal PT. A medical colleague brought into an emergency situation can be placed at risk for a malpractice suit if the primary provider is less than careful in the medical management of a patient.

Case 9

A 68-year-old patient with a history of atrial fibrillation had been taking warfarin, but it was discontinued while he underwent a course of epidural steroids for lumbar disk disease. Several weeks elapsed before the warfarin was restarted (PT 12.5/10). A dosage of 5 mg/day was ordered and arrangements were to be made for PTs to be drawn at a local hospital. Ten days after the initiation of the warfarin, the PT was 22/10. Approximately one week later, the patient suffered a fatal cerebral hemorrhage. A claim by the estate of the deceased alleged that the physician's inaccurate dose of warfarin caused the wrongful death of the patient.

Risk Management Issues

When a patient's warfarin is discontinued for any reason, a system should be in place to ensure that it is restarted.

Patients and/or families must be thoroughly educated in all aspects of oral anticoagulant management, including how long it is safe to discontinue the medication and to alert their providers when the safe period has been exceeded.

Noncompliance and Telephone Assessment

Case 10

A 69-year-old male, who had been on a maintenance dose of warfarin for several years subsequent to a mitral valve replacement, was monitored by a local physician in his community. His cardiac status was evaluated on a semiannual basis by the cardiologist at the university hospital where the surgery was performed. Six weeks after he had dental care, the patient telephoned his cardiologist to report that he had been experiencing a fever (T, 100°F–100.2°F) for three days, and that he was tired and did not have much pep. In his office notes, the cardiologist recorded the patient's telephone call and reported symptoms and then made the notation: "Imp [impression]: GOK [God only knows]: Rx: outpatient— FUO [fever of unknown origin]." Subsequently, he made arrangements for a series of laboratory tests, including a blood culture. All tests were within normal range except a sedimentation rate of 51, red blood cells in the urine, and a slightly elevated blood sugar. The cardiologist did not communicate with the patient again. One month later, the patient complained of chills, fever (T, 102°F), and headache. He was treated locally by telephone with penicillin for three days. Four days later, he was experiencing migrating muscle pains. Hospitalization was discussed, but no beds were available. Within a week, he was admitted on an emergency basis with headache, right-sided hemiparesis, visual field deficit, and aphasia. His PT was 27/11.8. Computed tomography confirmed an occipital intracerebral hematoma. The cardiologist was subsequently sued for failure to monitor the patient's PTs, with the result that the patient required surgery for an intracranial hemorrhage and long-term rehabilitation.

Risk Management Issues

Diagnosis and/or treatment by telephone is always risky. This patient did not have the benefit of a physical examination or a detailed review of his current status. If a thorough history had been taken, it might have been determined that his PTs were not being appropriately monitored; he was often noncompliant in getting tested and had been adjusting his warfarin dosage since his physician had died several months previously. It is good practice to question all patients taking oral anticoagulants about current warfarin dosage and most recent PT, regardless of their presenting symptoms. Such practice might prevent serious injury in patients who do not understand their treatment or are noncompliant for whatever reason. Care should be taken to document appropriately,

whether in hospital or office records. Unapproved abbreviations should be resisted because their explanations may create embarrassment for the physician in the courtroom and create a lack of credibility with the jury.

CONCLUSION

Clinical risk management has as its goal the identification and analysis of actual and potential human and financial losses in order to develop strategies that will reduce or prevent those losses. The staff of an anticoagulation clinic play an important role in the prevention, management, and control of losses. Patient education, design of clinical systems, communication, provider education, and appropriate documentation were among the most frequent lapses in the medical malpractice cases reviewed in this chapter.

Patient Education

This subject is presented in more detail in Chapter 10. In almost all of the cases reviewed, patient education was an issue. It is not enough to teach patients a series of facts about their therapy, such as medication use, effect, adverse reactions, PT target range, and importance of compliance, unless a system is in place to evaluate their knowledge periodically. Documentation of topics covered and patient response to the teaching effort is not only important, and can be lifesaving, but it is evidence of a high standard of care. Parents of children, family members, and significant others should be educated and that fact noted in patient records.

Design of Clinical Systems

Electronic monitoring systems that flag abnormal data, unreported laboratory results, and discontinued drugs with restart dates might have prevented several patient injuries reported in this chapter. Leape[18] suggests the development of an electronic system, such as bar codes, that will prevent dosage errors. Two major injuries in the case reports could have been prevented if such a system had been available. Patients who might be at risk because of sudden abnormal changes in PT should be contacted by telephone. Most institutions have policies for actions to be taken by staff when they are unable to contact patients at risk (including when to secure the assistance of the local police).

Communication

Goldhaber[19] states that "the need for detailed communication among practitioners from different disciplines cannot be overemphasized" in the management of anticoagulants. Anticoagulation clinics reduce the need for multiple providers and therefore the opportunity for lapses in communication. By ensuring patient safety and preventing loss as a result of patient injury, in addition to maintaining effective and efficient warfarin management, these clinics can be important strategies in loss prevention.

Malpractice attorneys report that 80% of malpractice suits are due to communication issues.[20] Communication breakdown between providers and patients creates a sense of dissatisfaction and anger in many patients. Devaluing patients' views, failing to understand patients' perspectives, desertion, and delivering information poorly are cited as four types of communication problems in a study by Beckman et al.[21] The first two communication problems were cited by the patient in one of the case reports. The same communication skills that lead to patient satisfaction and quality care are those that reduce risk of malpractice. Expressions of patient anger need to be dealt with immediately.

Effective patient/provider communication should ensure the opportunity to identify the noncompliant patient and the reasons for noncompliance. Anticoagulation clinics provide the necessary structure for accomplishing this communication.

Provider Education

The expertise of anticoagulation clinic staff should be utilized for provider education, particularly for providers who are infrequently involved in anticoagulant therapy. Continuing education should include the most recent concepts in the use of anticoagulant management, including use of the International Normalized Ratio for reporting PT. Additional topics suggested from the case analysis might include perioperative management of oral anticoagulants; indications for consultation; management of patients who are difficult to control; importance of medication history, particularly in the setting of trauma; and patient/family education.

Appropriate Documentation

A vital part of any risk management discussion is an emphasis on complete, concise, and appropriate documentation that not only is necessary for the delivery of quality care but is also a major factor in the successful defense of malpractice claims. The legal system is based on the presentation of evidence as legal proof, and juries are instructed to make their decisions in accordance with the evidence presented. In medical malpractice, documentation in patients' records is the major source of such evidence. Some cases, regardless of issues of negligence, are settled or result in verdicts on behalf of the plaintiffs only because of incomplete, lacking, inappropriate, or altered patient records.

A suit is often filed when there is a bad outcome but no deviation of standard, and proof of the appropriate standard of care must be substantiated. Such substantiation is most frequently accomplished through written documentation in the patient record.

In the cases cited, there were many instances of documentation lapses, including record gaps and no evidence of patient/family education regarding risks and benefits of treatment, consultations, and responsibility for PTs. Each clinic needs to develop carefully designed policies, protocols, and guidelines relating to documentation.

The final suggestion is that all clinic staff, both professional and support, know who their institutional risk manager is and what resources are available through his or her office. A copy of all institutional risk management policies and procedures that relate to reporting requirements for medication errors, adverse events, and patient dissatisfaction should be available. Education in basic risk management principles should be part of an ongoing continuing education program that is adapted to the individual needs of clinics and the institutions that support them.

REFERENCES

1. *St. Paul Insurance Company Report to Policyholders, Physicians and Surgeons Update.* St Paul, MN: St Paul Insurance Company; 1991.

2. California Medical Association. *Report of the Medical Insurance Feasibility Study.* San Francisco: California Medical Association; 1977.

3. Brown BL. *Risk Management for Hospitals: A Practical Approach.* Gaithersburg, MD: Aspen Publishers; 1979.

4. Hapsten LM. Introduction. In: Hapsten LM, Veach MS, eds. *Risk Management Handbook for Health Care Facilities.* Chicago, IL: American Hospital Publishing; 1990:3–8.

5. Orlinkoff JE. *Malpractice Prevention and Liability Control for Hospitals.* 2nd ed. Chicago, IL: American Hospital Publishing; 1988.

6. Orlinkoff JE, Lanham GB. Quality assurance and risk management: learning to live together. *J Qual Assurance.* 1980;2:8.

7. U.S. General Accounting Office. *Initiatives in Hospital Risk Management.* Washington, DC: U.S. General Accounting Office; 1989:1.

8. Troyer G, Salman SL. *Handbook of Health Care Risk Management.* Gaithersburg, MD: Aspen Publishers; 1986:153.

9. Brennan TA, Leape LL, Laird NM, et al. Incidence of adverse events and negligence in hospitalized patients—results of the Harvard Medical Practice Study I. *N Engl J Med.* 1991;324:370–376.

10. Leape LL, Brennan TA, Laird NM, et al. The nature of adverse events in hospitalized patients—results of the Harvard Medical Practice Study II. *N Engl J Med.* 1991;324:377–384.

11. Holoweiko M. What are your greatest malpractice risks? *Med Econ.* 1992;69:141–159.

12. Siders C. Medication errors in an acute care setting. *J Healthcare Risk Manage.* 1995;15:20–26.

13. Bates DW, Cullen DJ, Laird NM, et al. Incidence of adverse drug events. Implications for prevention. ADE Prevention Study Group. *JAMA.* 1995:274:29–34.

14. Bates DW. Anticoagulants: Errors in their use, and claims. *Forum.* 1994;15:12–14.

15. Landefeld CS, Goldman L. Major bleeding in outpatients treated with warfarin: incidence and prediction by factors known at the start of outpatient therapy. *Am J Med.* 1989;87:144–152.

16. Fihn SD, McDonell M, Martin D, et al. Risk factors for complications of chronic anticoagulation: a multicenter study. *Ann Intern Med.* 1993;118:511–520.

17. Hylek EM, Singer DE. Risk factors for intracranial hemorrhage in outpatients taking warfarin. *Ann Intern Med.* 1994;120:897–902.

18. Leape, LL. Errors in medicine. *JAMA.* 1994;272:1851–1857.

19. Goldhaber SZ. Outpatient monitoring of anticoagulation: an important component of risk management. *Forum.* 1994;15:14–15.

20. Avery JK. Lawyers tell what turns some patients litigious. *Med Malpractice Rev.* 1985;2:35–37.

21. Beckman HB, Markakis KM, Suchman AL, Frankel RM. The doctor–patient relationship and malpractice: lessons from plaintiff depositions. *Arch Intern Med.* 1994;154:1365–1370.

Medical-Legal Implications of Anticoagulation Therapy

William P. McCormick

INTRODUCTION

The management of anticoagulation therapy involves a high-wire balancing act in which clinical success is partially determined by avoidance of two equally serious clinical failures. In nonscientific jargon, these clinical failures are overanticoagulation and underanticoagulation. Both situations are life threatening, and they have been fertile ground for medical malpractice and professional negligence litigation in the United States. This chapter first explains the basic elements of a medical malpractice or professional negligence case so that anticoagulation clinicians can analyze their clinical choices from a medical-legal perspective as they "walk the high wire." The balance of this chapter consists of an in-depth review of one ongoing anticoagulation case that has been highly litigated and involves many important learning opportunities. This retrospective review illustrates the substantive anticoagulation management errors that are alleged to have been made in this case. The case also demonstrates the general timetable and unpredictability of civil litigation in the United States.

A TORT LAW PRIMER

Tort law concepts are the basis for the civil justice system in the United States. All negligence, malpractice, medical malpractice, professional negligence, and personal injury claims are based on a tort allegation of some kind. The traditional tort definition is as follows: *Tort*—(from Latin—torquere, to twist, tortus, twisted, wrested aside) A private or civil wrong or injury, other than breach of contract, for which the court will provide a remedy in the form of an action for damages.[1]

The three essential elements of any tort action are the (1) the existence of a legal duty from defendant to plaintiff, (2) a breach of that duty, and (3) damages as a proximate result.[2] Each of these elements must be established before an individual bringing a tort claim will prevail.

Legal Duty

A legal duty typically arises out of a relationship between two individuals and/or organizations that causes them to follow a particular standard of conduct during their interactions. A health care provider/patient relationship generally gives rise to a legal duty of the health care provider to conform to an acceptable standard of care while providing health care services to the patient. A health care provider can raise its minimum legal duty when it voluntarily assumes or creates a new duty on behalf of its patients. A pharmacy provider that advertises its expertise in detecting a Micronase®/Coumadin® drug interaction by using its branded software package was found to have voluntarily assumed a new duty to accurately screen for drug interactions.[3] This legal duty would not normally have been imposed on this pharmacy provider, but the pharmacy advertised its drug interaction detection program to the public and subsequently missed a Parnate®/Tavist D® drug interaction. The missed drug interaction caused the patient to have a stroke with resulting serious complications. The court that heard this case on appeal created a new theory of liability and legal duty for this pharmacy. The lesson from this case is that well-intentioned publicity may raise the legal duties a health care provider owes to its patients.

Breach of a Legal Duty

Once a legal duty is established, the facts need to be examined to determine whether there has been a breach of the legal duty. A breach of a legal duty can also be described as "substandard conduct" or conduct that is below what is expected of a "reasonable" person having the same professional qualifications and role. A pharmacist that inadvertently labels a Coumadin® prescription to be taken "every six hours" instead of "once each day" will be liable for the severe bleed that results.[4] This dispensing/labeling error by a pharmacist is a simple illustration of a breach of a pharmacist's duty to correctly label each prescription.

Damages as a Proximate Result

Damages are a fairly easy concept to understand, while proximate cause is not as intuitive. A stroke or a severe bleed are distinct events that are usually identified as part of the damages in an anticoagulation case. In addition to proving actual damages, a plaintiff must also prove that the damages were the proximate result of the substandard conduct to establish legal liability. When a plaintiff cannot establish a link between his or her injury and the alleged breach of a legal duty by the health care provider, he or she will not prevail in court. Proximate cause was the issue in a case where the wife of a deceased cardiac patient could not sufficiently prove that her husband's death due to hemorrhaging and/or cardiac disease was proximately caused by an emergency department visit three years earlier.[5] The patient was taking Coumadin® and was prescribed erythromycin in the emergency department because he was suffering from pneumonia at the time. The expert witness in the case admitted that he could not associate the patient's demise with the prior emergency department visit, and the case was dismissed for lack of proximate cause.

CASE STUDY

Understanding the above elements of a tort law matter should help with tough decisions and policy drafting in everyday clinical practice. Risk management is the proactive avoidance of liability exposure, and it should include an overlay of the above tort law analysis to determine whether a particular behavior may create tort liability. Basic risk management analysis encompasses three questions that can be asked about any clinical situation:

1. Is there a legal duty owing to the patient or patients in question?
2. If yes, will there be a breach of that legal duty (substandard conduct) if a certain course of conduct is undertaken or not undertaken?
3. Are damages a proximate result of the substandard conduct?

The following case, which illustrates these principles in context, has an interesting fact pattern and illustrates the various stages of a civil lawsuit. The case of *Austermiller vs. Dosick*, Lucas App. No. L-01-1223, 2001-Ohio-2910 (December 31, 2001), raises several interesting issues for clinicians who initiate anticoagulation therapy and then lose further contact with their patients. The case also illustrates the period of time a contentious tort action can take to fully litigate. The underlying medical treatment that gave rise to this case occurred in 1994, and the case is still not fully resolved as of this writing. The timeline for this case is as follows:

Austermiller Case Timeline

November 1992	Plaintiff has vein stripping and ligation performed by the Defendant.
January 1993	Plaintiff has Greenfield filter placed by the Defendant.
October 28, 1994– November 19, 1994	Plaintiff hospitalized for lower extremity graph surgery and discharged on Coumadin®.
November 17, 1994	Plaintiff misses follow-up visit with Defendant.
November 17, 1994– August 17, 1997	Plaintiff receives refills of his Coumadin® prescriptions at two different pharmacies.
September 19, 1997	Plaintiff dies from internal bleeding.
May 20, 1998	Administrator of Plaintiff's estate causes civil case No. CI98-2443 to be filed in the Court of Common Pleas, Lucas County, Ohio.
Sometime between May 20, 1998 and March 5, 2001	Plaintiff reaches settlement with pharmacy that filled Plaintiff's Coumadin® prescriptions.
March 5, 2001	Jury trial held in the Court of Common Pleas, Lucas County, Ohio. Trial court grants directed verdict, dismissing the case at Defendant's request on March 6, 2001.
July 5, 2001	Plaintiff files appeal No. L-01-1233 in the Sixth District Court of Appeals of Ohio, Lucas County.

December 31, 2001	The Sixth District Court of Appeals of Ohio, Lucas County, issues a Decision and Judgment Entry reversing the trial court's dismissal of this case.
May 1, 2002	Defendant's appeal No. 2002-0284 is not accepted for review by the Ohio Supreme Court.
Sometime in 2002 or 2003	A new jury trial will occur in the Lucas County Court of Common Pleas.

The Plaintiff was a 46-year-old male who worked as a quality control technician at a silica sand processing facility in northern Ohio. The Plaintiff had a multiyear history of alcohol abuse, smoking, serious venous and arterial disease, venous clotting, and pulmonary emboli. The Plaintiff initially presented at the Wound Care Center and/or the Jobst Vascular Center at Toledo Hospital with deep vein thrombosis. In 1992, the Plaintiff underwent a stripping and ligation of the greater saphenous vein due to a nonhealing ulceration of his right ankle, which was initially injured in a motor vehicle accident when the Plaintiff was 21 years old. In 1993, the Plaintiff had a Greenfield filter placed by the Defendant, a board-certified vascular surgeon, because the Plaintiff had experienced previous pulmonary emboli. At that time, the Plaintiff was started on Coumadin® because of a clotting defect, which retrospectively is suspected to have been a Factor V_{Leiden} genetic variant. In October of 1994, the Plaintiff underwent vascular surgery known as a right femoral popliteal bypass and enarterectomy for a totally blocked (knee to the groin area) right superficial femoral artery and blockage of the posterior tibia artery. Postsurgery, the Plaintiff had a good Doppler of his right leg and anticoagulation was indicated due to a history of a suspected clotting defect, pulmonary embolism, deep vein thrombosis, the very recent synthetic graft, and a suspected contraction of the Greenfield filter. During the procedure, the Plaintiff was placed on heparin and subsequently restarted on Coumadin® with daily prothrombin times. On November 10, 1994, the Plaintiff was discharged from the hospital by the Defendant, with instructions to take daily doses of Coumadin® and with instructions to return for a follow-up visit on November 14, 1994, to monitor the effects of the Coumadin® and for a postsurgical examination. Neither party disputed the fact that the Plaintiff failed to attend his follow-up visits, and the Defendant testified that he had no contact with the Plaintiff after his discharge from the hospital on November 10, 1994.

There is disputed testimony regarding whether Defendant or his office staff authorized the Plaintiff's Bowling Green, Ohio, pharmacy to refill his Coumadin® prescriptions over the 18 months after his discharge from the hospital. On March 11, 1996, a prescription for 60 Coumadin® tablets with six refills was recorded by the Bowling Green pharmacy. On December 20, 1996, the Bowling Green pharmacy transferred the prescription to a Napoleon, Ohio, pharmacy that was part of the same pharmacy chain operation as the Bowling Green, Ohio, pharmacy. The pharmacist at the Napoleon, Ohio, pharmacy erroneously recorded the original date of the prescription as December 20, 1996. As a result of this error, the prescription was filled for more than one year beyond the date it was originally written, which is a violation of Ohio pharmacy regulations. Refills of 60 tablets were dispensed by the Napoleon, Ohio, pharmacy on April 22, 1997, and August 14, 1997. The Plaintiff died of internal bleeding on September 19, 1997.

In May of 1998, a civil lawsuit was filed in Lucas County, Ohio, against the Defendant and the pharmacy chain. At some point before the case went to trial, the pharmacy chain settled on their behalf and the case proceeded against the Defendant.

The primary issue in this case is a factual discrepancy regarding the source of the ongoing prescriptions the Plaintiff received after the Plaintiff was discharged from the hospital on November 14, 1994. The Plaintiff's case included the following testimony by the Plaintiff's son who visited his father monthly from his home in Michigan where he lived with his mother. The testimony suggests an ongoing physician/patient relationship between the Defendant and the Plaintiff, well after the Plaintiff discharge from the hospital on November 10, 1994. This testimony also suggests that the Defendant authorized a Coumadin® dosing self-management technique, based on the frequency of the Plaintiff's nose bleeds. The testimony was as follows:

Q. Did your father ever talk to you about how often he took the Coumadin®?

A. I don't remember what he told me the exact dose was on it, but I know he did have to take it at least once a day every day.

Q. Did your father ever have nose bleeds?

A. Yeah.

Q. Did you ever see them or did he tell you about them?

A. He told me about them. And I also saw them. I was there for several of them.

Q. What did he attribute those nose bleeds to?

A. He told me it was the Coumadin®.

Q. And do you remember him telling you anything about whether he spoke to the doctor about that or not?

A. Yes.

Q. What did he tell you?

A. Well, he told me that when he started getting the nose bleeds, this was kind of a concern to him because he wasn't really the kind of person that would have a lot of nose bleeds when he was growing up or anything like that. And when he started getting them, it was kind of a concern to him, and he told me that he phoned the doctor's office, and the person there that he spoke with told him that all he would need to do was adjust the medication himself, and say that he were supposed to take one pill every day, and he would get a nose bleed, then the next day he could just take half a pill or perhaps skip the dosage altogether, and then if he wouldn't get a nosebleed that next day, then he would know the day after that he could go ahead and take his whole pill.

Q. Do you recall when you had that conversation with your father in relationship to when he died?

A. Oh, it was at least a year before he died.

Transcript of trial testimony of Plaintiff's son, March 5, 2001, page 74, line 7 through page 75, line 23.

The Plaintiff's brother gave similar testimony at the trial. He lived with the Plaintiff and was involved in his care. His testimony was as follows:

Q. You mentioned that your brother was taking Coumadin®. How did you know he was taking Coumadin®?

A. On occasion when he would get a prescription refilled, if he wasn't going to Napoleon, usually he would ask me to go and pick it up for him.

Q. Do you know who prescribed the Coumadin®?

A. [Defendant].

Q. How do you know that?

A. [Plaintiff] on occasion had showed me—well, he showed me the original prescription that was issued when he got out of the hospital, and after that all of those prescriptions were requested by telephone, so there wasn't actually any paper record that he could show me, but he would mention to my mother and I that he was running low on Coumadin® and he was going to call [Defendant], and usually that same day or the next day he would either go and pick it up himself or have me come and pick it up.

Q. Do you know if [Plaintiff] was seeing [Defendant] from the time he was released from the hospital in November of 1994, till his death?

A. I don't believe he ever saw him.

Q. Were you aware whether [Plaintiff] had any appointments scheduled to see [Defendant] after his discharge from the hospital that he did not keep?

A. I was not aware that there was any appointment.

Q. Did [Plaintiff] every talk to you about how often he was supposed to take the Coumadin®?

A. When he was released from the hospital, he said that his dosage prescribed by [Defendant] was 5 milligrams per day, and within about a month after starting to take the Coumadin®, he started to get numerous, almost daily nose bleeds. So he—I was not party to the phone call, but he said he was going to call [Defendant] and find out if he should cut this dosage back, and maybe a day or so later when the subject came up again, he said that he had talked to [Defendant] and [Defendant] had told him to cut those 5 milligram tablets in half, and one day to take a 5 milligram full capsule and the next day to take a half, and then one, and a half, and occasionally if a nose bleed would occur, he would—whatever one he was on, whether it was a full one or half one, he would just skip it for that day and then go back to the cycle again.

Transcript of trial testimony of Plaintiff's brother, March 6, 2001, page 134, line 11 through page 136, line 17.

The Defendant's testimony about the care he did and did not deliver to the Plaintiff after November 10, 1994, is in sharp contrast to the Plaintiff's witnesses. This type of contrast becomes the burden of the jury in the civil justice system. The jury must decide who to believe after hearing all of the testimony. The Defendant's testimony was as follows:

Q. Going back to this time period, again, 1993, was there a routine policy at your office in terms of monitoring a patient's protime if he was on Coumadin®?

A. Yes.

Q. Tell me about that.

A. The patients usually would have a protime done in a week. Then they would have it done every other week for the next three months usually, but depending on the patient. And then once a month was mandatory.

Q. Okay. And that was true for every patient that was on Coumadin® or only some of them?

A. All patients who are on Coumadin®.

Q. Okay. Do you have many patients in your practice who are on Coumadin®?

A. A large number.

Q. Back in 1993, 1994?

A. Since the inception of our practice. Coumadin® is a standard drug, yes.

Q. Now, is it your practice, and whether it's today or going back to 1993, to you or yourself personally pick up a phone and call a pharmacy to call in a prescription for Coumadin®?

A. As far as I know, I've never called a prescription for Coumadin®.

Q. Did you, Doctor, ever at any time call in a prescription to a pharmacy on [Plaintiff]?

A. None that I'm ever aware of.

Q. Okay. Now, if a patient was on Coumadin® but did not have any synthetic graft in place, under what circumstances could the medical assistants or the nurses at Toledo Vascular or Toledo Hospital authorize a refill on Coumadin®?

A. There are certain strict parameters, which the nurses have. They have to do with the numbers and where you are. We want that—the doctor tells the nurse by in the chart exactly where he wants the INR to be. If it is a patient who is such as [Plaintiff], you might want him higher, maybe more in the three or even four, now that our understanding of the clotting defects are.

Q. Now, when you say you want it higher?

A. The INR, we want it higher.

Q. Or the protime?

A. The protime. And but we give them parameters, and the parameters are usually written down in the chart, and if there's any question, they know the parameters. They know that two to three is where we go. Anything over three is our prerogative depending on the patient, but we want most people at least two.

Q. And there is any protocol or guideline for the medical assistants or nurses in terms of how frequently the patient should be getting the protimes?

A. The guidelines are written down, set up by the manager, but agreed by all the physicians. Again, we are a corporation, so everybody has to agree on that. But usually monthly is the standard.

Q. All right. Now, if a patient for whatever reason was not getting routine or regular protimes or INRs, as you talked about, what to your understanding would the medical assistants or your nurses at your office do?

A. They wouldn't give them the Coumadin®.

Q. Would they ever at any time contact you?

A. Oh, certainly, they could do that and say so-and-so is not getting the protimes, and we would say call them, tell them I'm not going to give them any more Coumadin®, we are not going to, they have to come in and get their blood test.

Q. Okay. And so assuming that a patient wasn't getting their regular protimes and you received a call from a nurse that a patient was requesting Coumadin® but hadn't had his regular protimes, what would your instructions be?

A. Not to give them any more Coumadin®.

Q. Would that be some of the time or routine?

A. No, that's routine.

Q. Why is that? Why wouldn't you do that?

A. Coumadin® is a very dangerous drug, and although it really—we use it so often that it doesn't always seem that way, but obviously it can cause bleeding and other problems, and we therefore keep a very close eye on it.

Transcript of trial testimony of Defendant, March 6, 2001, page 214, line 16 through page 218, line 18.

In addition, the Defendant testified regarding his Coumadin® prescribing habits as follows:

Q. Did you ever have contact with him (the Plaintiff) at any point in time after his discharge?

A. Not that I'm aware of.

Q. Now, from the time he was discharged in November of 1994 until the time of his death, did you ever authorize a prescription for Coumadin® for [Plaintiff]?

A. I did not.

Q. Why is that?

A. Because he didn't come back for his INR and protimes. And also never came back for follow-up. We wouldn't—I mean, I looked for his duplex records. I looked to see in the office. We'd say if you don't come back, you're not getting your prescription from us.

Q. Now, little bit different question. Assuming that [Plaintiff] at some point after November of 1994 had phoned your office asking for his prescription for Coumadin® to be refilled, and assuming someone from your office brought this to your attention, would you have authorized a refill on his prescription?

A. No.

Q. All right. And again, why not?

A. Because he is not following up with the situation. The most important thing is his protime, INR. If he's not getting them, then I'm not going to give him any prescription for Coumadin®.

Q. So, in other words, if someone at Toledo Vascular or someone at Toledo Hospital called in a prescription for Coumadin® for [Plaintiff] after November of 1994, would it have been under your direction or your authorization?

A. It would not. The prescriptions are in back of the time line.

Q. Can you see that?

A. I can. I can.

Q. Can the jury, can you see that okay? All right, Doctor, showing you a photocopy of a telephone prescription for [Plaintiff] that was issued March 11, 1996. Does this prescription indicate who allegedly phoned in this prescription?

A. No, I don't know what the name is next to there. If there's a name of anybody. Is that a name?

Q. My understanding from testimony we've had that says Toledo.

A. No, it does not say who phoned in, it just says the doctor's name.

Q. Now, and I think we've been through this. This is now 14 or 15 months after [Plaintiff's] bypass surgery. Would you under any condition have ever phoned this prescription into the pharmacy directly on [Plaintiff]?

A. Never.

Q. All right. The prescription is for 60 tablets with six refills. How much Coumadin® is that, assuming someone was taking a tablet a day?

A. That's a year's prescription.

Q. Would you under any circumstances ever prescribe or issue a prescription for Coumadin® on any of your patients for one year?

A. Never.

Q. Why not?

A. Because they could go along and never have their protime done again. That's why we usually give them only one month's supply. Occasionally they'll get a couple months because they have a pharmacy that they have to send away for, and we certainly don't want them to pay a large amount of money, so we might give them two month's supply. The maximum, three months. No more than that.

Q. All right. Would you under any circumstances authorize anyone at Toledo Vascular or any of the nurses at Toledo Hospital to issue a refill on Coumadin® for [Plaintiff] for one year's worth?

A. Never.

Transcript of trial testimony of Defendant, March 6, 2001, page 233, line 1 through page 236, line 18.

Before the end of the first jury trial in the Lucas County Court of Common Pleas, the Defendant's attorneys convinced the judge to dismiss the case by arguing that the prescription transfer error that gave the Plaintiff many unmonitored Coumadin® refills well after the allowable period under Ohio law, was the actual cause of the Plaintiff's death. They argued that the pharmacy's negligence was an intervening and superseding cause of the Plaintiff's injuries, thereby absolving the Defendant of any liability. The trial court judge agreed with this argument and dismissed the case before the jury had to determine which portions of the above testimony to believe.

The 6th District Court of Appeals of Ohio, Lucas County, disagreed with the trial court's decision and ruled that the jury, not the judge, must decide who to believe regarding the facts that were presented in this case. The Ohio Supreme Court chose not to review the 6th District Court of Appeals of Ohio, Lucas County's decision, so the case will go back to the Lucas County Court of Common Pleas for another jury trial approximately eight years after the plaintiff missed his follow-up appointment.

Using the risk management analysis method described earlier in this chapter, the jury will need to answer these key questions regarding the Defendant after hearing all of the testimony that is presented to them.

The jury of Lucas County citizens that hears this matter will most likely consist of lay people who have no formal medical training. Their decision will most likely be based on the perceived credibility of all of the witnesses.

CONCLUSION

Walking the "high wire" of anticoagulation management is a complex matter before any considerations are given to tort claims. The management of large populations of anticoagulated patients can be a scheduling, documentation, and communications challenge. Risk management strategies should be used based on comprehensive recordkeeping and documented, consistent decision-making protocols. Risk management is defined as an organized effort to identify, assess, and reduce, where appropriate, risk to patients, visitors, staff, and organizational assets.[6]

The pharmacy chain that settled with the Plaintiff before the first jury trial began could have prevented its involvement in this case by creating documentation policies that require complete information capture on oral prescriptions and retention of the original prescription date on all transferred prescriptions. Adequate patient counseling may have also detected the fact that the Plaintiff was not receiving any Coumadin® monitoring during the long period of time that he received Coumadin® from those pharmacies. An automatic "stop order" on Coumadin® prescriptions may have also served the Plaintiff's interests.

The American Society for Healthcare Risk Management in this case has suggested one risk management technique that may have prevented the Defendant's involvement in this matter. When a patient becomes uncooperative or noncompliant, the staff should thoroughly and objectively document the problem. Once a decision has been made that a patient either has constructively discharged him- or herself by failing to follow medical orders or is being proactively discharged for any other reason, the patient and/or family members should be advised orally, followed by a written notice. The written notice should be sent by certified mail, return receipt.[7] The written notice and proof of delivery should be retained as part of the medical record. In an anticoagulation management setting, the patient must be notified that he or she will no longer receive prescriptions for anticoagulation medications. The patient should also be advised to seek another medical provider to avoid serious consequences. This type of notification may have prevented the Defendant's involvement in this case. The use of this type of notification should be used after considering the administrative burden versus the potential claim avoidance value.

An understanding of the civil justice process, use of the basic risk management analysis described in this chapter, and implementation of published risk management techniques will help protect health care providers on a day-to-day basis. Health care providers who grasp these concepts will appropriately analyze patient care situations and make decisions that improve patient care while reducing litigation exposure.

REFERENCES

1. *Black's Law Dictionary*—Fifth Ed. 1355.
2. *Joseph vs. Husted Corp.*, 454 P.2d 916, 918.
3. *Baker vs. Arbor Drugs, Inc.*, 558 N.W. 2d 725; (1997).
4. *Earlie vs. Jacobs*, 745 F.2d 342.
5. *Armstrong vs. Weiland*, 225 S.E. 2d 851 (1976).
6. Kavaler F, Spiegel A. *Risk Management in Health Care Institutions, a Strategic Approach*, p. 3; 1997, Jones and Bartlett Publishers.
7. Carroll R, ed. *Risk Management Handbook for Health Care Organizations*, 3d ed., p. 417; 2001, Jossey-Bass, Inc.

Chapter 15

Developing a Business Plan for an Anticoagulation Clinic

Jennifer L. Wilson Norton

INTRODUCTION

What Is a Business Plan?

A business plan is a written document that describes the development and implementation needs of a new program or service. The standard format used in a business plan provides an organization with a consistent method for program evaluation. It summarizes a program's operational and administrative elements and compares its benefits with its expenses. The business plan also can be used to evaluate and analyze the feasibility and financial implications of a proposed program.

The business plan is based on information gathered from inside and outside the organization. As the plan is reviewed by multiple members of the organization, modifications are made. After the business plan is finalized and accepted, the proposed program is implemented.

Why Have a Business Plan?

A business plan serves many functions in an organization. A business plan provides a standard method to evaluate the appropriateness of allocating resources to a proposed program. It facilitates organizational approval and commitment toward program development and implementation. The summary of a plan of financial, operational, and clinical information provides appropriate prioritization of organizational resources. The business plan also serves as a reliable method to review programs, helping the organization to use scarce resources wisely.

Often the business plan is written in order to secure the approval of capital and other resources necessary to develop and implement the program. Last, a business plan provides a standardized mechanism for later evaluation of a new program or service.

Who Develops a Business Plan?

Any individual or team proposing a new program can develop the business plan. The individual or team with responsibility for implementing and making the program operational is the most appropriate originator, ensuring that the plan is attainable. For an anticoagulation clinic, the team may include individuals, such as a pharmacist, nurse, physician, administrator, and laboratory experts, or a program development group. The amount of time needed to develop and implement the business plan depends on the individuals driving the process. Reviews and modifications may be accelerated or delayed based on organizational development efforts being undertaken simultaneously.

KEYS TO BUSINESS PLAN DEVELOPMENT

Before writing the business plan, information must be gathered from internal and external sources. A simple format facilitates understanding by those who will be reviewing the plan. Business plans often are reviewed by administration, operations committees, and board of trustees members. The business plan, which must be well thought out and planned, should contain a description of the market and future trends.

Successful development of any business plan involves collaboration with everyone affected by the proposed program. In an anticoagulation clinic, personnel affected by the plan would include physicians, nurses, pharmacists, business office and billing staff, laboratory technicians, dietitians, patient registrars, administrators, and building services staff. Early involvement ensures needed buy-in and support throughout the development and implementation process.

For consistency and quicker development, a business plan for an anticoagulation clinic can be modeled after a previously successful plan from a different program within the organization. By reviewing a business plan for a previously approved program, the writer will gain insight as to what elements and style are appropriate. This practice also provides consistency in plan format and content, facilitating the work of the group approving business plans. Similarities and differences among programs being proposed and approved are readily apparent.

ELEMENTS OF A BUSINESS PLAN

In general, a business plan includes a business definition, a situational assessment that includes an internal and external assessment, a financial assessment, an objectives and outcome plan, evaluation criteria, and an executive summary. Many organizations and institutions have standard elements that must be addressed in a business plan. It is important to understand how an organization justifies new services or modifications of services, how programs are approved, and what model to follow. Each organization has a fixed amount of money and resources to invest in development of new programs. A business plan helps guide an organization's decisions regarding new investments.

Business Definition

The business definition describes the program's services and business functions. For an anticoagulation service, this definition describes a new method of coordinating care and managing patients. The following example presents a business definition for an anticoagulation clinic.

> A pharmacist-run outpatient anticoagulation clinic would provide a unique opportunity for the medical center to integrate with physicians currently affiliated with the institution. The service would partner and complement the cardiac nurse practitioners. The clinic would more efficiently utilize health care resources and fit well within a managed

care model. It would improve patients' quality of care, education, and compliance, leading to an improvement in outcomes. Services provided would include laboratory monitoring and review, patient assessment, dosage adjustment, patient education, and physician follow-up.

Figures 15–1 and 15–2 illustrate the change in practice that would occur. Figure 15–1 represents the centralized, point-of-care system of anticoagulation management that is being proposed. The model assumptions include improving the level of care through increased training and expertise of the anticoagulation therapy team, increasing productivity, centralizing patient management, and implementing a point-of-care testing system with quick turnaround times so that one-stop service can be achieved. The comparative model shown in Figure 15–2 is the existing telephone management model being used by multiple practitioners. By comparing these two figures, physicians and administrators can easily see that point-of-care testing improves patient management.

The business definition should also include a description of the services provided and how the service will work. These benefits have been documented in the literature and include improved patient outcomes through decreased bleeding and thromboembolic complications.[1–8] Additional benefits may include increased integration of the health care team, improved quality of patient care, more appropriate patient

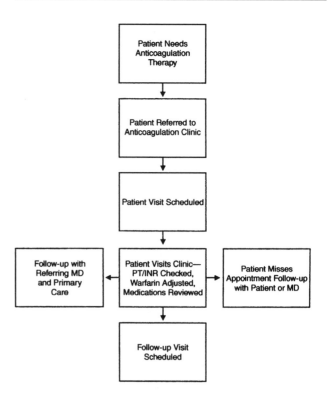

Figure 15–1 Proposed point-of-care testing system

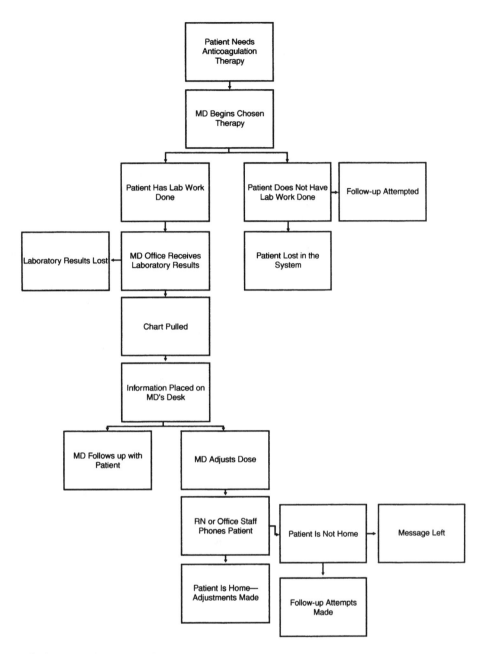

Figure 15–2 Existing telephone management system

utilization of the health care system, decreased nonreimbursable or lower reimbursable workload for physicians, a potential source of new revenue for nonphysician health care providers, decreased overall costs, and improved patient convenience.

Anticoagulation clinics serve patients who commonly have cardiac, rehabilitation, oncology, and general medicine needs. When developing the business definition, it is important to review the areas of care to which the organization provides significant amounts of routine service. Each care area is referred to as a product line, and if the organization is looking to expand or enhance product lines, an anticoagulation clinic is an excellent addition. Anticoagulation clinics have been successful in all types of hospitals, stand-alone clinics, and health maintenance organizations.[9]

The business definition should consider the current organizational goals. Table 15–1 displays a sample of an organization's goals and their relationship to an anticoagulation clinic. If current goals include areas in which an anticoagulation clinic would have an effect, a statement specifying the alignment between the goals and the proposed program can be very powerful. This business definition

Table 15–1 Benefits of an Anticoagulation Clinic and Relationship to Hospital Goals

Benefits of an Anticoagulation Clinic	Hospital Goals
Increased integration with medical staff	Develop programs and systems that increase integration and efficiency for the medical staff.
Increased quality of care for patients	Implement continuous quality improvement processes that lead to improvement in patient outcomes.
Decreased workload for physicians	Develop programs and systems that increase integration and efficiency for the medical staff.
Increased involvement in outpatient services	Increase percentage of hospital revenue gained from outpatient services.
Increased potential revenue	Increase financial strength of the hospital
Expanded professional practice	
Decreased hospital admissions due to inappropriate management of anticoagulation	Implement continuous quality improvement processes that lead to improvement in patient outcomes.
Increased usage of laboratory service	Increase financial strength of the hospital.
Increased prescription volume	Increase financial strength of the hospital.
Improved convenience in patient care	Be the preferred place for patients to receive health care.

should demonstrate to the various reviewers how the proposed program will add to achievement of organizational goals.

Situational Assessment: Internal and External Assessment

The situational assessment describes how an anticoagulation clinic fits into the organizational structure. Internal and external situations that will be affected by an anticoagulation clinic need to be evaluated to determine if the proposal is viable. The following list presents the critical meetings that must occur to develop these assessments.

- physician champion(s)
- medical director of laboratory
- key clinical laboratory personnel
- business office and finance departments

- patient registration
- administration
- current owners of warfarin management
- chairperson of internal medicine and cardiology medical sections
- medical staff section meetings
- key clinical leaders, including physicians, nurses, pharmacists, and dietitians

Physician support is a critical element of an anticoagulation clinic's success. A significant number of physicians must support the plan if it is to be successful. Early, active involvement is critical. A physician champion team or steering committee needs to be identified to serve as a liaison between the organization and other physicians and to act as a sounding board for development and implementation of the program. If the anticoagulation clinic concept is "owned" by the physicians, greater acceptance and success will result.

The internal assessment will vary depending on the health care system. The involvement of departments that have functions and processes that will be affected by an anticoagulation clinic is necessary. Typical involvement includes physicians, nurses, pharmacists, dietitians, clinical laboratory, patient financial services, contracting representatives, registration, facilities, and parking. In addition, the involvement of patients, insurers, and patient greeters is critical. Staffing standards and operations from these areas need to be studied and compared with projected patient impact estimates to see the requirements necessary to support the operation. From this assessment, needed buy-in will be gained as well as aligned goals and educational efforts. Projected workload and effect on each function will help further address needs for resources. Barriers to success will be identified and addressed.

The processes of operating an anticoagulation clinic need to be considered by all aspects of the organization that will be affected. From this analysis, estimates on staffing needs will be gathered. The following examples illustrate the effect of an anticoagulation clinic on various departments. These estimates should be included in the business plan.

1. Patient registration will increase by 50 patients/month
   - Average registration takes 5 minutes
   - Total time needed = 4.17 hours/month
2. Billing will handle 500 more patient visits/month
   - 10% of bills raise questions, and each question requires 5 minutes to address
   - Total time needed = 4.17 hours/month
3. Patient reception will increase by 500 visits/month
   - Each patient takes 1–2 minutes
   - Total reception time needed = 8.3–16.67 hours/month

In the external assessment, comparisons or benchmarks of similar organizations need to be gathered. A benchmark involves examining the operations of local and regional anticoagulation clinics. Operational benchmarks include hours of operation, after-hours procedures, space requirements, needed staffing, equipment, computer applications, facility location, parking, patient billing, reimbursement, organizational commitments, relationship with the laboratory, laboratory systems, and policies and procedures. Clinical benchmarks include protocol assessment, elements of patient care, continuum of care coordination, and staffing mix.

Benchmarking other organizations facilitates the staffing analysis as well as provides insight regarding gaining acceptance and overcoming barriers to implementation. This information can then be applied to the specific organizational resources available. Benchmarking helps indicate whether a realistic anticoagulation clinic model can be developed and implemented in a given organization and whether that organization can meet patient needs. It also helps the organization to decide if it is willing to commit the necessary space, capital, and expertise to manage and operate an anticoagulation clinic. An example of a hospital's situational assessment follows.

- External assessment
  - willingness of physicians to refer patients
  - internal medicine section support
  - family practice medical section support
  - orthopaedic section support
  - chief of staff support
  - projected patients on anticoagulation 500–1,000
  - known weaknesses in decentralized method of patient management
  - physicians not paid for management of warfarin
  - service provided in managed care environments
- Internal assessment
  - warfarin admissions for bleeding exceed national standards
  - collaborative interest by the lab
  - collaborative interest by the laboratory medical director
  - alignment with inpatient pharmacy-driven anticoagulation protocols
  - ability to collect revenue
  - support of developing new programs and services
  - complements comprehensive cardiac services product line

Financial Assessment

A financial analysis evaluates all cost implications of a program. It includes all expenses incurred (operational elements, labor expenses, nonlabor expenses, capital expenses, indirect costs), revenue earned from reimbursement and other sources, and expenditures not incurred on adverse outcomes. In many business plans, the financial section includes numerous charts, tables, and graphs.

Expenses

Operational Elements. Operational elements include all considerations that are related to the day-to-day operations of the anticoagulation clinic. *Patient volume* is the number of patients the anticoagulation clinic will be managing. It is important to calculate both the total number of patients and the estimated number of visits each month. Patients with a higher acuity will require more clinic time than medically stable patients. Estimates of new referrals each month must be made. New patients will take more time initially than established clients.

The patient management model will need to be decided. Will the anticoagulation clinic physically see as many patients as possible? Will the clinic do the laboratory work or will it be done by the laboratory? How much telephone management will be performed by the anticoagulation clinic? There are advantages and disadvantages to each type of anticoagulation clinic setup. Each patient mix is different and should be considered in the development of the clinic model.

Hours of operation will affect not only the staffing needs but also the success of the program. In addition to the hours when the clinic is fully staffed, an after-hours plan must be developed to address how staffing will cover clinical issues during nonclinic hours.

A computerized system of tracking may bring some efficiencies over a paper system. However, automation will require additional support resources in order to keep the system maintained and upgraded.

Labor Expenses. Labor expenses include salaries and benefits for individuals working in the anticoagulation clinic. This element is the most expensive aspect of operation. Both patient visit volume and organizational setup affect staffing, and the skill mix of the staff will affect labor expenses. It is important to address whether staffing will come from existing staff or whether new personnel will be hired. If new personnel are hired, the costs of recruitment need to be considered. Training costs are an additional startup cost. Until the anticoagulation clinic staff are proficient, extra hours will be needed for growth and development in this specialized area. Ongoing continuing education needs to be included in the operations budget to ensure an up-to-date, trained team.

The model chosen for operation of the anticoagulation clinic will affect the flexibility of staff. For example, if a point-of-care model is chosen, staff need to be available when patients are able to come to the clinic. If a telephone management model is selected, staff need to be available when the laboratory results are received. The effect of the clinic model on laboratory staff also needs to be examined.

Nonlabor Expenses. Ongoing expenses need to be calculated. They include laboratory supplies, paper, business cards, Medic Alert bracelets, patient brochures, pill splitters, medisets, and any other disposable items used in clinic operations.

Capital Expenses/Startup Expenses. One-time or infrequent expenses often are referred to as capital equipment needs. They make up part of the startup costs and include furniture items, rapid prothrombin time monitors, computers, printers, faxes, reference materials, and copy machines. Capital expenses may also include the remodeling costs associated with the clinic site.

Indirect Costs/Overhead. Overhead or indirect program costs include all of the services or portions of the organization that do not generate revenue but are required for operation. This expense category includes fees for the building, electricity, and telephones as well as the cost of support departments such as information services and human resources. How these expenses are put into profitability equations is organization dependent. Anticoagulation clinics that have generated revenue in the hospital setting have not been able to cover both their direct and indirect (or overhead) costs. This failure may be attributed to the technique used by the hospital to distribute overhead costs. Anticoagulation clinics do not utilize as many overhead departments and services as other, more traditional hospital departments.

Revenues

Reimbursement. Revenue is the amount of income generated by obtaining reimbursement from third-party payers and patients. Depending on the organization, this element can vary greatly. In a capitated environment the revenue will be part of the overall annual rate of reimbursement. This revenue will be paid in a lump sum and managed by the organization managing the capitated fee. In a fee-for-service or managed fee-for-service environment, revenue follows billing cycles. Based on contracting language, it may be a percentage of charges or a fee for the service provided.

Patient charges can be determined by many different mechanisms. Some considerations in determining patient charges include how the charges reflect the costs involved in providing the service, how the charges compare to other charges, and what is reasonable. In developing reimbursement strategies, collaborative work with a business office or reimbursement team is essential for financial success. Payer mix, the estimated number of patients coming from different third-party plans, must be estimated. This number will help determine which reimbursement strategy or setup is best utilized to optimize reimbursement levels from third-party payers. For example, if the clinic will have primarily a fee-for-service reimbursement base of Medicare patients, strategies for payment type should match that payer mix.

Additional Revenues. Patients will need other services in addition to the care provided by the anticoagulation clinic. Often, preference for an organization develops because of patients' impression of the people providing the care. Anticoagulation clinics can gain additional organizational revenue by filling prescriptions for patients. Laboratory revenue may also increase because of the coordination with invasive blood draws and because patients can receive all needed services at one location.

Outcome-Based Cost Avoidance. Hospitals and health maintenance organizations will want to evaluate as much retrospective outcome data as possible prior to implementing an anticoagulation clinic. This examination will help determine if there is a potential to improve patient outcomes. Analysis of the rates of admission for bleeding related to anticoagulation therapy should determine the potential decrease in rate of bleeding possible. Literature comparisons will help evaluate the potential for improvement in bleeding outcomes or incidence. Embolic admissions for patients on anticoagulation therapy can provide insight as to additional potential for improvement in patient management. Health maintenance organizations may wish to do an evaluation of the appropriate use of anticoagulation in specific disease states like atrial fibrillation. Evaluation of utilization of vitamin K may also be performed. After evaluating these data and reviewing the literature, projections on improvement of patient outcomes and savings to the hospital or health care organization can be developed and built into the financial assessment.

Additional Funding Sources

A financial analysis will also reveal potential outside sources of funding. Grants from a foundation may be a way to set up and fund an anticoagulation clinic. There may also be other departments or external funding sources that will support setup costs for an anticoagulation clinic.

Break-Even Analysis

A break-even analysis takes all of the revenue generated and the expenses incurred and determines at what level of volume costs will be covered by reimbursement gained. If it is unclear what level of reimbursement will be gained, assessments for different levels of reimbursement may be created. A graphic representation of these estimates can be used to show the best and worst case situations from a financial perspective. Table 15–2 presents a sample financial analysis for two different anticoagulation clinic models. It summarizes the direct costs and revenues gained by developing and implementing an anticoagulation clinic. Two estimates of the break-even analysis are presented in Figures 15–3 and 15–4. These graphs show the number of patients who must be seen in the anticoagulation clinic on a monthly basis in order for net revenue to meet expenses, using both low- and high-volume estimates. Presenting this information in both tables and graphs helps different people evaluate data in different ways.

Table 15–2 Financial Assessment

Variable	Low Volume (200 Visits/Month)	High Volume (500 Visits/Month)
Revenue		
Patient charge per visit*	$35	$35
Estimated annual gross revenue	$84,000	$210,000
Bad debt†	($1,260)	($3,150)
Contractual write-off	($24,822)	($62,055)
Billing service cost‡	($4,054)	($10,135)
Estimated annual net clinic revenue	$53,864	$134,660
Expenses		
Annual wages and benefits§	($60,000)	($90,000)
Supply cost	($12,000)	($30,000)
Expense reduction	$12,000	$30,000
Net loss or profit	($6,136)	$44,660

*Patient charge is clinic visit plus laboratory charge.
†Bad debt is based on average rate of 1.5%.
‡Billing cost is 7% of receivables.
§Low-volume staffing is one full-time clinician; high-volume staffing is one full-time clinician and one full-time technical support person.

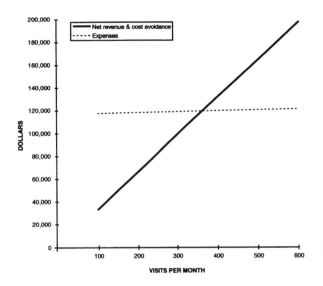

Figure 15–4 High volume break-even analysis

Objectives and Action Plan

The objectives and action plan summarize the recommendations to the organization for establishment of the service. A timeline for clinic implementation and one for ongoing program review are vital. This portion of the business plan may also address whether outside hiring will take place or if the organization has the internal resources to create and implement the new program. A sample timeline for implementation is presented in Exhibit 15–1. Depending on organizational demands, the timeline may be demanding or relaxed. It is important for implementation to be quick enough to maintain support and momentum yet slow enough to develop systems that work well for patients and physicians.

Evaluation Criteria

Clinical outcomes, including data related to bleeding and embolic rates, must be reviewed. Moreover, the information must be shared with the entire organization following clinic implementation. A good timeline for the first clinical outcomes review is one year after program implementation. Ongoing review of clinical outcomes is essential to ensure provision of high-quality care.

Operational outcomes also need to be reviewed in order to assess how well the anticoagulation clinic is working. A comparison between the projections made in the business plan and the actual operation needs to be made. Patient and physician satisfaction surveys also can assist in identifying the operational areas of strength and the areas in need of improvement. Evaluation can begin six months after implementation and should be completed on an ongoing basis.

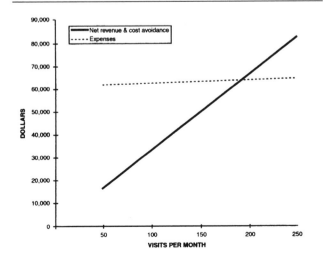

Figure 15–3 Low volume break-even analysis

Exhibit 15–1
SAMPLE TIMELINE FOR DEVELOPMENT OF OUTPATIENT ANTICOAGULATION CLINIC

MONTH	PROCESS UNDER DEVELOPMENT
September	• Casual conversation with physician discussing management of anticoagulation patients
October	• Survey of physicians to assess interest in anticoagulation services • Visit to a local anticoagulation clinic
October–March	• Multidisciplinary input/business plan development—medical staff, laboratory, business office, administration
December–January	• Prescriptive authority protocol development
January–February	• Prescriptive authority protocol approval
March	• Business plan approval
March–June	• Multidisciplinary coordination – Medical staff – Laboratory/phlebotomy, quality control, correlation studies, machine operation – Business office – Admissions – Information Services – Building services
May	• Initiation of clinic services
June	• Marketing of clinic
July	• Opening of clinic

Executive Summary

An executive summary is a one-page summary of the overall business plan. It is a concise document that capsulizes the most important information from each of the business plan sections and is understandable as a stand-alone summary. As the very first page of the business plan, the executive summary sets the tone for the remainder of the document. The chief executive officer and governing board often review the executive summary prior to granting final approval.

CONCLUSION

What happens once the business plan is developed? Business plans are generally reviewed by multiple committees, and modifications are made based on their input. Then the business plan is reviewed and either approved or rejected by the committee authorized to make these decisions within an organization. If the business plan is approved, program implementation begins.

A business plan combines clinical, operational, and organizational objectives to help companies in the decision-making process related to resource allocations for new programs. A collaborative, multidisciplinary approach is essential in developing the highest quality business plan. Moreover, realistic projections are critical to successful implementation of the plan. A simple, organized approach enhances understanding and facilitates support and approval. Reference books on writing business plans can provide helpful models.[10,11]

REFERENCES

1. Cortelazzo S, Finnzaai G, Vierol P, et al. Thrombotic and hemorrhagic complications in patients with mechanical heart valve prosthesis attending an anticoagulation clinic. *Thromb Haemost.* 1993;69:316–320.
2. Conte RR, Kehoe WA, Nielson N, et al. Nine-year experience with a pharmacist managed anticoagulation clinic. *Am J Hosp Pharm.* 1986;43:2460–2464.
3. Ellis FR, Stephens MA, Sharp GB. Evaluation of a pharmacist managed warfarin monitoring service to coordinate inpatient and outpatient therapy. *Am J Hosp Pharm.* 1992;49:387–394.
4. Engle JP. Anticoagulation: practice focus in ambulatory clinic. *J Pharm Pract.* 1990;3:349–357.
5. Garabedian-Ruffalo SM, Gray DR, Sax MJ, Ruffalo RL. Retrospective evaluation of a pharmacist-managed anticoagulation clinic. *Am J Hosp Pharm.* 1990;42:304–308.
6. Gray DR, Garbedian-Ruffalo SM, Chretien SD. Cost justification of a clinical pharmacist managed anticoagulation clinic. *Drug Intell Clin Pharm.* 1985;19:575–580.
7. Kornbilt P, Senderoff J, Davis-Erickson M, Zenk J. Anticoagulation therapy: patient management and evaluation of an outpatient clinic. *Nurs Pract.* 1990;15:21–32.
8. Wilt VM, Gums JG, Ahmed OI, Moore LM. Outcome analysis of a pharmacist-managed anticoagulation service. *Pharmacotherapy.* 1995;15:732–739.
9. Wilson Norton JL, Gibson DL. Establishing an outpatient anticoagulation clinic in a community hospital. *Am J Health Sys Pharm.* 1996;53:1151–1157.
10. Pinson L, Jinnett J. *Anatomy of a Business Plan.* 2nd ed. Chicago: Enterprise Dearborn: 1993.
11. Tiffany P, Pererson S. *Business Plans for Dummies.* Foster City, CA: IDG Books; 1997.

The Use of Oral Anticoagulants

Chapter 16

Physiology of Coagulation and the Role of Vitamin K

Scott H. Goodnight

INTRODUCTION

This chapter covers the physiology of blood coagulation and the role of vitamin K in hemostasis. Appreciation of this complex but fascinating biologic system has grown exponentially over the last century, and to summarize it in a few short pages is challenging indeed. The goal, therefore, must be to follow a dictum attributed to Albert Einstein: "Everything should be made as simple as possible, but not simple."

The dual role of the hemostatic system (ie, prompt cessation of hemorrhage from a wound and protection from lethal intravascular thrombosis) is a wonderful example of biologic regulation. Even though bleeding from an injury stops in just a few minutes, most people go through life without a pathologic venous or arterial thrombosis. These observations raise two important questions:

1. How does blood clot at a site of injury?
2. What keeps a thrombus from propagating into the normal vasculature?

CLOTTING AT AN INJURY SITE

Figure 16–1 illustrates a blood vessel with an injury that has destroyed an area of vascular endothelium and uncovered subendothelial tissues. The loss of endothelium and the exposure of tissue factor, phospholipids, and collagen triggers a group of biochemical reactions that culminates in the formation of a fibrin-containing blood clot (ie, soluble fibrinogen [a liquid] has been converted to insoluble fibrin [a gel]).[1,2]

Initiation of Coagulation by Exposure of Tissue Factor

Tissue factor is a potent clot-promoting protein that is usually not found on the surface of endothelial cells, but it can be expressed under certain pathologic circumstances, such as exposure to endotoxin or inflammatory cytokines.[3–5] Tissue factor, however, is constitutively expressed in other cell types located in the deeper layers of the blood vessel and in the tissues themselves. Following an injury, activated factor VII (VIIa) (a clotting factor present in small amounts in the circulating blood) binds to the tissue factor, which touches off a series of biochemical reactions that culminate in the formation of thrombin, the proteolytic enzyme that converts fibrinogen to fibrin (Figure 16–2).

Roles of Phospholipid Surfaces and Vitamin K

Coagulation reactions must take place on a phospholipid surface, a process that also targets clotting to the site of injury. As is the case with tissue factor, normal endothelial cells do not have negatively charged phospholipids (such as phosphatidylserine) available on their cell surfaces. Tissue injury damages cell membranes, however, which allows negatively charged phospholipids (normally present on the underside of cell membranes) to come into contact with the blood. The process of coagulation also activates platelets, which leads to the appearance of phospholipids on their surfaces as well (ie, platelet factor 3).[6]

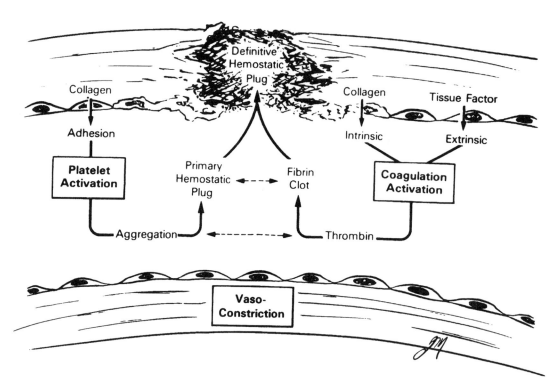

Figure 16–1 This diagram illustrates an injury site with an overlying thrombus in contact with a blood vessel lined with endothelial cells. The exposure of tissue factor, negatively charged phospholipids, and collagen serves to initiate thrombus formation and also to limit thrombosis to the site of injury. Regional blood flow dilutes and carries away activated blood coagulation factors that may have escaped the developing thrombus. Source: Reprinted with permission from JE Ansell, *Handbook of Hemostasis and Thrombosis*, p 4, © 1986, Little Brown & Company.

Several clotting factors critical to hemostasis bind directly to negatively charged phospholipids by means of specific sites that are part of these proteins after they have been formed in the liver.[7,8] This process, the addition of a dozen or more γ-carboxyglutamic acid (gla) residues to factors II, VII, IX, and X (and also protein C and protein S) requires the action of vitamin K (Figure 16–3). Therefore, the presence of the gla residues allows these vitamin K–dependent clotting factors to bind to negatively charged phospholipids, a process that requires calcium.

An appreciation of this process helps considerably in understanding important clinical phenomena related to hemostasis and thrombosis, such as the following examples:

- If vitamin K is lacking in the diet (eg, vitamin K deficiency in the newborn infant or in a patient with a poor diet who is treated with antibiotics), factors II, VII, IX, and X will not be fully carboxylated; the clotting factors cannot bind to phospholipids, and bleeding can occur.

- Oral anticoagulants block the action of vitamin K and prevent phospholipid binding by the vitamin K–dependent clotting factors. The blood is therefore less likely to clot, and, if warfarin is given in excessive doses, bleeding can occur.[9]

- The purpose of the anticoagulants used for blood tests (eg, sodium citrate) is to bind calcium, which in turn prevents the vitamin K–dependent clotting factors from binding to phospholipids in the test tube so that the blood won't clot. After the citrated plasma is separated by centrifugation, calcium is added in the laboratory so that coagulation (eg, prothrombin time [PT] or activated partial thromboplastin time [aPTT]) can proceed under controlled conditions.

- Both PT and aPTT require the addition of phospholipids. The phospholipid used in the PT is a component of the rabbit brain thromboplastin; newer thromboplastins that utilize recombinant or highly purified tissue factor require extra phospholipids. Negatively charged phospholipids are also added to the aPTT. When used in this way, the phospholipid is called a *partial* thromboplastin, whereas tissue factor plus phospholipid (for the PT) is designated a *complete* thromboplastin.

- Certain autoantibodies (eg, antiphospholipid antibodies, such as the lupus anticoagulant) interfere with the binding of clotting factors to phospholipid surfaces and therefore prolong the aPTT or other phospholipid-based coagulation assays, such as the Russell viper venom time or the dilute tissue thromboplastin inhibition test.[10,11]

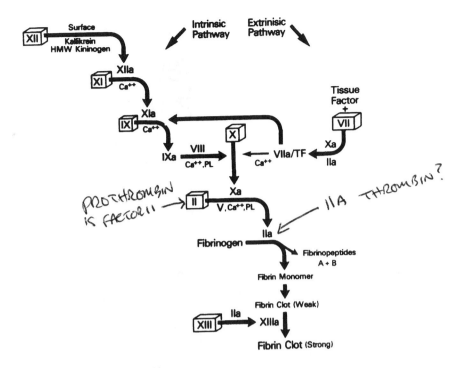

Key: Ca⁺⁺, calcium; HMW, high molecular weight; PL, phospholipid.

Figure 16–2 A schematic illustrating the biochemical reactions leading to the formation of fibrin. Note that tissue factor (**TF**) plus factor VIIa acts in vivo to convert factor IX to factor IXa. In contrast, coagulation reactions that occur in the test tube (eg, during performance of an activated partial thromboplastin time) activate factor X to factor Xa. Source: Adapted with permission from JE Ansell, *Handbook of Hemostasis and Thrombosis*, p 10, © 1986, Little Brown & Company.

Contribution of Collagen

A third factor present in the wound that initiates thrombus formation is the fibrillar protein, collagen. Collagen, like tissue factor and phospholipid, is not in contact with the flowing blood under normal circumstances. When it is exposed, however, collagen avidly binds and activates platelets, a process that also contributes to the formation of a clot.[12] Platelets adhere to collagen by binding von Willebrand factor, which in turn adheres to a specific receptor (glycoprotein Ib/IX) on the platelet surface (Figure 16–4).[13,14] Platelets also have receptors for collagen and thrombin that can initiate platelet activation, the release reaction, and the binding of fibrinogen that leads to aggregation of the platelets. Finally, as previously mentioned, platelet activation exposes platelet phospholipids, which can serve as a surface to support coagulation reactions.

Collagen and other negatively charged surfaces initiate the early intrinsic coagulation system by promoting activation of factor XII to factor XIIa and factor XI to factor XIa, both of which contribute to thrombin generation via the formation of intrinsic prothrombin activator.[15] The relative importance of factor XII activation by collagen versus the tissue factor/VIIa reaction for the initiation of coagulation is not entirely clear,

but it seems likely that the tissue factor pathway is dominant under most circumstances in vivo.

Formation of Thrombin

The initiation of coagulation by tissue factor, phospholipids, and collagen in the depths of the wound culminates in the generation of thrombin, the potent thrombogenic enzyme responsible for the conversion of fibrinogen to fibrin. The biochemistry underlying the conversion of prothrombin to thrombin is complex, but three broad principles should be kept in mind.

First, the tissue factor/VIIa complex preferentially converts factor IX to IXa in vivo, rather than directly activating factor X to factor Xa.[16] When coagulation occurs in vitro (eg, during performance of a coagulation test, such as PT), however, tissue factor/VIIa acts mainly on factor X and converts it to Xa, with the help of the cofactor for this reaction, factor V. This finding helps to explain the utility of the screening tests of hemostasis, the PT and the aPTT, for the identification of clotting factor defects or deficiencies in patients who are bleeding (Figure 16–5). Consequently, the aPTT reflects the activity of clotting factors XII, XI, IX, VIII, X, V, and II, and the PT is influenced by changes in factors VII, X, V,

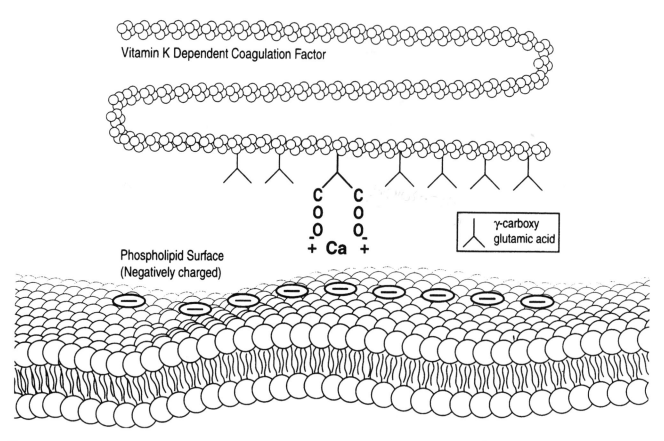

Figure 16–3 A rendition of the binding of a vitamin K–dependent clotting factor (eg, prothrombin) to negatively charged phospholipid via the g-carboxyglutamic acid (gla) residues near the N-terminal end of the molecule. Each clotting factor contains approximately 12 gla residues. Vitamin K converts the amino acid glutamine to γ-carboxyglutamic acid as a posttranslational event within the hepatocyte.

---

and II. *Note:* The PT is *not* prolonged in the presence of severe factor IX deficiency (eg, patients with hemophilia B).

Second, thrombin has many other actions besides the conversion of fibrinogen to fibrin.[17] Importantly, thrombin "feeds back" and changes factors V and VIII to their activated forms Va and VIIIa, which are much more efficient in augmenting the conversion of factor X to Xa and factor IX to IXa, respectively. Thrombin also promotes the activation of factor XI; aggregates platelets; stimulates fibrinolysis; activates fibrin-stabilizing factor (factor XIII); and, when bound to thrombomodulin, activates the natural anticoagulant, protein C.

Third, an enormous amount of biochemical amplification occurs following the generation of the first few molecules of tissue factor/VIIa.[2] A large quantity of thrombin is produced, which not only leads to the formation of fibrin at the wound site but also poses a major risk of pathologic thrombosis in adjacent undamaged blood vessels. Highly efficient inhibitors, such as antithrombin III, are poised to inhibit thrombin if it escapes the confines of the injury; this process is discussed in more detail below.

Conversion of Fibrinogen to Fibrin

The final common pathway in the coagulation of blood is the conversion of a soluble monomeric protein, fibrinogen, to an insoluble polymer, fibrin.[18,19] Thrombin initiates this process by enzymatically cleaving two small polypeptides, fibrinopeptide A and fibrinopeptide B, from native fibrinogen, which leads to the formation of fibrin monomer (Figure 16–6). The newly formed fibrin monomer spontaneously polymerizes into long chains and three-dimensional structures that characterize an insoluble fibrin clot. Initially, the monomers are weakly linked together by hydrogen bonds, but thrombin-activated factor XIIIa later creates stable amide bonds to produce fibrin that is physically strong and relatively resistant to fibrinolysis.

Role of Platelets

Platelets play a key role in promoting hemostasis, particularly in the cessation of bleeding from superficial wounds,

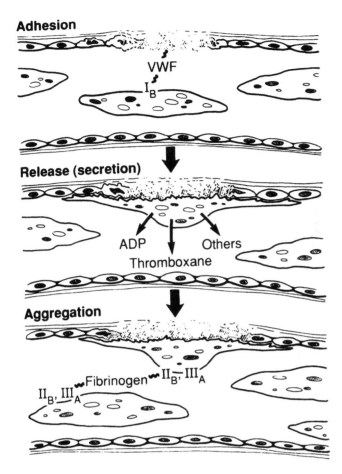

Figure 16–4 A diagram of platelet adhesion and aggregation at a site of vascular injury. Damage to the endothelial cell surface exposes collagen, which in turn binds von Willebrand factor (**VWF**) from the plasma or subendothelial surfaces. Platelets bind to the von Willebrand factor via glycoprotein I_B, a platelet membrane adhesion receptor. Activation of the platelet leads to the synthesis and release of thromboxane A_2 from membrane phospholipids, and storage granules release adenosine diphosphate (**ADP**). Both agents interact with receptors on adjacent platelets, allowing binding of fibrinogen by glycoprotein II_B/III_A.

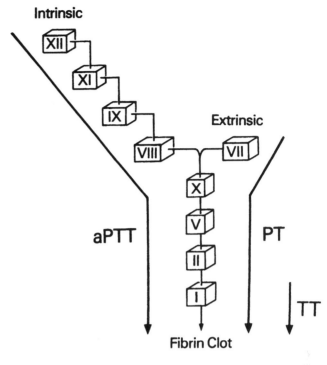

Figure 16–5 Diagram of the clotting factors studied in the most commonly used screening tests of coagulation—activated partial thromboplastin time (**aPTT**), prothrombin time (**PT**), and thrombin time (**TT**). Defects or deficiencies of clotting factors XII, XI, IX, or VIII will prolong the aPTT, whereas a defect or deficiency in factor VII will prolong the PT. A defect or deficiency of fibrinogen will prolong the TT. Disorders involving factor X, factor V, prothrombin, or fibrinogen will elevate both the aPTT and PT. Source: Reprinted with permission from JE Ansell, *Handbook of Hemostasis and Thrombosis*, p 20, © 1986, Little Brown & Company.

such as a shaving nick or a bleeding-time cut.[20,21] At the injury sites, aggregating platelets form primary hemostatic plugs that are later stabilized by the formation of fibrin strands after some thrombin has been generated. Platelets also contribute to blood coagulation by providing phospholipid surfaces and contributing to the coagulum some more clotting factors, such as factor V and fibrinogen, which are released from platelet alpha granules. In general, severe thrombocytopenia or platelet function defects promote superficial bleeding in contrast to coagulation disorders, such as hemophilia, which lead to hemorrhage in the muscles or joints.

ANTITHROMBOTIC MECHANISMS: PREVENTION OF THROMBOSIS

The presence of tissue factor, collagen, and phospholipid surfaces in the wound helps to limit clot formation to the area of injury. Once large amounts of thrombin are formed, however, powerful antithrombotic mechanisms slow coagulation and prevent extension of the clot into normal blood vessels. Blood flowing past the vascular defect plays an important role, along with potent antithrombotic forces closely linked to the normal endothelium (Figures 16–7 and 16–8).

Local blood flow tends to dilute any activated clotting factors (eg, factor Xa, thrombin) or activated platelets that might have escaped the injury site. These thrombogenic substances are flushed away into the general circulation, where they are easily neutralized by clotting factor inhibitors in the blood or microcirculation; cleared by the liver; or, in the case of activated platelets, removed by the reticuloendothelial system.

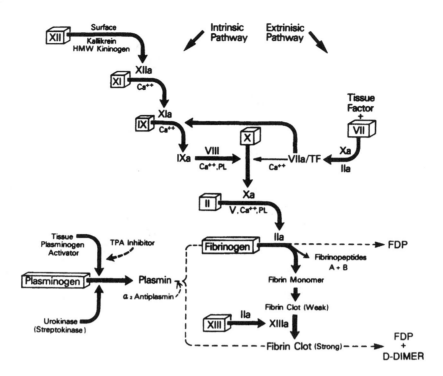

Figure 16–6 The conversion of fibrinogen to fibrin. Fibrinogen, a soluble protein, releases fibrinopeptide A and fibrinopeptide B when cleaved by the proteolytic enzyme thrombin. The loss of the fibrinopeptides produces fibrin monomer, which spontaneously forms a polymer held together by hydrogen bonds. The action of fibrin stabilizing factor (factor XIIIa) converts the fibrin to a stable clot bound together by amide bonds. The fibrinolytic system (at lower left) indicates that plasminogen is converted to plasmin by tissue plasminogen activator (**tPA**). tPA inhibitor is a principal inhibitor of tPA. Plasmin will act on either fibrinogen or fibrin clot to form fibrin(ogen) degradation products (**FDP**) or D-dimers.

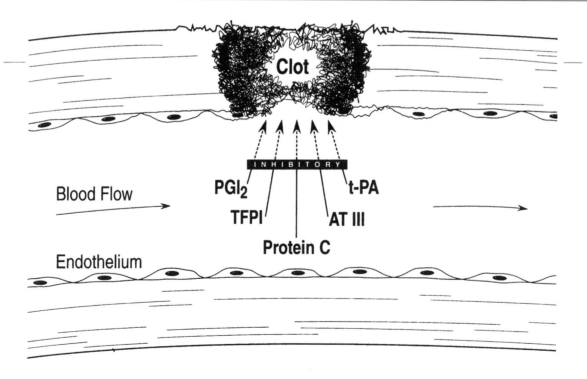

Figure 16–7 A diagram illustrating how the vascular endothelium acts to limit the formation of a thrombus to an injury site. Protein C, tissue factor pathway inhibitor (**TFPI**), antithrombin III (**AT-III**), prostacyclin (**PGI₂**), and tissue plasminogen activator (**t-PA**) each inhibit different aspects of thrombus formation. In addition, blood flow tends to dilute and remove activated clotting factors and other products of thrombosis.

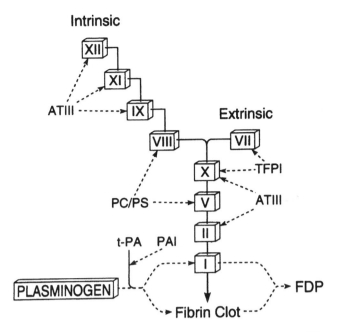

Key: ATIII, antithrombin III; FDP, fibrinogen degradation products; PAI, plasminogen activator inhibitor; PC, protein C; PS, protein S; TFPI, tissue factor pathway inhibitor; t-PA, tissue plasminogen activator.

Figure 16–8 Illustration of the various sites of coagulation factor interaction with inhibitors and fibrinolytic enzymes. Source: Reprinted with permission from J Rippe et al, *Intensive Care Medicine*, 3rd ed, p 1360. © 1996, Little Brown & Company.

Close to the injury, normal vascular endothelium contributes actively to the suppression of coagulation and platelet activation and stimulates local fibrinolysis. The endothelium is a rich source of natural anticoagulants (eg, antithrombin III, activated protein C). Endothelial cells also elaborate potent antiplatelet factors (eg, prostacyclin [PGI₂]) and stimulate clot breakdown (fibrinolysis) by releasing the profibrinolytic enzyme, tissue plasminogen activator (tPA).

Anticoagulant Systems

Antithrombin III

Antithrombin III is a powerful and direct inhibitor of thrombin.[22,23] It forms a 1:1 molecular complex with the enzyme and immediately neutralizes its clot-promoting activity. Antithrombin III circulates in the blood but also binds to heparin, a glycosaminoglycan present on the surface of normal endothelial cells. When bound to heparin, the ability of antithrombin III to neutralize thrombin is greatly enhanced. Large amounts of antithrombin III are associated with endothelial cells in the microcirculation, so that any circulating thrombin that escapes a distant injury site is rapidly neutralized.

In addition to neutralizing thrombin, antithrombin III also potently inhibits factors Xa and IXa. In high concentrations antithrombin III inhibits factor VIIa bound to tissue factor, but it is less effective against unbound VIIa.[24] The anticoagulant heparin owes its antithrombotic properties to augmentation of antithrombin III-induced neutralization of activated clotting factors.

Activated Protein C and Protein S

Protein C inhibits coagulation by a much different mechanism than that of antithrombin III.[25] After the zymogen, protein C, is converted to its enzymatic form, activated protein C (APC) destroys the coagulation cofactors, factor V and factor VIII, particularly after they have been stimulated by traces of thrombin (Figure 16–9). This important anticoagulant system is initially set in motion by thrombin, produced as a result of tissue injury. Thrombin binds to an endothelial cell surface glycoprotein, thrombomodulin, and, in the process, loses its procoagulant properties and gains the

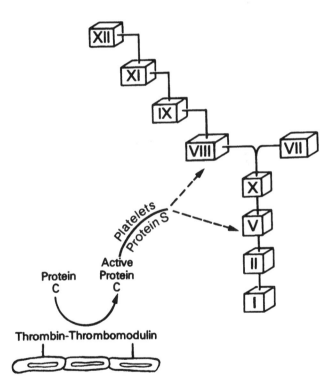

Figure 16–9 A model of the activation of protein C and the subsequent inhibition of factors Va and VIIIa. Thrombin binds to thrombomodulin, located on the endothelial cell surface, and acquires the ability to convert the zymogen, protein C, to its activated form—activated protein C. Activated protein C, with the help of its cofactor, protein S, and on the phospholipid surface of platelets, inactivates factors Va and VIIIa, thus making the blood less likely to clot. Source: Reprinted with permission from JE Ansell, *Handbook of Hemostasis and Thrombosis*, p 13, © 1986, Little Brown & Company.

ability to convert protein C to APC. In this instance, thrombin has been "turned" from a powerful prothrombotic to a potent anticoagulant enzyme. Protein S serves as a cofactor when APC destroys factor Va and factor VIIIa.

Protein S circulates in the blood in two forms: free (unbound) and attached to a complement-binding protein, C4b-BP.[26] Only the free form of protein S plays an active role in limiting coagulation. Inflammatory states (eg, systemic lupus erythematosus) can cause an increase in the binding protein that prompts a shift from the free to the bound form of protein S and thereby reduces the anticoagulant activity of protein S.

Both protein C and protein S are vitamin K–dependent proteins. They rely on the vitamin K–mediated γ-carboxylation reaction to allow binding to phospholipid surfaces and to ensure optimal interactions with their companion blood coagulation factors needed to prevent thrombosis. Vitamin K deficiency (eg, induced by oral anticoagulants) produces a fall in circulating protein C and protein S levels, although, under most circumstances, the reduction in clotting factors II, VII, IX, and X appears to be paramount so that bleeding is more likely to occur than thrombosis. An exception is the warfarin-induced skin necrosis syndrome, in which protein C–deficient (and occasionally protein S–deficient) patients can rapidly develop profound protein C deficiency (eg, <5%) during the early hours of anticoagulation with warfarin. The low levels of protein C can lead to thrombotic infarction of the skin and other organs, a condition similar to that of infants with homozygous protein C deficiency who develop neonatal purpura fulminans.[27,28]

Tissue Factor Pathway Inhibitor

A third anticoagulant system is also closely linked to the endothelial cell surface, but it inhibits coagulation by yet another mechanism.[29,30] As the name implies, tissue factor pathway inhibitor (TFPI) blocks tissue factor/VIIa but only after first binding to activated factor X generated during the course of thrombus formation. The TFPI-Xa complex is a potent inhibitor of tissue factor-mediated coagulation and serves to put a "brake" on this powerful procoagulant complex. Most of the TFPI is localized to vascular endothelial cells so that relatively little circulates in the blood, although it can be released into the circulation by injections of the anticoagulant heparin. To date, it is unclear whether deficiencies or molecular defects involving the TFPI molecule are associated with thrombosis in vivo.

Antiplatelet Actions of Endothelial Cells

Endothelial cells serve as a source of an important inhibitor of platelet aggregation—prostacyclin.[31] When endothelial cells are stimulated (eg, by thrombin), arachidonic acid, a 20-carbon polyunsaturated fatty acid, is liberated from membrane phospholipids and then enzymatically converted to prostacyclin, which is then released from the endothelial cell. Prostacyclin has a relatively short half-life (~30 minutes) but helps to limit hemostatic plug formation to sites of vascular injury, particularly in small blood vessels. Large doses of aspirin (eg, two tablets) inhibit both prostacyclin and the platelet proaggregatory substance thromboxane A_2, but the net effect is a mild tendency toward bleeding rather than vascular thrombosis.

Fibrinolysis: Limiting Clot Formation

The fibrinolytic system is activated in the regions of tissue injury and helps to limit the ultimate size and distribution of a thrombus[32] (Figure 16–6). Again, endothelial cells are an essential component of the reaction, serving as a site of synthesis of tPA, the enzyme responsible for the conversion of fibrin-bound plasminogen to the proteolytic enzyme plasmin. Plasmin breaks down (lyses) fibrin, which leads to dissolution of the clot and the formation of soluble fibrin degradation products that are ultimately removed from sites of tissue injury by local blood flow.

CONCLUSION

Hemostasis is a highly complex but finely tuned dynamic process that protects against both increased bleeding and unwanted vascular thrombosis. As might be expected in such a highly regulated system, hereditary and acquired defects occur rather frequently and can lead to hemorrhage or, all too often, pathologic arterial and venous thrombosis. Indeed, efforts have been made to alter this delicate balance in hopes of treating patients suffering from hemostatic or thrombotic defects. Included among these therapeutic options are the anticoagulants heparin and warfarin, which confer an increased likelihood of bleeding in exchange for protection against recurrent thromboembolism. Fortunately, the intensity of therapy with anticoagulants usually can be controlled to allow for safe and effective treatment of patients with most thrombotic disorders.

REFERENCES

1. Davie EW. Biochemical and molecular aspects of the coagulation cascade. *Thromb Haemost.* 1995;74:1–6.

2. Davie EW, Fujikawa K, Kisiel W. The coagulation cascade: initiation, maintenance, and regulation. *Biochem.* 1991;30:10363–10370.

3. Banner DW, D'Arcy A, Chene C, et al. The crystal structure of the complex of blood coagulation factor VIIa with soluble tissue factor. *Nature.* 1996;380:21–23.

4. Nemerson Y. The tissue factor pathway of blood coagulation. *Semin Hematol.* 1992;29:170–173.

5. Nemerson Y. Tissue factor: then and now. *Thromb Haemost.* 1995;74: 180–184.

6. Walsh PN. Platelet-coagulant protein interactions. In: Colman RW, Hirsh J, Marder VJ, Saizman EW, eds. *Hemostasis and Thrombosis: Basic Principles and Clinical Practice.* Philadelphia: JB Lippincott; 1994;629-651.

7. Stenflo J, Fernlund P, Egan W, Roepstorff P. Vitamin K–dependent modifications of glutamic acid residues in prothrombin. *Proc Natl Acad Sci USA.* 1974;71:2730–2733.

8. Nelsestuen GL, Zytkovicz TH, Howard JB. The mode of action of vitamin K. Identification of γ-carboxyglutamic acid as a component of prothrombin. *J Biol Chem.* 1974;249:6347–6350.

9. Zivelin A, Rao LVM, Rapaport SI. Mechanism of the anticoagulant effect of warfarin as evaluated in rabbits by selective depression of individual procoagulant vitamin K–dependent clotting factors. *J Clin Invest.* 1993;92:2131–2140.

10. Triplett DA. Protean clinical presentation of antiphospholipid-protein antibodies (APA). *Thromb Haemost.* 1995;74:329–337.

11. Smirnov MD, Triplett DA, Comp PC, Esmon NL, Esmon CT. On the role of phosphatidylethanolamine in the inhibition of activated protein C activity by antiphospholipid antibodies. *J Clin Invest.* 1995;95: 309–316.

12. Kroll MH. Mechanisms of platelet activation. In: Loscalzo J, Schafer AI, eds. *Thrombosis and Hemorrhage.* Boston: Blackwell Scientific Publications; 1994;247–277.

13. Sadler JE. von Willebrand factor. *J Biol Chem.* 1991;266:22777–22779.

14. Ruggeri ZM. The role of von Willebrand factor and fibrinogen in the initiation of platelet adhesion to thrombogenic surfaces. *Thromb Haemost.* 1995;74:460–463.

15. DeLa Cadena RA, Wachtfogel YT, Colman RW. Contact activation pathway: inflammation and coagulation. In: Colman RW, Hirsh J, Marder VJ, Saizman EW, eds. *Hemostasis and Thrombosis: Basic Principles and Clinical Practice.* Philadelphia: JB Lippincott; 1994: 219–240.

16. Rapaport SI. The activation of factor IX by the tissue factor pathway. *Prog Clin Biol Res.* 1981;72:57–76.

17. Fenton JW, Ofosu FA, Brezniak DV, Hassouna HI. Understanding thrombin and hemostasis. *Hematol Oncol Clin North Am.* 1993;7:1107–1119.

18. Mosesson MW. The roles of fibrinogen and fibrin in hemostasis and thrombosis. *Semin Hematol.* 1992;29:177–188.

19. Mosesson MW. Thrombin interactions with fibrinogen and fibrin. *Semin Thromb Hemost.* 1993;19:361–367.

20. Bennett JS. Mechanisms of platelet adhesion and aggregation: an update. *Hosp Pract.* 1992;27:124–126.

21. Ruggeri ZM. New insights into the mechanisms of platelet adhesion and aggregation. *Semin Hematol.* 1994;31:229–239.

22. Blajchman MA. An overview of the mechanism of action of antithrombin and its inherited deficiency states. *Blood Coag Fibrinolysis.* 1994;5:S5–S11.

23. Bauer KA, Rosenberg RD. Role of antithrombin III as a regulator of in vitro coagulation. *Semin Hematol.* 1991;28:10–13.

24. Rao LV, Rapaport SI, Hoang AD. Binding of factor VIIa to tissue factor permits rapid antithrombin III/heparin inhibition of factor VIIa. *Blood.* 1993;81:2600–2607.

25. Esmon CT, Fukudome K. Cellular regulation of the protein C pathway. *Semn Cell Biol.* 1995;6:259–268.

26. Comp PC. Laboratory evaluation of protein S status. *Semin Thromb Hemost.* 1990;16:177–181.

27. Comp PC. Coumadin-induced skin necrosis. Incidence, mechanisms. management and avoidance. *Drug Saf.* 1993;8:128–135.

28. Seligsohn U, Berger A, Abend M. et al. Homozygous protein C deficiency manifested by massive venous thrombosis in the newborn. *N Engl J Med.* 1984;310:559–562.

29. Le DT, Griffin JH, Greengard JS, Mujumdar V, Rapaport SI. Use of a generally applicable tissue factor–dependent factor V assay to detect activated protein C–resistant factor Va in patients receiving warfarin and in patients with a lupus anticoagulant. *Blood.* 1995;85: 1704–1711.

30. Broze GJ. Tissue factor pathway inhibitor. *Thromb Haemost.* 1995; 74:90–93.

31. Jaffe EA. Biochemistry, immunology, and cell biology of endothelium. In: Colman RW, Hirsh J, Marder VJ, Saizman EW, eds. *Hemostasis and Thrombosis: Basic Principles and Clinical Practice.* Philadelphia: JB Lippincott; 1994:718–744.

32. Verstraete M. The fibrinolytic system: from petri dishes to genetic engineering. *Thromb Haemost.* 1995;74:25–35.

Chapter 17

Thrombogenesis and Hypercoagulable States

Jeffrey I. Zwicker and Kenneth A. Bauer

Thrombosis is the leading cause of mortality and morbidity in developed countries. Although both arterial and venous thrombosis ultimately result from activation of the clotting system, the underlying mechanisms leading to thrombosis differ significantly. In the absence of arrhythmia or cardiomyopathy, arterial thrombosis is often the consequence of atherosclerotic disease, which is characterized by the subintimal accumulation of lipids and inflammatory cells leading to abnormal vascular endothelial function. Thrombosis occurs in the setting of acute plaque rupture and subsequent activation of platelets and clotting factors. Several conditions are known risk factors for atherosclerotic disease, including smoking, hypertension, diabetes, and hyperlipidemia. However, risk factors associated with atherosclerotic disease do not confer a similar increased risk of venous thromboembolism.

Venous thromboembolism occurs in approximately one per 1,000 people annually.[1] Underlying risk factors associated with venous thrombosis can be classified as either acquired or hereditary. Acquired risk factors for venous thrombosis consist of a heterogeneous group of disorders that lead to a prothrombotic state through various mechanisms. In cases of trauma or surgery, activation of the coagulation system through exposure to tissue factor and a depressed

fibrinolytic response results in a significantly higher incidence of deep venous thrombosis. Venous thrombosis is also a common complication in many disease states including sepsis and cancer whereby several mechanisms for thrombosis have been implicated including elaboration of inflammatory cytokines and augmented expression of tissue factor. However, venous thrombosis commonly occurs in the absence of clearly identified precipitants. For many years researchers suspected that hereditary defects of coagulation were responsible for a large number of idiopathic venous thromboembolic events, but only recently with the discovery of the Factor V Leiden and prothrombin G20210A mutations have a significant number of cases been identified as familial (Exhibit 17–1). This chapter details several hereditary and acquired conditions known to be associated with venous thromboembolic disease.

HEREDITARY THROMBOPHILIA

Antithrombin III Deficiency

Antithrombin is a protein that inactivates several clotting factors including thrombin, a property that is markedly accelerated in the presence of heparin. First described in a Norwegian family with history of recurrent thrombosis, heterozygous antithrombin deficiency has been demonstrated in approximately 4% of families with inherited thrombophilia and in 1% of consecutive patients with a first episode of deep vein thrombosis.[2,3]

Dr. Zwicker is a Clinical Fellow in Medicine at Harvard Medical School and Beth Israel Deaconess Medical Center. Dr. Bauer is an Associate Professor of Medicine, Harvard Medical School, Chief, Hematology Section, VA Boston Healthcare System, and Director, Thrombosis Clinical Research at Beth Israel Deaconess Medical Center, Boston, Massachusetts.

Supported in part by the Medical Research Service of the Department of Veterans Affairs.

Exhibit 17–1
PREVALENCE OF DEFECTS IN PATIENTS WITH IDIOPATHIC DEEP VENOUS THROMBOSIS

Factor V Leiden	12–40%
Prothrombin G20210A mutation	6–18%
Deficiencies of antithrombin, protein C, or protein S	5–15%
Hyperhomocysteinemia	10–20%
Antiphospholipid antibody syndrome	10–20%

Researchers have identified many mutations that cause antithrombin deficiency either through decreased synthesis or altered functional activity. Acquired antithrombin deficiency is found in several disease states including liver disease, nephrotic syndrome, sepsis, and disseminated intravascular coagulation.[4–7] Modest reductions are also found in users of oral contraceptives or estrogens.[8–9] In addition, the administration of heparin decreases plasma antithrombin levels by accelerating its clearance.[10] Thus, evaluation of plasma samples from individuals during a period of heparinization can potentially lead to an erroneous diagnosis of antithrombin deficiency.

Due to the number of clinical disorders that can be associated with reductions in the plasma concentration of antithrombin, definitive diagnosis of the hereditary deficiency is often difficult. Whereas antithrombin level in the normal range is usually sufficient to exclude the disorder, low levels should be confirmed at a later date. This determination is ideally performed when the individual is no longer receiving warfarin because plasma antithrombin levels can occasionally be elevated into the normal range in individuals in the deficiency state.[11]

Protein C Deficiency

Protein C is a vitamin K–dependent protein synthesized by the liver that exerts its anticoagulant function after activation to the serine protease, activated protein C (APC). In 1981, Griffin et al[12] described low levels of protein C in a family with recurrent thrombotic events. In subsequent large cohort studies, protein C deficiency was documented in 2–9% of individuals with a history of venous thrombosis.[13] Screening for protein C deficiency can be performed by clotting assay (based on prolongation of the aPTT), and low levels reflect a reduced ability of activated protein C to be activated or interact with the platelet membrane and its substrates such as factor Va or factor VIIIa. Because the levels of protein C in the heterozygous deficiency state overlap with the normal population, measurements that are between 60% and 70% of normal represent borderline values and warrant repeat testing. Protein C antigen levels can also vary depending on age: newborns have 20-40% normal adult levels; in adults, protein C levels typically increase 4% per decade.[14,15] Homozygous or doubly heterozygous deficiencies can lead to significant perinatal thrombosis (purpura fulminans).

Acquired protein C deficiency is found in numerous disease states, including liver disease, DIC, and sepsis. Similarly, anticoagulation with warfarin lowers protein C levels; thus patients should be investigated only after oral anticoagulation has been discontinued for at least one week. Alternatively, individuals can be studied while receiving heparin therapy, which does not alter plasma protein C levels.

Protein S Deficiency

Protein S is a vitamin K–dependent protein that enhances the anticoagulant effect of APC. Protein S deficiency is reported in approximately 10% of families with inherited thrombophilia,[16,17] but the prevalence is much lower (around 1%) among consecutive patients with a first episode of deep venous thrombosis.[18] There are multiple causes of acquired protein S deficiency, including pregnancy, oral contraception, acute thrombosis, and disseminated intravascular coagulation. Protein S levels also increase with age and are influenced by sex; females in the general population have a lower mean plasma protein S level than males. Thus it is often difficult to diagnose heterozygous protein S deficiency based on a single assay measurement; repeat sampling and family studies are often required to make the diagnosis with certainty.

Factor V Leiden

Prior to 1993, hereditary deficiencies were infrequently identified in patients with familial thromboembolic disease. Researchers then identified families in which the plasma of affected members demonstrated resistance to APC in an activated partial thromboplastin (aPTT)-based clotting assay and found that a single point mutation of the factor V gene was responsible for the defect.[19,20] This arginine-506 substitution by glutamine renders factor Va relatively resistant to inactivation by APC. Many studies have identified the factor V gene mutation (or Factor V Leiden) as a common abnormality in Caucasian populations, occurring in approximately 5% of the general population and in 20% of individuals with a first deep venous thrombosis.[21,22] The U.S. Physician's Health Study confirmed the high prevalence of heterozygosity for Factor V Leiden.[23] In this nested, case-control study of 14,916 healthy men older than 40 years, heterozygosity was identified in 12% of individuals with a first episode of deep venous thrombosis and in 6% of controls, corresponding to a 3.5-fold increased risk of venous thrombosis. The risk of thrombosis increases dramatically in the homozygous state or in the presence of a second hereditary defect.[24,25]

Factor V Leiden can be accurately identified using a screening coagulation assay; after an individual's plasma is diluted with factor V–deficient plasma, an aPTT is measured. This assay limits the influence of other coagulation factor levels on clotting time determinations and thus is useful even when an individual is treated with anticoagulants. Abnormal results should then be confirmed by genotyping for the Factor V Leiden mutation.

Prothrombin G20210A Mutation

Prothrombin (factor II) is the precursor of thrombin, the end product of the coagulation cascade. A single base pair mutation in the prothrombin gene has been identified as an independent risk factor for hereditary venous thromboembolic disease and is the second most common hereditary defect after Factor V Leiden. Originally described in 1996, the G to A substitution at position 20210 was identified in 18% of individuals among 28 probands with a personal and familial history of thrombosis.[26] Large population studies have shown an overall prevalence of about 2% in the general Caucasian population, but it is very infrequent among individuals of Asian or African descent.[27] In the Leiden Thrombophilia Study, which investigated individuals with an idiopathic first deep venous thrombosis, the prevalence of the prothrombin

G20210A mutation was 6.2% versus 2.3% of healthy matched controls.[26] This corresponded to a 2.8-fold increased risk of a first episode of deep venous thrombosis in carriers of the mutation, an effect that was seen in both sexes and all age groups.

Polymerase chain reaction methods have been used to detect the prothrombin G20210A mutation. Although plasma prothrombin activity and antigen levels are significantly higher in individuals with the prothrombin G20210A mutation, prothrombin levels cannot be used to screen for the defect due to significant overlap with the normal population.[28]

Hyperhomocysteinemia

Homocysteine is a sulfur-containing amino acid involved in metabolic pathways leading to the formation of other amino acids. As shown in Figure 17–1, methionine is generated through the remethylation of homocysteine or metabolized to cysteine via trans-sulfuration. Elevated levels of homocysteine are seen in a variety of disorders that affect either the concentration of substrates or the activity of enzymes involved in its metabolism.

The association between severe hyperhomocysteinemia and thrombosis was initially described in infants with homocystinuria. Homocystinuria results from several rare inborn errors involving homocysteine metabolism (ie,

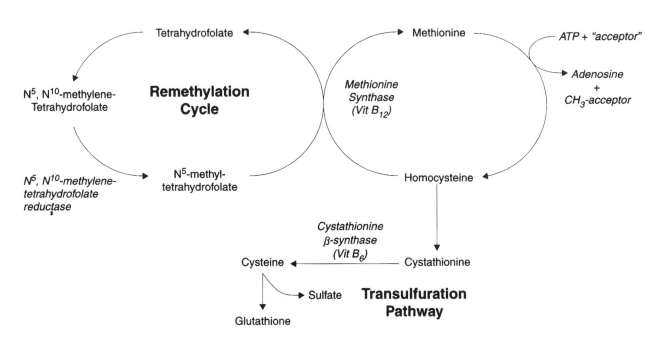

Figure 17–1 Metabolism of homocysteine. Homocysteine is an amino acid that is generated through the catabolism of methione. Methione serves as a methyl donor to different acceptors (eg, choline, creatine, etc.) and is regenerated through a remethylation cycle via the vitamin B$_{12}$-dependent enzyme N$_5$, N$_{10}$, methylenetretrahydrofolate reductase. Excess homocysteine is metabolized to other amino acids via the transulfuration pathway, which is catalyzed by a vitamin B$_6$-dependent enzyme, cystationine β-synthase.

cystathione β-synthase deficiency) leading to premature arterial and venous thrombosis as well as mental retardation and skeletal abnormalities. Cross-sectional studies noted an association between even mild elevations in plasma homocysteine and atherosclerotic or venous thromboembolic disease.[29,30] In a large cohort study of over 5,000 British men, among the 107 subjects who suffered a stroke, there was a graded increase in relative risk based on increasing homocysteine concentrations.[31] The Leiden Thrombophilia Study showed that individuals with homocysteine levels above the 95th percentile (>18 μmol/L) were 2.5 times more likely to suffer an initial episode of deep venous thrombosis.[29]

Several genetic and acquired abnormalities can lead to mild or moderate elevations in serum homocysteine concentrations. The most common genetic defects include heterozygous cystathione β-synthase deficiency, which occurs in approximately 0.3% of the population, and homozygosity for a methylenetetrahydrofolate reductase mutation is present in approximately 20% of Italian and U.S. Hispanic populations, but less than 1% of African Americans.[32] The most common causes of acquired hyperhomocysteinemia include mild to moderate deficiencies in vitamin B_{12} folate, or vitamin B_6, which serve as cofactors in homocysteine metabolism. Other associations include advanced age, smoking, medications, and disease states such as liver or renal failure.

Hyperhomocysteinemia is usually diagnosed by measuring fasting plasma levels of homocysteine by high pressure liquid chromatography. Hyperhomocysteinemia is classified as mild (15–30 μmol/L), moderate (30–100 μmol/L), or severe (>100 μmol/L). Because individuals with heterozygous cystathione β-synthase deficiency may have normal levels of fasting homocysteine, the methionine oral load has been used to diagnose these heterozygous individuals.

Factor XII Deficiency

Factor XII initiates the contact activation reactions and intrinsic blood coagulation *in vitro*. Subjects with severe factor XII deficiency (less than 1% of normal) have markedly prolonged aPTT but do not exhibit a bleeding diathesis;[33] however, there have been a number of case reports of venous thromboembolism or myocardial infarction in factor XII-deficient individuals.[34] The frequency with which severe factor XII deficiency leads to thrombosis is uncertain; one review found that 8% had a history of thromboembolism.[34] In another study of 14 Swiss families with factor XII deficiency, 2 of 18 homozygous or doubly heterozygous patients suffered deep vein thrombosis; however, each episode occurred in association with predisposing thrombotic risk factors.[35] It remains unproven if factor XII deficiency is associated with an increased risk of thrombosis.

Elevated Levels of Factors VIII, IX, XI, and Thrombin Activatable Fibrinolysis Inhibitor

Recently, investigators have focused on the presence of supranormal levels of clotting factors and their role in venous thrombosis. In the Leiden Thrombophilia Study, 25% of patients with a first episode of venous thrombosis and 11% of healthy controls had factor VIII coagulant activity (VIII:C) greater than 150% of normal (>150 IU/dl). Individuals with VIII:C levels greater than 150 IU/dl had a five-fold increased risk of a first episode of deep venous thrombosis compared to individuals with lower VIII:C levels (<100 IU/dl).[36] An Austrian study prospectively followed 360 patients for an average of 30 months and found that among 38 patients who developed recurrent thromboembolism, the mean VIII:C level was greater than among those without recurrences.[37] Among those individuals with levels above the 90th percentile, the likelihood of recurrence at two years was 37% versus 5% with lower VIII:C levels (relative risk 6.7). Corroborating studies are required prior to recommending routine measurement of VIII:C levels in patients with prior venous thrombotic events. Elevated antigenic levels of several other coagulation factors including factor XI, factor IX, and thrombin-activatable fibrinolysis inhibitor also confer a modest, albeit significantly increased risk for an initial episode of deep venous thrombosis.[38–40]

ACQUIRED THROMBOPHILIA

The acquired hypercoagulable state consists of a heterogeneous group of disorders that are associated with an increased tendency toward thrombotic complications. In a case control study of 1,272 outpatients with deep venous thrombosis, pregnancy was associated with the greatest risk of thrombosis (or 11.4) followed by muscle trauma (7.6), immobilization (5.6), venous insufficiency (4.5), chronic heart failure (2.9), and long-distance travel (2.3).[41] Although commonly considered a risk factor, the issue of extended travel is controversial; a recent study of 788 patients found no association with deep venous thrombosis and travel greater than 5 hours.[42]

Thrombosis is commonly associated with several disease states (Exhibit 17–2). It may represent the presence of an underlying malignancy (especially carcinomas of the gastrointestinal tract, ovary, prostate, and lung), which in some populations is later diagnosed in over 10% of individuals after an initial episode of idiopathic deep venous thrombosis.[43] Antiphospholipid antibodies can lead to both arterial and venous thrombosis; they are associated with autoimmune disorders such as systemic lupus erythematosus, exposure to medications, or malignancies, or can occur in some

Exhibit 17–2
ACQUIRED CONDITIONS AND DISORDERS ASSOCIATED WITH HYPERCOAGULABLE STATES

Pregnancy
Immobilization
Trauma
Postoperative state
Advancing age
Estrogen
Antiphospholipid syndrome
Malignancy
Nephrotic syndrome
Heparin-induced thrombocytopenia
Thrombotic thrombocytopenic purpura
Myeloproliferative disorders
Paroxysmal nocturnal hemoglobinuria
Hyperlipidemia
Diabetes mellitus
Hyperviscosity
Congestive heart failure

individuals without any underlying disease. The development of thrombosis and thrombocytopenia with concurrent heparin administration should always prompt consideration of heparin-induced thrombocytopenia. Nephrotic syndrome is characterized by large amounts of protein in the urine and is often complicated by thrombosis, especially in the renal veins.

LABORATORY IDENTIFICATION OF HYPERCOAGULABLE STATES

The laboratory evaluation of individuals with thrombosis should begin with a complete blood count and review of peripheral smear, which may show morphologic changes suggestive of a myeloproliferative disorder, microangiopathic hemolytic anemia in association with disseminated intravascular coagulation, or leukoerythroblastosis indicative of marrow infiltration by tumor. Abnormalities of serum chemistries such as liver and renal tests may reflect thrombosis within the hepatic circulation (Budd-Chiari syndrome) or the presence of nephrotic syndrome, respectively.

Given the lack of consensus regarding the optimal treatment for hereditary thrombophilia, coupled with the cost of performing a complete laboratory evaluation, a targeted approach to the laboratory diagnosis of hereditary thrombophilic disorders is prudent. In general, laboratory investigation is not routinely recommended in instances of acquired hypercoagulability such as major surgery, malignancy, systemic lupus erythematosus, or myeloproliferative disorders. In contrast, acquired states such as oral contraception, the puerperium, and pregnancy frequently trigger throm-

botic events in women with hereditary thrombophilia and thus warrant further investigation.[44]

In order to guide laboratory evaluation, it is useful to classify patients as *strongly* or *weakly* thrombophilic. An individual can be labeled *strongly* thrombophilic based on three historical features (see Exhibit 17–3):

1. First thromboembolic event occurring prior to age 50
2. History of recurrent thrombotic episodes
3. A first-degree relative with a documented venous thromboembolic event prior to age 50

In those individuals who meet any of the above criteria, full laboratory investigation is warranted, including testing for the Factor V Leiden and prothrombin G20210A mutations and deficiencies of antithrombin, protein C, and protein S. On the other hand, a more focused diagnostic approach should be conducted in *weakly* thrombophilic patients. The frequency of the Factor V Leiden or prothrombin G20210A remains significant even in weakly thrombophilic patients,

Exhibit 17–3
A TARGETED EVALUATION OF INITIAL IDIOPATHIC THROMBOSIS BASED ON THROMBOPHILIA HISTORY

Strongly thrombophilic refers to the presence of any of the following historical features: venous thromboembolism prior to 50 years of age, two or more venous thrombotic episodes, or a family history of venous thromboembolic events.

Arterial: Homocysteine, lupus anticoagulant/antiphospholipid antibodies

Venous: Thrombophilia History?
1. DVT prior to 50 years
2. recurrent events
3. positive family history

Strongly (one or more strongly thrombophilic features):
- Antiphospholipid antibodies
- Hyperhomocysteinemia
- Factor V Leiden
- Prothrombin G20120A
- Protein C deficiency
- Protein S deficiency
- Antithrombin III deficiency

Weakly (no strongly thrombophilic features):
- Lupus (anticoagulant/antiphospholipid antibodies
- Hyperhomocysteinemia
- Factor V Leiden
- Prothrombin G20120A

and thus screening for these defects is reasonable; however, the diagnosis of antithrombin, protein C, or protein S deficiencies is rare in individuals without a "strongly" thrombophilic history. Both strongly and weakly thrombophilic patients should also undergo laboratory testing for the presence of antiphospholipid antibody syndrome and hyperhomocysteinemia. These defects should also be investigated in individuals with unexplained arterial thrombosis.

The levels of antithrombin, protein C, or protein S can be affected by acute thrombosis, anticoagulation, or disease states. Consequently, evaluation for a hereditary abnormality should be conducted at least one week after completing the initial 3- to 6-month course of anticoagulation. If, upon acute presentation, levels of antithrombin, protein C, or protein S are obtained that are well within the normal range, then the diagnosis of deficiency can be reliably excluded. However, a low value will require confirmation after anticoagulation is discontinued. In those in whom temporary discontinuation of anticoagulation is not practical, confirmation in first-degree relatives can be helpful.

REFERENCES

1. Nordstrom M, Lindblad B, Bergqvist D, Kjellstrom T. A prospective study of the incidence of deep-vein thrombosis within a defined urban population. *J Intern Med.* 1992 Aug;232(2):155–160.

2. Heijboer H, Brandjes DPM, Buller HR, Sturk A, ten Cate JW. Deficiencies of coagulation-inhibiting and fibrinolytic proteins in outpatients with deep venous thrombosis. *N Engl J Med.* 1990;323: 1512–1516.

3. Lane DA, Mannucci PM, Bauer KA, et al. Inherited thrombophilia: Part 1. *Thromb Haemost.* 1996;76:651–662.

4. von Kaulla E, von Kaulla KN. Antithrombin III and diseases. *Am J Clin Path.* 1967;48:69–80.

5. Kauffman RH, Vetlkamp JJ, Van Tilburg NH, Van Es LA. Acquired antithrombin III deficiency and thrombosis in the nephrotic syndrome. *Am J Med.* 1978,65:607–613.

6. de Boer AC, van Riel LAM, den Ottolander GJH. Measurement of antithrombin III, -$_2$-macroglobulin and -$_1$-antitrypsin in patients with deep venous thrombosis and pulmonary embolism. *Thromb Res.* 1979;15:17–25.

7. Damus PS, Wallace GA. Immunologic measurement of antithrombin III-heparin cofactor and -$_2$-macroglobulin in disseminated intravascular coagulation and hepatic failure coagulapathy. *Thromb Res.* 1989;6: 27–38.

8. Weenink GH, Kahle LH, Lamping RJ, ten Cate JW, Treffers PE. Antithrombin III in oral contraceptive users and during normotensive pregnancy. *Acta Obstet Gynecol Scand.* 1984;63:57–61.

9. Caine YG, Bauer KA, Barzegar S, et al. Coagulation activation following estrogen administration to postmenopausal women. *Thromb Haemost.* 1992;68:392–395.

10. Marciniak E, Gockemen JP. Heparin-induced decrease in circulating antithrombin III. *Lancet.* 1978;2:581–584.

11. O'Brien JR, Etherington MD. Effect of heparin and warfarin on antithrombin III. *Lancet.* 1977 Dec 10;2(8050):1231.

12. Griffin JH, Evatt B, Zimmerman TS, Kleiss AJ, Wideman C. Deficiency of protein C in congenital thrombotic disease. *J Clin Invest.* 1981;68: 1370–1373.

13. Horellou MH, Conard J, Bertina RM, Samama M. Congenital protein C deficiency and thrombotic disease in nine French families. *Br Med J.* 1984;289:1285–1287.

14. Manco-Johnson MJ, Marlar RA, Jacobson LJ, Hays T, Warady BA. Severe protein C deficiency in newborn infants. *J Pediatr.* 1988; 113:359–363.

15. Miletich JP, Sherman L, Broze GJ Jr. Absence of thrombosis in subjects with heterozygous protein C deficiency. *N Engl J Med.* 1987; 317:991–996.

16. Martinelli I, Mannucci P, DeStefano V, et al. Different risks of thrombosis in four coagulation defects associated with inherited thrombophilia: a study of 150 families. *Blood.* 1998;92: 2353–2358.

17. Gandrille S, Borgel D, Ireland H, et al. Protein S deficiency: a database of mutations. For the Plasma Coagulation Inhibitors Subcommittee of the Scientific and Standardization Committee of the International Society on Thrombosis and Haemostasis. *Thromb Haemost.* 1997;77:1201.

18. Koster T, Rosendaal FR, Briet E, et al. Protein C deficiency in a controlled series of unselected outpatients: an infrequent but clear risk factor for venous thrombosis (Leiden Thrombophilia Study). *Blood.* 1995;85:2756–2761.

19. Dählback B, Carlsson M, Svensson PJ. Familial thrombophilia due to a previously unrecognized mechanism characterized by poor anticoagulant response to activated protein C: prediction of a cofactor to activated protein C. *Proc Natl Acad Sci. USA* 1993;90:1004–1008.

20. Bertina RM, Koeleman BPC, Koster T, et al. Mutation in blood coagulation factor V associated with resistance to activated protein C. *Nature.* 1994;369:64–67.

21. Svensson PJ, Dahlback B. Resistance to activated protein C as a basis for venous thrombosis. *N Engl J Med.* 1994;330:517–522.

22. Koster T, Rosendaal FR, de Ronde H, Briet E, Vandenbroucke JP, Bertina RM. Venous thrombosis due to poor anticoagulant response to activated protein C: Leiden thrombophilia study. *Lancet.* 1993; 342:1503–1506.

23. Ridker PM, Hennekens CH, Lindpaintner K, Stampfer MJ, Eisenberg PR, Miletich JP. Mutation in the gene coding for coagulation factor V and the risk of myocardial infarction, stroke, and venous thrombosis in apparently healthy men. *N Engl J Med.* 1995;332:912–917.

24. Rosendaal FR, Koster T, Vandenbroucke JP, Reitsma PH. High-risk of thrombosis in patients homozygous for factor V Leiden (APC-resistance). *Blood.* 1995;85:1504–1508.

25. Ridker PM, Hennekens CH, Selhub J, Miletich JP, Malinow MR, Stampfer MJ. Interrelation of hyperhomocyst(e)inemia, factor V Leiden, and risk of future venous thromboembolism. *Circulation.* 1997;95:1777–1782.

26. Poort SR, Rosendaal FR, Reitsma PH, Bertina RM. A common genetic variation in the 3'-untranslated region of the prothrombin gene is associated with elevated prothrombin levels and an increase in venous thrombosis. *Blood.* 1996;88:3698–3703.

27. Rosendaal FR, Doggen CJM, Zivelin A, et al. Geographic distribution of the 20210 G to A prothrombin variant. *Thromb Haemost.* 1998;79:706–708.

28. Soria J, Almasy L, Souto J, et al. Linkage analysis demonstrates that the prothrombin G2121 0A mutation jointly influences plasma prothrombin levels and risk of thrombosis. *Blood.* 2000;95:2780–2785.

29. Den Heijer M, Koster T, Blom HJ, et al. Hyperhomocysteinemia as a risk factor for deep-vein thrombosis. *N Engl J Med.* 1996;334:759–762.

30. Ridker PM, Hennekens CH, Selhub J, Miletich JP, Malinow MR, Stampfer MJ. Interrelation of hyperhomocyst(e)inemia, factor V Leiden, and risk of future venous thromboembolism. *Circulation.* 1997;95:1777–1782.

31. Perry IJ, Refsum H, Morris RW, Ebrahim SB, Ueland PM, Shaper AG. Prospective study of serum total homocysteine concentration and risk of stroke in middle-aged British men. *Lancet.* 1995;346:1395–1398.

32. Botto L, Yang Q. 5,10 Methylenetetrahydrofolate reductase gene variants and congenital anomalies. *Am J Epidemiol.* 2000;151:862–877.

33. Saito H. Contact factors in health and disease. *Semin Thromb Haemostas.* 1987;13:36–49.

34. Goodnough LT, Saito H, Ratnoff OD. Thrombosis or myocardial infarction in congenital clotting factor abnormalities and chronic thrombocytopenias: a report of 21 patients and a review of 50 previously reported cases. *Medicine.* 1983;62:248–255.

35. Lammle B, Wuillemin WA, Huber I, et al. Thromboembolism and bleeding tendency in congenital factor XII deficiency—a study on 74 subjects from 14 Swiss families. *Thromb Haemost.* 1991;65:117–121.

36. Koster T, Blann AD, Briët E, Vandenbroucke JP, Rosendaal FR. Role of clotting factor VIII in effect of von Willebrand factor on occurrence of deep-vein thrombosis. *Lancet.* 1995;345:152–155.

37. Kyrle PA, Minar E, Hirschi M, et al. High plasma factor VIII and the risk of recurrent venous thromboembolism. *N Engl J Med.* 2000;343:457–462.

38. van Tilburg NH, Rosendaal FR, Bertina RM. Thrombin activatable fibrinolysis inhibitor and the risk for deep vein thrombosis. *Blood.* 2000;95:2855–2859.

39. Meijers JCM, Tekelenberg W, Bouma BN, Bertina RM, Rosendaal FR. High levels of coagulation factor XI as a risk factor for venous thrombosis. *N Engl J Med.* 2000;342:696–701.

40. van Hylckama A, van der Linden IK, Bertina RM, Rosendaal FR. High levels of factor IX increase the risk of venous thrombosis. *Blood.* 2000;95:3678–3682.

41. Samama M. An epidemiologic study of risk factors for deep vein thrombosis in medical outpatients. *Arch Intern Med.* 2000;160:3415–3420.

42. Kraaijenhagen R, Haverkamp D, Koopman MM, et al. Travel and risk of venous thrombosis. *Lancet.* 2000;356:1492.

43. Schulman S, Lindmarker P. Incidence of cancer after prophylaxis with warfarin against recurrent venous thromboembolism. *N Engl J Med.* 2000;342:1953–1958.

44. Vandenbroucke JP, Koster T, Briët E, Reitsma PH, Bertina RM, Rosendaal FR. Increased risk of venous thrombosis in oral-contraceptive users who are carriers of factor V Leiden mutation. *Lancet.* 1994;344:1453–1457.

Cardiovascular Indications for Anticoagulation Therapy

Richard C. Becker and Frederick Spencer

INTRODUCTION

Anticoagulants are used widely in the treatment of arterial thrombotic disorders of the cardiovascular system. In some clinical circumstances, effectiveness and management guidelines already have been established, but further investigation is required for others before firm recommendations can be made. This chapter provides the rationale, benefits, limitations, and management strategies for patients with cardiovascular indications for anticoagulation therapy. The discussion covers the following areas of cardiovascular pathology:

- coronary artery disease
- unstable angina/non-ST segment elevation myocardial infarction (non-ST segment elevation, acute coronary syndromes)
- acute myocardial infarction (MI)
- fibrinolytic therapy and coronary revascularization
- valvular heart disease
- prosthetic heart valves
- cardiomyopathies

Alternative and conjunctive antithrombotic therapies are included to provide a comprehensive overview and scientific basis for current management recommendations.

CORONARY ARTERY DISEASE

Coronary artery disease and its accompanying clinical manifestations remain the leading cause of death and health care expenditures among men and women in the United States. Based on recent estimates, ten million individuals have symptomatic atherosclerotic coronary artery disease.

Pathobiology

The collagenous portion of advanced atherosclerotic plaques, although most prevalent, is also the most stable. In distinct contrast, the soft atheromatous lipid core is vulnerable to fissuring and rupture.[1,2] Most plaques that are responsible for abrupt clinical symptoms (unstable angina, MI, sudden cardiac death) are relatively small when rupture occurs; however, the sudden exposure of circulating blood to plaque components and subendothelial connective tissues is a strong stimulus for intravascular thrombosis.

Epidemiologic studies show that individuals with coronary artery disease are at risk for sudden thrombotic events. Accordingly, considerable investigation has focused not only on the atherosclerotic plaque itself but on the potential role of coagulation factors that, conceivably, could be modified. In the Northwick Park Heart Study,[3,4] factor VII coagulant activity correlated with cardiovascular mortality. Fibrinogen was also found to correlate strongly, as did factor VIII, although less strongly than other hemostatic markers. The Framingham[5] and Caerphilly[6] studies both identified an association between fibrinogen levels and coronary artery disease—related events in men and women.

Clinical Trials of Anticoagulation Therapy

Primary Prevention

The Thrombosis Prevention Trial[7] is the largest clinical trial performed to date of warfarin anticoagulation therapy among patients at risk for cardiac events. The design, unique from several perspectives, identified high-risk patients on the basis of factor VII activity.[8,9] The initial screening phase identified 13,500 potential candidates for study inclusion, from which slightly greater than 6,100 were invited to selected screening clinics. Only men in the top 20% of the risk scale were considered eligible, of whom 5,499 were enrolled and followed for, on average, six years. The final protocol, based on rapidly emerging support for aspirin administration among individuals at risk for cardiac events, compared warfarin (target international normalized ratio [INR], 1.5), aspirin (75 mg controlled-release preparation daily), combination aspirin and warfarin, and placebo. Overall, aspirin was shown to prevent three ischemic heart disease events (per 1,000 patients treated), as was warfarin. The combination strategy prevented five ischemic heart disease events per 1,000 patients treated, but at a cost of an increased risk for major hemorrhage, including intracranial bleeding (fourfold increase compared with aspirin alone).

Clinical Trials of Platelet Antagonists

Aspirin has been evaluated in several trials of primary prevention,[7,10–12] and the large Women's Health Initiative is currently evaluating the effects of low-dose aspirin (100 mg every other day) prophylaxis in 40,000 healthy women.

Considered collectively, the data show that aspirin reduces the risk of fatal and non-fatal MI, but at a cost of bleeding complications, including hemorrhagic stroke.

Management Recommendations

Platelet inhibition with aspirin (160 to 325 mg daily) should be considered for individuals with established coronary artery disease or those greater than 50 years of age with one or more risk factors (see Figure 18–1). Combination

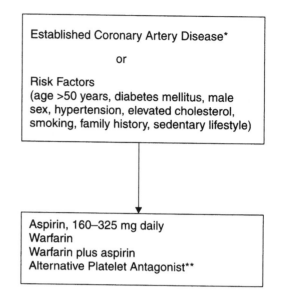

*Abnormal exercise tolerance test (or equivalent functional study) or documentation by coronary angiography

**Clopidogrel or ticlopidine

Figure 18–1 Primary prevention management algorithm

pharmacotherapy with warfarin (low to moderate intensity) and low-dose aspirin may provide maximal protection for patients of highest risk for an ischemic/thrombotic event; however, further investigation is needed. The role of alternative platelet antagonists (eg, clopidogrel 75 mg qd/ticlopidine 250 mg bid) in primary prevention has not yet been established, but should be entertained in patients at risk who cannot be treated with aspirin because of either true allergy or intolerance. In this situation, warfarin alone (target INR 1.5) is also an acceptable treatment alternative.

UNSTABLE ANGINA/NON-ST SEGMENT ELEVATION MI

Unstable angina is an acute coronary syndrome responsible for nearly 600,000 hospital admissions yearly in the United States. Its importance in the evolution of atherosclerotic coronary artery disease is signified by the transition from a stable to an unstable condition.

The advent of sensitive markers (Troponin I and T) for detecting myocardial necrosis has determined that upward of 30% of patients with a clinical diagnosis of unstable angina have, in fact, non-ST segment elevation MI. Accordingly, it is considered appropriate to consider unstable angina and non-ST segment elevation MI as non-ST segment elevation acute coronary syndromes.

Pathobiology

As its name implies, unstable angina represents an important change within the atherosclerotic plaque from being relatively quiescent to active, and with this transition comes an increased risk for clinical events, including MI and cardiac death.

Plaque rupture is common among patients with unstable angina and is typically accompanied by varying degrees of mural thrombus, coronary vasospasm, and intracoronary thromboembolism.[13–15] Interestingly, careful microscopic examination of coronary thrombi often reveals a layered structure, suggesting strongly that repeated mural deposits and episodic growth cause a progressive decrease in cross-sectional luminal dimension.

Within the spectrum of unstable angina, ranging from minimally active to very active plaques and procoagulant potential, lies a varying contribution of platelets and thrombin as the major thrombogenic substrate.[16,17] An ability to identify and differentiate these mechanisms among individual patients has important treatment implications.

Clinical Trials of Anticoagulation Therapy and Platelet Antagonists

The treatment of unstable angina has been investigated in a number of large-scale clinical trials. Théroux and colleagues[18] randomized 479 patients to treatment with aspirin, heparin, both, or neither. The incidence of fatal and non-fatal MI in aspirin-treated patients was reduced from 6.3% to 2.6% (risk reduction, 63%; p = 0.04) and with heparin-treated patients from 7.5% to 1.2% (risk reduction, 85%; p = 0.007). Heparin more effectively reduced the incidence of refractory angina than aspirin. There was no added benefit derived from combining heparin and aspirin.

The RISC study group[19] randomized 949 men with unstable angina (or non-ST segment elevation MI) to treatment with aspirin or heparin (double-blind, placebo-controlled study). Aspirin, compared with no aspirin, significantly reduced 5-, 30-, and 90-day event rates (MI and death). Although heparin therapy did not yield a benefit, the combination of heparin and aspirin had the greatest impact on in-hospital events (risk reduction, 72%; p = 0.02).

A potential limitation that applies to both Théroux's study and the RISC trial was the *short-term* use of anticoagulant therapy. Indeed, recurrent events were common following the discontinuation of intravenous heparin.[20] Accordingly, the ATACS trial[21] randomized 214 patients either to aspirin alone (162.5 mg) or to the combination of aspirin and unfractionated heparin (target activated partial thromboplastin time [aPTT] 2.0 times control). Intravenous heparin was continued until adequate anticoagulation with warfarin was achieved. At 14 days, there was a significant reduction in the combined end-point of recurrent ischemia, MI, and death favoring the combination group (10.5% versus 27%; p = 0.004).

Low Molecular Weight Heparin

The pivotal role played by factor X in the sequence of thrombin generation, coupled with predictable pharmacokinetics, consistent pharmacodynamics, subcutaneous, fixed-dose administration, and their lack of need for routine coagulation-monitoring have made low molecular weight heparin (LMWH) preparations attractive alternatives for treating thrombotic disorders, including acute coronary syndromes. In several large-scale randomized trials, LMWH has been proven superior to unfractionated heparin in reducing the combined occurrence of death, MI, and refractory angina.[22,23]

Glycoprotein IIb/IIIa Receptor Antagonists

Platelet aggregation, mediated by fibrinogen binding to the GP IIb/IIIa receptor, is a key event in coronary arterial thrombosis. Inhibition of the glycoprotein (GP) IIb/IIIa receptor has been shown to reduce the risk of death, MI, and refractory ischemia among high-risk patients with unstable angina/non-ST segment elevation MI, particularly those undergoing percutaneous coronary interventions.[24]

Warfarin

The question of long-term anticoagulation therapy with warfarin and its potential benefit among patients with non-ST segment elevation acute coronary syndromes was the basis for the OASIS (Organization to Assess Strategies for Ischemic Syndromes) Pilot[25] and Phase 2[26] Trials. The OASIS Pilot Study compared a fixed dosage of warfarin (3 mg daily) and moderate intensity treatment to achieve an INR of 2.0 to 2.5. Although low intensity warfarin was not beneficial, moderate intensity treatment reduced the six-month incidence of death, MI, or refractory ischemia by 58%. The larger OASIS-2 Study of 3,712 patients randomized to moderate intensity warfarin (plus aspirin) or aspirin alone failed to identify a benefit in favor of combination therapy. Compliance to therapy may have influenced the trials outcome.

Management Recommendations

Patients with unstable angina/non-ST segment elevation MI should receive aspirin (160–325 mg) upon serious consideration of the diagnosis. Those unable to take aspirin should be treated with clopidogrel (300 mg) or ticlopidine (500 mg). The combined use of aspirin and clopidogrel may provide added benefit. Anticoagulation therapy with either unfractionated heparin (60 U/kg bolus; 15 U/kg/h to target aPTT 50–70 sec) or LMWH (enoxaparin 1.0 mg/kg SC q 12 h) should be added once a diagnosis is confirmed. Patients at greatest risk for adverse cardiac events (eg, troponin I or T positive, dynamic ST segment shifts, hemodynamic instability, refractory symptoms, and/or prior coronary interventions) should also receive an intravenous GP IIb/IIIa antagonist. In this setting, early coronary angiography and revascularization are strongly encouraged.

Long-term management, in addition to aggressive risk factor modification, should include aspirin (160–325 mg daily) and/or an alternative platelet antagonist (clopidogrel 75 mg daily).

Anticoagulation therapy with warfarin (target INR 2.5) should be considered in patients unable to take aspirin or clopidogrel and in those with specific indications (eg, mechanical heart valve, atrial fibrillation, and high-risk features). See Figure 18–2.

ACUTE MYOCARDIAL INFARCTION

Acute MI, occurring in more than 1.25 million individuals yearly in the United States, is a major cause of morbidity, mortality, and health care expenditures.

Pathobiology

In a majority of cases, MI is caused by occlusive thrombosis developing at a site of vessel wall injury and atheromatous plaque rupture. The predisposition to thrombosis is multifactorial:

- Vascular thromboresistance is impaired.
- Following plaque rupture, there is a sudden change in vessel wall geometry, which favors platelet-vessel wall interactions.

Thrombogenic components within the plaque are directly exposed to circulating blood cells and coagulant proteins.

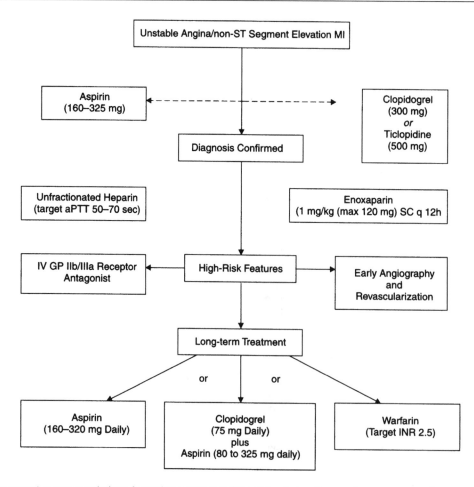

Figure 18–2 Management recommendations for patients with non-ST segment elevation acute coronary syndromes

The thrombotic properties of the atheromatous plaque's lipid core have not been unraveled completely. Potential contributors include phospholipids, crystalline lipids, tissue factor, matrix thrombin, and collagen degradation products.[27-29] Because tissue factor contributes significantly to coronary arterial thrombogenesis, the extrinsic coagulation pathway is considered a strong determinant in the natural history and ultimate clinical expression of atheromatous plaque rupture.

Unlike unstable angina and non-ST segment elevation MI, which are characterized by platelet-dominant thrombosis and microvascular thromboembolism, ST segment elevation MI is a fibrin-dominant coronary occlusive event characterized by large areas of jeopardized myocardium.

Clinical Trials of Anticoagulation Therapy

During the mid-1970s, Chalmers and coworkers[30] pooled the results from 37 published reports examining the role for anticoagulation therapy among patients with acute MI and concluded that treatment reduced mortality by approximately 20%. Reanalyzing the data with the use of more rigorous statistical methods, Peto[31] later confirmed their conclusions.

It is important to recognize, however, that many of the anticoagulation therapy studies performed over the years have been nonrandomized, poorly controlled, and either historic or observational in design. As a result, and in the final analysis, they have provided limited information for practicing clinicians. Overall, only three trials included in Chalmers and coworkers' and Peto's original analyses were randomized, controlled, and of sufficient sample size to draw meaningful conclusions; the British Medical Research Council trial[32] the Bronx Municipal Hospital study,[33] and the Veterans Administration Cooperative study[34] (Table 18–1).

The Medical Research Council (MRC) study was a single-blind, controlled trial of 1,427 patients with MI.[32] Patients were randomized to unfractionated heparin (15,000 U intravenous bolus, followed by 10,000 U every six hours for five doses) or no-heparin. Heparin-treated patients received an oral anticoagulant (phenindione) simultaneously, adjusted to maintain the INR between 1.6 and 2.1, whereas the no-heparin group received low-dose phenindione (maintenance dose 0.5 mg twice daily). In the high-dose anticoagulation group, mortality (all cause) decreased from 18.2% to 16.2%, reinfarction decreased from 13% to 9.7%, and the composite end point of death or reinfarction decreased from 31% to 29.5% (risk reduction, 16%). In addition, a significant reduction in overall thromboembolic events, including deep vein thrombosis, pulmonary embolism, and stroke, was observed. Although hemorrhagic events were more common in the high-dose anticoagulation group, there were no deaths.

The Bronx Municipal Hospital study[33] randomized 1,136 men and women with acute MI either to anticoagulation (heparin 5,000 U bolus, followed by 10,000 U subcutaneously every eight hours for five doses and phenindione [INR 2.0–2.5]) or to placebo. Treatment was continued throughout the hospital stay. Mortality (all cause) decreased in the anticoagulation group, and reinfarction also decreased. A reduction in mortality was particularly evident in women older than 55 years, in whom a reduction from 31% to 14.9% was observed. As in the MRC trial, thromboembolic events were lower and hemorrhagic events were higher in the anticoagulation group. There were, however, no fatal hemorrhagic events.

The Veterans Administration Cooperative study[34] included 999 men with acute MI. Patients randomized to anticoagulation received heparin (10,000 U subcutaneously every 8 to 12 hours, adjusted to clotting time of twice normal) and warfarin (prothrombin time 25–30 seconds), whereas control patients received matching placebo. The observation period on treatment was 28 days. Among anticoagulated patients, in-hospital mortality (all cause) decreased from 11.2% to 9.6%,

Table 18–1 Clinical Trials of Short-Term Anticoagulation Therapy for Myocardial Infarction

Study	Group	Patients (n)	Mortality (%)	p	Reinfarction (%)	p	Thromboembolism (%)	p
Medical Research Council	High-dose OA	712	16.2		9.7		2.2	
	Low-dose OA	715	18.0	NS	13.0	NS	5.6	<0.01
Bronx Municipal Hospital	OA	745	14.8		12.5		0.1	
	Placebo	391	21.2	<0.01	18.7	<0.05	0.2	NS
Veterans Administration Cooperative	OA	500	9.6		4.0		3.6	
	Placebo	499	11.2	NS	6.0	NS	10.8	0.005

Key: NS, not significant; OA, oral anticoagulant.

and reinfarction decreased from 4% to 2%. The rate of pulmonary embolism and stroke was substantially decreased—2.6% to 0.2% and 3.8% to 0.8%, respectively. Although anticoagulation therapy was discontinued because of bleeding in five patients, major hemorrhage was uncommon and there were no deaths.

Thus, the early use of anticoagulation therapy following MI is associated with a modest reduction in thromboembolic-related morbidity and mortality.

Long-Term Administration

At least 26 clinical trials examining the safety and efficacy of oral anticoagulants in the secondary prevention of cardiac events have been conducted during the past three decades.[35–37] As with studies investigating the benefits of anticoagulation in the early postinfarction phase,[38,39] many of these trials were poorly designed, which precluded firm conclusions being drawn from them. Pooled data from several studies with acceptable designs, however, suggest that long-term anticoagulant therapy reduces the combined end point of death and reinfarction by approximately 20% (Table 18–2).

In the 60-Plus Reinfarction study,[40] 878 patients older than 60 years (mean 67.6 years), who had experienced a prior ST segment elevation MI at least six months earlier (mean 6 years) and were receiving oral anticoagulant therapy (acenocoumarin or phenprocoumon), were randomly allocated to either continued treatment (INR 2.7–4.5) or no treatment (placebo). Mortality among patients randomized to continue oral anticoagulation therapy decreased from 13.4% to 7.6% (risk reduction, 43%). Recurrent MI decreased from 15.7% to 11.6% (risk reduction, 26%). Stroke rates were also decreased with active treatment. There were no fatal hemorrhagic events.

In the Warfarin Reinfarction study (WARIS),[41] researchers recruited 1,214 patients who had sustained an MI (mean 27 days previously). They were randomized in a double-blind fashion to receive either warfarin (INR 2.8–4.8) or placebo. During an average follow-up of 37 months, mortality (all cause) decreased from 20% to 15.5% (risk reduction, 24%), reinfarction decreased from 20.4% to 13.5% (risk reduction, 34%), and stroke decreased from 7.2% to 3.3% (risk reduction, 55%). Serious bleeding was observed in 0.6% of warfarin-treated patients per year. In a study conducted by the Anticoagulation in the Secondary Prevention of Events in Coronary Thrombosis research group,[42] 3,404 patients with MI were randomized (double-blind, placebo-controlled study) to treatment with nicoumalone or phenprocoumon (INR 2.8–4.8) or with placebo. During a mean follow-up of 37 months, reinfarction decreased from 5.1% to 2.3% per year (risk reduction, 53%), stroke decreased from 1.2% to 0.7% per year (risk reduction, 40%), and mortality (all cause) decreased from 3.6% to 3.2% per

year (risk reduction, 10%). Event-free survival (death, non-fatal MI, nonfatal cerebrovascular events, major bleeding) was significantly higher in the treatment group (83% versus 76%, p = <0.001).

As with early-outcome experience, the long-term beneficial effects of anticoagulation (moderate to high intensity) following MI are present but modest. Patients at moderate to high risk for experiencing a thromboembolic event derive the greatest overall benefit.

Clinical Trials of Platelet Antagonists

The Antiplatelet Trialists Collaboration[43] provides convincing evidence in support of aspirin administration for patients with acute MI, reducing non-fatal MI, stroke, and vascular death. Although the greatest benefit is observed during the first 30 days of treatment, reduced event rates have been documented following several years of therapy.

Clinical Trials of Combination Pharmacotherapy

The contribution of platelets and coagulation factors to coronary arterial thrombosis provides the basis for interest in combination pharmacotherapy (Table 18–3). The disappointing results of the Coumadin Aspirin Reinfarction Study[44] and Combined Hemotherapy and Mortality Prevention trial suggests that low-intensity warfarin therapy (in combination with aspirin) is not beneficial. The potential benefit (and safety) of moderate intensity anticoagulation has also been challenged with preliminary observations made in WARIS-II.

Cardiac Chamber Thromboembolism

Left ventricular mural thrombosis is diagnosed either echocardiographically or at the time of the autopsy among patients with MI,[45,46] especially in those with anterior infarction involving the ventricular apex.[47,48] In large clinical trials of anticoagulation therapy, researchers have reported an incidence of cerebral embolism of 2% to 4% among control patients, which frequently causes either severe neurologic deficits or death.[32,33] Two of these trials showed a statistically significant reduction in stroke with early anticoagulation, whereas a third trial demonstrated a positive trend.

A meta-analysis performed by Vaitkus and Barnathan[49] supports the findings of three previous studies published during the early 1980s.[50–52] The odds ratio for increased risk of systemic embolism in the presence of echocardiographically demonstrated mural thrombus was 5.45 (95% confidence interval [CI] 3.02 to 9.83), and the event rate difference was 0.09 (95% CI 0.003 to 0.14). The odds ratio of anticoagula-

Table 18–2 Clinical Trials of Long-Term Anticoagulation Therapy for Myocardial Infarction

Study	Group	Patients	Follow-Up	Target INR	Mortality (%)	p	Reinfarction (%)	p	Hemorrhage (%)	p
60-Plus Reinfarction	OA	439	2 yr	2.7–4.5	51 (11.6)	0.07	29 (6.6)	0.0005	84 (19.1)	<0.05
	Placebo	439			69 (15.7)		64 (14.5)		10 (2.2)	
Warfarin Reinfarction	OA	607	37 mo	2.8–4.8	94 (15.5)	0.02	82 (13.5)*	0.0007	52 (8.5)*	<0.005
	Placebo	607			123 (20.3)		124 (20.4)		25 (4.1)	
Anticoagulation in the Secondary Prevention of Events in Coronary Thrombosis (ASPECT)	OA	1,700	37 mo	2.8–4.8	170 (10.0)	NS	114 (6.7)	<0.001	24 (6.7)	<0.001
	Placebo	1,704			189 (11.1)		189 (11.1%)		40 (14.2)	<0.001

*Intention to treat.
Key: INR, international normalized ratio; NS, not significant; OA, oral anticoagulant.

Table 18–3 Clinical Trials of Combination Pharmacotherapy

	CARS	CHAMPS	WARIS-2	ASPECT-2
Patients	9,000	4,000	6,000	9,000
Strategies	Aspirin 160 mg/d or Aspirin 80 mg/d + Coumadin 1 mg/d or Aspirin 80 mg/d + Coumadin 3 mg/d	Aspirin 160 mg/d or Aspirin 80 mg/d + Coumadin (INR 1.5–2.5)	Aspirin 75 mg/d or Aspirin 75 mg/d + OA (INR 2.0–2.5) or OA (INR 2.8–4.2)	Aspirin 80 mg/d or Aspirin 80 mg/d + OA (INR 2.0–2.5) or OA (INR 2.8–4.8)
End Points	Nonfatal MI Nonfatal ischemic Cardiovascular death	Mortality	Mortality	Mortality
Follow-up	4 years	4 years	2 years	3 years

Key: INR, international normalized ratio; OA, oral anticoagulant.

tion versus no anticoagulation in preventing embolism was 0.14 (95% CI 0.04 to 0.52), with an event rate difference of –0.33 (95% CI –0.50 to –0.16). The odds ratio of anticoagulation versus control in preventing mural thrombus formation was 0.32 (95% CI 0.20 to 0.52), and the event rate difference was –0.19 (95% CI –0.09 to –0.28). The available data support the following three conclusions:

1. Mural thrombosis following acute MI increases the risk of systemic embolism.
2. Anticoagulation can reduce mural thrombus formation.
3. The risk of systemic embolism can be substantially reduced by anticoagulation.

Management Recommendations

All patients with MI should receive aspirin (initial dose, 160–325 mg) as soon as possible after the diagnosis is made, and it should be repeated daily for an indefinite period of time. In the setting of true aspirin allergy or severe intolerance, clopidogrel (300 mg initially followed by 75 mg daily) should be considered. Patients at an increased risk of systemic or pulmonary embolism because of anterior site of infarction, severe left ventricular dysfunction (ejection fraction <35%), congestive heart failure, history of systemic or pulmonary embolism, echocardiographic evidence of mural thrombosis, or atrial fibrillation should initially receive heparin, followed by warfarin (target INR 2.5; range 2.5–3.0) for up to three months. Anticoagulation therapy should be continued for persisting risk factors, including atrial fibrillation (target INR 2.5; range 2.0–3.0), recurrent thromboembolic events, and poor cardiac performance. Although the combined administration of aspirin and warfarin leads to a slight increase of hemorrhagic complication, patients with recurrent events might benefit from combination therapy; an aspirin dose of 80 mg is recommended. Full-dose aspirin (160–325 mg/day) can be restarted when the planned course of warfarin is completed. Patients with contraindications to aspirin should be considered for long-term therapy with an oral anticoagulant (target INR 3.0; range 2.5–3.5). The ideal duration of treatment is unknown but should probably be at least one to two years (Figure 18–3).

FIBRINOLYTIC THERAPY AND CORONARY REVASCULARIZATION

The prevalence of atherosclerotic coronary artery disease and its clinical manifestations, including angina pectoris and MI, although decreasing over the past two decades, remains unacceptably high. The speed of coronary arterial reperfusion correlates directly with the overall extent of myocardial salvage, which in turn determines clinical outcome. Thus, improvements in the efficacy, stability, and duration of reperfusion have a significant impact on patient morbidity and mortality.

Among patients with advanced coronary artery disease, treatment options to reduce symptoms and, in some cases, lower mortality include coronary angioplasty, stent placement, and bypass grafting. As with reperfusion therapy in more acute circumstances, successful revascularization is influenced significantly by long-term maintenance of coronary arterial blood flow and myocardial perfusion.

Pathobiology

While novel strategies designed to achieve earlier and more complete coronary arterial reperfusion are being investigated, it is important to recognize that coronary reocclusion is a major contributor to poor clinical outcome. In most instances, a platelet-fibrin rich, occlusive thrombus develops at the original site of plaque rupture.

An early complication of coronary angioplasty is vessel wall dissection, with or without overlying thrombosis and distal embolization, whereas the major late complication is atrial restenosis. The latter, predominantly caused by reactive hyperplasia in response to vessel wall injury, occurs in 30–40% of angioplasty sites.

Coronary stents were introduced originally to prevent abrupt vessel closure following vessel wall dissection and late restenosis. Unfortunately, subacute thrombosis can occur, particularly if the stent is not properly placed and adequately expanded to full intracoronary dimensions. Similarly, coronary bypass grafts, particularly harvested veins exposed to trauma and high flow (shearing) rates after placement in the arterial circulation, can thrombose.

Thus coronary arterial thrombosis represents a major obstacle to achieving optimal patient outcome following fibrinolytic therapy and coronary revascularization.

Fibrinolytic Therapy Clinical Trials

Intravenous unfractionated heparin and oral aspirin are mainstays of early treatment after fibrinolytic therapy. Heparin appears to be particularly important as an adjunct to tissue plasminogen activator (tPA) treatment. In the Antithrombotics in the Prevention of Reocclusion in Coronary Thrombolysis study,[53] 300 patients with angiographically validated infarct-related artery patency after fibrinolytic therapy were assigned randomly to treatment with warfarin (INR 2.8–4.0), aspirin (300 mg/d), or placebo. Patency of the infarct-related artery was assessed three months later. The rate of reocclusion was 25% with aspirin, 39% with warfarin, and 32% with

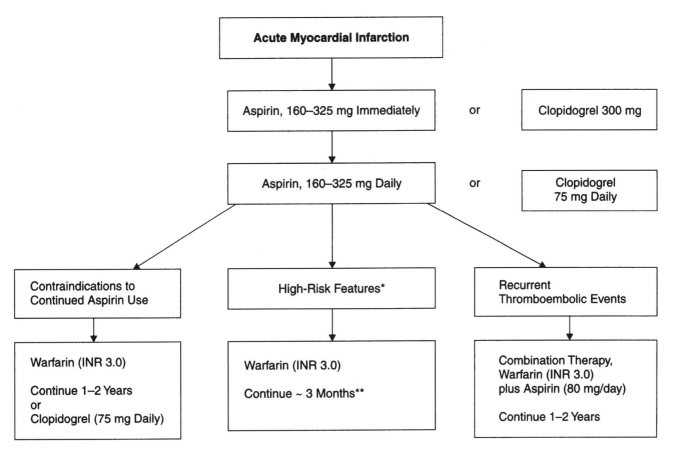

*Anterior site of infarction, severe left ventricular dysfunction, congestive heart failure, history of systemic or pulmonary embolism, echocardiographic mural thrombosis, atrial fibrillation.
**A more prolonged course of treatment should be considered if one or more high-risk features persist.

Figure 18–3 Management recommendations for acute myocardial infarction

placebo (p = NS). In coronary lesions with less than 90% stenosis (determined by the original angiogram), the reocclusion rate was lower with aspirin (17%) than with warfarin (25%) or placebo (30%) (p = 0.001). The combination of moderate intensity warfarin (INR 2.0 to 3.0) and low dose aspirin (80 mg) may be more effective than either used alone.

Aspirin (325 mg starting dose, followed by 160–325 mg daily) should be given to all patients with acute MI, including those receiving fibrinolytic therapy. Clopidogrel should be substituted in cases of true aspirin allergy or severe intolerance. Unfractionated heparin (60 U/kg–4000 U maximum, followed by an infusion of 12 U/kg/h–1000 U maximum, to target aPTT 50–70 sec) should be administered for 48 hours (or longer in patients at high risk for thromboembolism) when tPa, r-PA, or TNK-tPA is the fibrinolytic chosen. Unfractionated heparin (initiated 6 hours after fibrinolytic

administration when aPTT <70 sec) is also recommended for patients at increased risk for thromboembolism (large or anterior site of infarction; atrial fibrillation, prior embolism, known left ventricular mural thrombus) when streptokinase or antistreplase is the chosen fibrinolytic. The use of Enoxaporin in conjunction with tPA is being investigated.

Coronary Angioplasty

Clinical Trials of Anticoagulation Therapy

Procedural outcome following coronary angioplasty is compromised by several events, including death (1%). MI (3%–4%), and vessel occlusion (6%). Over the past several years procedure-related major complications have progressively declined as a result of improved technology, operator experience, and antithrombotic strategies. Oral anticoagulation therapy has not been extensively investigated as a pretreatment or post-treatment strategy.

Management Recommendations

All patients undergoing coronary angioplasty should receive aspirin (325 mg) at least two hours before the procedure. For patients unable to take aspirin, clopidogrel (75 mg daily) should be substituted beginning at least two and preferably four days before the procedure. (An oral loading dose of 300 mg is recommended to initiate therapy.) Intravenous unfractimated heparin is recommended during the procedure to achieve an activated clotting time (ACT) of 250–300 seconds. Bivalirudin, a direct thrombin inhibitor, should be considered in patients at risk for hemorrhagic complications and those with renal insufficiency. The use of an IV GP IIb/IIIa receptor antagonist is recommended for patients with acute coronary syndromes undergoing percutaneous coronary interventions. The combined administration of LMWH (enoxaparin) and GP IIb/IIIa receptor antagonists is currently undergoing clinical trial investigation. The preliminary results are encouraging.

Coronary Arterial Stents

Clinical Trials of Anticoagulation Therapy

Emerging evidence supports the use of intracoronary stents for the prevention of abrupt closure (early benefit) and restenosis (late benefit). In the early experience, subacute stent thrombosis (average, six days) occurred in 4% to 5% of stented patients.[54,55] Accordingly, aggressive anticoagulation regimens, including intravenous heparin, dextran, dipyridamole, aspirin, and postprocedure warfarin (INR 2.0–3.5) were employed for one to three months. Unfortunately, this "kitchen sink" approach caused a high incidence of vascular and hemorrhagic complications. It is now clear that underdilation of the stent, proximal/distal vessel wall dissections, small vessel caliber, and reduced inflow/outflow, rather than suboptimal anticoagulation regimens, are the major causes of stent thrombosis.

Clinical Trials of Platelet Antagonists

The results of several large-scale comparative trials establish the superiority of platelet inhibition over anticoagulation therapy in preventing peri-procedural coronary arterial thrombotic events in patients undergoing stent deployment.[56,57] The addition of an intravenous GP IIb/IIIa receptor antagonist provides benefit in high-risk settings.

Management Recommendations

Aspirin (325 mg) in combination with either clopidogrel (300 mg starting dose, 75 mg daily for 30 days) or ticlopidine (500 mg starting dose, 250 mg twice daily for 30 days) should be given to all patients with treatment preferably initiated four to six hours before stent deployment. Intravenous unfractionated heparin (target ACT 250–300 seconds) is the current standard; however, LMWH preparations appear promising in the setting of percutaneous coronary interventions. Glycoprotein IIb/IIIa receptor antagonists should be administered to patients with acute coronary syndromes who are undergoing coronary arterial stenting. The benefit of long-term LMWH and/or oral anticoagulation therapy after successful stent placement has not been established; therefore, warfarin should be considered only when concomitant indications for anticoagulation (e.g., mechanical heart valve, atrial fibrillation) exist. Several clinical trials in progress will determine the role of clopidogrel treatment beyond 30 days from stent deployment (Figure 18–4).

Saphenous Vein Coronary Bypass Grafts

Clinical Trials of Anticoagulation Therapy and Platelet Antagonists

Information regarding the use of oral anticoagulants in the prevention of saphenous vein graft occlusion is available. In a majority of studies,[58–60] oral anticoagulants were started two to three days after surgery. One of the trials revealed improved patency over placebo (Table 18–4).[61–63] Unfortunately, bleeding complications were increased. Similar patency rates have been observed when comparing oral anticoagulants and low-dose aspirin (50–100 mg) for both saphenous vein and internal mammary artery bypass grafts (Table 18–5).[62,63] There have been no trials directly comparing standard-dose aspirin (325 mg or higher) and oral anticoagulants. Similarly, trials of anticoagulation therapy started the day of surgery have not been conducted. In contrast, there is convincing evidence that aspirin (325 mg) initiated six hours after surgery and continued daily for at least one year reduces the frequency of saphenous vein graft closure.[64]

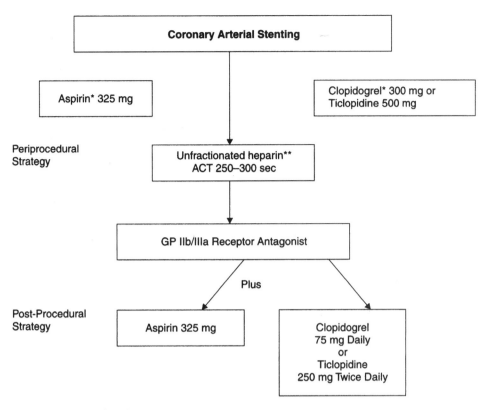

*Clopidogrel is the preferred agent.
**Low molecular weight heparin (enoxaparin) may be an acceptable alternative.

Figure 18–4 Antithrombotic therapy management algorithm for coronary arterial stenting

Table 18–4 Saphenous Vein Graft Patency with Oral Antithrombotic Therapy

Author	Treatment Strategy	Duration	Patency N (%) Aspirin	Patency N (%) Aspirin + Persantine	Patency N (%) Oral Anticoagulant	p
Weber et al[61]	Aspirin 100 mg *or* Heparin, OA (INR 2.4–4.8)	2–3 months	91/123 (74)	—	132/166 (80)	NS
Yli-Mayry et al[62]	Aspirin 50 mg + Persantine 400 mg *or* OA (PT 5%–15% activity)	12 months	—	239/311 (77)	203/275 (74)	NS
Van der Meer et al[63]	Aspirin 50 mg *versus* Aspirin 50 mg + Persantine 400 mg *or* OA (INR 2.8–4.8)	12 months	352/440 (80)	392/461 (85)	363/448 (81)	NS

Key: INR, international normalized ratio; OA, oral anticoagulant; PT, prothrombin time.

Table 18–5 Internal Mammary Artery Graft Patency with Oral Antithrombotic Therapy

Author	Treatment Strategy	Duration	Aspirin	Patency N (%)		p
				Aspirin + Persantine	Oral Anticoagulant	
Van der Meer et al[63]	Aspirin 50 mg *or* Aspirin 50 mg + Persantine 400 mg *or* OA (INR 2.8–4.8)	12 months	14/157 (94)	132/139 (95)	115/126 (91)	NS
Yli-Mayry et al[62]	Aspirin 250 mg + Persantine 225 mg *or* OA (PT 5%–15% activity)	3 months	—	64/68 (94)	40/44(91)	NS

Key: INR, international normalized ratio; OA, oral anticoagulant; PT, prothrombin time.

Management Strategies

Aspirin (325 mg daily) is recommended for all patients who undergo saphenous vein coronary bypass grafting. In patients with aspirin allergy, clopidogrel should be substituted (300 mg started six hours post-op, followed by 75 mg daily). Patients with a separate indication for anticoagulation therapy (eg, mechanical heart valve, atrial fibrillation) should receive warfarin (target INR 2.5) in combination with low-dose aspirin (80 mg daily). Although aspirin treatment is optional in the setting of internal mammary (thoracic) arterial grafting, it is strongly encouraged for patients with documented coronary artery disease to reduce cardiac and vascular events.

VALVULAR HEART DISEASE

Systemic embolism, frequently involving the central nervous system, is the most devastating complication of valvular heart disease. Mounting evidence suggests that antithrombotic therapy can reduce the likelihood of embolic events.

Clinical Trials of Anticoagulant Therapy and Platelet Antagonists

The support for antithrombotic therapy among patients with valvular heart disease is derived, for the most part, from large clinical series, case-control studies, and autopsy studies, rather than from randomized trials.

Rheumatic Mitral Valve Disease

The incidence of systemic thromboembolism is greater in rheumatic heart disease than in any other common cardiac disorder, particularly in the presence of advanced age and concomitant atrial fibrillation. Available evidence suggests that anticoagulant therapy can reduce thromboembolic event rates by 50% to 80%.[65–67]

Mitral Annular Calcification

The occurrence of thromboembolism in mitral annular calcification is variable because of varying substrate that includes fibrin clots, calcified spicules, and atrial thrombus from concomitant atrial fibrillation. Data from the Framingham Heart Study, however, suggest that mitral annular calcification, in and of itself, is a risk factor for systemic embolization.[68]

Mitral Valve Prolapse

Mitral valve prolapse is the most common valvular abnormality in adults and can be complicated by thromboembolism,[69] although the overall incidence is low.[70]

Aortic Valve Disease

Although pathologic studies have demonstrated fibrin thrombi on the surface of calcified aortic valves, the majority of emboli are probably calcific in nature. Many patients with aortic valve disease have concomitant mitral valve disease, atrial fibrillation, and/or atheromatous disease of the aortic root, however, which places them at increased risk for thromboembolism.

Patent Foramen Ovale and Atrial Septal Aneurysm

Paradoxical embolism through a patent foremen ovale is not common; however, cases have been reported, and a true association is strengthened by demonstration of right to left shunting with the Valsalva maneuver (during echocardiography) and/or concomitant venous thrombosis.[71-73] Thrombus within an atrial septal aneurysm can also be a source for systemic embolism.[74]

Management Recommendations

Patients with rheumatic mitral valve disease should receive long-term warfarin therapy (target INR 2.5; range 2.0–3.0), particularly those with atrial fibrillation, prior thromboembolism, or an enlarged left atrium (55 mm). Aspirin (80–100 mg) can be added if recurrent events develop despite adequate anticoagulation therapy with warfarin.

Aortic valve disease, unless there is accompanying mitral valve disease, prior thromboembolism, or separate indications, does not warrant treatment with anticoagulants.

Mitral annular calcification, in and of itself, is not an indication for warfarin therapy. Patients with atrial fibrillation or prior thromboembolism should receive warfarin (target INR 2.5; range 2.0–3.0).

Documented transient ischemic attacks (TIAs) among patients with mitral valve prolapse is an indication for antiplatelet therapy (aspirin, 160–325 mg). Oral anticoagulation with warfarin (target INR 2.5; range 2.0–3.0) is suggested for patients with any of the following:

- documented systemic embolism
- atrial fibrillation
- recurrent TIAs despite aspirin (antiplatelet) therapy

Anticoagulation therapy (target INR 2.5; range 2.0–3.0) is recommended for patients with either a patent foramen ovale or an atrial septal aneurysm in the presence of either of the following:

- unexplained TIA or systemic embolism
- demonstrable deep vein thrombosis or pulmonary embolism

Mobile aortic atheromas and aortic plaques >4 mm (measured by transesophageal echocardiography) are associated with an increased risk of systemic thromboembolism, including stroke. Accordingly, warfarin therapy (target INR 2.5; range 2.0–3.0) should be considered, particularly in patients with documented thromboembolic events.

Routine aspirin (160–325 mg) administration for all patients with these anatomic abnormalities is controversial. (See Figure 18–5.)

PROSTHETIC HEART VALVES

Patients with prosthetic heart valves are at risk for thromboembolism, and many require long-term (lifelong) anticoagulation therapy. It is recognized that the risk of thromboembolism is particularly high with mechanical prosthetic heart valves in descending order of risk—caged-ball, tilting disk, and bileaflet valves. Prosthetic valves in the mitral position also pose greater risk than those in the aortic or other positions. Although biologic (tissue) valves inherently carry less risk, it is important to consider all associated risk factors for thromboembolism when decisions regarding anticoagulation are being made (eg, atrial fibrillation, prior thromboembolic events, dilated [>55 mm] left atrium, poor left ventricular performance).

Clinical Trials of Anticoagulation Therapy

A wealth of information is available from clinical trials and clinical experience gained during the past several decades. The incidence of thromboembolism ranges from less than 1% to 4% per year, with higher rates occurring with mechanical mitral valves and multiple site mechanical valves. The rate of major hemorrhage varies from 0.7% to 5% per year and is highest among older individuals, in those with an INR >4.0, and in the presence of concomitant aspirin use. In a study of 1,608 patients with mechanical heart valves followed during 6,475 patient years,[75] cerebral embolism occurred at a rate of 0.68 per 100 patient years and peripheral embolism at a rate of 0.03 per 100 patient years. The rate of intracranial bleeding was 0.57 per 100 patient years, and the rate of major extracranial bleeding was 2.1 per 100 patient years. The optimal level of anticoagulation, with a low incidence of both complications, was an INR between 2.5 and 4.9. As anticipated, the risk of adverse events (combined thromboembolism and hemorrhage) increased with age, valve position (aortic plus mitral >mitral >aortic), and valve type (caged ball or caged disk >tilting disk >bileaflet).

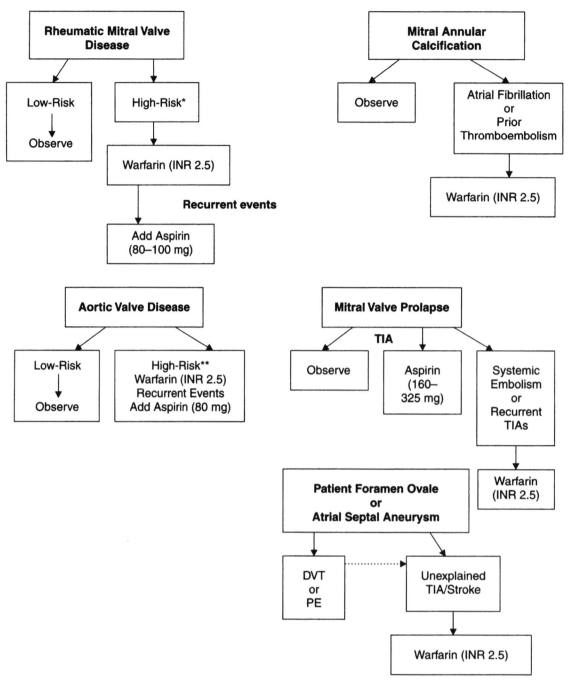

*Atrial fibrillation, dilated (>55mm) left atrium, prior thromboembolism.
**Concomitant mitral valve disease, atrial fibrillation, prior thromboembolism.

Figure 18–5 Antithrombotic management strategies for valvular heart disease

Management Recommendations

All patients with mechanical prosthetic heart valves should receive oral anticoagulation therapy indefinitely to a target INR of 3.0; range 2.5–3.5. A higher intensity of anticoagula-

tion (INR 4.0) might be beneficial among patients at high-risk for thromboembolism (caged-ball valve, caged-disk valve, multiple site mechanical valves, recurrent thromboembolism, mitral position, left atrium >55 mm, atrial fibrillation); however, it is preferable to maintain a target

INR of 3.0 and add low-dose (80–100 mg) aspirin daily. Low-risk patients (bileaflet prosthetic valve in the aortic position without additional thromboembolic risk factors) can be maintained at an INR of 2.5 (range 2.0–3.0). The combination of oral anticoagulants and aspirin (80–100 mg/d) might reduce thromboembolism but is unlikely to offer added benefit among low-risk patients. Patients with bioprosthetic valves in the mitral position should receive oral anticoagulants (INR 2.5) for at least three months after insertion. A more prolonged duration of therapy should be considered strongly for those at continued risk (atrial fibrillation, prior thromboembolism, documented atrial thrombus at the time of surgery, dilated [>55 mm] left atrium, poor ventricular performance). Patients with bioprosthetic valves in the aortic position should receive anticoagulation therapy (INR 2.5) for the initial three months after insertion. Therapy beyond three months should be considered for patients with atrial fibrillation, concomitant mitral valve disease, or poor ventricular performance. Long-term therapy with aspirin (80 mg) is recommended for low-risk patients (Figures 18–6 and 18–7).

CARDIOMYOPATHIES

Cardiac mural thrombosis is a potential complication of dilated cardiomyopathies characterized by left ventricular dilation and systolic dysfunction. There is an inherent risk for thromboembolism, although the incidence has been difficult to quantitate.

Clinical Experience with Anticoagulation Therapy

Autopsy and case series form the basis for current clinical practice. There has not been a large-scale, randomized, controlled trial of anticoagulation therapy among patients with dilated cardiomyopathy. A widely quoted retrospective study of 104 patients followed for a minimum of six years cites an overall embolic event rate of 3.5 per 100 patient years in the absence of anticoagulant therapy.[76] Slightly lower event rates of 2.7 and 2.2 per 100 patient years were reported in the Veterans Affairs Cooperative Vasodilator Heart Failure trials, phases 1 and 2, respectively.[77]

The role of antiplatelet therapy with aspirin and/or clopidogrel is currently being evaluated in a large-scale clinical trial.

Management Recommendations

Patients with dilated cardiomyopathy (ejection fraction <35%), particularly if there is clinical heart failure, should be considered for anticoagulation therapy (INR 2.5). Careful consideration should be given to individuals with prior thromboembolic events, echocardiographic evidence of mural thrombosis, and decreased apical flow velocity by Doppler studies. In the presence of high-risk features that persist, long-term treatment is suggested.

CONCLUSION

Cardiovascular disease is associated with a heightened propensity toward thrombosis that can manifest in the form of acute MI, cardiac death, and stroke. Similarly, valvular heart disease, by altering blood flow dynamics, and the insertion of prosthetic materials, which stimulate localized thrombosis on foreign surfaces, is associated with platelet aggregation and thrombin-mediated bioamplification of the coagulation cascade. Physiologic principles and pathobiologic mechanisms strongly influence the preferred means to prevent or attenuate thrombosis and subsequent cardiovascular events. Only carefully designed clinical trials can establish safe and effective antithrombotic therapies for wide-scale implementation.[78]

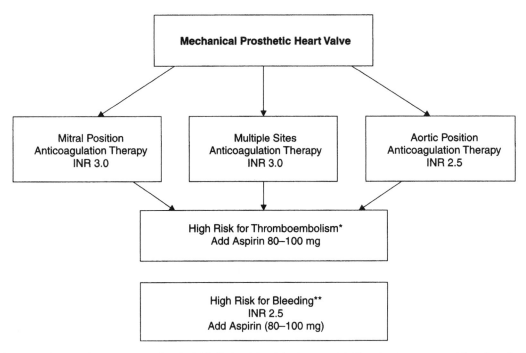

*Patients at high risk for thromboembolism (atrial fibrillation, left atrial enlargement (>55 mm), prior or recurrent thromboembolism, reduced left ventricular function (ejection fraction <35%).
**Hemorrhagic events requiring hospitalization, surgical intervention, transfusion, or transient discontinuation of anticoagulation therapy.

Figure 18–6 Clinical approach to patients with mechanical prosthetic heart valves

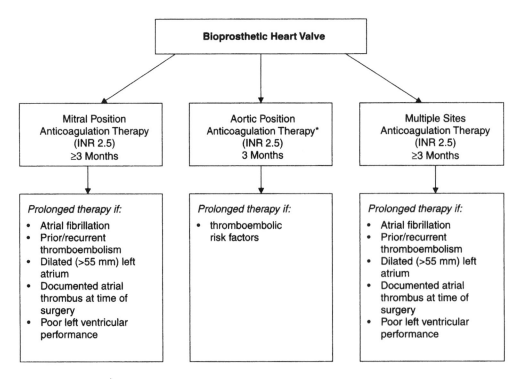

*Anticoagulation therapy is strongly recommended in the presence of concomitant mitral valve disease, atrial fibrillation, prior thromboembolism, or poor left ventricular performance.

Figure 18–7 Management algorithm for patients with bioprosthetic heart valves

REFERENCES

1. Davies MJ, Thomas AC. Plaque fissuring: the cause of acute myocardial infarction, sudden ischaemic death, and crescendo angina. *Br Heart J.* 1985;53:363–373.

2. Forrester JS, Litvack F, Grundfest W, et al. A perspective of coronary disease seen through the arteries of living man. *Circulation.* 1987; 75:505–513.

3. Brozovic M, Stirling Y, Harricks C. Factor VII in an industrial population. *Br J Haematol.* 1974;28:381–391.

4. Meade TW, Mellows S, Brozovic M, et al. Hemostatic functions and ischaemic heart disease: principal results of the Northwick Park Heart Study. *Lancet.* 1986;2:533–537.

5. Kannel WB, Castelli WP, Meeks SL. Fibrinogen and cardiovascular disease. Presented at 34th Annual Scientific Session of the American College of Cardiology; March 1985; Anaheim, CA.

6. Yarnell JWG, Baker IA, Sweetnam PM, et al. Fibrinogen, viscosity and white blood cell count are major risk factors for ischemic heart disease. *Circulation.* 1991;83:836–844.

7. MRC general practice research framework. Thrombosis prevention trial: randomized trial of low intensity oral anticoagulation with warfarin and low-dose aspirin in the primary prevention of ischemic heart disease in men at risk. *Lancet.* 1998;351:233–241.

8. Meade TW, Roderick PJ, Brennan PJ, et al. Extracranial bleeding and other symptoms due to low dose aspirin and low intensity oral anticoagulation. *Thromb Haemost.* 1992;1:1–6.

9. Meade TW, Wilkes HC, Stirling Y, et al. Randomized controlled trial of low dose warfarin in the primary prevention of ischaemic heart disease in men at high risk: design and pilot study. *Eur Heart J.* 1988;9:836–843.

10. The Steering Committee of the Physicians' Health Study Research Group. Final report on the aspirin component of the ongoing Physicians' Health Study. *N Engl J Med.* 1989;321:129–135.

11. Peto R, Gray R, Collins R, et al. Randomized trial of prophylactic daily aspirin in British male doctors. *BMJ.* 1988;296:313–316.

12. Hansson L, Zanchetta A, Carruthers SG, et al. Effects on intensive blood pressure-lowering and low-dose aspirin in patients with hypertension: principal results of the Hypertension Optimal Treatment (HOT) randomized trial. *Lancet.* 1998;351:1755–1762.

13. Falk E. Unstable angina with fatal outcome: dynamic coronary thrombosis leading to infarction and/or sudden death: autopsy evidence of recurrent mural thrombosis with peripheral embolization culminating in total vascular occlusion. *Circulation.* 1985;71:699–708.

14. Davies MJ, Thomas AC, Knapman PA, et al. Intramyocardial platelet aggregation in patients with unstable angina suffering sudden ischemic cardiac death. *Circulation.* 1986;73:418–427.

15. Davies MJ, Thomas A. Thrombosis and acute coronary artery lesions in sudden cardiac ischemic death. *N Engl J Med.* 1984;310:1137–1140.

16. Fitzgerald DJ, Roy L, Catella F, et al. Platelet activation in unstable coronary disease. *N Engl J Med.* 1986;315:983–989.

17. Théroux P, Latour JG, Léger-Gauthier C, et al. Fibrinopeptide A and platelet factor levels in unstable angina pectoris. *Circulation.* 1987;75:156–162.

18. Théroux P, Waters D, Qui S, et al. Aspirin versus heparin to prevent myocardial infarction during the acute-phase unstable angina. *Circulation.* 1993;88:2045–2048.

19. Research Group on Instability in Coronary Artery Disease. Risk of myocardial infarction and death during treatment with low-dose aspirin and intravenous heparin in men with unstable coronary artery disease. *Lancet.* 1990;336:827–830.

20. Théroux P, Waters D, Lam J, et al. Reactivation of unstable angina following discontinuation of heparin. *N Engl J Med.* 1992;327:141–145.

21. Cohen M, Adams PC, Parry G, et al. Combination antithrombotic therapy in unstable rest angina and non-Q-wave infarction: primary end point analysis from the ATACS trial. *Circulation.* 1994;89:81–88.

22. Cohen M, Demers C, Gurfinkel EP for the ESSENCE Investigators. A comparison of low molecular weight heparin with unfractionated heparin for unstable coronary artery disease. *N Engl J Med.* 1997; 337:447–452.

23. Antman EM for the TIMI 11B Investigators. Enoxaparin prevents death and cardiac ischemic events in unstable angina-non-Q wave MI. *Circulation.* 1999;100:1593–1601.

24. Kong DF, Califf RM, Miller DP, et al. Clinical outcomes of therapeutic agents that block the platelet glycoprotein IIb/IIIa integrin in ischemic heart disease. *Circulation.* 1998;98:2829–2835.

25. Anand SS, Tusuf S, Pogue J, Weitz JI, Flather M. Long-term oral anticoagulant therapy in patients with unstable angina or suspected non-Q wave myocardial infarction: OASIS Pilot Study Results. *Circulation.* 1998;98:1064–1070.

26. OASIS-2 Investigators. Effects of recombinant Hirudin (lepirudin) compared with heparin on death, myocardial infarction, refractory angina and revascularization procedures in patients with acute myocardial ischemia without ST segment elevation: a randomized trial. *Lancet.* 1999;353:429–438.

27. Van der Wal AC, Becker AE, van der Loos CM, et al. Site of intimal rupture or erosion of thrombosed coronary atherosclerotic plaques is characterized by an inflammatory process irrespective of the dominant plaque morphology. *Circulation.* 1994;89:36–44.

28. Fuster V, Badimon JJ, et al. The pathogenesis of coronary artery disease and the acute coronary syndromes. *N Engl J Med.* 1992;362:242–250, 310–318.

29. Farrell M, Fuster V. Mechanisms of acute myocardial infarction. In: Becker RC, ed. *The Modern Era of Coronary Thrombolysis.* Boston: Kluwer Academic Publishers; 1994:1–13.

30. Chalmers TC, Matta RJ, Smith H, Kunzler A-M. Evidence favoring the use of anticoagulants in the hospital phase of acute myocardial infarction. *N Engl J Med.* 1977;297:1091–1096.

31. Peto R. Clinical trial methodology. *Biomed Pharmacol Ther.* 1978; 28:24–36.

32. Medical Research Council Group. Assessment of short term anticoagulant administration after cardiac infarction: report of the working party on anticoagulant therapy in coronary thrombosis. *Br Med J.* 1969;1:335–342.

33. Drapkin A, Merskey C. Anticoagulant therapy after acute myocardial infarction. *JAMA.* 1972;222:541–548.

34. Veterans Administration Cooperative Study. Anticoagulants in acute myocardial infarction: results of cooperative clinical trial. *JAMA.* 1973;225:724–729.

35. Wright IS, Marple CD, Beck DF. Anticoagulant therapy of coronary thrombosis with myocardial infarction. *JAMA.* 1948;1074–1079.

36. Gifford RH, Feinstein AR. A critique of methodology in studies of anticoagulant for acute myocardial infarction. *N Engl J Med.* 1969; 280:351–357.

37. Carleton RA, Sanders CA, Burack WR. Heparin administration after acute myocardial infarction. *N Engl J Med.* 1960;263:1002–1005.

38. Loeliger EA, Hensen A, Kroes F, et al. A double blind trial of long term anticoagulant treatment after myocardial infarction. *Acta Med Scand.* 1967;182:549–566.

39. Meuwissen OJAT, Vervoorn AC, Cohen O, et al. Double blind trial of long term anticoagulant treatment after myocardial infarction. *Acta Med Scand.* 1969;186:361–368.

40. 60-Plus Reinfarction Study Research Group. A double blind trial to assess long term oral anticoagulant therapy in elderly patients after myocardial infarction. *Lancet.* 1980;2:989–993.

41. Smith P, Arnesen H, Holme I. The effect of warfarin on mortality and reinfarction after myocardial infarction. *N Engl J Med.* 1990;323: 147–152.

42. Anticoagulation in the Secondary Prevention of Events in Coronary Thrombosis Research Group. Effect of long-term oral anticoagulant treatment on mortality and cardiovascular morbidity after myocardial infarction. *Lancet.* 1994;343:499–503.

43. Antiplatelet Trialists Collaboration. Collaborative overview of randomized trials of antiplatelet therapy. I. Prevention of death, myocardial infarction and stroke by antiplatelet therapy in various categories of patients. *Br Med J.* 1994;308:81–106.

44. Coumadin Aspirin Reinfarction Study (CARS) Investigators. Randomized double-blind study of fixed low dose warfarin with aspirin after myocardial infarction. *Lancet.* 1997;350:389–396.

45. Tulloch JA, Gilchrist AR. Anticoagulants in treatment of coronary thrombosis. *Br Med J.* 1950;2:965–971.

46. Burton CR. Anticoagulant therapy of recent cardiac infarction. *Can Med Assoc J.* 1954;70:404–408.

47. Davis MJ, Ireland MA. Effect of early anticoagulation on the frequency of left ventricular thrombi after anterior wall acute myocardial infarction. *Am J Cardiol.* 1986;57:1244–1247.

48. Arvan S, Boscha K. Prophylactic anticoagulation for left ventricular thrombi after acute myocardial infarction: a prospective randomized trial. *Am Heart J.* 1987;113:688–693.

49. Vaitkus PT, Barnathan ES. Embolic potential, prevention and management of mural thrombus complicating anterior myocardial infarction: a meta-analysis. *J Am Coll Cardiol.* 1993;22:1004–1009.

50. Weinreich DJ, Burke JF, Pauletto FJ. Left ventricular mural thrombi complicating acute myocardial infarction: long term follow up with serial echocardiography. *Ann Intern Med.* 1984;100:789–794.

51. Keating EC, Gross SA, Schlamowitz RA, et al. Mural thrombi in myocardial infarctions: prospective evaluation of two dimensional echocardiography. *Am J Med.* 1983;74:989–995.

52. Friedman MF, Carlson K, Marcus FI, et al. Clinical correlation in patients with acute myocardial infarction and left ventricular thrombus detected by two dimensional echocardiography. *Am J Med.* 1982;72: 894–898.

53. Veen G, Meyer A, Verheugt FWA, et al. Culprit lesion morphology and stenosis severity in the prediction of reocclusion after coronary thrombolysis: angiographic results of the APRICOT study. *J Am Coll Cardiol.* 1993;22:1755–1762.

54. Hearn JA, King SB, Douglas JS, et al. Clinical and angiographic outcomes after coronary stenting for acute or threatened closure after percutaneous coronary angioplasty: initial results with a balloon-expandable, stainless steel stent. *Circulation.* 1993;88:2455–2457.

55. Roubin GS, Cannon AD, Agrawal SK, et al. Intracoronary stenting for acute and threatened closure complicating percutaneous transluminal coronary angioplasty. *Circulation.* 1992;85:916–927.

56. Urban P, Macaya C, Rupprecht H-J for the MATTIS Investigators. Randomized evaluation of anticoagulation versus antiplatelet therapy after coronary stent implantation in high risk patients. *Circulation.* 1998;98:2126–2132.

57. Schömig A, Neuman F-J, Kastrati A. et al. A randomized comparison of antiplatelet and anticoagulant therapy after placement of coronary artery stems. *N Engl J Med.* 1996;334:1084–1089.

58. McEnany MT, Saizman EW, Mundth ED, et al. The effect of antithrombotic therapy on patency rates of saphenous vein coronary artery bypass grafts. *J Thorac Cardiovasc Surg.* 1982;83:81–89.

59. Pantely GA, Goodnight SH Jr, Rahimtoola SH, et al. Failure of antiplatelet and anticoagulant therapy to improve patency of grafts after coronary artery bypass: a controlled, randomized study. *N Engl J Med.* 1979;301:962–966.

60. Sanz G, Pajaron A, Alegria E, et al. Prevention of early aortocoronary bypass occlusion by low-dose aspirin and dipyridamole. *Circulation.* 1990;82:765–773.

61. Weber MAJ, Hasford J, Taillens C, et al. Low dose aspirin versus anticoagulants for prevention of coronary graft occlusion. *Am J Cardiol.* 1990;66:1464–1468.

62. Yli-Mayry S, Huikuri HV, Korhonen UR, et al. Efficacy and safety of anticoagulant therapy started preoperatively in preventing coronary vein graft occlusion. *Eur Heart J.* 1992;13:1259–1264.

63. Van der Meer J, Hillege HL, Koofstria GJ, et al. Prevention of 1 year graft occlusion after aorto coronary bypass surgery. *Lancet.* 1993;342: 257–264.

64. Goldman S, Copeland J, Moritz J, et al. Improvement in early saphenous vein graft patency after coronary artery bypass surgery with antiplatelet therapy: results of a Veterans Administration cooperative study. *Circulation.* 1988;77:1324–1332.

65. Szekely P. Systemic embolism and anticoagulant prophylaxis in rheumatic heart disease. *BMJ.* 1964;1:209–212.

66. Daley R, Mattingly TW, Holt C, et al. Systemic arterial embolism in rheumatic heart disease. *Am Heart J.* 1951;42:566–581.

67. Adams GF, Merrett JD, Hutchinson WM, et al. Cerebral embolism and mitral stenosis: survival with and without anticoagulants. *J Neurol Neurosurg Psychiatry.* 1974;37:378–383.

68. Benjamin EJ, Plehn JF, D'Agostino RB, et al. Mitral annular calcification and the risk of stroke in an elderly cohort. *N Engl J Med.* 1992;327:374–379.

69. Barnett HJM, Boughner DR, Taylow DW. Further evidence relating mitral valve prolapse to cerebral ischemic events. *N Engl J Med.* 1980; 302:139–144.

70. Hart RG, Easton JD. Mitral valve prolapse and cerebral infarction. *Stroke.* 1982;13:429–430.

71. Thompson T, Evans W. Paradoxical embolism. *Q J Med.* 1930;23: 135–150.

72. Hagen PT, Scholtz DG, Edwards WD. Incidence and size of patent foramen ovale during the first 10 years of life: an autopsy study of 965 normal hearts. *Mayo Clin Proc.* 1984;59:17–20.

73. Lynch JJ, Schuchand GH, Gross CM, et al. Prevalence of right-to-left shunting in the healthy population: detection by Valsalva maneuver contrast echocardiography. *Am J Cardiol.* 1984;53:1478–1480.

74. Schneider B, Hanrath P, Vogel P, et al. Improved morphologic characterization of atrial septal aneurysm by transesophogeal echocardiography: relation to cerebral events. *J Am Coll Cardiol.* 1990;16:1000–1009.

75. Cannegieter SC, Rosendaal FR, Wintzen AR, van der Meer FJM, Vandenbroucke JP, Briet E. Optimal oral anticoagulant therapy in patients with mechanical heart valves. *N Engl J Med.* 1995;333:11–17.

76. Fuster V, Gersh BJ, Guiliani ER, et al. The natural history of idiopathic dilated cardiomyopathy. *Am J Cardiol.* 1981;47:525–530.

77. Dunkman WB, Johnson GR, Carson PE, et al. Incidence of thromboembolic events in congestive heart failure. *Circulation.* 1993;87(suppl 6):VI94–VI101.

78. Dalen JE, Hirsh J. Sixth ACCP Consensus Conference on Antithrombotic Therapy. *Chest.* 2001;119:1S–370S.

Chapter 19

Atrial Fibrillation, Stroke, and the Role of Anticoagulation

Daniel E. Singer

INTRODUCTION

Atrial fibrillation (AF) is one of the most common cardiac rhythm disorders and also a potent risk factor for stroke. A consistent set of randomized trials clearly demonstrates that long-term anticoagulation removes most of the risk of stroke posed by AF and can do so with acceptable safety. The challenge is to translate the findings of the randomized trials into effective clinical practice. In particular, clinicians need to identify those patients with AF who are at high enough risk of thromboembolism to merit the inconvenience and potential toxicity of anticoagulant therapy, and they need to develop systems for managing anticoagulation that optimize control of the intensity of anticoagulation as well as patient compliance.

ATRIAL FIBRILLATION AS A RISK FACTOR FOR STROKE

Until relatively recently, the relationship between nonrheumatic AF, the predominant category of AF in the United States, and stroke and the likely benefit of anticoagulation in patients with AF were controversial. AF occurs as people get older and as they develop other cardiac diseases. Although AF simply might be a marker of these other risk factors for stroke and not a true cause of stroke itself, epidemiologic studies provide support for AF as an independent cause of stroke. Perhaps the strongest such evidence comes from the Framingham Heart Study.[1] In the Framingham

study, the prevalence of AF increased strikingly with age, from 2% for those in their 60s to 10% for those over the age of 80. The incidence of stroke in those without AF rose from 4.5 per 1,000 person years in individuals in their 60s to 14.3 per 1,000 person years for those in their 80s. The rate of stroke among individuals with AF, however, was fivefold greater across this entire range of ages. This persistence of effect into the oldest age groups is different from the most common risk factor for stroke, hypertension, where the effect diminishes among the oldest individuals.[2] The percentage of all strokes in a given population that are due to a given risk factor is measured as the population-attributable risk percentage and is a function of the prevalence of the risk factor and the strength of the risk factor, measured as the relative risk. From such a calculation, one can estimate that about 14% of all strokes in the United States, or 75,000 strokes per year, are due to AF.

RANDOMIZED TRIALS OF ANTITHROMBOTIC THERAPY IN ATRIAL FIBRILLATION

Despite the epidemiologic evidence that AF is a risk factor for stroke, there remained uncertainty whether warfarin would actually prevent stroke in AF and, even if it did, whether anticoagulation would be adequately safe for the predominantly older population with AF. Five randomized trials began to address these issues during the 1980s:

1. Atrial Fibrillation, Aspirin, Anticoagulation Study (AFASAK)
2. Boston Area Anticoagulation Trial for Atrial Fibrillation (BAATAF)
3. Canadian Atrial Fibrillation Anticoagulation Study (CAFA)
4. Stroke Prevention in Atrial Fibrillation Study (SPAF)
5. Veterans Affairs Stroke Prevention in Nonrheumatic Atrial Fibrillation Study (SPINAF)

Table 19–1 summarizes the findings of these primary prevention trials, as well as the findings of the secondary prevention European Atrial Fibrillation Trial (EAFT).[3–8]

Only a small fraction of potentially eligible patients entered the trials at participating sites. Nonetheless, participants had characteristics common to patients with AF. In particular, they were older individuals, with an average age of 69; about one-fifth were older than age 75. The majority of subjects were male, although a substantial proportion (27%) were women. Most patients had had AF for more than one year, and only a small percentage had intermittent, or paroxysmal AF. Nearly 50% had hypertension, 15% had diabetes, and more than 20% had coronary artery disease and/or congestive heart failure. It stands to reason that participants in the trials were not the frailest patients with AF and that they were viewed as relatively safe anticoagulation candidates, but it is likely that the results of the trials can be confidently applied to many patients with AF.

The results of these randomized trials were dramatic and consistent (see Table 19–1). Each of the five primary prevention trials stopped early because of the marked efficacy of warfarin (the CAFA trial stopped early because of the results of other trials). This efficacy, measured as the relative risk reduction, ranged from 35% to 86%. In the EAFT secondary prevention trial, where subjects had AF and a recent minor stroke or transient ischemic attack, the control group experienced a remarkably high 12% annual rate of stroke. Nonetheless, the relative risk reduction that was due to anticoagulants seen in EAFT was essentially the same as that for the primary prevention trials.

Two additional points about the results of these trials are worth nothing. First, the efficacy values were estimated according to the "intention to treat" principle. In fact, a large fraction of the strokes counted in the warfarin category occurred among patients randomized to warfarin who were not taking warfarin at the time of their strokes. Ischemic strokes are unusual in patients with AF who are truly anticoagulated. Second, the lowest intensity of anticoagulation tested in these trials was as effective as higher intensities. BAATAF and SPINAF used the lowest target, a prothrombin time ratio (PTR) range of 1.2-1.5, roughly corresponding to an International Normalized Ratio (INR) target of 2.0-3.0, and the efficacies observed in these two trials were actually somewhat higher than in the other trials.

The first five trials pooled their original data.[9] The pooled relative risk reduction for the five primary prevention trials was 68% with a 95% confidence interval ranging from 50% to 79%. The EAFT results demonstrating a relative risk reduction of 66% were remarkably consistent with the first set of trials. Because AF raises the risk of stroke fivefold, a complete reversal of the effect of AF would result in a relative risk reduction of 80% (ie, reduce the risk from fivefold to onefold). The observed relative risk reduction that is due to anticoagulants in AF is close to such a complete reversal.

Clinical decisions hinge on absolute, rather than relative, benefits and risks. For the primary prevention trials, the

Table 19–1 Overview of the Randomized Trials of Anticoagulation for Atrial Fibrillation: Efficacy

Trial	AFASAK	BAATAF	CAFA	SPAF	SPINAF	EAFT
Anticoagulation:						
Target	INR 2.8–4.2	PTR 1.2–1.5	INR 2.0–3.0	PTR 1.3–1.8	PTR 1.2–1.5	INR 2.5–4.0
No. of subjects	335	212	187	210	260	225
No. of emboli	10	2	7	6	4	20
Annual rate	2.3%	0.41%	3.0%	2.3%	0.88%	3.9%
Control:						
No. of subjects	336	208	191	211	265	214
No. of emboli	22	13	11	18	19	50
Annual rate	5.6%	3.0%	4.6%	7.4%	4.3%	12.3%
Preventive efficacy	59%	86%	35%	69%	79%	66%
95% confidence interval	15–81%	51%–96%	(–64)–75%	27%–85%	52%–90%	43%–80%

Note: Preventive efficacy is the relative risk reduction calculated as (1 – RR) × 100, where RR is the annual rate in the anticoagulation group divided by the annual rate in the control group.

Source: Reprinted with permission from DE Singer et al, Preventing Stroke in Atrial Fibrillation, *Coronary Artery Disease*, Vol 3, pp 753–760, © 1992, Rapid Science Publishers.

average absolute risk reduction was 3.1% per year. In cardiovascular prevention trials, this magnitude of effect is large. For example, 3% per year is about five times the impact of treating hypertension in the elderly.[10] Of course, anticoagulation is more difficult than taking antihypertensives. For the secondary prevention EAFT study, the absolute risk reduction of 8% per year is a powerful reason for using anticoagulants.

In these trials, and coagulation was also quite safe. The only hemorrhagic complication of warfarin comparable in impact to ischemic stroke is intracranial hemorrhage. The increase in intracranial hemorrhage in the five primary prevention trials was only 0.25% per year, and no intracranial hemorrhages were reported in the EAFT study. Aggregate major hemorrhage (eg, intracranial hemorrhage plus hemorrhage leading to hospitalization and/or transfusion) was higher, but the highest rate observed (in the EAFT study) was only 1.8% per year.

In summary, the randomized trials demonstrate that warfarin at low intensity is very effective and can be safe. It is likely that the bleeding results seen in the trials were better than those observed in general practice. Patients were probably better than average candidates for safe anticoagulation, and the management of anticoagulation was probably better organized than in many practices. Nonetheless, the record of the first six randomized trials stands as strong evidence that warfarin can be used safely among older patients with AF. At least one study has shown that the efficacy and safety seen in the trials can be approached in clinical practice.[11]

ASPIRIN: AN EFFECTIVE ALTERNATIVE TO ANTICOAGULATION?

Despite the dramatic results of the randomized trials, warfarin remains a risky and burdensome therapy. Some clinicians have expressed enthusiasm for using aspirin to prevent strokes in AF and thereby avoid anticoagulation. The currently available evidence, however, indicates that aspirin's efficacy is small, at best. There have been four separately randomized trials of aspirin in AF: AFASAK, which used 75 mg per day[4]; two separately randomized trials, within SPAF I, using 325 mg per day[12]; and EAFT, using 300 mg per day.[8] The SPAF I Group 1 trial included patients who could be randomized to warfarin and compared groups treated with aspirin or aspirin-placebo, as well as warfarin. Group 2 of the SPAF I trial included patients with AF who would not or could not take warfarin and simply compared groups assigned to aspirin versus placebo.

In AFASAK, the rate of outcome events was not significantly lower in the aspirin group. In SPAF I Group 2, there were 28 events in control patients versus 25 events in aspirin patients for a nonsignificant reduction of 8%. There was, as well, no significant effect of aspirin seen in the EAFT study,

which observed 88 events in the aspirin category versus 90 events in the control group. Interest in aspirin as an antithrombotic in AF stems almost entirely from the SPAF I Group 1 trial, where there were 18 events in the control group versus only 1 event in the aspirin group for the highest efficacy seen for any therapy—95%. No explanation has been found to account for the disparate results of SPAF I Group 1. A pooled analysis of these aspirin trials provided a summary relative risk reduction due to aspirin of 21%, with a 95% confidence interval that included 0% efficacy.[13] A subsequent large trial, SPAF3, tested anticoagulation targeted at INR values between 2.0 and 3.0 versus very low intensity anticoagulation, INR 1.2 to 1.5, plus aspirin 325 mg per day, in AF patients who were at high risk for stroke.[14] Full anticoagulation targeted at INR 2.0 to 3.0 was much more effective with a relative risk reduction of 74%. Taken together, these studies indicate that aspirin's effect in AF is small, and that its use should be limited to AF patients at very low risk of stroke.

RISK FACTORS FOR STROKE IN PATIENTS WITH ATRIAL FIBRILLATION

It is reasonable to limit the use of anticoagulants to those patients with AF who are at heightened risk of stroke. The pooled analysis of the first five trials provides the most powerful assessment of putative clinical risk factors.[9] In this analysis, prior stroke, hypertension, older age, and diabetes were independent risk factors for subsequent stroke in AF. Patients in the first five trials were categorized according to age and the presence of at least one of the other risk factors—hypertension, diabetes, or prior stroke (Table 19–2). For patients in the control group who were younger than age 65 and had none of these risk factors, the rate of stroke was 1% per year. Similar patients treated with warfarin had the same incidence rate of 1% per year. Such findings support the conclusion that younger patients with so-called "lone" AF do not need to be anticoagulated. For the other categories of patients with AF, however, the rates of stroke were substantial and the benefit of warfarin so dramatic that warfarin was strongly indicated. Subsequent reports from the pooled analysis revealed that left ventricular dysfunction on echocardiograms was also an additional independent risk factor for stroke.[15]

Another risk stratification scheme has been provided by the SPAF investigators.[14,16] The SPAF risk factors also include prior stroke or transient ischemic attack (TIA) and hypertension. However, the SPAF group did not confirm diabetes as a risk factor and viewed age 75, rather than age 65, as the threshold for heightened risk of stroke. In consideration of these two prominent risk analyses, the guidelines from the American College of Chest Physicians stated that warfarin was indicated for all patients with AF who were

Table 19–2 Pooled Analysis of the First Five Atrial Fibrillation Trials: Efficacy of Warfarin by Risk Category

Risk Category	Control		Warfarin	
	No. of Strokes	Rate (95% CI)	No. of Strokes	Rate (95% CI)
Age <65 years:				
No risk factor	3	1.0% (0.3–3.1)	3	1.0% (0.3–3.0)
≥1 Risk factor	16	4.9 (3.0–8.1)	6	1.7% (0.8–3.9)
Age 65–75 years:				
No risk factor	16	4.3% (2.7–7.1)	4	1.1% (0.4–2.8)
≥1 Risk factor	27	5.7 (3.9–8.3)	7	1.7% (0.9–3.4)
Age >75 years:				
No risk factor	6	3.5% (1.6–7.7)	3	1.7% (0.5–5.2)
≥1 Risk factor	13	8.1 (4.7–13.9)	2	1.2% (0.3–5.0)

Note: The first five trials are listed in Table 19–1. Risk factors are history of hypertension, diabetes, or prior stroke or transient ischemic attack. Rate is annual rate; CI is Confidence interval.

Source: Reprinted with permission from Atrial Fibrillation Investigators. Risk Factors for Stroke and Efficacy of Anti-Thrombotic Therapy in Atrial Fibrillation, *Archives of Internal Medicine*, Vol 154, pp 1449–1457, © 1994, American Medical Association.

older than 75 years or who had an additional risk factor. For patients younger than 65 without risk factors, aspirin was recommended. For patients age 65–75 without risk factors, either warfarin or aspirin was recommended (Figure 19–1).[17]

RISK OF BLEEDING WITH ANTICOAGULATION

Several studies have highlighted the importance of excessive anticoagulation in causing major hemorrhage on antico-

agulants.[18–22] This problem was evident in a study of intracranial hemorrhage among Massachusetts General Hospital patients taking warfarin. A total of 121 consecutive cases of intracranial hemorrhage in hospitalized patients on warfarin was assembled during an 11-year period, and each case was compared with three calendar-matched controls selected from the hospital's large anticoagulant therapy unit.[21] There were 77 cases of intracerebral hemorrhage and 44 cases of subdural hemorrhage. Outcome was very poor—46% of patients with intracerebral hemorrhage died, and only 9% left the hospital without disability; 20% of patients with subdural

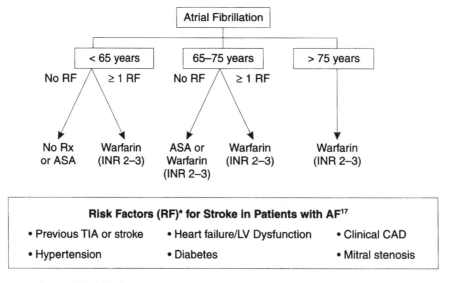

Figure 19–1 Clinical approach to atrial fibrillation

*Consistently demonstrated RFs include previous TIA or stroke, hypertension, and heart failure/LV dysfunction. Less consistently demonstrated RFs include diabetes and clinical CAD. Mitral stenosis representing rheumatic AF is widely accepted as a powerful RF. AF patients with prosthetic heart valves should take anticoagulants. The INR target should be appropriate for the valve.

hemorrhage died, and only 20% left the hospital without major disability. The presence of cerebrovascular disease and of a prosthetic heart valve were independent risk factors for intracranial hemorrhage. Increasing age also was a significant risk factor, with a 1.4-fold increase in risk for each ascending decade. The most potent risk factor emerging from the analysis, however, was the intensity of anticoagulation, a risk factor that physicians can control. The relative odds for intracranial hemorrhage increased dramatically for PTRs above 2.0, roughly corresponding to INR levels above 4.0. Prospective follow-up of patients with prosthetic heart valves by Dutch Thrombosis Centers demonstrated a similar relationship with risk of intracerebral hemorrhage rising rapidly with INR values above 5.0.[23]

LOWEST EFFECTIVE INTENSITY OF ANTICOAGULATION

A critically important question not answered by the randomized trials relates to the lowest possible intensity of anticoagulation that still can be effective in preventing strokes in AF. The lower the target INR, the less likely is major hemorrhage. The lowest intensities tested in the initial randomized trials remained fully effective, thus raising the possibility that very low INRs might work. Analysis of a small number of events in the EAFT suggested that INRs less than 2.0 might not be effective in AF.[24] The SPAF III trial clearly established that INR values between 1.3 and 1.5 were ineffective.[14] A large case-control analysis demonstrated a sharp loss of efficacy at INR levels less than 2.0, a finding that has been repeatedly confirmed.[14,25]

The clinical implications of these findings are clear. Anticoagulant efficacy in AF can be obtained at INRs targeted between 2.0 and 3.0. INRs above 4.0 are not necessary and should be avoided; INRs less than 2.0 raise the risk of stroke. The key to safe and effective anticoagulation in AF is consistent control of the INR in the range of 2.0 to 3.0.

PHYSICIAN PRACTICES REGARDING ANTICOAGULATION

Despite the striking evidence favoring use of anticoagulants, more than two-thirds of patients with AF are not anticoagulated. Precisely what percentage should be anticoagulated is not known, but clinical experience and a report from a large health maintenance organization suggest that more than 50% of patients with AF are suitable for safe anticoagulation.[11] Surveys also have indicated that physicians frequently favor low-target INRs (eg, 1.5), particularly in elderly patients, to avoid bleeding complications.[27] Such a low intensity of anticoagulation raises the risk of stroke.

Many physician practices are not optimally organized to manage anticoagulation. The needed recordkeeping and pa-tient follow-up pose substantial burdens, with the result that physicians lose enthusiasm for this effective therapy. It is clear that dedicated anticoagulation services remove these burdens from the prescribing physician and probably better control anticoagulation.

ANTICOAGULATION FOR CARDIOVERSION

The epidemiologic studies and randomized trials discussed above deal with chronic AF, either sustained or paroxysmal. A related issue is anticoagulation to prevent stroke in the context of cardioversion of AF. Here, the data are very sparse, and no randomized trial results are available. Observational series of electrical cardioversion appear to indicate that cardioversion increases the risk of stroke in AF, and that anticoagulation is quite effective in preventing such thromboembolic events.[28] Published guidelines recommend three weeks of anticoagulation, targeted at INR 2.0–3.0, before attempting cardioversion.[17] Patients who have been in AF for periods shorter than 48 hours might be cardioverted without anticoagulation because of the presumed lessened time for formation of intracardiac thrombi. Rarely, however, can a physician be confident of the exact duration of the AF episode. Anticoagulation should be continued until normal sinus rhythm has been established for more than four weeks. Reports suggest that patients who have a transesophageal echocardiogram revealing *no* atrial thrombi can safely undergo electrical cardioversion without prior anticoagulation.[29] It has become clear, however, that anticoagulation after cardioversion is still necessary for patients with no atrial thrombi evident prior to cardioversion.[30] Without anticoagulation, such patients are at heightened risk of stroke in the period following cardioversion. Anticoagulation targeted at INR 2.0–3.0 should be maintained for four weeks after normal sinus rhythm has been established.[17] The use of transesophageal echocardiography prior to cardioversion is an area of ongoing research. For the time being, guidelines for anticoagulation for cardioversion of AF remain those given in Table 19–3.[17]

CONCLUSION

The primary result of anticoagulation research conducted over the past 15 years is the clear demonstration of its striking efficacy in AF. By contrast, current evidence makes it unlikely that aspirin has a sizable effect. Warfarin at an INR target of 2.0–3.0 can be safe. Patients with AF who are younger than age 65 and have no other risk factors are at sufficiently low risk of stroke to avoid warfarin. For all other patients with AF, anticoagulation is indicated although aspirin may be acceptable for patients ages 65–75 without any risk factor. All patients undergoing elective cardioversion

Table 19–3 Recommendations for Anticoagulation for Patients with Atrial Fibrillation Undergoing Elective Cardioversion

Patient Group	Recommendation
1. Duration of AF > 2 days or unknown	Anticoagulation, INR 2.0–3.0 3 weeks prior to cardioversion and for 4 weeks after sinus rhythm established
2. Duration of AF confidently known to be < 2 days	Consider forgoing anticoagulation

Source: Data from A Laupacis, G Albers, J Dallen, et al, Antithrombotic therapy in atrial fibrillation, *Chest*, Vol 114, pp 579S–589S, © 1998.

Source: Adapted from A. Laupacis, G. Albers, J. Dallen et al., Antithrombotic Therapy in Atrial Fibrillation, *Chest*, Vol. 114, pp. 579S–589S, © 1998, American College of Chest Physicians.

should have several weeks of anticoagulation both before cardioversion and after sinus rhythm has been established. The target INR for cardioversion of AF is also 2.0–3.0 (Table 19–3). In the unusual circumstance when the duration of AF is clearly less than 48 hours, anticoagulation may be avoided.

Formal cost-effectiveness analyses demonstrate that anticoagulation for AF actually can be cost saving, as well as beneficial in terms of health outcomes.[31,32] More widespread and more consistently accurate anticoagulation for AF will need better organized systems to manage anticoagulation. Dedicated anticoagulation services using computerized support systems can meet this need. Such units should prove attractive to managed care organizations serving large numbers of older patients. In this way, the remarkable benefits of anticoagulation demonstrated in the randomized trials can be effectively extended to the growing number of patients with AF.

REFERENCES

1. Wolf PA, Abbott RD, Kannel WB. Atrial fibrillation: a major contributor to stroke in the elderly. *Arch Intern Med.* 1987;147:1561–1564.

2. Wolf PA, Abbott RD, Kannel WB. Atrial fibrillation as an independent risk factor for stroke: the Framingham Study. *Stroke.* 1991;22:983–988.

3. Boston Area Anticoagulation Trial for Atrial Fibrillation Investigators. The effect of low-dose warfarin on the risk of stroke in patients with nonrheumatic atrial fibrillation. *N Engl J Med.* 1990;323:1505–1511.

4. Petersen P, Godtfredsen J, Boysen G, Andersen ED, Andersen B. Placebo-controlled, randomised trial of warfarin and aspirin for prevention of thromboembolic complications in chronic atrial fibrillation: the Copenhagen AFASAK study. *Lancet.* 1989;1:175–179.

5. Stroke Prevention in Atrial Fibrillation Investigators. Stroke prevention in atrial fibrillation study: final results. *Circulation.* 1991;84:527–539.

6. Connolly SJ, Laupacis A, Gent M, Roberts RS, Caims JA, Joyner C. Canadian atrial fibrillation anticoagulation (CAFA) study. *J Am Coll Cardiol.* 1991;18:349–355.

7. Ezekowitz MD, Bridgers SL, James KE, et al. Warfarin in the prevention of stroke associated with nonrheumatic atrial fibrillation. *N Engl J Med.* 1992;327:1406–1412.

8. European Atrial Fibrillation Trial Study Group. Secondary prevention in nonrheumatic atrial fibrillation after transient ischaemic attack or minor stroke. *Lancet.* 1993;342:1256–1262.

9. Atrial Fibrillation Investigators. Atrial fibrillation: risk factors for embolization and efficacy of antithrombotic therapy. *Arch Intern Med.* 1994;154:1449–1457.

10. Mulrow CD, Cornell JA, Herrera CR, Kadri A, Farnett L, Aguilar C. Hypertension in the elderly: implications and generalizability of randomized trials. *JAMA.* 1994;272:1932–1938.

11. Gottlieb LK, Salem-Schatz S. Anticoagulation in atrial fibrillation: does efficacy in clinical trials translate into effectiveness in practice? *Arch Intern Med.* 1994;154:1945–1953.

12. Stroke Prevention in Atrial Fibrillation Investigators. A differential effect of aspirin on prevention of stroke in atrial fibrillation. *J Stroke Cerebrovasc Dis.* 1993;3:181–188.

13. Atrial Fibrillation Investigators. The efficacy of aspirin in patients with atrial fibrillation: analysis of pooled data from three randomized trials. *Arch Intern Med.* 1997;157:1237–1240.

14. Stroke Prevention in Atrial Fibrillation Investigators. Adjusted-dose warfarin versus low-intensity, fixed-dose warfarin plus aspirin for high-risk patients with atrial fibrillation: Stroke Prevention in Atrial Fibrillation III randomized clinical trial. *Lancet.* 1996;348:633–638.

15. Atrial Fibrillation Investigators. Echocardiographic predictors of stroke in patients with atrial fibrillation: a prospective study of 1,066 patients from three clinical trials. *Arch Intern Med.* 1998;158:1316–1320.

16. SPAF III Writing Committee for the Stroke Prevention in Atrial Fibrillation Investigators. Patients with nonvalvular atrial fibrillation at low risk of stroke during treatment with aspirin: Stroke Prevention in Atrial Fibrillation III Study. *JAMA.* 1998;279:1273–1277.

17. Laupacis A, Albers G, Dalen J, Dunn MI, Jacobson AK, Singer DE. Antithrombotic therapy in atrial fibrillation. *Chest.* 1998;114:579S–589S.

18. Landefeld CS, Goldman L. Major bleeding in outpatients treated with warfarin: incidence and prediction by factors known at the start of outpatient therapy. *Am J Med.* 1989;87:144–152.

19. Gurwitz JH, Avorn J, Ross-Degnan D, Choodnovsky I, Ansell J. Aging and the anticoagulant response to warfarin therapy. *Ann Intern Med.* 1992;116:901–904.

20. Fihn SD, McDonell M, Martin D, et al. Risk factors for complications of chronic anticoagulation: a multicenter study. *Ann Intern Med.* 1993;118:511–520.

21. Hylek EM, Singer DE. Risk factors for intracranial hemorrhage in outpatients taking warfarin. *Ann Intern Med.* 1994:120:897–902.

22. Cannegieter SC, Rosendaal FR, Wintzen AR, Van der Meer FJM, Vandenbroucke JP, Briet E. Optimal oral anticoagulant therapy in patients with mechanical heart valves. *N Engl J Med.* 1995;333: 11–17.

23. van der Meer FJM, Rosendaal FR, Vandenbroucke JP, Briet E. Assessment of a bleeding index in two cohorts of patients treated with oral anticoagulants. *Thromb Haemost.* 1996;96:12–16.

24. European Atrial Fibrillation Trial Study Group. Optimal anticoagulant therapy in patients with nonrheumatic atrial fibrillation and recent cerebral ischemia. *N Engl J Med.* 1955;333:5–10.

25. Hylek EM, Skates SJ, Sheehan MA, Singer DE. An analysis of the lowest effective intensity of prophylactic anticoagulation for patients with nonrheumatic atrial fibrillation. *N Engl J Med.* 1996;335: 540–546.

26. Brass LM, Krumholz HM, Scinto JM, Radford M. Warfarin use among patients with atrial fibrillation. *Stroke.* 1997;28:2382–2389.

27. McCrory DC, Matchar DB, Samsa G, Sanders LL, Pritchett ELC. Physician attitudes about anticoagulation for nonvalvular atrial fibrillation in the elderly. *Arch Intern Med.* 1995;155:277–281.

28. Bjerkelund C, Orning O. The efficacy of anticoagulant therapy in preventing embolism related to DC cardioversion of atrial fibrillation. *Am J Cardiol.* 1969;23:208–216.

29. Manning WJ, Silverman DL, Gordon SPF, Krumholz HM, Douglas PS. Cardioversion from atrial fibrillation without prolonged anticoagulation with use of transesophageal echocardiography to exclude the presence of atrial thrombi. *N Engl J Med.* 1993;328: 750–755.

30. Black IW, Fatkin D, Sagar KB, et al. Exclusion of atrial thrombus by transesophageal echocardiography does not preclude embolism after cardioversion of atrial fibrillation. *Circulation.* 1994;89:2509–2513.

31. Gage BF, Cardinalli AB, Albers GW, Owens DK. Cost-effectiveness of warfarin and aspirin for prophylaxis of stroke in patients with nonvalvular atrial fibrillation. *JAMA.* 1995;274:1839–1845.

32. Gustafsson C, Asplund K, Britton M, Norrving B, Olsson B, Marke L-A. Cost effectiveness of primary stroke prevention in atrial fibrillation: Swedish national perspective. *BMJ.* 1992;305:1457–1460.

Prevention and Treatment of Venous Thromboembolism

Graham F. Pineo and Russell D. Hull

INTRODUCTION

Pulmonary embolism results in death in approximately 150,000 patients per year in the United States and contributes to death in another 150,000 patients.[1,2] After acute myocardial infarction and stroke, pulmonary embolism is the third most common cause of cardiovascular death. It is the most common preventable cause of death in hospitalized patients.[3] Venous thromboembolism (pulmonary embolism and/or venous thrombosis) frequently develops in hospitalized patients with one or more co-morbid disorders, but this condition can also develop in otherwise healthy individuals who have undergone orthopaedic surgery or trauma or who are pregnant.[4] Although effective prophylaxis is available for most of these situations, venous thromboembolism can occur unexpectedly in ambulant patients, particularly if they have been exposed to risk factors during the preceding months.[5-8] When venous thromboembolism occurs, it is important that appropriate objective testing be performed so that an accurate diagnosis can be established and treatment can be instituted immediately. A massive pulmonary embolus might be the first indication that venous thromboembolism has occurred, and, unfortunately, it can be fatal within a short time in up to one-third of patients. This chapter highlights practical approaches to the diagnosis, prevention, and treatment of venous thromboembolism, including the use of anticoagulants, thrombolysis, embolectomy, and vena cava filters.

PATHOGENESIS OF VENOUS THROMBOEMBOLISM

Factors that predispose an individual to the development of venous thromboembolism are listed in Exhibit 20–1. Deep venous thrombosis (DVT) usually arises in the deep veins of the calf muscles or, less commonly, in the proximal deep veins of the leg.[9-12] When DVT remains confined to the calf veins, it is associated with a low risk of clinically important pulmonary embolism. Without treatment, however, approximately 20% of calf-vein thrombi extend into the proximal venous system, where they can pose a serious threat for a potentially life-threatening disorder.[13,14] Untreated proximal venous thrombosis is associated with a 10% risk of fatal pulmonary embolism and at least a 50% risk of pulmonary embolism or recurrent venous thrombosis.[11,12,15] In addition, the postphlebitic syndrome is associated with extensive proximal venous thrombosis and carries its own long-term morbidity. Pulmonary emboli in most cases (90%) originate from thrombi in the deep venous system of the legs.[16-20] Less common sources of pulmonary embolism include the deep pelvic veins or renal veins, the inferior vena cava, the right heart, and occasionally the axillary veins. The clinical significance of pulmonary embolism depends on the size of the embolus and the cardiorespiratory reserve of the patient.

Venous thromboembolism is generally considered to be a single disorder.[21-23] Therefore, the diagnostic approach might begin at the legs or the lungs, and testing starts with the least

Exhibit 20–1
FACTORS PREDISPOSING TO THE DEVELOPMENT OF VENOUS THROMBOEMBOLISM

- Clinical risk factors
  - surgical and nonsurgical trauma
  - previous venous thromboembolism
  - immobilization
  - malignant disease
  - heart disease
  - leg paralysis
  - age (> 40)
  - obesity
  - estrogens
  - parturition
- Inherited or acquired abnormalities
  - activated protein C resistance
  - protein C deficiency
  - protein S deficiency
  - antithrombin III deficiency
  - anticardiolipin syndrome
  - heparin-induced thrombocytopenia

invasive methods and proceeds to the more invasive methods. The treatment of venous thrombosis or pulmonary embolism is basically the same.

CLINICAL FEATURES

The clinical features of venous thrombosis include leg pain, tenderness and swelling, a palpable cord, discoloration, venous distention and prominence of the superficial veins, and cyanosis. None of the symptoms or signs is unique, and each can be caused by nonthrombotic disorders. This makes the clinical diagnosis of venous thrombosis highly nonspecific. Some patients with relatively minor symptoms and signs have extensive deep venous thrombi. Other patients have florid leg pain and swelling suggestive of extensive DVT, but objective testing might produce negative results.[24,25] Thus, objective testing is mandatory to confirm or exclude a diagnosis of venous thrombosis.

Pulmonary embolism presents clinically in various ways, depending on the size, location, and number of emboli and on the patient's underlying cardiorespiratory reserve. In general, the clinical manifestations of acute pulmonary embolism can be divided into four syndromes that overlap considerably:

1. transient dyspnea and tachypnea in the absence of other associated clinical manifestations
2. the syndrome of pulmonary infarction or congestive atelectasis (also known as ischemic pneumonitis or

incomplete infarction), including pleuritic chest pain, cough, hemoptysis, pleural effusion, and pulmonary infiltrates on the chest X-ray
3. an assortment of less common and highly nonspecific clinical features, such as confusion and coma, pyrexia, wheezing, resistant cardiac failure, and unexplained arrhythmia
4. acute massive pulmonary embolism[25]

In patients with acute massive pulmonary embolism, there is usually a dramatic presentation: a sudden onset of severe shortness of breath, hypoxemia, and right ventricular failure. Symptoms include central chest pain (often identical to angina), severe dyspnea, and, frequently, syncope, confusion, or coma. Examination reveals a patient in severe distress with tachypnea, cyanosis, and hypotension. The marked increase in pulmonary vascular resistance leads to acute right ventricular failure with the presence of large A waves in the jugular veins and a right ventricular diastolic gallop. When pulmonary hypertension is present, there is marked right ventricular dilatation with a shift of the intraventricular septum, decreasing cardiac output, and further decreasing coronary perfusion. This frequently results in cardiorespiratory arrest. If patients with a massive pulmonary embolus survive, they are acutely threatened by any further pulmonary thromboembolism.

It is now widely accepted that the clinical diagnosis of pulmonary embolism is highly nonspecific. Multiple studies indicate that this diagnosis is not confirmed by objective testing in more than half of all patients with clinically suspected pulmonary embolism.

In prospective studies, patients presenting with the clinical diagnosis of either DVT or pulmonary embolism have been assessed for clinical probabilities of the diagnosis before undergoing objective testing.[26–28] Although such pretest probabilities have been useful for experienced clinical investigators, they will require further assessment in prospective studies before their use can be generalized. Therefore, investigative algorithms that use objective tests still must be used to establish the diagnosis for a large proportion of patients with suspected venous thromboembolism.

LABORATORY FEATURES

A number of laboratory abnormalities have been associated with venous thromboembolism. These include increased levels of fibrinopeptide A and fibrinogen degradation products, thrombin-antithrombin complexes, prothrombin fragment 1.2, and D-dimer. Patients with venous thromboembolism frequently have other co-morbid conditions, including cancer, recent surgery or trauma, infection, and inflammation. Also, many of the laboratory changes associated with venous thromboembolism are highly nonspecific.

The D-dimer assay has been evaluated in several studies of patients who had clinically suspected DVT that was later confirmed by objective testing. The D-dimer can be measured by the enzyme-linked immunosorbent assay or by a latex agglutination assay.[29–31] When the appropriate cutoff is used, the negative predictive value of these tests is quite high in patients with suspected venous thromboembolism.[29–31] Several of these assays have a rapid turnaround time,[30] and some of them are quantitative, so that now they can be studied in a prospective fashion in patients with suspected venous thromboembolism.

OBJECTIVE TESTS FOR THE DIAGNOSIS OF VENOUS THROMBOEMBOLISM

Ancillary Tests

Various ancillary tests, such as chest X-ray, arterial blood gas measurement, and electrocardiogram, as well as laboratory tests for fibrinopeptide A, D-dimer, and serum lactate dehydrogenase, have a role in the diagnosis of venous thromboembolism, but they all lack sensitivity and specificity. The main role of these tests is to rule out other conditions that can mimic pulmonary embolism. Such conditions are acute myocardial infarction, pneumonia, and pneumothorax. In the case of venous thrombosis, objective tests include B-mode ultrasound, duplex ultrasonography, color flow ultrasonography, impedance plethysmography (IPG), and ascending venography. For the diagnosis of pulmonary embolism, the objective tests include ventilation-perfusion lung scanning and pulmonary angiography.

Ultrasonography

Venous imaging using real time B-mode ultrasound, with or without Doppler assessment, is a promising technique for evaluating patients with clinically suspected DVT.[32–39] As shown in prospective studies, the single criterion of vein compressibility is highly sensitive and specific for proximal venous thrombosis (sensitivity and specificity both greater than 95%).[32–35] Other criteria, such as echogenicity or change in venous diameter during a Valsalva maneuver, are less useful. The visualization of an echogenic band is highly sensitive but nonspecific (specificity 50%). The percentage of change in venous diameter during a Valsalva maneuver is both insensitive and nonspecific. Real time B-mode venous ultrasound is insensitive for isolated calf-vein thrombosis, and, as with IPG, serial testing is required to detect patients who develop proximal extension.[36–39] B-mode venous ultrasound can fail to detect isolated iliac-vein thrombi. This is a practical clinical limitation in patient groups in whom isolated iliac-vein thrombosis is not uncommon, such as the pregnant patient with clinically suspected venous thrombosis. Color flow imaging and other technologic advances have improved the ability of B-mode venous imaging to detect isolated iliac-vein thrombi and calf-vein thrombi.[39]

Doppler ultrasound is highly sensitive and specific for diagnosing proximal venous thrombosis in symptomatic patients. It is more sensitive than IPG for symptomatic calf-vein thrombosis and more reliable than IPG for detecting proximal venous thrombosis in patients with increased central venous pressure or with arterial insufficiency. Doppler ultrasound can be used in the patient who has a leg in a plaster cast, who has external fixation, who is in traction, or who has had a leg amputated. Ultrasonography lacks both sensitivity and specificity for the detection of asymptomatic venous thrombosis in postoperative patients.[40–44] Ascending venography remains the only reliable test for the detection of venous thrombosis in the high-risk patient or for clinical trials.

Impedance Plethysmography

IPG is sensitive and specific for proximal venous thrombosis in symptomatic patients, but it is insensitive for calf-vein thrombosis.[45–48] In patients with clinically suspected venous thrombosis, positive IPG results can be used to make therapeutic decisions as long as no clinical conditions known to produce false-positive results are present.[47–49] A normal result essentially excludes the diagnosis of proximal venous thrombosis, but it does not exclude calf-vein thrombosis. This potential limitation can be overcome by performing serial IPG. The use of serial IPG is based on the concept (now confirmed by clinical observation) that calf-vein thrombi are clinically important only when extension into the proximal veins occurs; at this point, detection with IPG becomes possible. The effectiveness and safety of IPG have been evaluated by prospective clinical trials in patients with clinically suspected venous thrombosis.[9,10,12,23] From these studies, two recommendations can be made:

1. A positive result by IPG is highly predictive of acute proximal vein thrombosis (positive predictive value greater than 90%).
2. It is safe to withhold anticoagulant therapy in symptomatic patients who remain negative by serial IPG for 10 to 14 days.

As in the case of ultrasonography, IPG lacks sensitivity for the detection of asymptomatic venous thrombosis after surgery.[50,51] False-positive results can occur in disorders that interfere with arterial inflow or venous outflow. Such disorders include severe congestive cardiac failure, constrictive pericarditis, severe arterial insufficiency, hypotension, and external compression of the veins. Most of these disorders are readily recognized on clinical grounds.

Venography

Venography is accepted as the standard objective method for the diagnosis of venous thrombosis.[52–54] Venography is a difficult technique to perform well, and accurate interpretation requires considerable experience. A number of venographic abnormalities have been defined as criteria for the diagnosis of acute DVT.[24] The most reliable of these is the presence of an intraluminal filling defect that is constant on all films and can be seen in a number of projections. Other venographic abnormalities, such as nonfilling of a segment of the deep venous system or nonfilling of the entire deep venous system above the knee, can be caused by technical artifacts, particularly if the dye is injected too far proximally into the dorsal foot vein. Such artifacts then could be interpreted to indicate either a thrombus because the vein is not filled or a normal vein because a filling defect is not seen. The common femoral, external iliac, and common iliac veins might not be adequately filled by ascending venography, which can lead to an incorrect diagnosis as the result of inadequate venography. In the case of nonfilling of an entire segment of the deep venous system, the diagnosis of acute or recurrent venous thrombosis must depend on the use of other tests, such as IPG or ultrasound.

A number of problems are related to venography. Even in the best of circumstances, it might be impossible to cannulate a vein on the dorsum of the foot and so make ascending venography impossible on one or both legs. If there is inadequate filling of the common femoral or iliac systems, it might be necessary to perform a femoral venogram.

Venography is associated with a number of clinically troublesome side effects. Pain can occur in the foot while dye is being injected, or delayed pain can occur in the calf one or two days after injection. The procedure can be complicated by superficial phlebitis and even DVT in a small percentage of patients with normal venograms (1 to 2%).[45] Other, less common complications of venography include hypersensitivity to the radiopaque dye and local skin or tissue necrosis resulting from extravasation of dye at the site of injection. Both nonionic and high-ionic contrast media can cause or aggravate renal insufficiency in patients at high risk for these complications (eg, patients with established renal disease, hypertension, heart failure, diabetes, or multiple myeloma).[55,56] The risks of venography must be carefully weighed in such circumstances and reviewed with patients before venography is performed.

Ventilation-Perfusion Lung Scanning

Perfusion lung scanning is the key diagnostic test for patients with suspected pulmonary embolism.[57] A normal perfusion scan excludes important pulmonary embolism. An abnormal perfusion scan, however, is nonspecific and can occur in conditions that produce either increased radiographic density (eg, pneumonia, atelectasis, pleural effusion) or a regional reduction in ventilation (eg, chronic obstructive lung disease, acute asthma, bronchial mucous plugs, bronchitis—conditions frequently associated with normal radiography).

Ventilation imaging improves the specificity of an abnormal perfusion scan by differentiating between embolic occlusion of the pulmonary vasculature and perfusion defects occurring secondary to a primary disorder of ventilation.[58] Recent prospective clinical trials show the basic premise—perfusion defects that ventilate normally (ventilation-perfusion mismatch) are due to pulmonary embolism but that matching ventilation-perfusion abnormalities are due to other conditions—to be incorrect.

Ventilation lung scanning is helpful only if the perfusion defect is segmental or greater and is associated with ventilation mismatch. Pulmonary angiography shows that such patients have a high probability ($\geq$86%) of pulmonary embolism.[57] Other abnormal findings on lung scans, such as matching ventilation-perfusion defects (either segmental or subsegmental), subsegmental defects with ventilation mismatch, or perfusion defects that correspond to an area of increased density on the chest radiograph (nondiagnostic perfusion scan), are associated with a 20%–40% frequency of pulmonary embolism. Therefore, further investigations, including pulmonary angiography and objective tests for venous thrombosis, must be carried out in patients with nondiagnostic ventilation-perfusion scan findings. Pulmonary angiography and/or venography should be used when other approaches are unavailable or inconclusive. The morbidity associated with these tests is substantially less than that arising from unnecessary anticoagulant therapy and inappropriate hospitalization.

At least 80% of patients with pulmonary embolism have thrombi that originate in the lower leg veins.[11] Prospective studies in patients with nondiagnostic lung scan findings who have adequate cardiorespiratory reserve indicate that serial noninvasive leg testing is a simple and safe alternative to pulmonary angiography.[59,60] If the noninvasive leg test is positive initially or on serial screening, anticoagulant treatment can be instituted. On the other hand, if noninvasive leg testing remains negative for 10 to 14 days, anticoagulant therapy can be safely withheld. Pulmonary angiography is required in patients with decreased cardiopulmonary reserve and nondiagnostic lung scan findings.

Pulmonary Angiography

Pulmonary angiography is the accepted diagnostic reference standard for pulmonary embolism.[61] The diagnosis is established if an intraluminal filling defect is a constant finding on multiple films or if abrupt termination (cutoff) of a vessel greater than 2–5 mm in diameter is a constant finding on multiple films. Other abnormalities, such as oligemia, vessel pruning, and loss of filling of small vessels, are nonspecific and occur in a variety of conditions, including pneumonia, atelectasis, bronchiectasis, emphysema, and pulmonary carcinoma.[61]

In recent years, the diagnostic resolution of pulmonary angiography has been markedly improved and the risk to the patient decreased by the use of selective catheterization with repeated injections of small volumes of dye. This is a safe technique in the absence of severe chronic pulmonary hypertension or severe cardiac or respiratory decompensation. Clinically significant complications, including tachyarrhythmias, endocardial or myocardial injury, cardiac perforation, cardiac arrest, and hypersensitivity reactions to contrast medium, occur in fewer than 3% to 4% of patients.[61]

RECOMMENDED APPROACHES TO THE DIAGNOSIS OF VENOUS THROMBOEMBOLISM

Deep Vein Thrombosis

In patients with symptoms of DVT, both IPG and compression ultrasound (CUS) have been reported to have a high degree of accuracy. The negative predictive value of both tests is high so that either test can be used to exclude the diagnosis. Recent studies indicate that CUS has a higher sensitivity when compared with IPG using venography as the gold standard for the diagnosis of proximal venous thrombosis.[26] Both CUS and IPG have relatively low sensitivities when the distal popliteal veins are involved with small thrombi. Therefore, in patients with suspected venous thrombosis who have a negative CUS or IPG, serial testing will detect thrombi that extend and become more occlusive. If a diagnosis is more urgently required, ascending venography can be performed.

An algorithm describing an approach to the diagnosis of venous thrombosis is shown in Figure 20–1, in which CUS is used as the main screening test.

Pulmonary Embolism

The ventilation-perfusion lung scan is the main screening test for patients with suspected pulmonary embolism. Using the Prospective Investigation of Pulmonary Embolism Diagnosis criteria, if the lung scan shows a high probability pattern, the patient is treated with anticoagulants. If the pattern is normal, the patient requires no further testing and no treatment. In patients with a nondiagnostic lung scan pattern and poor cardiorespiratory reserve, pulmonary angiography should be performed; however, in patients with nondiagnostic lung scan patterns and normal cardiorespira-

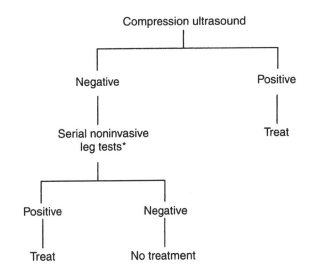

*Ascending venography can be used in place of serial noninvasive leg testing.

Figure 20–1 Approach to the diagnosis of suspected deep vein thrombosis

tory reserve, a noninvasive leg test (eg, CUS) should be performed. If the test is positive, the patient is treated. If the test is negative, the patient can be followed with serial noninvasive leg tests for a period of two weeks. For patients whose tests remain negative during this period, it is considered safe to withhold anticoagulants. If a diagnosis is more urgently required, pulmonary angiography would be the test of choice. Algorithms showing the approaches to the diagnosis of suspected pulmonary embolism are presented in Figures 20–2 and 20–3.

PREVENTION OF VENOUS THROMBOSIS IN GENERAL SURGERY AND ORTHOPAEDICS

Unless prophylaxis against DVT is applied, the frequency of fatal pulmonary embolism ranges from 0.1% to 0.8% in patients undergoing elective general surgery,[62] from 2% to 3% in patients undergoing elective hip replacement,[63] and from 4% to 7% in patients undergoing surgery for fractured hip.[64] Many physicians and surgeons still do not comply with recommendations for prophylaxis of venous thromboembolism, despite the fact that there is convincing evidence for the efficacy and safety of a number of agents.[5–8,64,65] A retrospective audit of hospitals in Massachusetts indicated that prophylaxis of venous thromboembolism, even in high-risk patients, was grossly underutilized, particularly in nonteaching hospitals.[66] In orthopaedic surgery, as shown in surveys conducted in England and Sweden, some form of prophylaxis, usually in the form of drugs, is used in the majority of cases.[67,68]

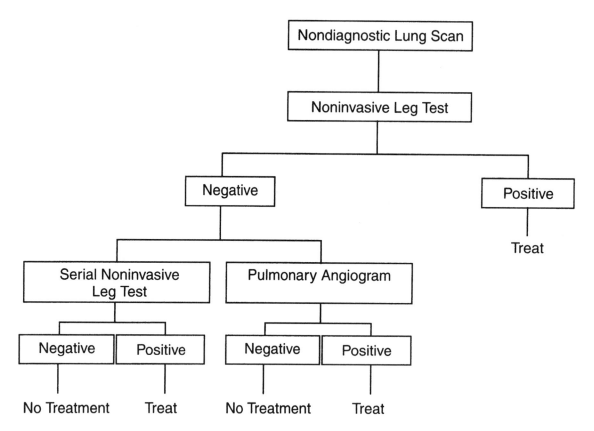

Figure 20–2 Approach to the diagnosis of suspected pulmonary embolism in patients with adequate cardiorespiratory reserve and nondiagnostic lung scan

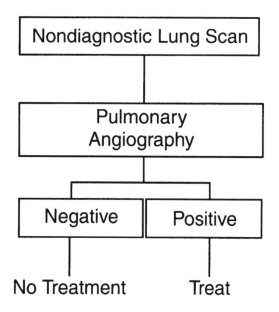

Figure 20–3 Approach to the diagnosis of suspected pulmonary embolism in patients with inadequate cardiorespiratory reserve and nondiagnostic lung scan

Two approaches can be taken to prevent fatal pulmonary embolism:

1. primary prophylaxis, using either drugs or physical methods that are effective for preventing DVT.
2. secondary prevention by the early detection and treatment of subclinical venous thrombosis by screening postoperative patients with objective tests that are sensitive for venous thrombosis.

Primary prophylaxis is preferred in most clinical circumstances. Prevention of DVT and pulmonary embolism is more cost-effective than treating the complications where they occur.[69–71] Secondary prevention by case-finding studies should never replace primary prophylaxis. It is reserved for patients in whom primary prophylaxis is either contraindicated or relatively ineffective.

The recommended primary prophylactic approach depends on the patient's risk category and the type of surgery. The risk for calf-vein thrombosis, proximal vein thrombosis, and fatal pulmonary embolism has been assessed by objective tests for patients undergoing a variety of surgical procedures.[8] The risk of postoperative DVT can be identified as low, moderate, or high, depending on the surgical procedure and the presence or absence of additional risk factors.

The ideal primary prophylactic method is described as:

- effective compared with placebo or active approaches
- safe
- good compliance with patient, nurses, and physicians
- ease of administration
- no need for laboratory monitoring
- cost-effective

The prophylactic measures most commonly used are low-dose or adjusted-dose unfractionated heparin, low–molecular-weight heparin, oral anticoagulants (International Normalized Ratio, 2.0–3.0), and intermittent pneumatic leg compression.[72] Ideally, prophylaxis should be started before the operation and continued until the patient is fully ambulant. Studies are currently underway to assess the need for continued prophylaxis following discharge in patients at high risk of developing DVT, such as those who have total hip replacement.

SPECIFIC PROPHYLACTIC MEASURES

Low-Dose Heparin

Low-dose subcutaneous heparin is usually given in a dose of 5,000 units 2 hours preoperatively and then postoperatively every 8 or 12 hours (Exhibit 20–2). The effectiveness of low-dose heparin for preventing DVT has been established by multiple randomized clinical trials. Most of the patients in these trials underwent abdominothoracic surgery, particularly for gastrointestinal disease, but also included were patients who had gynecologic and urologic surgery, as well as some who had mastectomy or vascular procedures. Pooled data from meta-analyses confirm that low-dose heparin reduces the incidence of all DVTs, proximal deep vein thrombosis, and all pulmonary emboli.[5–8] The International Multicentre Trial also established the effectiveness of low-dose heparin for preventing fatal pulmonary embolism with a clinically striking reduction from 0.7%–0.1%.[62]

The incidence of major bleeding complications is not increased by low-dose heparin, but there is an increase in minor wound hematomas. The platelet count should be monitored regularly in all patients on low-dose heparin to detect the rare but significant development of heparin-induced thrombocytopenia. Low-dose heparin has the advantages of being relatively inexpensive and easily administered and not requiring anticoagulant monitoring.

Adjusted-Dose Heparin

Adjusted-dose subcutaneous heparin was shown to be an effective approach for prophylaxis when compared with low-dose heparin or low–molecular-weight heparin in patients undergoing total hip replacement or when compared with low-dose heparin in patients with spinal cord injury.[73–75] Bleeding occurred more commonly in the latter group with

---

Exhibit 20–2
HEPARIN PROTOCOL

- Initial intravenous heparin bolus: 5,000 units
- Continuous intravenous heparin infusion: commence at 42 mL/hour of 20,000 units (1,680 units/hour) in 500 mL of two-thirds dextrose and one-third saline (a 24-hour heparin dose of 40,320 units), except in the following patients, in whom heparin infusion will be commenced at a rate of 31 mL/hour (1,240 units/hour) (ie, a 24-hour dose of 29,760 units):
  - patients who have undergone surgery within the previous two weeks
  - patients with a previous history of peptic ulcer disease or gastrointestinal or genitourinary bleeding
  - patients with recent stroke (ie, thrombotic stroke within two weeks previously)
  - patients with a platelet count <150 × 10^9 per liter
  - patients with miscellaneous reasons for a high risk of bleeding (eg, hepatic failure, renal failure, or vitamin K deficiency)
- Heparin dose adjusted by using the activated partial thromboplastin time (aPTT). The aPTT is performed in all patients as outlined below:
  - The aPTT is performed 4–6 hours after commencing heparin; the heparin dose is then adjusted according to information presented in Table 20–1.
  - The aPTT is performed 4–6 hours after implementing the first dosage adjustment.
  - The aPTT is then performed as indicated by the nomogram for the first 24 hours of therapy.
  - Thereafter, the aPTT will be performed once daily, unless the patient is subtherapeutic, in which case the aPTT will be repeated 4–6 hours after increasing the heparin dose.

Source: Reprinted with permission from RD Hull, GE Raskob, D Rosenbloom et al, Optimal Therapeutic Level of Heparin Therapy in Patients with Venous Thrombosis, *Archives of Internal Medicine*, Vol 152, pp 1589–1595, © 1992, American Medical Association.

adjusted-dose heparin, however, than in patients with fixed-dose heparin.[75] Adjusted-dose heparin has not become popular because of the time and expense required for laboratory monitoring.

Low–Molecular-Weight Heparin

Several low–molecular-weight heparin fractions have been evaluated by randomized clinical trials in moderate-risk general surgical patients.[76–80] The heparin fractions most extensively evaluated include daltaparin, fraxiparine, enoxaparin, and tinzaparin. In randomized clinical trials comparing low–molecular-weight heparin with unfractionated heparin, the low–molecular-weight heparins given once or twice daily have been shown to be as effective or more effective in preventing thrombosis.[76–80] Most of the trials documented similarly low frequencies of bleeding for low–molecular-weight heparin and low-dose unfractionated heparin, although the incidence of bleeding was somewhat higher with unfractionated heparin when various bleeding end points were combined.[76]

During the past several years, there have been a few large randomized clinical trials in patients undergoing total joint replacement (hip or knee).[81–87] Various low–molecular-weight heparins have been compared with placebo, unfractionated heparin, adjusted-dose heparin, dextran 70, and warfarin sodium. Compared with placebo, low–molecular-weight heparin significantly decreased the rates of both distal and proximal DVTs with no significant increase in bleeding rates.[81–87] Low–molecular-weight heparins were at least as effective as low-dose unfractionated heparin given two or three times daily. Bleeding rates were comparable in the unfractionated heparin and low–molecular-weight heparin groups, with the exception of one study using unfractionated heparin, 7,500 units twice daily.[84] Studies comparing low–molecular-weight heparin with dextran 70 showed a significant improvement in thrombosis rates with low–molecular-weight heparin and no significant differences in bleeding rates.

In a meta-analysis, low–molecular-weight heparin is shown to be somewhat more effective than unfractionated heparin in the prevention of venous thrombosis following general surgery or orthopaedic surgery, but it is associated with a slightly higher risk of bleeding.[88] The low–molecular-weight heparins have the advantage that they can be given once a day at a constant dose without any laboratory monitoring. Studies comparing the cost-effectiveness of low–molecular-weight heparin with either warfarin or unfractionated heparin are currently underway.

Oral Anticoagulants

Prophylaxis with oral anticoagulants can be commenced 12 hours preoperatively, at the time of operation, or during the early postoperative period. Although oral anticoagulants might not prevent the development of venous thrombi during surgery, these agents are effective in inhibiting the extension of thrombi that might form and can thereby prevent clinically important venous thromboembolism.

Warfarin started postoperatively has been compared with low–molecular-weight heparin[86,87] or intermittent pneumatic compression in patients undergoing total hip or knee replacement.[89–91] Little or no difference was noted in the incidence of postoperative venous thrombosis or bleeding.[89–91] Very–low-dose warfarin did not provide protection against DVT following hip replacement.[92]

In patients suffering hip fractures, warfarin was superior to aspirin or placebo in the prevention of venous thrombosis.[93] Very–low-dose oral anticoagulants (warfarin, 1 mg/day), when compared with placebo, was shown to decrease postoperative thrombosis rates in patients undergoing gynecologic surgery or major general surgery[94] and to decrease the thrombosis rate in indwelling central line catheters.[95]

Intermittent Pneumatic Compression

Intermittent pneumatic compression (IPC) prevents venous thrombosis by enhancing blood flow in the deep veins of the legs and by increasing blood fibrinolytic activity. IPC is effective in preventing venous thrombosis in moderate-risk general surgical patients[96] and patients undergoing neurosurgery.[97–99] In patients undergoing hip surgery, IPC involving either calf compression or both calf and thigh compression effectively decreases calf-vein thrombosis, but the incidence of proximal venous thrombosis remains moderately high.[100] In patients undergoing total knee replacement, IPC of the calf decreased distal venous thrombosis, but proximal thrombosis remained high.[101] Combined calf and thigh compression reduced the incident rate of both distal and proximal venous thromboses.

Intermittent pneumatic leg compression is virtually free of clinically important side effects, and it offers a valuable alternative in patients who have a high risk of bleeding. Various well-accepted, comfortable, and effective IPC devices are currently available for applying preoperatively, at the time of operation, or in the early postoperative period. IPC should be continued for the entire postoperative period until the patient is fully ambulatory.

Graduated Compression Stockings

Graduated compression stockings reduce venous stasis in the limb by applying a graded degree of compression to the ankle and the calf with greater pressure being applied more distally in the limb. Clinical trials demonstrate graduated compression stockings to be effective for preventing postoperative venous thrombosis in low-risk general surgical patients and in selected moderate-risk patients.[102–104] A more recent meta-analysis confirmed the reduction of venous thrombosis following moderate risk surgery with the use of graduated compression stockings.[105] There is inadequate information to verify whether graduated compression stockings used in combination with other forms of prophylaxis result in any further risk reduction.

SPECIFIC RECOMMENDATIONS

Recommendations for the prevention of venous thrombosis are derived from the Fourth American College of Chest Physicians Consensus Conference on Antithrombotic Therapy.[72]

Low-Risk Patients

Low-risk general surgery patients with no added risk factors require no prophylaxis apart from early ambulation.

Moderate-Risk Patients

When undergoing major operations, moderate-risk general surgery patients who are older than 40 years but have no additional risk factors can receive graduated compression stockings, low-dose heparin, or IPC. In all moderate-risk patients, the use of subcutaneous low dose heparin (5,000 units every 8 or 12 hours) or subcutaneous low–molecular-weight heparin is recommended. An alternative recommendation is intermittent pneumatic compression used continuously until the patient is ambulatory. This method is indicated in patients at a high risk of bleeding. In some countries, it is routine clinical custom to combine the pharmacologic methods with graduated compression stockings in selected patients.

High-Risk Patients

- *Higher-Risk General Surgery.* Patients older than 40 years who undergo major operations and have additional risk factors should receive low-dose heparin or low–molecular-weight heparin. Those patients who are prone to wound complications, such as hematomas and infection, should receive IPC. High-risk general surgery patients with multiple risk factors should receive low-dose heparin or low–molecular-weight heparin combined with IPC. Perioperative warfarin therapy can be used in selected, very–high-risk general surgery patients.
- *Total Hip Replacement.* Recommended prophylactic measures include low–molecular-weight heparin, low-

intensity oral anticoagulation (INR 2.0–3.0), or adjusted-dose heparin.
- *Total Knee Replacement Surgery.* Recommended prophylaxis includes low–molecular-weight heparin and IPC.
- *Hip Fracture Surgery.* Recommended prophylaxis is either low–molecular-weight heparin started preoperatively or oral anticoagulation started postoperatively.
- *Intracranial Neurosurgery.* IPC with or without graduated compression stockings should be used. In very-high-risk neurosurgical patients, IPC can be combined with low-dose heparin.
- *Acute Spinal Cord Injury.* Recommended prophylaxis is adjusted-dose heparin or low–molecular-weight heparin.
- *Multiple Trauma.* Recommendations include IPC, warfarin, and low–molecular-weight heparin.

Effective prophylaxis is available for patients undergoing general surgery, although it is disappointing that such measures are not applied more uniformly. Low-dose subcutaneous unfractionated heparin or low–molecular-weight heparin is used most extensively, with sequential intermittent compression being recommended in selected cases. For orthopaedic surgery, the options include low–molecular-weight heparin, warfarin, and IPC. In the future, studies will include the use of combined modalities and the use of newer antithrombotic agents. The ultimate goal for clinicians is to minimize the incidence of fatal pulmonary embolism in all patients undergoing surgical procedures.

TREATMENT OF VENOUS THROMBOEMBOLISM

The three objectives of treatment in patients with venous thromboembolism are

1. to prevent death from pulmonary embolism
2. to prevent recurrent venous thromboembolism
3. to prevent the postphlebitic syndrome

The accepted anticoagulant therapy for venous thromboembolism is a combination of continuous intravenous heparin and oral warfarin sodium.[106–110] The use of heparin and warfarin simultaneously has become standard clinical practice for all patients with venous thromboembolism who are medically stable.[109,110] Exceptions include patients who require immediate medical or surgical intervention, such as thrombolysis or insertion of a vena cava filter, and patients at high risk for bleeding. The length of the initial intravenous heparin therapy has been reduced to five days, thus shortening the hospital stay and leading to significant cost savings.[110]

Heparin Therapy

The anticoagulant activity of unfractionated heparin depends on a unique pentasaccharide that binds to antithrombin III (AT-III) and potentiates the inhibition of thrombin and activated factor X (Xa) by AT-III.[111,112] Heparin also catalyzes the inactivation of thrombin by another plasma cofactor, heparin cofactor II, which acts independently of AT-III. Other effects of heparin include

- the release of tissue factor inhibitor
- the binding to numerous plasma and platelet proteins, endothelial cells, and leukocytes
- an increase in vascular permeability

The anticoagulant response to a standard dose of heparin varies widely among patients. It is necessary, therefore, to monitor the anticoagulant response of heparin either by measuring the activated partial thromboplastin time (aPTT) or heparin levels and to titrate the dose to the individual patient.[106,107]

The laboratory test most commonly used to monitor heparin therapy is the aPTT. The traditional approach has been to adjust the heparin infusion dose to maintain the aPTT within a defined "therapeutic range."[112] Over the years, this therapeutic range has evolved as a result of clinical custom to the use of upper and lower limits (an aPTT ratio of 1.5 to 2.5 times control). The clinical practice of adjusting the heparin dose to maintain the aPTT response within this range is based on two concepts:

1. Maintaining the aPTT ratio above the lower limit of 1.5 will minimize recurrent venous thromboembolic events.
2. Maintaining the aPTT ratio below the upper limit of 2.5 will minimize the risk of bleeding complications.

It has been established from experimental studies and clinical trials that the efficacy of heparin therapy is dependent on achieving a critical therapeutic level of heparin within the first 24 hours of treatment.[113–115] Patients receiving heparin, either by continuous intravenous infusion or intermittent subcutaneous injection, who do not achieve therapeutic aPTT values during initial therapy, have an increased risk of recurrent venous thromboembolism during follow-up over the subsequent 3 to 12 weeks. The critical therapeutic level of heparin, as measured by the aPTT, is 1.5 times the mean of the control value or the upper limit of the normal aPTT range. This corresponds to a heparin blood level of 0.2 to 0.4 units/mL by the protamine sulfate titration assay and 0.35 to 0.70 u/mL by the anti-factor Xa assay.[116] When using reagents from different manufacturers or even using different batches of the same reagent, however, the aPTT and heparin blood levels vary widely. Therefore, it is vital for each laboratory to establish the minimal therapeutic level of heparin, as measured by the aPTT, that provides a heparin blood level of at least 0.2 units/mL, as measured by the protamine sulfate titration assay, for each batch of thromboplastin reagent being used, particularly for reagents provided by different manufacturers.[116]

Although there is a strong correlation between sub-therapeutic aPTT values and recurrent thromboembolism, the relationship between supratherapeutic aPTT and bleeding (aPTT ratio 2.5 or more) is less definite. Indeed, bleeding during heparin therapy is more closely related to underlying clinical risk factors than to aPTT elevation above the therapeutic range.[110] Recent studies confirm that age greater than 65 years and female gender increase the risk of bleeding while on heparin.

Numerous audits of heparin therapy indicate that administration of intravenous heparin is fraught with difficulty and that the clinical practice of using an ad hoc or intuitive approach to heparin dose-titration frequently results in inadequate therapy.[117–119] For example, an audit of physician practices at three university-affiliated hospitals shows that 60% of patients failed to achieve an adequate aPTT response (ratio 1.5) during the initial 24 hours of therapy.[118] Further 30% to 40% of patients remained subtherapeutic over the next three to four days.

Two clinical trials evaluated the use of a prescriptive protocol for administering intravenous heparin therapy in patients with venous thromboembolism.[114,120] In one trial, patients with proximal venous thrombosis were given either intravenous heparin alone, followed subsequently by warfarin sodium, or intravenous heparin and simultaneous warfarin sodium. This heparin nomogram is summarized in Table 20–1. Only 2% and 1% of the patients were subtherapeutic for more than 24 hours in the heparin and warfarin group and in the group initially receiving only heparin, respectively. Recurrent venous thromboembolism, objectively documented, occurred in both groups infrequently, for a rate of 7%, which is similar to trials previously reported. These findings demonstrate that subtherapy was avoided in most patients and that the heparin protocol resulted in effective delivery of heparin therapy in both groups.[120]

In the second clinical trial, a weight-based heparin-dosing nomogram was compared with a standard care nomogram (Table 20–2).[114] In the weight-adjusted group, 89% of patients achieved the therapeutic range within 24 hours, compared with 75% in the standard care group. The risk of recurrent thromboembolism was more frequent in the standard care group. This trial included patients with unstable angina and arterial thromboembolism in addition to venous thromboembolism, thus indicating that the principles applied to a heparin nomogram for the treatment of venous thromboembolism might be generalizable to other clinical conditions.[114]

Table 20–1 Intravenous Heparin Dose–Titration Nomogram for aPTT

aPTT	IV Infusion		Additional action
	Rate Change (mL/hour)	Dose Change (U/24 hours*)	
≤45	+6	+5,760	Repeat aPTT[†] in 4–6 hours
46–54	+3	+2,880	Repeat aPTT in 4–6 hours
55–85	0	0	None[‡]
86–110	−3	−2,880	Stop heparin sodium treatment for 1 hour; repeat aPTT 4–6 hours after restarting heparin treatment
>110	−6	−5,760	Stop heparin treatment for 1 hour; repeat aPTT 4–6 hours after restarting heparin treatment

*Heparin sodium concentration, 2000 U in 500 mL = 40 U/mL.
[†]With the use of actin-FS thromboplastin reagent.
[‡]During the first 24 hours, repeat aPTT in 4 to 6 hours. Thereafter, the aPTT will be determined once daily, unless subtherapeutic.

Key: aPTT, activated partial thromboplastin time; IV, intravenous.

Source: Reprinted with permission from RD Hull, GE Raskob, D Rosenbloom et al, Optimal Therapeutic Level of Heparin Therapy in Patients with Venous Thrombosis, *Archives of Internal Medicine*, Vol 152, pp 1589–1595, © 1992, American Medical Association.

Complications of Heparin Therapy

The main side effects of heparin therapy include bleeding, thrombocytopenia, and osteoporosis, with rarer complications being hypersensitivity, hypoaldosteronism, and elevated liver enzymes. Approximately 5% of patients on continuous intravenous heparin experience major bleeding. Patients at particular risk are those who have had recent surgery or trauma, or who have other predisposing clinical factors, such as peptic ulcer, occult malignancy, liver disease, or hemostatic defects. Age greater than 65 years and female gender predispose to bleeding on heparin.

The management of bleeding on heparin will depend on the location and severity of bleeding, the risk of recurrent venous thromboembolism, and the level of the aPTT. Heparin should be discontinued temporarily or permanently. Patients with recent venous thromboembolism might be candidates for insertion of an inferior vena cava filter. If urgent reversal of the heparin effect is required, protamine sulfate can be administered.

Heparin-induced thrombocytopenia is a well-recognized complication of heparin therapy; it usually occurs within 5 to 10 days after the start of heparin treatment.[121–124] Approximately 1%–2% of patients receiving unfractionated heparin experience a fall in platelet count to less than the normal range or a 50% fall in the platelet count within the normal range. In the majority of cases, this mild to moderate thrombocytopenia appears to be a direct effect of heparin on platelets and is of no consequence. Approximately 0.1%–0.2% of patients receiving heparin, however, develop an

Table 20–2 Weight-Based Nomogram

Initial dose	80 U/Kg bolus, then 18 U/kg/hour
aPTT, <35s (<1.2 × control)	80 U/kg bolus, then 4 U/kg/hour
aPTT, 35–45s (1.2–1.5 × control)	40 U/kg bolus, then 2 U/kg/hour
aPTT, 46–70s (1.5–2.3 × control)	No change
aPTT, 71–90s (2.3–3.0 × control)	Decrease infusion rate by 2 U/kg/hour
aPTT >90s (>3.0 × control)	Hold infusion 1 hour, then decrease infusion rate by 3 U/kg/hour

Key: aPTT, activated partial thromboplastin time; s, seconds.

Source: Reprinted with permission from RA Raschke, BM Reilly, JR Guidry et al, The Weight-Based Heparin Dosing Nomogram Compared with a "Standard Care" Nomogram, *Annals of Internal Medicine*, Vol 119, pp 874–881, © 1993, American College of Physicians.

immune thrombocytopenia mediated by IgG antibody directed against a complex of PF4 and heparin.[125–128] The development of thrombocytopenia might be accompanied by arterial or venous thrombosis, which can lead to serious consequences, such as death or limb amputation. The diagnosis of heparin-induced thrombocytopenia, with or without thrombosis, must be made on clinical grounds because the assays with the highest sensitivity and specificity are not readily available and have a slow turnaround time.[122–124]

When the diagnosis of heparin-induced thrombocytopenia is made, heparin in all forms must be stopped immediately.[122] For patients requiring ongoing anticoagulation, several alternatives exist: warfarin therapy; insertion of an inferior vena cava filter; or use of the defibrinogenating extract of snake venom Arvin,[129] the heparinoid Danaparoid sodium,[130] and, more recently, the specific antithrombins hirudin or argatroban. Most of the reports in case series have included the use of Arvin or Danaparoid, but clinical trials are currently underway to assess the efficacy and safety of the specific antithrombin agents.

Osteoporosis has been reported in patients receiving unfractionated heparin in doses of 20,000 units or more per day for more than 6 months.[112] Demineralization can progress to the fracture of vertebral bodies or long bones, and the defect might not be entirely reversible.

Other complications of heparin therapy, such as hypersensitivity, elevated liver enzymes, and hyperkalemia secondary to hypoaldosteronism, are rare and of little clinical consequence.

Low–Molecular-Weight Heparin

In recent years, there has been an increasing trend to manage medical and surgical conditions in the outpatient setting. Furthermore, the downsizing of hospitals in North America has made bed availability a constant problem, thereby encouraging the development of outpatient management programs to ensure proper use of the limited number of beds. At the same time, the treatment of venous thromboembolism has been facilitated by the advent of the low–molecular-weight heparins. This section reviews the evidence supporting outpatient treatment of venous thromboembolism and discusses some of the logistic problems that such programs create.

Advantages of Low–Molecular-Weight Heparin over Unfractionated Heparin

The low–molecular-weight heparins differ from unfractionated heparin in numerous ways.[131,132] Important differences include the following: increased bioavailability (>90% after subcutaneous injection); prolonged half-life and predictable clearance, enabling once- or twice-day injection; and predictable antithrombotic response based on body weight, permitting treatment without laboratory monitoring.[131,132] Patients or other caregivers in the home can be readily taught to inject low–molecular-weight heparin, particularly from prefilled syringes. Other possible advantages include an ability to inhibit platelet bound factor Xa, resistance to inhibition by platelet factor IV, and decreased effect on platelet function and vascular permeability (possibly accounting for less hemorrhagic effects at comparable antithrombotic doses).[131,132] The use of low–molecular-weight heparins also is associated with a lower incidence of heparin-induced thrombocytopenia and osteoporosis when compared with unfractionated heparin.[132]

Treatment of Venous Thromboembolism with Low–Molecular-Weight Heparin

In a number of early clinical trials, some of which were dose finding, low–molecular-weight heparin given by subcutaneous or intravenous injection was compared with continuous intravenous unfractionated heparin with repeat venography at day 7 to 10 being the primary end point.[133–141] These studies demonstrated that low–molecular-weight heparin is at least as effective as unfractionated heparin in preventing extension or increasing resolution of thrombi on repeat venography.

A number of recent level I clinical trials[142] used the more useful end points of recurrence of venous thromboembolism on follow-up and major bleeding during initial therapy.[133–137,143,144] Most of these studies compared the once- or twice-daily subcutaneous injection of low–molecular-weight heparin with a continuous infusion of unfractionated heparin in patients presenting with proximal and, in some cases, distal venous thrombosis.[133–137,144] However, one study specifically addressed patients presenting with acute pulmonary embolism.[143] The outcomes of these inpatient trials, in terms of recurrent venous thromboembolism, major bleeding, and mortality, are summarized in Table 20–3.

Outpatient Treatment of DVT and Pulmonary Embolism with Low–Molecular-Weight Heparin

Three level I clinical trials[142] compared the use of low–molecular-weight heparin given primarily in the outpatient setting with continuous, intravenous, unfractionated heparin given in-hospital to patients with proximal venous thrombosis.[140,141,145] The outcomes relative to recurrent venous thromboembolism and major bleeding are shown in Table 20–4. All studies found that outpatient treatment of select patients with proximal venous thrombosis with low–molecular-weight heparin is as effective and safe as treatment with continuous, intravenous unfractionated heparin in-hospital.[140,141,145] However, it is important to emphasize that these patients were carefully selected, and not all eligible patients entered the study. Thus the results may not be entirely generalizable. Also, many patients with proximal venous thrombosis will

Table 20–3 Randomized Trials of Low–Molecular-Weight Heparin versus Unfractionated Heparin for the In-Hospital Treatment of Proximal Deep Vein Thrombosis or Acute Pulmonary Embolism: Results of Long-Term Follow-Up

Reference	Treatment	Recurrent Venous Thromboembolism, no. (%)	Major Bleeding, no. (%)	Mortality, no. (%)
Hull et al[133]	Tinzaparin	6/213 (2.8)	1/213 (0.5)	10/213 (4.7)
	Heparin	15/219 (6.8)	11/219 (5.0)	21/219 (9.6)
Prandoni et al[134]	Nadroparin	6/85 (7.1)	1/85 (1.2)	6/85 (7.1)
	Heparin	12/85 (14.1)	3/85 (3.5)	12/85 (14.1)
Lopaciuk et al[135]	Nadroparin	0/74 (0)	0/74	0/74
	Heparin	3/72 (4.2)	1/72 (1.4)	1/72 (1.4)
Simonneau et al[136]	Enoxaparin	0/67	0/67	3/67 (4.5)
	Heparin	0/67	0/67	2/67 (3.0)
Lindmarker et al[137]	Dalteparin	5/101 (5.0)	1/101	2/101 (2.0)
	Heparin	3/103 (2.9)	0/103	3/103 (2.9)
Simonneau et al[143]	Tinzaparin	5/304 (1.6)	3/304 (1.0)	12/304 (3.9)
	Heparin	6/308 (1.9)	5/308 (1.6)	14/308 (4.5)
Decousus et al[144]	Enoxaparin	10/195 (5.1)	7/195 (3.6)	10/195 (5.1)
	Heparin	12/205 (5.9)	8/205 (3.9)	15/205 (7.3)

require in-hospital treatment, with either intravenous heparin or low–molecular-weight heparin.

In the study by Levine et al,[141] patients were excluded if they had one or two previous episodes of DVT or pulmonary embolism, had concurrent symptomatic pulmonary embolism, were at high risk of bleeding, or had a known inhibitor deficiency state. They also were excluded if they were considered unable to be treated with low–molecular-weight heparin as an outpatient because of a coexisting condition, the likelihood of noncompliance, or geographic inaccessibility. Of the 2,230 consecutive patients with proximal DVT who were screened, 1,491 were excluded. Of the remaining 739 patients, 500 (68%) gave informed consent; 247 were randomized to receive low–molecular-weight heparin. Of these patients, 120 were not hospitalized at all (29 were admitted to the hospital at night or on a weekend before randomization, and 22 were hospitalized for other reasons).

The 127 patients who were admitted spent an average of 2.2 days in the hospital.

In the study by Koopman et al,[140] the exclusion criteria were less stringent. They included previous venous thromboembolism within 2 years, suspected pulmonary embolism at presentation, geographic inaccessibility, life expectancy of less than 6 months, or overt postthrombotic syndrome. Of 692 eligible patients, 216 (31%) were excluded. Of the 476 eligible patients, 76 (16%) did not consent to participate, and 200 of the remaining 400 patients were randomized to receive low–molecular-weight heparin. Of these patients, 72 (36%) were never admitted, 50 (25%) were treated entirely in the hospital, 44 (22%) were discharged in less than 48 hours, and 36 (18%) were discharged after more than 48 hours.

In the Columbus study,[145] patients were excluded if anticoagulant therapy was contraindicated; if thrombolytic therapy was planned; if a recent episode of gastrointestinal bleeding,

Table 20–4 Predominantly Outpatient Treatment of Proximal Deep Vein Thrombosis with Low–Molecular-Weight Heparin versus Inpatient Treatment with Intravenous Heparin

Study	Treatment	Recurrent DVT	Major Bleeding
Levine et al[141]	Enoxaparin	13/247 (5.3%)	5/247 (2.0%)
	Heparin	17/253 (6.7%)	3/253 (1.2%)
Koopman et al[140]	Nadroparin	14/202 (6.9%)	1/202 (0.5%)
	Heparin	17/198 (8.6%)	4/198 (2.0%)
Columbus Investigators[145]	Reviparin	27/510 (5.3%)	16/510 (3.1%)
	Heparin	24/511 (4.7%)	12/511 (2.3%)

surgery, or stroke had occurred; or if thrombocytopenia was evident. Eligibility criteria included symptomatic DVT, pulmonary embolism, or both. Of the 1,745 consecutive patients who met the eligibility criteria, 425 were excluded. Of the eligible patients, 1,021 gave informed consent; 510 patients were assigned to the low–molecular-weight heparin group. In the low–molecular-weight heparin treatment group, 138 presented with pulmonary embolism. Of 372 patients with DVT, 100 (27%) were never admitted to the hospital, and 56 (15%) were discharged during the first 2 days of treatment.

The Cost-Effectiveness of Low–Molecular-Weight Heparin in the Treatment of Proximal Venous Thrombosis

Based on a prospective randomized clinical trial, a cost-effectiveness analysis comparing the treatment of proximal venous thrombosis with subcutaneous low–molecular-weight heparin and intravenous heparin was performed.[146] The total cost and effects per 100 patients of the two alternative approaches to antithrombotic therapy of proximal venous thrombosis are shown in Table 20–5. This cost-effectiveness analysis showed that low–molecular-weight heparin, which is at least as effective and safe as continuous intravenous heparin, is less costly. The use of low–molecular-weight heparin in this setting both reduced cost and improved health care outcomes—a win-win situation. In the cost analysis, it was defined a priori that treatment could be given on an outpatient basis to patients without co-morbid conditions.[146] A total of 70 of the 231 patients who were treated with low–molecular-weight heparin had uncomplicated proximal venous thrombosis and could have been treated out-of-hospital. The effect of treating 79 patients as outpatients with discharge from hospital on day 2 was examined. The potential use of outpatient therapy with low–molecular-weight heparin in 37% of patients increased the Canadian cost

savings from $15,252.00 to $95,736.00, and it increased the US cost savings from $40,149.00 to $91,332.00 in the treatment of 100 patients with proximal venous thrombosis.[146] Thus, it is clear that the outpatient management of acute proximal venous thrombosis with the use of low–molecular-weight heparin will be more cost effective than treatment using intravenous heparin in-hospital.

The economic effect of replacing inpatient treatment of DVT with intravenous heparin with outpatient treatment with low–molecular-weight heparin was evaluated using data from a perspective randomized clinical trial.[147] The data were collected from case record forms, complemented by a prospective questionnaire in 78 consecutive patients, from interviews with health care providers, and from hospital databases. The use of low–molecular-weight heparin reduced the average number of hospital days during initial treatment by 59% and this reduction was accompanied by a limited increase in outpatient and professional domiciliary care. A cost-minimization analysis that focused on resource utilization directly related to the treatment of DVT and associated costs (in one center in Amsterdam) demonstrated a cost reduction of 64% with the use of outpatient treatment.[147] This study provides further evidence that outpatient management of patients with proximal venous thrombosis with the use of low–molecular-weight heparin reduces hospital utilization and total treatment costs.

Prerequisites for Outpatient Treatment of Venous Thrombosis with Low–Molecular-Weight Heparin

Many patients with proximal venous thrombosis will require hospitalization because of co-morbid conditions and thus will receive either unfractionated heparin or low–molecular-weight heparin in-hospital. The use of out-of-hospital low–molecular-weight heparin along with warfarin has

---

Table 20–5 Total Costs and Effects per 100 Patients of the Alternative Approaches for Antithrombotic Therapy for Proximal Vein Thrombosis

Approach	Recurrent Venous Thromboembolism	Death	Major Bleeding Complications	Cost ($ Canadian)	Cost ($ USA)
Intravenous heparin	7	10	5	414,655	375,836
Low–molecular-weight heparin	3	5	3	399,403	335,687
				(15,252)[†]	(40,149)[*]
				(95,736)[†]	(91,332)[†]

*Cost saving per 100 patients treated with low–molecular-weight heparin.
[†]Cost saving per 100 patients treated with low–molecular-weight heparin and discharged on day 2.

Source: Adapted with permission from RD Hull et al, Treatment of Proximal Vein Thrombosis with Subcutaneous Low Molecular Weight Heparin vs Intravenous Heparin: An Economic Perspective, *Archives of Internal Medicine*, Vol 157, pp 289–294, © 1997, American Medical Association.

created a number of logistic problems, however. So far there are no easy solutions. Many of the exclusion criteria in the clinical trials apply in clinical practice as well. Therefore, exclusion criteria for the outpatient treatment of venous thromboembolism will include the following: proximal DVT with vascular compromise, pulmonary embolism with hemodynamic instability, patients at high risk of bleeding, patients with significant co-morbid conditions requiring hospitalization, geographic inaccessibility, noncompliant patients, and patients with a previous history of heparin-induced thrombocytopenia.

The outpatient treatment of venous thromboembolism with low–molecular-weight heparin and warfarin necessitates certain changes that must be in place before such treatment can be broadly applied. These requirements include appropriate clinical space with adequate staffing for patient education and care, a seamless transition from hospital to clinic and back to hospital again (if required), and adequate funding. The payment for low–molecular-weight heparin, particularly in patients with no third party insurance, remains an unresolved problem.

The advent of the low–molecular-weight heparins and the clinical trials demonstrating that the outpatient treatment of proximal venous thrombosis and acute pulmonary embolism with subcutaneous low–molecular-weight heparin is as safe and effective as continuous intravenous heparin in select patients have provided a strong impetus to shift initial treatment of these disorders from the hospital setting to the outpatient clinic. In addition to increased patient satisfaction and more rapid mobilization with outpatient treatment, economic evaluations have demonstrated that the outpatient management of venous thromboembolism with low–molecular-weight heparin is cost effective. Before the outpatient management of these disorders can become widespread, certain administrative requirements must be satisfied with respect to patient selection and to the infrastructure of the outpatient clinic. A number of demonstration models have been described, enabling treatment centers to develop outpatient management clinics specific to their own needs.

LONG-TERM TREATMENT OF VENOUS THROMBOEMBOLISM

Patients with venous thromboembolism (proximal venous thrombosis or pulmonary embolism) require oral anticoagulants for a period of 3 months to prevent recurrent disease.[148] Attempts have been made to shorten the treatment period to 12 or 6 weeks, but recurrent disease outcomes are superior when oral anticoagulants are used for 3 to 6 months.[149–151] There may be an exception in patients who develop venous thromboembolism in association with an obvious and transient risk factor, such as trauma, orthopaedic surgery, or bed rest. In these patients, the recurrence rate is lower than in

patients who have idiopathic venous thromboembolism, even when shorter courses of anticoagulants are used. Patients with continuing risk factors, such as malignancy, paralysis, or prolonged bed rest, might require long-term therapy until the risk has decreased. Patients with irreversible risk factors, such as deficiency of AT-III or activated protein C resistance, might need anticoagulant treatment indefinitely after an episode of venous thromboembolism.[152] Patients with a first recurrence of venous thromboembolism are treated empirically for 12 months, whereas those with a second recurrence usually receive lifelong anticoagulants. Clinical trials are currently underway to establish the most appropriate duration of anticoagulation in some of these clinical situations.

TREATMENT OF ACUTE MASSIVE PULMONARY EMBOLISM

The emergency management of massive pulmonary embolism includes the use of intravenous heparin, the use of oxygen (with or without mechanical ventilation), volume resuscitation, and the use of inotropic agents and vasodilators. In addition to these supportive measures, specific treatment options for acute massive pulmonary embolism include thrombolysis and insertion of an inferior vena caval filter.

THROMBOLYTIC THERAPY

Randomized clinical trials demonstrate that the mortality rate from venous thromboembolism can be decreased by anticoagulant treatment.[153–155] A mortality rate of less than 5% can be achieved with intravenous heparin and oral anticoagulants.[133] This rate can be further reduced with the use of low–molecular-weight heparin. Patients who present with acute massive pulmonary embolism and hypotension, however, have a mortality rate of approximately 20%, even though anticoagulants and other supportive measures are used. For such patients, the appropriate use of thrombolytic agents has a role. A high percentage of acute pulmonary emboli occur within 10 to 14 days of surgery, and the patients are therefore excluded from treatment protocols that include thrombolytic agents.[156–159] These patients might be candidates for local infusion of low-dose thrombolytic agents.[159]

In several randomized clinical trials, thrombolytic drugs have been compared with heparin for the treatment of pulmonary embolism.[160–165] These trials compared urokinase (UK) with heparin,[160] streptokinase (SK) with heparin,[161,162] or tissue plasminogen activator (TPA) with heparin.[163,164] The dosage regimens used either a bolus or chronic infusion up to 72 hours. Outcome measures for accelerated thrombolysis included quantitative measures on repeat pulmonary angiograms, quantitative scores on repeat pulmonary perfusion scans, and measures of pulmonary vascular resistance. Although all studies demonstrated the superiority of thrombolysis (in particular with TPA) in terms of resolution of both radiographic and hemodynamic abnormalities when measured within the first 24 hours, this advantage was short-lived. Repeat perfusion scans at 5 to 7 days revealed no significant difference between the patients treated with thrombolytic agents or with heparin. Further, the trials demonstrated neither a difference in mortality rate nor in resolution of symptoms. Measurement of diffusion capacity and capillary volumes at 2 weeks and 1 year after treatment showed that those receiving thrombolytic therapy had higher diffusion capacity and lung capillary volumes compared with patients receiving heparin.[166] Follow-up of the same group of 23 patients an average of 7 years after thrombolytic treatment showed that patients who had been treated with thrombolytic therapy had lower pulmonary artery pressure and pulmonary vascular resistance compared with patients who had received heparin.[167] The clinical relevance of these findings, however, must await further prospective studies.

Several randomized clinical trials have compared various thrombolytic agents used in different treatment protocols: SK versus UK,[168] UK with UK,[169] TPA with TPA,[170] and TPA with UK.[171] These studies, again, demonstrate resolution of angiographic, echocardiographic, and perfusion scan abnormalities, as well as reduction of pulmonary pressure, but there was little or no difference between the regimens being compared. Again, the clinical relevance of the changes requires further study.

In weighing the risks and benefits of thrombolytic therapy, the main concern is bleeding. The incidence of major bleeding has decreased, particularly with the use of bolus or short-term infusions and with the use of newer thrombolytic agents. Intracerebral hemorrhage, however, continues to occur more frequently than with heparin.[156,165,172]

At this time, the role of thrombolytic agents in the management of acute massive pulmonary embolism remains controversial. Although there is a more rapid dissolution of venous thromboemboli, the risk of serious bleeding is still a concern. Until reductions in both morbidity and mortality are clearly demonstrated in well-controlled prospective, randomized clinical trials, the question of risk/benefit will remain.[173] In the meantime, the use of thrombolytic agents has become simpler as a result of the following:

- the use of high-probability ventilation/perfusion scans or echocardiography to confirm the diagnosis
- the use of short-term or bolus infusion of thrombolytic agents into peripheral veins, rather than into the pulmonary artery
- the elimination of monitoring by the use of laboratory tests
- treatment in the medical unit, rather than in the intensive care unit

The fact that a high percentage of acute massive pulmonary emboli still occur after surgery, even though effective prophylactic regimens are available against venous thromboembolism,[158,159] indicates that greater efforts must be taken to ensure that these prophylactic measures are being applied in a more uniform fashion.

Thrombolytic therapy can benefit selected patients with acute massive venous thrombosis, such as those with phlegmasia cerulea dolens. For the majority of patients with acute DVT, however, the indication for thrombolytic therapy remains controversial, and most of these patients do well with unfractionated heparin or low–molecular-weight heparin. At present, randomized clinical trials have yielded no definitive evidence that thrombolytic therapy is associated with improved benefit through the prevention of postphlebitic syndrome.

OTHER EMERGENCY PROCEDURES FOR ACUTE MASSIVE PULMONARY EMBOLISM

Pulmonary embolectomy with the use of cardiopulmonary bypass support has been a lifesaving procedure in selected patients with massive pulmonary embolism who have severe cardiovascular decompensation with severe hypotension, oliguria, and hypoxia refractory to aggressive treatment.[174–176] The mortality rate is high, however, and the procedure is also dependent on the ready availability of a cardiovascular surgical team. Patients who are not candidates for thrombolysis or who have not responded to maximum medical therapy might be candidates for pulmonary embolectomy.[174–176]

In patients who have contraindications to anticoagulants or thrombolysis, pulmonary embolectomy via a catheter suction device inserted into the jugular or femoral vein under local anesthetic has been used in the treatment of acute massive pulmonary embolism.[177–179] Catheter clot extraction is currently confined to a few centers with the required expertise.

INFERIOR VENA CAVAL INTERRUPTION IN THE TREATMENT OF PULMONARY THROMBOEMBOLISM

The insertion of an inferior vena caval filter is indicated in:

- the patient with acute venous thromboembolism and an absolute contraindication to anticoagulant therapy
- the rare patient with massive pulmonary embolism who survives but in whom recurrent embolism might be fatal

• the very rare patient who has objectively documented recurrent venous thromboembolism during adequate anticoagulant therapy

Characteristics of an ideal filter include one that is easily and safely placed percutaneously, is biocompatible and mechanically stable, is able to trap emboli without causing occlusion of the vena cava, does not require anticoagulation, and is not ferromagnetic (does not cause artifacts on magnetic resonance images).[180,181] Although there is at present no ideal filter, several of the available devices have proved useful. These include the Greenfield stainless steel filter, titanium Greenfield filter, bird's nest filter. Vena Tech filter, and Simon-Nitinol filter.[182] In experienced hands, these devices can be quickly and safely inserted under fluoroscopic control. One novel filter can be inserted temporarily when needed, used in conjunction with thrombolytic therapy, and then removed.[183] With the available follow-up to date, the Greenfield filter has had the best performance record, and any future comparative studies should use this filter as the standard.[184]

REFERENCES

1. Dismuke SE, Wagner EH. Pulmonary embolism as a cause of death. The changing mortality in hospitalized patients. *JAMA*. 1986; 255:2039–2042.

2. Dalen JE, Alpert JS. Natural history of pulmonary embolism. *Prog Cardiovasc Dis*. 1975;17:257–270.

3. Anderson FA, Wheeler HB, Goldberg RJ, et al. A population-based perspective of the hospital incidence and case-fatality rates of deep vein thrombosis and pulmonary embolism. *Arch Intern Med*. 1991; 151:933–938.

4. Donaldson GA, Williams C, Scanell J, et al. A reappraisal of the application of the Trendelenburg operation to massive fatal embolism. *N Engl J Med*. 1963;268:171–174.

5. Clagett GP, Reisch JS. Prevention of venous thromboembolism in general surgical patients. Results of meta-analysis. *Ann Surg*. 1988;208:227–240.

6. Collins R, Scrimgeour A, Yusef S, et al. Reduction in fatal pulmonary embolism and venous thrombosis by perioperative administration of subcutaneous heparin. *N Engl J Med*. 1988;318:1162–1173.

7. Colditz GA, Tuden RL, Oster G. Rates of venous thrombosis after general surgery: combined results of randomized clinical trials. *Lancet*. 1986;19:143–146.

8. Nicolaides AN, Arcelus J, Belcaro G, et al. Prevention of venous thromboembolism. *Int Angiol*. 1992;11(3):151–158.

9. Hull RD, Hirsh J, Carter CJ, et al. Diagnostic efficacy of impedance plethysmography for clinically suspected deep vein thrombosis: a randomized trial. *Ann Intern Med*. 1985;102:21–28.

10. Huisman MV, Büller HR, ten Cate JW, et al. Serial impedance plethysmography for suspected deep venous thrombosis in outpatients. The Amsterdam General Practitioner Study. *N Engl J Med*. 1986; 314:823–828.

11. Moser KM, Le Moine JR. Is embolic risk conditioned by location of deep venous thrombosis? *Ann Intern Med*. 1981;94:439–444.

12. Huisman MV, Büller HR, ten Cate JW, et al. Management of clinically suspected acute venous thrombosis in outpatients with serial impedance plethysmography in a community hospital setting. *Arch Intern Med*. 1989a;149:511–513.

13. Kakkar VV, Flanc C, Howe CT, et al. Natural history of postoperative deep vein thrombosis. *Lancet*. 1969;2:230–233.

14. Lagerstedt CI, Fagher BO, Olsson CG, et al. Need for long-term anticoagulant treatment in symptomatic calf-vein thrombosis. *Lancet*. 1985;2:515–518.

15. Hull RD, Delmore T, Genton E, et al. Warfarin sodium versus low-dose heparin in the long-term treatment of venous thrombosis. *N Engl J Med*. 1979;301:855–858.

16. Huisman MV, Büller HR, ten Cate JW, et al. Unexpected high prevalence of silent pulmonary embolism in patients with deep venous thrombosis. *Chest*. 1989;95:498–502.

17. Sevitt S, Gallagher N. Venous thrombosis and pulmonary embolism. A clinicopathological study in injured and burned patients. *Br J Surg*. 1961;48:475–489.

18. Mavor GE, Galloway JMD. The iliofemoral venous segment as a source of pulmonary emboli. *Lancet*. 1967;1:871–874.

19. Hull RD, Hirsh J, Carter CJ, et al. Diagnostic value of ventilation-perfusion lung scanning in patients with suspected pulmonary embolism. *Chest*. 1985;88:819–828.

20. A collaborative study by the PIOPED investigators. Value of the ventilation/perfusion scan in acute pulmonary embolism: results of the Prospective Investigation of Pulmonary Embolism Diagnosis (PIOPED). *JAMA*. 1990;263:2753–2769.

21. Bone RC. Ventilation/perfusion scan in pulmonary embolism. "The emperor is incompletely attired." *JAMA*. 1990;263:2794–2795.

22. Secker-Walker RH. On purple emperors, pulmonary embolism, and venous thrombosis. *Ann Intern Med*. 1983;98:1006–1008.

23. Stein PD, Hull RD, Saltzman HA, et al. Strategy for diagnosis of patients with suspected acute pulmonary embolism. *Chest*. 1993;103:1553–1559.

24. Rabinov K, Paulin S. Roentgen diagnosis of venous thrombosis in the leg. *Arch Surg*. 1972;104:134–144.

25. Stein PD. Clinical features of deep vein thrombosis and pulmonary embolism. In: Hull RD, Pineo GF, eds. *Disorders of Thrombosis*. Philadelphia: WB Saunders; 1996:234–238.

26. Wells P, Hirsh J, Anderson D, et al. Accuracy of clinical assessment of deep-vein thrombosis. *Lancet*. 1995;345:1326–1330.

27. Tourassi GD, Floyd CE, Sostman HD, Coleman RE. Artificial neural network for the diagnosis of acute pulmonary embolism: effect of case and observer selection. *Radiology*. 1995;194:889–893.

28. Patil S, Henry JW, Rubenfire M, Stein PD. Neural network in the clinical diagnosis of acute pulmonary embolism. *Chest*. 1995; 104:1685–1689.

29. Ginsberg JS, Wells PS, Brill-Edwards P, et al. Application of a novel and rapid whole blood assay for D-dimer in patients with clinically suspected pulmonary embolism. *Thromb Haemost*. 1995;73:35–38.

30. Wells PS, Brill-Edwards P, Stevens P, et al. A novel and rapid whole-blood assay for D-dimer in patients with clinically suspected deep vein thrombosis. *Circulation*. 1995;91:2184–2187.

31. Heijboer H, Ginsberg JS, Büller HR, et al. The use of the D-dimer test in combination with non-invasive testing versus serial non-invasive

testing alone for the diagnosis of deep-vein thrombosis. *Thromb Haemost.* 1992;67:510–513.

32. Cronan JJ, Dorfman GS, Scola FH, et al. Deep venous thrombosis: US assessment using vein compressibility. *Radiology.* 1987;162: 191–194.

33. Lensing AWA, Prandoni P, Brandjes D, et al. Detection of deep-vein thrombosis by real-time B-mode ultrasonography. *N Engl J Med.* 1989;320:342–345.

34. Heijboer H, Jongbloets LMM, Büller HR, et al. The clinical utility of real-time compression ultrasound in the diagnostic management of patients with recurrent venous thrombosis. *Acta Radiol.* 1992; 33:297–300.

35. Heijboer H, Büller HR, Lensing AWA, et al. A comparison of real-time compression ultrasonography with impedance plethysmography for the diagnosis of deep-vein thrombosis in symptomatic outpatients. *N Engl J Med.* 1993;329:1365–1369.

36. Baxter GM, McKechnie S, Duffy P. Colour Doppler ultrasound in deep venous thrombosis: a comparison with venography. *Clin Radiol.* 1990;42:32–36.

37. Rose SC, Zwiebel WJ, Nelson BD, et al. Symptomatic lower extremity deep venous thrombosis: accuracy, limitations, and role of colour duplex flow imaging in diagnosis. *Radiology.* 1990;175:639–644.

38. Mitchell DC, Grasty MS, Stebbings WSL, et al. Comparison of duplex ultrasonography and venography in the diagnosis of deep venous thrombosis. *Br J Surg.* 1991;78:611–613.

39. Mattos MA, Londey GL, Leutz DW, et al. Color-flow duplex scanning for the surveillance and diagnosis of acute deep venous thrombosis. *J Vasc Surg.* 1992;15:366–375.

40. Ginsberg JS, Caco CC, Brill-Edwards P, et al. Venous thrombosis in patients who have undergone major hip or knee surgery: detection with compression US and impedance plethysmography. *Radiology.* 1991;181:651–654.

41. Borris LC, Christiansen HM, Lassen MR, et al. Comparison of real-time B-mode ultrasonography and bilateral ascending phlebography for detection of postoperative deep vein thrombosis following elective hip surgery. *Thromb Haemost.* 1989;61:363–365.

42. Davidson B, Elliott GC, Lensing AWA. Low accuracy of color Doppler ultrasound to detect proximal leg vein thrombosis during screening of asymptomatic high-risk patients. *Ann Intern Med.* 1992; 117:735–738.

43. Rose SC, Zwiebel WJ, Murdock LE, et al. Insensitivity of color Doppler flow imaging for detection of acute calf deep venous thrombosis in asymptomatic postoperative patients. *J Vasc Intern Radiol.* 1993;4:111–117.

44. Elliott GC, Suchyta M, Rose SC, et al. Duplex ultrasonography for the detection of deep vein thrombi after total hip or knee arthroplasty. *Angiology.* 1993;44:26–32.

45. Hull RD, Hirsh J, Sackett DL, et al. Replacement of venography in suspected venous thrombosis by impedance plethysmography and ^{125}I-fibrinogen leg scanning: a less invasive approach. *Ann Intern Med.* 1981;94:12–15.

46. Hull RD, Carter C, Jay R, et al. The diagnosis of acute recurrent deep-vein thrombosis: a diagnostic challenge. *Circulation.* 1983;67: 901–906.

47. Prandoni P, Lensing AWA, Huisman MV, et al. A new computerized impedance plethysmograph: accuracy in the detection of proximal deep vein thrombosis in symptomatic outpatients. *Thromb Haemost.* 1991;65:229–232.

48. Heijboer H, Cogo A, Büller HR, et al. Detection of deep vein thrombosis with impedance plethysmography and real-time

compression ultrasonography in hospitalized patients. *Arch Intern Med.* 1992;152:1901–1903.

49. Hull RD, Hirsh J, Sackett DL, et al. Combined use of leg scanning and impedance plethysmography in suspected venous thrombosis: an alternative to venography. *N Engl J Med.* 1977;296:1497–1500.

50. Paiement GD, Wessinger SJ, Waltman AC, et al. Surveillance of deep vein thrombosis in asymptomatic total hip replacement patients. Impedance plethysmography and fibrinogen scanning versus roentgenographic phlebography. *Am J Surg.* 1988;155: 400–404.

51. Cruickshank MK, Levine MN, Hirsh J, et al. An evaluation of impedance plethysmography and ^{125}I-fibrinogen leg scanning in patients following hip surgery. *Thromb Haemost.* 1989;62: 830–834.

52. Lensing AWA, Prandoni P, Büller HR, et al. Lower extremity venography with iohexol: results and complications. *Radiology.* 1990;177:503–505.

53. Lensing AWA, Büller HR, Prandoni P, et al. Contrast venography, the gold standard for the diagnosis of deep vein thrombosis: improvement in observer agreement. *Thromb Haemost.* 1992;67: 8–12.

54. McLachlan MSF, Thomson JG, Taylor DW, et al. Observer variation in the interpretation of lower limb venograms. *Am J Radiol.* 1979; 132:227–229.

55. Parfrey PS, Griffiths SM, Barrett BJ, et al. Contrast material-induced renal failure in patients with diabetes mellitus, renal insufficiency or both. *N Engl J Med.* 1989;320:143–149.

56. Schwab SJ, Hlarky MA, Pieper KS, et al. Contrast nephrotoxicity: a randomized controlled trial of a non-ionic and an ionic radiographic contrast agent. *N Engl J Med.* 1989;320:149–153.

57. Gottschalk A, Bisesi MA, Stein PD. Ventilation-perfusion lung scan for the diagnosis of acute pulmonary embolism. In: Hull RD, Pineo GF, eds. *Disorders of Thrombosis.* Philadelphia: WB Saunders; 1996;258–271.

58. Alderson PO, Biello DR, Gottschalk A, et al. Tc-99m-DTPA aerosols and radioactive gases compared as adjuncts to perfusion scintigraphy in patients with suspected pulmonary embolism. *Radiology.* 1984; 153:515–521.

59. Hull RD, Raskob GE, Ginsberg JS, et al. A noninvasive strategy for the treatment of patients with suspected pulmonary embolism. *Arch Intern Med.* 1994;154:289–297.

60. Stein PD, Hull RD, Pineo GF. Strategy that includes serial noninvasive leg tests for diagnosis of thromboembolic disease in patients with suspected acute pulmonary embolism based on data from PIOPED. *Arch Intern Med.* 1995;155:2101–2104.

61. Sharma GVRK, Sashara AA. Pulmonary angiography. In: Hull RD, Raskob GE, Pineo GF, eds. *Venous Thromboembolism: An Evidence Based Atlas.* New York: Futura Publishing Co; 1996;183–191.

62. International Multicentre Trial: prevention of fatal postoperative pulmonary embolism by low doses of heparin. *Lancet.* 1975;2: 45–64.

63. Coventry MB, Nolan DR, Beckenbaugh RD. "Delayed" prophylactic anticoagulation: a study of results and complications in 2,012 total hip arthroplasties. *J Bone Joint Surg Am.* 1973;55:1487–1492.

64. Eskeland G, Solheim K, Skhorten F. Anticoagulant prophylaxis, thromboembolism and mortality in elderly patients with hip fracture: a controlled clinical trial. *Acta Chir Scand.* 1986;131:16–29.

65. Kakkar V, Stamatakis JD, Bentley PG, et al. Prophylaxis for post-operative deep-vein thrombosis. *JAMA.* 1979;241:39–42.

66. Anderson FA, Wheeler HB, Goldberg RJ, et al. Physician practices in the prevention of venous thromboembolism. *Ann Intern Med.* 1991;115:581–595.

67. Bergqvist D. Prevention of postoperative deep vein thrombosis in Sweden: results of a survey. *World J Surg.* 1980;4:489–495.

68. Laverick MD, Croak SA, Molian RA. Orthopedic surgeons and thromboprophylaxis. *Br Med J.* 1991;303:549–550.

69. Salzman EW, Davies GC. Prophylaxis of venous thromboembolism. Analysis of cost-effectiveness. *Ann Surg.* 1980;191:207–218.

70. Hull R, Hirsh J, Sackett DL, et al. Cost-effectiveness of primary and secondary prevention of fatal pulmonary embolism in high-risk surgical patients. *Can Med Assoc J.* 1982;127:990–995.

71. Oster G, Tuden RL, Colditz GA. A cost-effectiveness analysis of prophylaxis against deep vein thrombosis in major orthopedic surgery. *JAMA.* 1987;257:203–208.

72. Clagett GP, Anderson FA, Heit J, Levine M, Wheeler HB. Prevention of venous thromboembolism. *Chest.* 1995;108(suppl 4):312S–334S.

73. Leyvraz PF, Richard J, Bachmann F, et al. Adjusted versus fixed dose subcutaneous heparin in the prevention of deep vein thrombosis after total hip replacement. *N Engl J Med.* 1983;309:954–958.

74. Leyvraz PF, Bachmann F, Hoek J, et al. Prevention of deep vein thrombosis after hip replacement: randomised comparison between unfractionated heparin and low molecular weight heparin. *Br Med J.* 1991;303:543–548.

75. Green D, Lee MY, Ito VY, et al. Fixed vs adjusted dose heparin in the prophylaxis of thromboembolism in spinal cord injury. *JAMA.* 1988;260:1255–1258.

76. Kakkar VV, Cohen AT, Edmonson RA, et al. Low molecular weight versus standard heparin for prevention of venous thromboembolism after major abdominal surgery. *Lancet.* 1993;341:259–265.

77. Bergqvist D, Matzsch T, Brumark U, et al. Low–molecular-weight heparin given the evening before surgery compared with conventional low-dose heparin in prevention of thrombosis. *Br J Surg.* 1988;75:888–891.

78. Samama M, Bernard P, Bonnardot JP, et al. Low–molecular-weight heparin compared with unfractionated heparin in prevention of postoperative thrombosis. *Br J Surg.* 1988;75:128–131.

79. European Fraxiparin Study Group. Comparison of a low–molecular-weight heparin and unfractionated heparin for the prevention of deep vein thrombosis in patients undergoing abdominal surgery. *Br J Surg.* 1988;75:1058–1063.

80. Leizorovicz A, Picolet H, Peyrieux JC, et al. Prevention of perioperative deep vein thrombosis in general surgery: a multicentre double-blind study comparing two doses of logiparin and standard heparin. *Br J Surg.* 1991;78:412–416.

81. Turpie AGG, Levine MN, Hirsh J, et al. A randomized controlled trial of low–molecular-weight heparin (enoxaparin) to prevent deep vein thrombosis in patients undergoing elective hip surgery. *N Engl J Med.* 1986;315:925–929.

82. Lassen MR, Borris LC, Christiansen HM, et al. Prevention of thromboembolism in 190 hip arthroplasties. *Acta Orthop Scand.* 1991;62(1):33–38.

83. Danish Enoxaparin Study Group. Low–molecular-weight heparin (enoxaparin) vs dextran 70. *Arch Intern Med.* 1991;151:1621–1624.

84. Levine MN, Hirsh J, Gent M, et al. Prevention of deep vein thrombosis after elective hip surgery: a randomized trial comparing low molecular weight heparin with standard unfractionated heparin. *Ann Intern Med.* 1991;114:545–551.

85. Planes A, Vochelle N, Fagola M, et al. Prevention of deep vein thrombosis after total hip replacement: the effect of low–molecular-weight heparin with spinal and general anesthesia. *J Bone Joint Surg Br.* 1991;73:418–423.

86. Hull RD, Raskob GE, Pineo GF, et al. A comparison of subcutaneous low–molecular-weight heparin with warfarin sodium for prophylaxis against deep-vein thrombosis after hip or knee implantation. *N Engl J Med.* 1993;329:1370–1376.

87. LeClerc JR, Geerts WH, Desjardins L, et al. Prevention of venous thromboembolism after knee arthroplasty—a randomized, double-blind trial comparing a low molecular weight heparin fragmin (enoxaparin) to warfarin. *Ann Intern Med.* 1996;124(7):619–626.

88. Nurmohamed MT, Rosendaal FR, Büller HR, et al. Low molecular weight heparin in the prophylaxis of venous thrombosis: a meta-analysis. *Lancet.* 1992;340:152–156.

89. Francis CW, Pellegrini VD, Marder VJ, et al. Comparison of warfarin and external pneumatic compression in prevention of venous thrombosis after total hip replacement. *JAMA.* 1992;267:2911–2915.

90. Paiement GD, Wessinger SJ, Waltman WC, et al. Low-dose warfarin versus external pneumatic compression for prophylaxis against venous thromboembolism following total hip replacement. *J Arthroplasty.* 1987;2:23–26.

91. Kaempffe FA, Lifeso RM, Meinking C. Intermittent pneumatic compression versus Coumadin: prevention of deep vein thrombosis in lower-extremity total joint arthroplasty. *Clin Orthop.* 1991;269:89–97.

92. Dale C, Gallus A, Wycherley A, et al. Prevention of venous thrombosis with minidose warfarin after joint replacement. *Br Med J.* 1991;303:224.

93. Powers PJ, Gent M, Jay R, et al. A randomized trial of less intense postoperative warfarin or aspirin therapy in the prevention of venous thromboembolism after surgery for fractured hip. *Arch Intern Med.* 1989;149:771–774.

94. Poller L, McKernan A, Thomson JM, et al. Fixed minidose warfarin: a new approach to prophylaxis against venous thrombosis after major surgery. *Br Med J.* 1987;285:1309–1312.

95. Bern MM, Lokich JJ, Wallach SR, et al. Very low doses of warfarin can prevent thrombosis in central venous catheters. *Ann Intern Med.* 1990;112:423–428.

96. Roberts VC, Sabri S, Beely AH, et al. The effect of intermittently applied external pressure on the hemodynamics of the lower limb in man. *Br J Surg.* 1972;59:233–236.

97. Turpie AGG, Gallus A, Beattie WS, et al. Prevention of venous thrombosis in patients with intracranial disease by intermittent pneumatic compression of the calf. *Neurology.* 1977;27:435–438.

98. Turpie AGG, Delmore T, Hirsh J, et al. Prevention of venous thrombosis by intermittent sequential calf compression in patients with intracranial disease. *Thromb Res.* 1979;16:611–616.

99. Skillman JJ, Collins RR, Coe NP, et al. Prevention of deep vein thrombosis in neurosurgical patients: a controlled, randomized trial of external pneumatic compression boots. *Surgery.* 1978;83:354–358.

100. Hull RD, Raskob G, Gent M, et al. Effectiveness of intermittent pneumatic leg compression for preventing deep vein thrombosis after total hip replacement. *JAMA.* 1990;263:2313–2317.

101. Hull RD, Delmore TJ, Hirsh J, et al. Effectiveness of intermittent pulsatile elastic stockings for the prevention of calf and thigh vein thrombosis in patients undergoing elective knee surgery. *Thromb Res.* 1979;16:37–45.

102. Turner GM, Cole SE, Brooks JH. The efficacy of graduated compression stockings in the prevention of deep vein thrombosis after major gynaecological surgery. *Br J Obstet Gynaecol.* 1984;91:588–591.

103. Ishak MA, Moreley KD. Deep venous thrombosis after total hip arthroplasty: a prospective controlled study to determine the prophylactic effect of graded pressure stockings. *Br J Surg.* 1981;68:429–432.

104. Allan A, Williams JT, Bolton JP, et al. The use of graduated compression stockings in the prevention of postoperative deep vein thrombosis. *Br J Surg.* 1983;70:172–174.

105. Wells PS, Lensing AWA, Hirsh J. Graduated compression stockings in the prevention of postoperative venous thromboembolism. *Arch Intern Med.* 1994;154:67–72.

106. Colvin BT, Barrowcliffe TW. The British Society for Haematology Guidelines on the use and monitoring of heparin 1992: second revision. *J Clin Pathol.* 1993;46:97–103.

107. Hirsh J, van Aken WG, Gallus AS, et al. Heparin kinetics in venous thrombosis and pulmonary embolism. *Circulation.* 1976;53:691–695.

108. Moser KM. Venous thromboembolism. *Am Rev Respir Dis.* 1990;141:235–249.

109. Gallus A, Jackaman J, Tillett J, Mills W, Wycherley A. Safety and efficacy of warfarin started early after submassive venous thrombosis or pulmonary embolism. *Lancet.* 1986;2:1293–1296.

110. Hull RD, Raskob GE, Rosenbloom D, et al. Heparin for 5 days as compared with 10 days in the initial treatment of proximal venous thrombosis. *N Engl J Med.* 1990;322:1260–1264.

111. Bjork I, Lindahl U. Mechanism of the anticoagulant action of heparin. *Mol Cell Biochem.* 1982;48:161–182.

112. Hirsh J, Raschke R, Warkentin TE, et al. Heparin: mechanism of action, pharmacokinetics, dosing consideration, monitoring, efficacy, and safety. *Chest.* 1995;108(suppl 4):258S–275S.

113. Hull RD, Raskob GE, Hirsh J, et al. Continuous intravenous heparin compared with intermittent subcutaneous heparin in the initial treatment of proximal-vein thrombosis. *N Engl J Med.* 1986;315:1109–1114.

114. Raschke RA, Reilly BM, Guidry JR, et al. The weight-based heparin dosing nomogram compared with a "standard care" nomogram. *Ann Intern Med.* 1993;119:874–881.

115. Brandjes DPM, Heijboer H, Büller HR, et al. Acenocoumarol and heparin compared with acenocoumarol alone in the initial treatment of proximal-vein thrombosis. *N Engl J Med.* 1992;327:1485–1489.

116. Brill-Edwards P, Ginsberg S, Johnston M, et al. Establishing a therapeutic range for heparin therapy. *Ann Intern Med.* 1993;119:104–109.

117. Fennerty A, Thomas P, Backhouse G, et al. Audit of control of heparin treatment. *Br Med J.* 1985;290:27–28.

118. Wheeler AP, Jaquiss RD, Newman JH. Physician practices in the treatment of pulmonary embolism and deep venous thrombosis. *Arch Intern Med.* 1988;148:1321–1325.

119. Cruickshank MK, Levine MN, Hirsh J, Roberts R, Siguenza M. A standard heparin nomogram for the management of heparin therapy. *Arch Intern Med.* 1991;151:333–337.

120. Hull RD, Raskob GE, Rosenbloom DR, et al. Optimal therapeutic level of heparin therapy in patients with venous thrombosis. *Arch Intern Med.* 1992;152:1589–1595.

121. Kelton JG. Heparin-induced thrombocytopenia. *Haemostasis.* 1986;16(2):173–186.

122. Warkentin TE, Kelton JG. Heparin-induced thrombocytopenia. *Prog Hemost Thromb.* 1991;10:1–34.

123. Boshkov LK, Warkentin TE, Hayward CP, Andrew M, Kelton JG. Heparin-induced thrombocytopenia and thrombosis: clinical and laboratory studies. *Br J Haematol.* 1993;84:322–328.

124. Warkentin TE, Levine MN, Hirsh J, et al. Heparin-induced thrombocytopenia in patients treated with low–molecular-weight heparin or unfractionated heparin. *N Engl J Med.* 1995;332:1330–1335.

125. Greinacher A, Michels I, Kiefel V, Mueller-Eckhardt C. A rapid and sensitive test for diagnosing heparin-associated thrombocytopenia. *Thromb Haemost.* 1991;66:734–736.

126. Chong BH, Burgess J, Ismail F. The clinical usefulness of the platelet aggregation test for the diagnosis of heparin-induced thrombocytopenia. *Thromb Haemost.* 1993;69:344–350.

127. Arepally G, Reynolds C, Tomaski A, et al. Comparison of PF4/heparin ELISA assay with the (14)C-serotonin release assay in the diagnosis of heparin-induced thrombocytopenia. *Am J Clin Pathol.* 1995;104:648–654.

128. Kelton JG. The laboratory diagnosis of heparin-induced thrombocytopenia: still a journey, not yet a destination. *Am J Clin Pathol.* 1995;104:611–613. Editorial.

129. Demers C, Ginsberg JS, Brill-Edwards P, et al. Rapid anticoagulation using ancrod for heparin-induced thrombocytopenia. *Blood.* 1991;78:2194–2197.

130. Magnani HN. Heparin-induced thrombocytopenia (HIT): an overview of 230 patients treated with Orgaran (Org 10172). *Thromb Haemost.* 1993;70:554–561.

131. Hirsh J, Levine MN. Low molecular weight heparin. *Blood.* 1992;79:1–17.

132. Pineo GF, Hull RD. Low molecular weight heparin: prophylaxis and treatment of venous thromboembolism. *Annu Rev Med.* 1997;48:79–91.

133. Hull RD, Raskob GE, Pineo GF, et al. Subcutaneous low–molecular-weight heparin compared with continuous intravenous heparin in the treatment of proximal-vein thrombosis. *N Engl J Med.* 1992;326:975–988.

134. Prandoni P, Lensing AW, Büller HR, et al. Comparison of subcutaneous low–molecular-weight heparin with intravenous standard heparin in proximal deep-vein thrombosis. *Lancet.* 1992;339:441–445.

135. Lopaciuk S, Meissner AJ, Filipecki S, et al. Subcutaneous low–molecular-weight heparin versus subcutaneous unfractionated heparin in the treatment of deep vein thrombosis: a Polish multicentre trial. *Thromb Haemost.* 1992;68:14–18.

136. Simonneau G, Charbonnier B, Decousus H, et al. Subcutaneous low–molecular-weight heparin compared with continuous intravenous unfractionated heparin in the treatment of proximal deep vein thrombosis. *Arch Intern Med.* 1993;153:1541–1546.

137. Lindmarker P, Holmstrom M, Granqvist S, Johnsson H, Locner D. Comparison of once-daily subcutaneous fragmin with continuous intravenous unfractionated heparin in the treatment of deep venous thrombosis. *Thromb Haemost.* 1994;72:186–190.

138. Lensing AW, Prins MH, Davidson BL, Hirsh J. Treatment of deep venous thrombosis with low–molecular-weight heparins. *Arch Intern Med.* 1995;155:601–607.

139. Meyer G, Brenot F, Pacouret G, et al. Subcutaneous low–molecular-weight heparin fragmin versus intravenous unfractionated heparin in the treatment of acute non massive pulmonary embolism: an open randomized pilot study. *Thromb Haemost.* 1995;74:1432–1435.

140. Koopman MMW, Prandoni P, Piovella F, et al. Treatment of venous thrombosis with intravenous unfractionated heparin administered in the hospital as compared with subcutaneous low–molecular-weight heparin administered at home. *N Engl J Med.* 1996;334:682–687.

141. Levine M, Gent M, Hirsh J, et al. A comparison of low–molecular-weight heparin administered primarily at home with unfractionated heparin administered in the hospital for proximal deep-vein thrombosis. *N Engl J Med.* 1996;334:677–681.

142. Cook DJ, Guyatt GH, Laupacis A, et al. Clinical recommendations using levels of evidence for antithrombotic agents. *Chest.* 1995;10(4): 227S–230S.

143. Simonneau G, Sors H, Charbonnier B, et al. A comparison of low molecular weight heparin with unfractionated heparin for acute pulmonary embolism. *N Engl J Med.* 1997;337:663–669.

144. Decousus H, Leizorovicz A, Parent F, et al. A clinical trial of vena caval filters in the prevention of pulmonary embolism in patients with proximal deep vein thrombosis. *N Engl J Med.* 1998;338: 409–415.

145. The Columbus Investigators. Low molecular weight heparin in the treatment of patients with venous thromboembolism. *N Engl J Med.* 1997;337:657–662.

146. Hull RD, Raskob G, Rosenblood D, et al. Treatment of proximal vein thrombosis with subcutaneous low molecular weight heparin vs. intravenous heparin. An economic perspective. *Arch Intern Med.* 1997;157:289–294.

147. Van den Belt AGM, Bossuyt PMM, Prins MH, et al. Replacing inpatient care by outpatient care in the treatment of deep vein thrombosis—an economic evaluation. *Thromb Haemost.* 1998;79: 259–263.

148. Hirsh J, Dalen JE, Deykin D, Poller L, Bussey HI. Oral anticoagulants: mechanism of action, clinical effectiveness, and optimal therapeutic range. *Chest.* 1995;108(suppl 4):231S–246S.

149. Research Committee of the British Thoracic Society. Optimum duration of anticoagulation for deep-vein thrombosis and pulmonary embolism. *Lancet.* 1992;340:873–876.

150. Schulman S, Rhedin AS, Lindmarker P, et al. A comparison of six weeks with six months of oral anticoagulant therapy after a first episode of venous thromboembolism. *N Engl J Med.* 1995;332: 1661–1665.

151. Levine MN, Hirsh J, Gent M, et al. Optimal duration of oral anticoagulant therapy: a randomized trial comparing four weeks with three months of warfarin in patients with proximal deep vein thrombosis. *Thromb Haemost.* 1995;74:606–611.

152. Hyers TN, Hull RD, Weg JG. Antithrombotic therapy for venous thromboembolic disease. *Chest.* 1995;108(suppl 4):335S–351S.

153. Barritt DW, Jordon SC. Anticoagulant drugs in the treatment of pulmonary embolism: a controlled trial. *Lancet.* 1960;1:1309–1312.

154. Sevitt S, Gallagher NG. Venous thrombosis and pulmonary embolism: a clinicopathologic study in injured and burned patients. *Br J Surg.* 1961;48:475–489.

155. Hull RD, Delmore T, Genton E, et al. Warfarin sodium versus low-dose heparin in the long-term treatment of venous thrombosis. *N Engl J Med.* 1979;301:855–858.

156. Goldhaber SZ, Morpurgo M. Diagnosis, treatment, and prevention of pulmonary embolism. Report of the WHO/International Society and Federation of Cardiology Task Force. *JAMA.* 1992;268:1727–1733.

157. Goldhaber SZ. Thrombolytic therapy in venous thromboembolism. Clinical trials and current indications. *Clin Chest Med.* 1995;16: 307–320.

158. Markel A, Manzo RA, Strandness E, Jr. The potential role of thrombolytic therapy in venous thrombosis. *Arch Intern Med.* 1992; 152:1265–1267.

159. Molina JE, Hunter DW, Yedlicka JW, et al. Thrombolytic therapy for postoperative pulmonary embolism. *Am J Surg.* 1992;163:375–381.

160. The Urokinase Pulmonary Embolism Trial: a natural cooperative study. *Circulation.* 1973;47(suppl 2):1–108.

161. Tibbutt DA, Davies JA, Anderson JA, et al. Comparison by controlled clinical trial of streptokinase and heparin in treatment of life-threatening pulmonary embolism. *Br Med J.* 1974;1:343–347.

162. Ly B, Arnesen H, Eie H, et al. A controlled clinical trial of streptokinase and heparin in the treatment of major pulmonary embolism. *Acta Med Scand.* 1978;203:465–470.

163. Prospective Investigation of Pulmonary Embolism Diagnosis investigators. Tissue plasminogen activator for the treatment of acute pulmonary embolism. *Chest.* 1990;97:528–533.

164. Levine M, Hirsh J, Weitz J, et al. A randomized trial of a single bolus dosage regimen of recombinant tissue plasminogen activator in patients with acute pulmonary embolism. *Chest.* 1990;98:1473–1479.

165. Dalla-Volta S, Palla A, Santolicandro A, et al. PAIMS 2: alteplase combined with heparin versus heparin in the treatment of acute pulmonary embolism. Plasminogen activator Italian multicentre study 2. *J Am Coll Cardiol.* 1992;20:520–526.

166. Sharma GVRK, Burleson VA, Sasahara AA. Effect of thrombolytic therapy on pulmonary-capillary blood volume in patients with pulmonary embolism. *N Engl J Med.* 1980;303:842–845.

167. Sharma GVRK, Folland ED, McIntyre KM, et al. Longterm hemodynamic benefit of thrombolytic therapy in pulmonary embolic disease. *J Am Coll Cardiol.* 1990;15:65A. Abstract.

168. Urokinase-streptokinase embolism trial. Phase 2 results. *JAMA.* 1974;229:1606–1613.

169. UKEP Study Research Group. The UKEP study: multicentre clinical trial on two local regimens of urokinase in massive pulmonary embolism. *Eur Heart J.* 1987;8:2–10.

170. Verstraete M, Miller GAH, Bounameaux H, et al. Intravenous and intrapulmonary recombinant tissue-type plasminogen activator in the treatment of acute massive pulmonary embolism. *Circulation.* 1988;77:353–360.

171. Goldhaber SZ, Kessler CM, Heit JA, et al. Recombinant tissue-type plasminogen activator versus a novel dosing regimen of urokinase in acute pulmonary embolism: a randomized controlled multicentre trial. *J Am Coll Cardiol.* 1992;20:24–30.

172. Goldhaber SZ. Evolving concepts in thrombolytic therapy for pulmonary embolism. *Chest.* 1992;101:183S–185S.

173. Goldhaber SZ. Pulmonary embolism thrombolysis: a clarion call for international collaboration. *J Am Coll Cardiol.* 1992;19:246–247.

174. delCampo C. Pulmonary embolectomy: a review. *Can J Surg.* 1985; 28:111–113.

175. Sasahara AA, Sharma GVRK, Barsamian EM, et al. Pulmonary thromboembolism: diagnosis and treatment. *JAMA.* 1983;249:2945–2950.

176. Meyer G, Tamisier D, Sors H, et al. Pulmonary embolectomy: a 20-year experience at one center. *Ann Thorac Surg.* 1991;51: 232–236.

177. Greenfield LJ. Vena caval interruption and pulmonary embolectomy. *Clin Chest Med.* 1984;5:495–505.

178. Timsit J-F, Reynaud P, Meyer G, et al. Pulmonary embolectomy by catheter device in massive pulmonary embolism. *Chest.* 1991;100:655–658.

179. Brady AJB, Crake T, Oakley CM. Percutaneous catheter fragmentation and distal dispersion of proximal pulmonary embolus. *Lancet.* 1991;338:1186–1189.

180. King JN, Champlin AM, Ashby RN. Vena cava filters. *West J Med.* 1992;156:295–296.

181. Grassi CJ. Inferior vena caval filters: analysis of five currently available devices. *Am J Roentgenol.* 1991;156:813–821.

182. Ballew KA, Philbrick JT, Becker DM. Vena cava filter devices. *Clin Chest Med.* 1995;16:295–305.

183. Thery C, Asseman P, Amrouni N, et al. Use of a new removable vena cava filter in order to prevent pulmonary embolism in patients submitted to thrombolysis. *Eur Heart J.* 1990;11:334–341.

184. Greenfield LJ. Evolution of venous interruption for pulmonary thromboembolism. *Arch Surg.* 1992;127:622–626.

Chapter 21

Prevention and Treatment of Thromboembolic Disease in Childhood

Velma Marzinotto, Michael Leaker, Patricia Massicotte, and Maureen Andrew

INTRODUCTION

The prevalence of thromboembolic events in adult patients and the necessity for antithrombotic therapy resulted in the formation of a new medical specialty approximately 20 years ago. Thromboembolism programs for adults optimize the provision of clinical care and the advancement of knowledge through both basic and clinical research. The clinical component of this comprehensive system is an inpatient and outpatient anticoagulation service. A team of health care personnel provides consultations, utilizes objective tests to prove or disprove the presence of a thromboembolic event, involves the coagulation laboratory in the detection of prothrombotic disorders, monitors antithrombotic agents, and provides long-term follow-up.

Until recently, the same need for an anticoagulation service for pediatric patients did not exist because of the relative rarity of thromboembolic events requiring treatment and the paucity of high-risk conditions requiring prophylactic anticoagulation. Tertiary care pediatrics, however, is rapidly changing and improving, with the result that most children with serious primary problems are cured or successfully treated. Paradoxically, these successes are associated with numerous secondary problems, of which thromboembolic events constitute one of the most serious and frequent. Most congenital prothrombotic disorders now can be diagnosed during infancy and childhood, thus providing a new patient population that requires counseling and, in some circumstances, intermittent prophylactic anticoagulation therapy. In addition, large numbers of children are requiring prophylactic anticoagulation to prevent thromboembolic events in such conditions as prosthetic heart valves, cardiopulmonary bypass, extracorporeal membrane oxygenation, stents, and central venous lines, and other children require thrombolytic therapy. The term commonly used in adult patients, *anticoagulation service*, does not fully describe the breadth of services required for children. The term *thrombophilia* encompasses both the diagnosis and treatment of thromboembolic events, in addition to the use of antithrombotic agents in several other clinical settings.

The emergence of a new medical discipline in pediatrics is usually unexpected and without immediate resources or expertise within a group of health care providers. Childhood thrombophilia is clearly a new field in pediatrics and a natural component of pediatric hematology/oncology programs. One approach to the rapid development of childhood thrombophilia programs is to model them on adult thromboembolism programs and pediatric hemophilia programs. In 1991, the Hospital for Sick Children (HSC) in Toronto, Canada, sponsored an institutional childhood thrombophilia program (now part of a broader institutional hemostasis program). The childhood program at HSC has three goals:

1. to provide optimal clinical service to children with or at risk for thromboembolic events
2. to conduct clinical research

Note: Dr. M. Andrew was a Career Investigator of the Heart and Stroke Foundation of Canada. This work was supported by a grant in aid from the Medical Research Council of Canada.

3. to provide a training program for pediatric hematologists in this new field of pediatrics

At the same time as the initiation of the HSC program, national registries were established with all 16 pediatric centers in Canada participating. This chapter is based on a comprehensive review of the literature on antithrombotic therapy for children, the Canadian registries, and an analysis of the first five years of the HSC childhood thrombophilia program.

CHILDHOOD THROMBOPHILIA PROGRAM

The literature review failed to find any publications describing thrombophilia programs in children. Therefore, the HSC childhood thrombophilia program is described in some detail. Hopefully, it will serve as a template for the development of other childhood thrombophilia programs.

Initiation of the Program

The need for a thrombophilia program was identified because of the number and complexity of patients referred to the hospital's hematology division for evaluation for thromboembolic events and/or antithrombotic therapy. Prior to initiating the thrombophilia program, meetings were held with division heads of all subspecialty services to identify conditions in which thrombotic problems occurred and antithrombotic therapy was required, either prophylactically or therapeutically. Based on the available information for children and adults, standardized protocols for heparin, oral anticoagulants, antiplatelet therapy, and thrombolytic therapy were developed. The protocols were approved by institutional regulatory committees and incorporated into the hospital's handbook for residents and fellows. The use of uniform protocols provided cohort studies that were analyzed yearly by the clinical research arm of the thrombophilia program.

Operational Aspects of the Program's Clinical Service

The thrombophilia program's clinical service is the responsibility of one full-time nurse and three physicians who work in conjunction with an inpatient hematology consult service. Two mechanisms were established for inpatient referral to the program's clinical service. First, several indications were identified in which heparin and/or oral anticoagulation therapy were indicated, but a consult from the hematology service was not necessary for the initiation of therapy (eg, mechanical heart valves, Blalock-Taussig shunts). For these patients, the responsible physician, following standardized protocols, orders anticoagulant therapy. If long-term therapy with oral anticoagulants is indicated, the program nurse provides an educational service for hospitalized patients, books appointments for follow-up care in the thrombophilia clinic, and arranges outpatient blood testing. The second mechanism for patient accrual is through an in-hospital consult to the hematology service. These consults request assistance with diagnoses and management of pediatric patients with or at risk for thromboembolic complications. In either case, the nurse-practitioner from the anticoagulation service works with the inpatient hematology consultative service by providing protocols, taking a comprehensive history, and initiating an in-hospital educational program. All children admitted to the hospital who require anticoagulation therapy at home are comprehensively evaluated in an outpatient clinic shortly after discharge from the hospital.

Outpatient Clinical Services

The childhood outpatient program provides consultations, diagnostic evaluation, and management of children with or at risk for thromboembolic events and their families. A comprehensive dedicated clinic is in place on a weekly basis with physicians and a nurse-practitioner responsible for the program in attendance. A specialized stroke clinic, held monthly, is attended by a pediatric neurologist in addition to the program's physicians and nurse. A weekly clinic also provides an educational experience for pediatric hematologists in training and a resource to the clinical trial arm of the program. Subsequent complete evaluations by physicians occur at a minimum of once per year or more frequently, depending on individual circumstances.

For each clinic visit, information on anticoagulation therapy and thrombotic risk is collected through the use of standardized forms. Extensive demographic information is also collected. Other outpatient services are also provided by the same dedicated nurse-practitioner on a daily basis for numerous issues. A significant proportion of the nurse-practitioner's time is spent in monitoring oral anticoagulant therapy. Most frequently, children have International Normalized Ratio (INR) measurements at community laboratories, which send results directly, via computer linkup, to the nurse-practitioner on the same day. Dose adjustments of oral anticoagulant therapy are conducted by the nurse-practitioner with the use of predefined protocols, and physician backup is available at all times.

Educational Program

The nurse-practitioner of the thrombophilia program develops and provides a uniform educational program for each family. Issues discussed with the family include the need for anticoagulant therapy, type of anticoagulant, monitoring with blood tests, symptoms to watch for in case of bleeding or recurrent thrombotic disease, and how to access the nurse-practitioners during working hours and physician assistance at any time. Specific pamphlets for pediatric patients on heparin, oral anticoagulants, thrombolytic therapy, and mechanical heart valves are provided to families. If a whole blood monitor is to be used by the parents or the patient at home, a separate educational session includes a video developed for pediatric patients and a calendar for entering daily doses of anticoagulant and laboratory values. For many children, Medic-Alert bracelets are indicated, and families are provided with the necessary forms.

Home Program

A whole blood prothrombin time (PT) monitor, Ciba Corning 512 Coagulation Monitor (Ciba Corning Diagnostics), was evaluated by the thrombophilia program's clinical research arm for use in outpatient clinics and the home setting. Figure 21–1 shows the correlation between INR values measured on the whole blood monitor compared with laboratory INR values. The correlation is excellent at:

$$y = 0.76x + 0.37; r = 0.93; p = <0.001$$

Whole blood monitor INR values are now routinely used in the thrombophilia clinic. Home use of whole blood INR monitors by parents and patients also has been validated.[1] Figure 21–2 shows INR values for two children, with different INR target ranges, who used whole blood monitors at home.[1] Whole blood PT/INR monitors provide one solution to patients with different venous access, geographical distance from a laboratory, or the need for frequent testing. Prior to home use, parents (in some cases, patients) have to demonstrate their ability to use the whole blood PT/INR monitor successfully on at least three separate occasions. In addition to the hospital record, families record all PTs/INRs in a calendar, along with any changes in dose of the oral anticoagulant. The nurse-practitioner is responsible for teaching parents and patients, remains in close contact with the families, and talks with them at least weekly by telephone and after every home test. The medical team (nurse-practitioner/physician) adjusts the dose of oral anticoagulant based on the

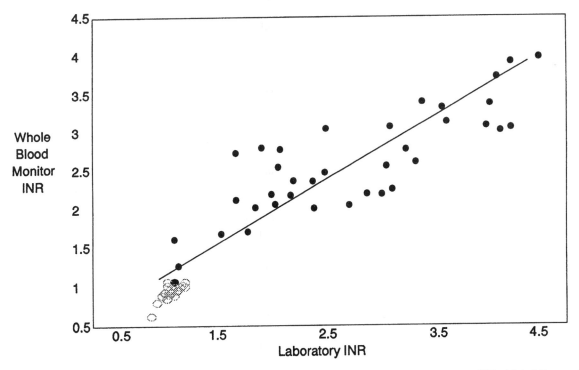

Figure 21–1 Accuracy of the whole monitor INR plotted against the laboratory INR value. The agreement at an INR of 2.0–3.5 was within 0.8 INR unit for 90% of values. The healthy control subjects are represented by empty circles. The clinic patients are represented by solid circles. Source: Reprinted with permission from P Massicotte et al, Home Monitoring of Warfarin Therapy in Children with a Whole Blood Prothrombin Time Monitor, *Journal of Pediatrics*, Vol 127, pp 389–394, © 1995, Mosby-Year Book, Inc.

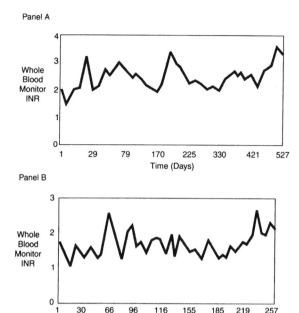

Figure 21–2 INR values for two children with different INR target ranges. **Panel A**, INR values of a child with a therapeutic range of 2.0 to 3.0. **Panel B**, INR values of a child with a therapeutic range of 1.3 to 2.0. Source: Reprinted with permission from P Massicotte, et al, Home Monitoring of Warfarin Therapy in Children with a Whole Blood Prothrombin Time Monitor, *Journal of Pediatrics*, Vol 127, pp 389–394, © 1995, Mosby-Year Book, Inc.

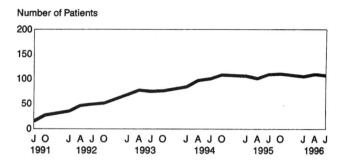

Figure 21–3 The number of active patients who have received anticoagulants at the Hospital for Sick Children's thrombophilia outpatient program, July 1991–June 1996

whole blood monitor PT/INR values.[2] The family is instructed when to perform the test and asked to call results to the nurse-practitioner. If the INR is not in the therapeutic range, the test is repeated, and an appropriate clinician decision is made. If the INR is above 4.5 on repeat testing, the child is brought to the hospital for laboratory confirmation of the INR results.

Home programs are also used for the outpatient administration of low–molecular-weight heparin. Usually, a subcutaneous catheter is placed weekly by the nurse-practitioner or visiting nurse and parents are taught to inject the heparin through the catheter twice daily. Some children prefer subcutaneous injections for each dose. In these instances, a topical anesthetic can be used and the injection of heparin with a 27-gauge needle is usually painless.

Patient Population

The patient population attending the HSC children's thrombophilia outpatient program was analyzed for this report, and 350 children were evaluated in the outpatient setting. The number of active patients receiving anticoagulants for any given month is rapidly increasing and shows no signs of leveling off (Figure 21–3). The age

distribution shows a predominance of young infants and teenagers (Figure 21–4). The indications for antithrombotic therapy are shown in Figure 21–5. The majority of patients require long-term or lifelong anticoagulant therapy. The incidence of serious bleeding problems is very low at less than 1%.[2]

INDICATIONS FOR ANTITHROMBOTIC THERAPY FOR PEDIATRIC PATIENTS

Several recent reviews[3–6] discuss the indications for antithrombotic therapy in detail. The most common indications for such therapy in pediatric patients are briefly considered here.

Venous Thromboembolic Disease

The incidence of venous thromboembolic complications (deep venous thrombosis [DVT] and pulmonary embolism [PE]) is estimated at 0.07/10,000 in the general pediatric population and at 5.3/10,000 in hospital admissions.[7–9] Comparable incidences of DVT/PE in the adult population are approximately 2.5%–5.0%.[10–12] Idiopathic DVT/PE, in contrast to adults, is rare in children.[13] In pediatric patients, 95% of DVT/PE is secondary to such problems as prematurity, cancer, trauma/surgery, congenital heart disease, and systemic lupus erythematosus.[13–17] The thrombus is in the upper venous system in more than 50% of pediatric patients and is due to a central venous line.[13,18] The age groups of greatest risk for DVT/PE are infants younger than one year of age and teenagers.[13,16,17] The clinical presentations and treatment of DVT/PE are similar to those for adults.[9,13,16,19]

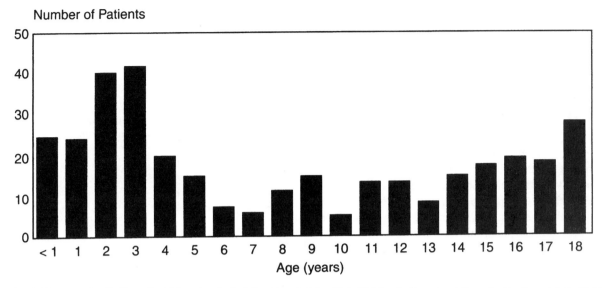

Figure 21–4 The age distribution of children treated at the Hospital for Sick Children's thrombophilia outpatient program. There is a predominance of young infants and teenagers.

Inherited Prothrombotic Complications

The most common inherited prothrombotic disorders include activated protein C resistance (APCR); deficiencies of antithrombin, protein C, protein S, and plasminogen; and dysfibrinogenemias. More rare disorders include heparin cofactor II deficiency, hyperhomocystinemia, inherited hypofibrinolytic states, and some forms of hyperlipidemia. The contribution of congenital prethrombotic disorders is uncertain, as the effect of APCR, present in approximately 5% of the population, has not been fully assessed.[4,20,21] In general, patients with heterozygous deficiencies are protected during childhood except in the presence of a secondary challenge. Exceptions include children with homozygous or double heterozygous states.

Arterial Thromboembolic Disease

The most common etiology of arterial thromboembolic disease in children is a catheter, either as part of cardiac catheterization or in the intensive care setting. Noncatheter-related arterial thrombotic complications are rare and occur in Takayasu's arteritis,[22–24] arteries from transplanted organs,[25–29] and giant coronary aneurysms secondary to Kawasaki's disease,[30–32] or as complications of some forms of congenital heart disease and cerebral vessels from local lesions or emboli from cardiac or other locations.

The response to anticoagulation therapy has been assessed in many disorders characterized by arterial thrombotic complications. Prophylaxis with 100–150 units/kg of heparin reduces the incidence of thrombotic complications from 40%

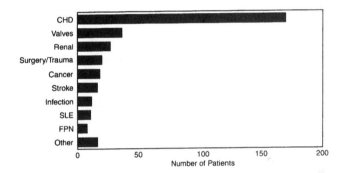

Figure 21–5 The most common indications for antithrombotic therapy in children treated at the Hospital for Sick Children's thrombophilia outpatient program

to 6% following cardiac catheterization.[33] Low-dose prophylactic therapy with heparin (3–5 units/hour) significantly prolongs umbilical artery catheter patency in newborns and likely reduces the incidence of catheter-related thrombosis.[34–39] For patients who develop the giant aneurysms of Kawasaki's disease, a combination of warfarin and low-dose aspirin might prevent subsequent occlusion and ischemic infarction. Warfarin in doses that sustain an INR of 2.5–3.5 is indicated as prophylaxis for children with mechanical heart valves.[3,4]

Other Disorders

Antithrombotic therapy is used in several other disorders in pediatric patients that are not discussed here. Readers are referred to other references for antithrombotic therapy in cardiopulmonary bypass,[40–43] extracorporeal membrane oxygenation,[44–46] Fontan procedures,[47–49] endovascular stents,[50] atrial fibrillation, myocardial infarction,[51] and continuous veno-venous hemoperfusion.[52–54]

GUIDELINES FOR ANTITHROMBOTIC THERAPY IN PEDIATRIC PATIENTS

Current recommendations for antithrombotic therapy in children are based on clinical trials in adults and cohort studies in pediatric patients. Although the general indications for antithrombotic therapy in pediatric patients are similar to those for adults, the frequency of specific disease states and underlying pathologies differs. For example, myocardial infarction and cerebrovascular accidents are two of the more common indications for antithrombotic therapy in adults but the least common in children.[55] The current indications for antithrombotic therapy in children are provided in Exhibit 21–1.

Optimal treatment of children with thromboembolic events likely differs from adults because of important ontogenic features of hemostasis that influence both the pathophysiology of the thrombotic processes and the response to antithrombotic agents. Clinical trials currently in progress will undoubtedly change the recommendations for antithrombotic therapy in children and help to define optimal treatment. Pediatric thrombophilia programs can and should assume responsibility for rapid implementation of new recommendations and monitoring of antithrombotic therapy.

Heparin Therapy

General Information

Heparin is the most commonly used anticoagulant in pediatric patients. Heparin's activities can be considered as anticoagulant (the inhibition of coagulation enzymes in vitro) and antithrombotic (the prevention of thromboembolic events in vivo). Heparin's activities are mediated by antithrombin (AT-III), a major inhibitor of several coagulation enzymes, particularly thrombin.[56–59]

Plasma concentrations of AT-III are age dependent, with values less than 0.50 unit/mL being common during early infancy (Figure 21–6).[60] At the same time, plasma concentrations of prothrombin are approximately 0.60 unit, which results in a decreased capacity to generate thrombin (Figure 21–6).[61] Heparin's activities are directly influenced by the ratio of AT-III to prothrombin (Figures 21–7 and 21–8).[61] The latter strongly suggests that heparin's antithrombotic potential will differ in pediatric patients, particularly young infants. Clearly, clinical trials with the objective of determining optimal use of heparin in children are required.

Exhibit 21–1
INDICATIONS FOR ANTITHROMBOTIC AGENTS IN PEDIATRIC PATIENTS

Treatment

- Venous thromboembolic complications
- Arterial thromboembolic complications

Treatment: Probable

- Myocardial infarction
- Some forms of stroke

Prophylaxis

- Mechanical prosthetic heart valves
- Biologic prosthetic heart valves
- Cardiac catheterization
- Central arterial catheters

Prophylaxis: Probable

- Endovascular stents
- Blalock-Taussig shunts
- Fontan procedures
- Central venous catheters
- Atrial venous fibrillation

Other

- Kawasaki's disease
- Cardiopulmonary bypass
- Extracorporeal membrane oxygenation
- Hemodialysis
- Continuous veno-venous hemoperfusion

Source: Reprinted with permission from AD Michelson, E Bovill, and M Andrew, Antithrombotic Therapy in Children, *Chest*, Vol 108, No 4, pp 506S-522S, © 1995, American College of Chest Physicians.

Therapeutic Range and Monitoring

Heparin therapy is most commonly monitored by the activated partial thromboplastin time (aPTT). The therapeutic range reflects a minimum aPTT value above which new thromboembolic events rarely occur and a maximum level that minimizes the risk of bleeding.[62–64] Unfortunately, differing sensitivities of aPTT reagents to heparin adversely affect the consistency of the aPTT.[65] To circumvent this problem, coagulation laboratories should standardize aPTT values to reflect heparin levels of 0.2–0.4 U/mL by protamine sulfate assay or 0.30 to 0.70 U/mL by anti-factor Xa assay.[62,66–68] The historical use of an aPTT ratio of 1.5 to 2.0

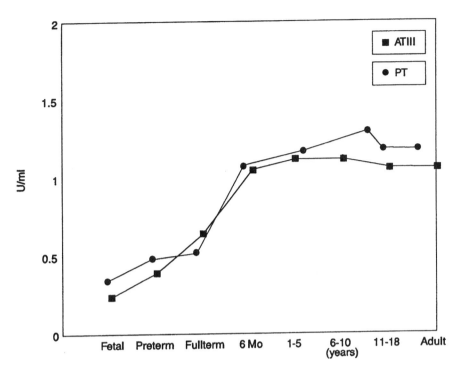

Figure 21–6 The plasma concentration of antithrombin III is age dependent, with values less than 0.50 unit/mL being common during early infancy

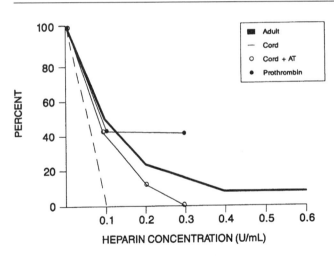

Figure 21–7 Dose response curves of thrombin activity (expressed as area under the curve) versus standard heparin concentration. Source: Reprinted from *Thrombosis Research*, Vol 63, A Vieira, F Ofosu, and M Andrew, Heparin Sensitivity and Resistance in the Neonate: An Explanation, pp 85–99, Copyright 1991, with kind permission from Elsevier Science Ltd, The Boulevard, Langford Lane, Kidlington 0X5 1GB, UK.

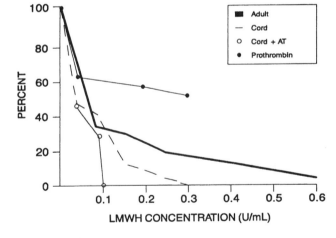

Figure 21–8 Dose response curves of thrombin activity (expressed as area under the curve) versus the concentration of the low–molecular-weight heparin (LMWH) Choay 222. Source: Reprinted from *Thrombosis Research*, Vol 63, A Vieira, F Ofosu, and M Andrew, Heparin Sensitivity and Resistance in the Neonate: An Explanation, pp 85–99, Copyright 1991, with kind permission from Elsevier Science Ltd, The Boulevard, Langford Lane, Kidlington 0X5 1GB, UK.

times the baseline value is no longer adequate for monitoring heparin.[68] In pediatric patients, aPTT values correctly predict heparin concentrations 70% of the time.[69] If the baseline aPTT is prolonged (as in the presence of a nonspecific inhibitor) or short (as in the presence of high factor VIII

levels), aPTT values might not reflect heparin concentrations. One approach is to measure at least one simultaneous aPTT and heparin level for a patient to ensure that the aPTT value accurately reflects the heparin concentration. When aPTT values and heparin levels are discordant, heparin levels should be preferentially used because they are a better predictor of heparin's antithrombotic effect in vivo.[70,71]

Dose Response

Doses of heparin required in pediatric patients to achieve adult therapeutic aPTT values for DVT/PE have been assessed using a weight-based nomogram (Exhibit 21–2).[69] Bolus doses of 75–100 units/kg result in therapeutic aPTT values in 90% of children. Maintenance heparin doses are age dependent, with infants having the highest requirements (28 units/kg/hour) and children over one year of age having lower requirements (20 units/kg/hour), similar to adults (18 U/kg/hour).[66,72] The clearance of heparin is faster in the young than in the adult.[73,74] The duration of heparin therapy for the treatment of DVT is a minimum of 5 days and 7–10 days for extensive DVT or PE.[75,76] Oral anticoagulation therapy can be initiated on day 1 of heparin therapy except for extensive DVT or PE, when oral anticoagulant therapy should be delayed.[77] At least 2 days of a therapeutic INR are required prior to discontinuing heparin therapy. A validated nomogram for rapidly adjusting heparin dosing in children is presented in Exhibit 21–2.[69,78] Heparin-dosing nomograms can be adapted into preprinted order sheets to facilitate rapid and effective anticoagulation.

Adverse Effects

There are at least three clinically important adverse effects of heparin:

1. *Bleeding*—although the complication of greatest concern, bleeding is not frequent in children treated for DVT/PE.[69,79]
2. *Osteoporosis*—although there is no information for children, it seems prudent to avoid long-term use of heparin because of the convincing relationship between heparin and osteoporosis in pregnant women.[80–83]
3. *Heparin-induced thrombocytopenia*—in the absence of an alternative etiology for thrombocytopenia, pediatric patients should be evaluated for heparin-induced thrombocytopenia (HIT) and alternative therapy employed.[84–86]

Use of Heparin in Childhood Programs

An inpatient thrombophilia program can facilitate the optimal use of heparin through ongoing educational programs for parents and caregivers, as well as provide supervision of heparin therapy in the hospital. Six common mistakes are

1. interruption of a dedicated heparin line for other medications
2. use of the aPTT value, instead of a heparin level, to monitor heparin therapy when the two are discordant
3. early discontinuation of heparin therapy when warfarin therapy is initiated
4. lack of recognition of HIT
5. inappropriate dilutions of heparin or infusion rate
6. inappropriate timing of aPTT values and dose adjustments

Exhibit 21–2
PROTOCOL FOR SYSTEMIC HEPARIN ADMINISTRATION AND ADJUSTMENT FOR PEDIATRIC PATIENTS

1. Loading dose: heparin 75 units/kg IV over 10 minutes.
2. Initial maintenance dose: 28 units/kg/hour for infants less than one year.
3. Initial maintenance dose: 20 units/kg/hour for children over one year.
4. Adjust heparin to maintain aPTT 60–85 seconds (assuming this reflects an anti–factor Xa level of 0.30 to 0.70):

aPTT (sec)	Bolus (units/kg)	Hold (min)	% Rate (units/kg/hr)	Repeat aPTT
<50	50	0	+10%	4 hrs
50–59	0	0	+10%	4 hrs
60–85	0	0	0	Next day
86–95	0	0	−10%	4 hrs
96–120	0	30	−10%	4 hrs
>120	0	60	−15%	4 hrs

5. Obtain blood for aPTT four hours after administration of the heparin loading dose and four hours after every change in the infusion rate.
6. When aPTT values are therapeutic, a daily CBC, and aPTT.

Source: Reprinted with permission from AD Michelson, E Bovill, and M Andrew, Antithrombotic Therapy in Children, *Chest*, Vol 108, No 4, pp 506S–522S, © 1995, American College of Chest Physicians.

Relatively age-specific problems, such as poor venous access, which limits the administration and monitoring of heparin, also can arise. The subcutaneous use of heparin and a whole blood aPTT monitor can circumvent many of these problems.

Low–Molecular-Weight Heparin

General Information

Numerous clinical trials in adult patients convincingly demonstrate that low–molecular-weight heparin (LMWH) has several significant advantages over heparin.[87–93] For many disorders in adult patients, LMWH is recommended ahead of heparin for the following four reasons:

1. The risk of bleeding with LMWH is significantly less than with heparin[94–99] (perhaps the most important reason).
2. LMWH is at least as effective and, in some conditions, more effective than heparin.[97,98,100–102]
3. The pharmacokinetics of LMWH are predictable, thereby minimizing the frequency of monitoring, a particularly important consideration for pediatric patients. The marked variability in the anticoagulant response to heparin necessitates close monitoring.[103,104]
4. LMWH can be administered subcutaneously every 12 hours, which eliminates the need for continuous venous access devoted to heparin administration, another significant advantage for children. The number of needle pokes can be further reduced by the use of a subcutaneous catheter that can be accessed twice daily and remain in place for seven days.[105]

In summary, LMWH is particularly attractive in clinical situations where the use of heparin is problematic. Pediatric patients requiring anticoagulation therapy are frequently problematic because of the seriousness of their underlying disorders, increased risk of bleeding, and poor venous access that limits monitoring.[69] Similar to heparin, LMWH's activities are directly influenced by the ratio of AT-III to prothrombin (see Figure 21–8). This observation suggests that LMWH's antithrombotic potential will differ in pediatric patients, particularly in young infants.

Therapeutic Range and Monitoring

In vitro, LMWH possesses a very high specific activity against factor Xa and considerably less activity against thrombin in contrast to heparin, which has equivalent activity against Xa and thrombin.[90,91,106,107] The explanation for the reduced inhibition of thrombin is that the inhibition of thrombin requires that both AT-III and thrombin bind to the heparin polysaccharides, with a minimum requirement of approximately 18 monosaccharide units.[105] In contrast, the inhibition of factor Xa requires that only AT-III bind to heparin, thus reducing the required length of the polysaccharide to amounts present in LMWH preparations.[105] Because of this property, LMWH must be monitored with an anti-factor Xa assay. The target range for treatment with LMWH for DVT/PE is extrapolated from adult clinical trials and is an anti-factor Xa level between 0.50 and 1.0, four to six hours following subcutaneous administration.[105] The aPTT is not prolonged by LMWH within this therapeutic range.[105]

Dose Response

Newborns have increased dose requirements with an average of 1.6 units/kg subcutaneous twice a day (enoxaparin) to achieve therapeutic heparin levels.[105] For older children, an initial dose of 1.0 mg/kg subcutaneous twice a day (enoxaparin) is usually sufficient to achieve therapeutic heparin levels.[105]

Adverse Effects

The three clinically important adverse effects of heparin are considerably reduced for LMWH[108]:

1. Based on several adult trials and a meta-analysis of these same trials, the risk of bleeding is estimated to be reduced by 2.3%[108] in comparison with standard heparin. The decreased risk of bleeding will likely apply to children as well as to adults.[105]
2. The risk of osteoporosis appears to be reduced with LMWH, based on animal models[80,82,109] and osteoclast and osteoblast cell culture experiments[110–115] as well as studies in pregnant women.[110,116–118] Preliminary data from two young girls treated with LMWH for severe protein C deficiency (levels of approximately 3%)[119] show normal bone development, based on sensitive measurements of bone density.[119]
3. The risk of HIT is considerably decreased with LMWH in comparison with standard heparin.[110,120–123] In fact, in some situations, LMWH is used to treat HIT.[124–127]

In addition, a potentially adverse effect of LMWH is the inability to neutralize completely LMWH's anticoagulant activity by protamine sulphate.[124]

Use of LMWH in Childhood Programs

One of the functions of childhood thrombophilia programs is the rapid and safe introduction of new therapies for pediatric patients when appropriate. LMWH therapy is an example of this function. Most pediatricians will not be familiar with LMWH and will require assistance in the dosing and monitoring of its activities.

Oral Anticoagulation Therapy

General Information

Warfarin (4-hydroxycoumarin) is the oral anticoagulant most commonly used in pediatric patients. It functions by competitively interfering with vitamin K metabolism. Vitamin K is an essential cofactor for the posttranslational carboxylation of glutamic acid (gla) residues on specific coagulation proteins (factors II, VII, IX, and X). The gla residues serve as calcium-binding sites, which are essential for these coagulation proteins to interact on phospholipid surfaces and thrombin generation to occur. Plasma concentrations of the vitamin K–dependent coagulant proteins are significantly reduced during early infancy (Figure 21–9), similar to those in adults who are receiving therapeutic amounts of warfarin.[128] This makes the use of oral anticoagulants problematic. When possible, warfarin should be avoided in children, particularly during early infancy.

Somewhat unexpectedly, the in vitro capacity of plasmas from children on oral anticoagulants to generate thrombin is delayed and decreased by 25% in comparison with plasmas from adults.[129] Concurrently, plasma concentrations of prothrombin fragment 1.2, one index of thrombin generation in vivo, are significantly lower in children compared with those in adults receiving warfarin.[130] These two observations suggest that optimal therapeutic ranges for oral anticoagulation therapy in children might differ from adults. Clinical trials are urgently needed to test this hypothesis.

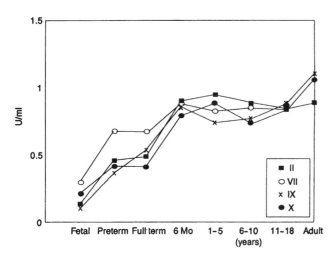

Figure 21–9 Plasma concentrations of the vitamin K–dependent factors, which are significantly reduced during early infancy. Source: Reprinted with permission from M Andrew, Developmental Hemostasis: Relevance to Thromboembolic Complications in Pediatric Patients, *Thrombosis and Haemostasis*, Vol 74, Suppl 1, pp 415–425, © 1995, International Society of Haemostasis.

Therapeutic Range

The PT is sensitive to plasma concentrations of three vitamin K–dependent coagulant proteins, factors II, VII, and X, and is the most commonly used test for monitoring warfarin therapy in North America.[55,131] Unfortunately, thromboplastin reagents for PT assays have widely varying sensitivities to low plasma concentrations of vitamin K–dependent proteins.[132–136] The INR provides a mechanism to correct for differing sensitivities of PT reagent.[134–136] Laboratories involved in monitoring warfarin therapy need to provide INR values to clinicians in order to facilitate optimal management. Currently, therapeutic INR ranges for pediatric patients are directly extrapolated from recommendations for adult patients because no clinical trials have assessed optimal INR ranges for pediatric patients based on clinical outcomes. The usual therapeutic range for children with DVT/PE is an INR of 2.0–3.0[2,18] and for those with mechanical prosthetic heart valves, 2.5–3.5.[2]

Monitoring

Monitoring oral anticoagulant therapy in pediatric patients is difficult and requires close supervision with frequent dose adjustments.[2] In contrast to adults, only 10%–20% of children can be safely monitored monthly.[2] Contributing causes to the need for close monitoring include the following:

- *Diet*—Vitamin K content in breast milk is very low, with the result that breastfed infants have a relative sensitivity to warfarin.[137–142] In contrast, nutrient formulas are heavily supplemented with vitamin K (4.2–100 μg/L)[139,143] to protect against hemorrhagic disease of the newborn and result in a relative resistance to medication.[144,145]
- *Medications*—Because of the seriousness of their primary problems, most children requiring oral anticoagulation are receiving multiple medications, both long term and intermittently. Table 21–1 provides a list of the most commonly prescribed medications and their effects on warfarin dosing.[55]
- *Primary medical problems*—Most pediatric patients requiring oral anticoagulants have serious primary problems that influence the biologic effect and clearance of warfarin, as well as the risk of bleeding.[2,146]
- *Age distribution*—Unfortunately, the two largest pediatric populations requiring oral anticoagulants are infants less than one year of age and teenagers.[2] Teenagers are not necessarily compliant with their medication,[147–148] and infants are a difficult group of patients to monitor because of poor venous access, as well as complicated medical problems.[148–156]

Table 21–1 Commonly Used Drugs in Children That Affect Their INR Value

Drug	Effect on INR
Amiodarone	Increase
Amoxil	Slight Increase
Ceclor	Slight Increase
Co-trimoxazole	Increase
Dilantin	Decrease
Phenobarbital	Decrease
Prednisone	Increase
Tegretol	Decrease

Source: Reprinted with permission from M Andrew et al, Oral Anticoagulant Therapy in Pediatric Patients: A Prospective Study, *Thrombosis and Haemostasis*, Vol 71, No 3, pp 265–269, © 1994, International Society of Haemostasis.

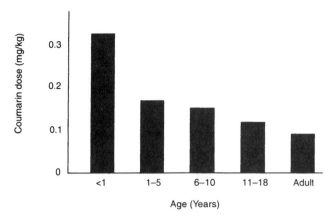

Figure 21–10 The effect of age on the dose of Coumadin required to sustain an INR of 2.0–3.0. Younger children required significantly more Coumadin than older children (p<0.001). Vertical bars describe ±2 standard error of the mean. Source: Reprinted with permission from M Andrew et al, Oral Anticoagulant Therapy in Pediatric Patients: A Prospective Study, *Thrombosis and Haemostasis*, Vol 71, No 3, pp 265–269, © 1994, International Society of Haemostasis.

Dose Response

If the baseline INR is less than 1.3, oral anticoagulant therapy can be initiated with a dose of 0.2 mg/kg.[2] Maintenance doses for oral anticoagulants are age dependent, with infants having the highest (0.32 mg/kg) and teenagers the lowest (0.09 mg/kg) requirements (Figure 21–10). For adults, weight-adjusted doses for oral anticoagulants are not precisely known but are in the range of 0.04 to 0.08 mg/kg for an INR of 2.0–3.0.[55] The mechanisms responsible for the age dependency of oral anticoagulant doses are not completely clear. Exhibit 21–3 provides a nomogram for loading and monitoring oral anticoagulants in children.[2] Guidelines for the duration of therapy with oral anticoagulants in children reflect recommendations for adults with similar disorders.[2,13] Patients with a first venous thromboembolic event are treated for three months, whereas those with mechanical prosthetic heart valves are treated for life.

Adverse Effects

Bleeding is the main complication of oral anticoagulants. Minor bleeding, which is of limited clinical consequence (eg, bruising, minor nosebleeds, heavy menses, microscopic hematuria, slightly prolonged bleeding from cuts and loose teeth), occurs in approximately 20% of children receiving oral anticoagulants.[2] The risk of serious bleeding in children receiving oral anticoagulants for mechanical prosthetic valves is similar to adults at less than 3.2/100 patient years.[148,151,154–163] Nonhemorrhagic complications of oral anticoagulants, such as tracheal calcification or hair loss, have been described on rare occasions in young children.[164] Although oral anticoagulants do not affect bone density in adults,[165,166] the effects on children have not been assessed. At this time, there

are no other serious complications of oral anticoagulants reported in the pediatric population.

Use of Oral Anticoagulation in Childhood Programs

The problems with monitoring oral anticoagulants in children and concerns over serious bleeding have limited their use, even in cases where they are strongly indicated. Childhood thrombophilia programs provide part of the solution for this problem. Specialized clinics,[2] educational programs for families, use of whole blood PT/INR monitors used in the clinic, and home programs with parents and patients measuring INR values with whole blood monitors[1] are mechanisms for safely using oral anticoagulants in children.

Antiplatelet Agents

Therapeutic Range and Monitoring

In contrast to other anticoagulants, there is no therapeutic range or a need to monitor antiplatelet agents.

Dose Response

Doses of aspirin used as adjunctive therapy for mechanical prosthetic heart valves range from 6 to 20 mg/kg/day.[149,151–153,157,161,167,168] Doses of dipyridamole used for mechanical prosthetic heart valves range from 2 to 5 mg/kg/day.[149,151,157,167,168] High-dose aspirin (80–100 mg/kg/day) is indicated for

Exhibit 21–3
PROTOCOL FOR PEDIATRIC ORAL ANTICOAGULATION THERAPY TO MAINTAIN AN INR OF 2.0–3.0

1. Day 1—if the baseline INR is 1.0–1.3, dose = 0.2 mg/kg orally; maximum initial dose limit = PO 10 mg od.
2. Loading days 2–4—if the INR is:

INR	Action
1.1–1.3	Repeat loading dose
1.4–1.9	50% of loading dose
2.0–3.0	50% of loading dose
3.1–3.4	25% of loading dose
>3.5	Hold until INR <3.5, then restart at 50% less than previous dose

3. Maintenance oral anticoagulation dose guidelines:

INR	Action
1.1–1.4	Increase by 20% of dose
1.5–1.9	Increase by 10% of dose
2.0–3.0	No change
3.1–3.4	Decrease by 10% of dose
>3.5	Hold until INR <3.5, then restart at 20% less than previous dose

Source: Reprinted with permission from M Andrew et al, Oral Anticoagulant Therapy in Pediatric Patients: A Prospective Study, *Thrombosis and Haemostasis*, Vol 71, No 3, pp 265–269, © 1994, International Society of Haemostasis.

the initial treatment of children with Kawasaki's disease (up to 14 days) and then a lower dose of 3–5 mg/kg/day for seven weeks or longer if there is echocardiographic evidence of coronary artery abnormalities.[32] The effects of antiplatelet agents persist for the life span of the platelet.

Adverse Effects

In general, antiplatelet agents rarely cause clinically important bleeding except in patients with underlying hemostatic defects or in the presence of anticoagulation with heparin or warfarin. A specific potential adverse effect of aspirin in young children lies in its relationship to Reye's syndrome. First described as a distinct clinical and pathologic entity in 1963, Reye's syndrome is characterized by a mild prodromal viral-like illness, followed abruptly by vomiting and encephalopathy, with symptoms ranging from a hyperexcitable state of delirium or lethargy to coma with dysfunction of the lower brain stem.[169] Eleven case control studies link Reye's syndrome to aspirin.[169–179] The relationship between aspirin and Reye's syndrome appears to be a dose-dependent effect of aspirin.[169,172,175] The relatively low doses of aspirin used as antiplatelet therapy, however, seldom cause other adverse effects.

Thrombolytic Therapy

General Information

Three thrombolytic agents are used in pediatric patients: streptokinase (SK), urokinase (UK), and tissue plasminogen activator (tPA). Each mediates its activities through the conversion of endogenous plasminogen to plasmin. Unfortu-

nately, plasma concentrations of plasminogen during early infancy and in many older children requiring thrombolytic therapy are decreased.[180,181] Low plasma levels of plasminogen slow the generation of plasmin[182] and reduce fibrin clot lysis in response to all three thrombolytic agents (Figure 21–11).[183–185] Supplementation of plasmas with plasminogen increases their thrombolytic effects.[183–185]

Patient Population Receiving Thrombolytic Therapy

A MEDLINE search of the literature (177 patients)[181] and a single institutional study (88 patients)[186] form the basis for the following information. The age distribution was similar for all three agents, with newborns and infants less than one year of age comprising 35% of treated children.[181] The most common underlying primary disease was congenital heart disease (51% of patients). Catheterization, either short term or long term, was the single most frequent cause of thrombotic events treated with thrombolytic therapy. Catheterizations could be grouped as short-term cardiac catheterizations, central venous lines, and umbilical arterial lines. Of these, cardiac catheterization was the single most frequent indication for thrombolytic therapy. UK and tPA were used to treat thrombi in all locations, whereas SK was used primarily to treat arterial occlusion in the femoral artery secondary to cardiac catheterization.

Therapeutic Range and Monitoring

At this time, there is no single laboratory test that can be used to delineate a therapeutic range for thrombolytic agents; however, a variety of coagulation tests can and should be

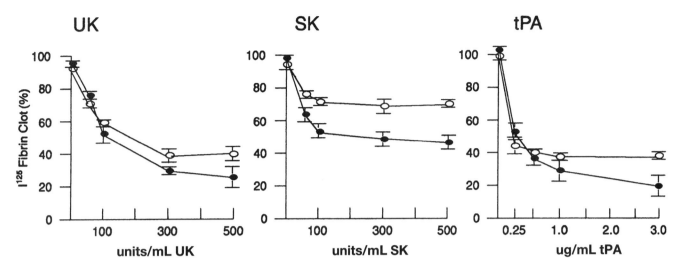

Figure 21–11 The remaining ^{125}I-fibrin in a clot system (washed cord ^{125}I-fibrin clots in cord plasma, ○—○) compared with a similar adult system (●—●) in the presence of increasing amounts of urokinase (**UK**), streptokinase (**SK**), and tissue plasminogen activator (**tPA**). The cord system (○—○) was resistant to the effects of all three thrombolytic agents compared with the adult system (●—●) (mean ± standard error of the mean, p <0.01). Source: Reprinted with permission from M Andrew, et al, Fibrin Clotlysis by Thrombolytic Agents Is Impaired in Newborns Due to a Low Plasminogen Concentration, *Thrombosis and Haemostasis*, Vol 68, No 3, pp 325–330, © 1992, International Society of Haemostasis.

used to monitor the activities of thrombolytic agents to ensure that a fibrinogen/fibrinolytic effect is present. These tests include fibrinogen concentration, thrombin clotting time, fibrin/fibrinogen degradation products, and D-dimer. Because of the substantial risk of bleeding, concurrent hemostatic problems, such as vitamin K deficiency, should be corrected prior to the use of thrombolytic therapy.

Dose Response

Thrombolytic therapy is used in low doses to restore central line patency and in higher doses in children with extensive DVT or massive PE. SK should not be used to reestablish central venous line patency because of the possibility of allergic reactions with repeated doses. For central venous line patency, one commonly used low-dose protocol is to instill 2–3 mL of UK (5,000 u/mL) for two to four hours.[187–190] Short infusions of low-dose UK also have been used if direct instillation of UK did not reestablish patency. One approach is to infuse UK at 150 U/kg/hour for eight hours and reassess with objective tests.

A wide range of higher doses has been used for systemic therapy with each of these thrombolytic agents. The most commonly used protocols are summarized in Table 21–2. The choice of agent reflects the decade and indication. During the 1970s and 1980s, SK was most commonly used for thrombotic complications of cardiac catheterization, but tPA has become the preferred agent during the 1990s. In

contrast, UK is the most commonly used agent for thromboembolic events because of central venous lines and umbilical arterial thrombi.[181]

Delivery of the thrombolytic agent is agent specific. UK is usually administered locally through an indwelling catheter, whereas tPA and SK are usually each administered from a peripheral site. The duration of tPA therapy is 12 hours or less in 91% of patients, compared with a minimum of 48 hours in 66% of patients treated with UK and a median of 24 hours for SK therapy in 78% of patients.[181]

Efficacy and Adverse Effects

Resolution of thrombosis is difficult to assess accurately because objective testing has not been uniformly applied or reported. The literature[181] and an institutional study[186] suggest that resolution was accomplished in more than 80% of patients with all three agents but with vastly different durations of therapy (Figure 21–12). Bleeding at local sites was frequent and required transfusion in 54% of children. Severe bleeding, such as into the central nervous system, however, was rare (<1%).[191] Treatment of mild bleeding secondary to thrombolytic therapy consisted of local measures (eg, pressure, topical thrombin preparations) and transfusion of packed red blood cells, when necessary. Treatment of major bleeding consists of stopping the thrombolytic therapy, plasma and/or cryoprecipitate, and consideration for an antifibrinolytic agent.

Table 21–2 Thrombolytic Therapy for Pediatric Patients

Low Dose for Blocked Catheters

	Regimen	Monitoring
Instillation	UK (5,000 U/mL) 1.5–3 mL/lumen, 2–4 hours	None
Infusion	UK (150 U/kg/hr) per lumen, 12–48 hours	Fibrinogen, TCT, PT, aPTT

Systemic Thrombolytic Therapy*

	Load	Maintenance	Monitoring
UK	4,400 U/kg	4,400 U/kg/hr, 6–12 hours	Fibrinogen, TCT, PT, aPTT
SK	2,000 U/kg	2,000 U/kg/hr, 6–12 hours	Same
TPA	None	0.1–0.6 mg/kg/hr, for 6 hours	Same

*Start heparin therapy either during or immediately upon completion of thrombolytic therapy. A loading dose of heparin can be omitted. The length of time for optimal maintenance is uncertain. Values provided are starting suggestions; some patients might respond to longer or shorter courses of therapy.

Key: aPTT, activated partial thromboplastin time; PT, prothrombin time; TCT, thrombin clotting time; UK, urokinase.

Source: Reprinted with permission from AD Michelson, E Bovill, and M Andrew, Antithrombotic Therapy in Children, *Chest*, Vol 108, No 4, pp 506S–522S, © 1995, American College of Chest Physicians.

Use of Thrombolytic Therapy in Childhood Programs

Childhood thrombophilia programs can assist physicians administering thrombolytic therapy to circumvent some of the most common problems, such as:

- the effect of low plasminogen levels on either a physiologic basis or an acquired basis by early replacement with plasma
- the prolonged use of thrombolytic therapy (days) when the patient has become refractory and requires concurrent anticoagulant therapy, as well as plasminogen replacement

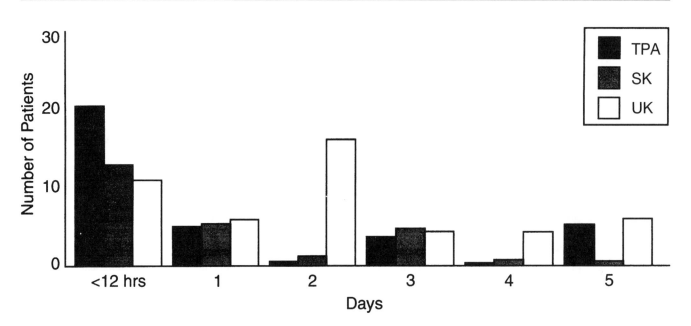

Figure 21–12 Duration of therapy for the three thrombolytic agents, tissue plasminogen activation (tPA), streptokinase (SK), and urokinase (UK). The duration was similar for SK and UK, but shorter for tPA.

- local and generalized bleeding
- effective utilization of the coagulation laboratory for the monitoring of thrombolytic therapy and its side effect of excessive bleeding

RECOMMENDATIONS

The Fourth Consensus Conference on Antithrombotic Therapy by the American College of Chest Physicians was published in *Chest,* October 1995.[3] For the first time, a chapter focusing on antithrombotic therapy in pediatric patients was included. The basis for the chapter was a MEDLINE search of the literature from 1966 to 1995 that used combinations of key words. It was supplemented by additional references located through the bibliographies of listed articles. All articles were graded as levels I to V and recommendations classified into grades A, B, and C (Table 21–3).[192] The following recommendations are reproduced, with approval, from the *Chest* supplement.[3]

Treatment of Venous Thromboembolism in Children

1. Children (over two months of age) with deep vein thrombosis or pulmonary embolism should be treated with intravenous (IV) heparin sufficient to prolong the aPTT to a range that corresponds to an anti-factor Xa level of 0.3–0.7 units/mL. This grade C recommendation is based on grade A recommendations for adults and one level IV study in children.[69]
2. It is recommended that treatment with heparin should be continued for 5 to 10 days and that oral anticoagulation should be overlapped with heparin for 4 to 5 days. For many patients, heparin and warfarin can be started together and heparin discontinued on day 6 if the PT (INR) is therapeutic. For massive pulmonary embolism or extensive deep vein thrombosis, a longer period of heparin therapy should be considered. This grade C

Table 21–3 Levels of Evidence and Grades of Recommendations for Therapy

Level of Evidence	Grade of Recommendation
Level I	**Grade A**
Level I	Results come from a single RCT, in which the lower limit of the CI for the treatment effect exceeds the minimal clinically important benefit.
Level I+	Results come from a meta-analysis of RCTs, in which the treatment effects from individual studies are consistent and the lower limit of the CI for the treatment effect exceeds the minimal clinically important benefit.
Level I–	Results come from a meta-analysis of RCTs, in which the treatment effects from individual studies are widely disparate but the lower limit of the CI for the treatment effect still exceeds the minimal clinically important benefit.
Level II	**Grade B**
Level II	Results come from a single RCT, in which the CI for the treatment effect overlaps the minimal clinically important benefit.
Level II+	Results come from a meta-analysis of RCTs, in which the treatment effects from individual studies are consistent and the CI for the treatment effect overlaps the minimal clinically important benefit.
Level II–	Results come from a meta-analysis of RCTs, in which the treatment effects from individual studies are widely disparate and the CI for the treatment effect overlaps the minimal clinically important benefit.
Level III	**Grade C**
Level III	Results come from nonrandomized concurrent cohort studies.
Level IV	**Grade C**
Level IV	Results come from nonrandomized historic cohort studies.
Level V	**Grade C**
Level V	Results come from case series.

Key: CI, confidence interval; RCT, randomized controlled trial.

recommendation is based on grade A recommendations for adults and one level IV study in children.[69]

3. Long-term anticoagulant therapy should be continued for at least three months with oral anticoagulants to prolong the INR to 2.0–3.0. This grade C recommendation is based on grade A recommendations for adults and one level IV study[2] and six level V studies[146,156,157,193–195] in children.

4. Either indefinite oral anticoagulant therapy with an INR of 2.0–3.0, low-dose oral anticoagulant therapy (INR <2.0), or close monitoring should be considered for children with a first recurrence of venous thrombosis or a continuing risk factor, such as a central venous line, antithrombin ID deficiency, protein C or S deficiency, activated protein C resistance, and lupus anticoagulants in the antiphospholipid antibody syndrome or systemic lupus erythematosus. This grade C recommendation is based on grade C recommendations for adults and one level V study in children.[2]

5. Indefinite oral anticoagulant therapy with an INR of 2.0–3.0 should be considered for children with a second recurrence of venous thrombosis or a continuing risk factor, such as a central venous line, antithrombin III deficiency, protein C or S deficiency, activated protein C resistance, and lupus anticoagulants in the antiphospholipid antibody syndrome or systemic lupus erythematosus.

6. The use of thrombolytic agents in the treatment of venous thromboembolism continues to be highly individualized. Further clinical investigation is needed before more definitive recommendations can be made.

7. Children with congenital prethrombotic disorders should receive short-term prophylactic anticoagulation in high-risk situations, such as immobility, significant surgery, or trauma.

Treatment of Venous and Arterial Thromboembolism in Newborns

1. The use of anticoagulation therapy in the treatment of newborns with DVT, PE, or arterial thrombosis continues to be highly individualized. Further clinical investigation is needed before more definitive recommendations can be made.

2. If short-term anticoagulation therapy is not used, the thrombus should be closely monitored with objective tests and, if extending, anticoagulation therapy instituted.

3. If anticoagulation is used, there should be a short course (10 to 14 days) of IV heparin, sufficient to prolong the aPTT to the therapeutic range that corresponds to an anti–factor Xa level of 0.3–0.7 units/mL. The thrombus should be closely monitored with objective tests for

evidence of extension or recurrent disease. This grade C recommendation is based on unpublished data.[196] If the thrombus extends following discontinuation of heparin therapy, oral anticoagulation therapy should be considered.

4. The use of thrombolytic agents in the treatment of venous thromboembolism continues to be highly individualized. Further clinical investigation is needed before more definitive recommendations can be made. Supplementation with plasminogen might be helpful.[183,196]

Prophylaxis for Cardiac Catheterization in Children and Newborns

Newborns and children requiring cardiac catheterization via an artery should be prophylaxed with IV heparin in doses of 100–150 units/kg as a bolus. This grade B recommendation is based on one level II study in children less than 10 years of age.[33] Aspirin alone cannot be recommended (one level II study).[197]

Mechanical Prosthetic Heart Valves in Children

1. It is strongly recommended that children with mechanical prosthetic heart valves receive oral anticoagulation therapy. This grade C recommendation is based on grade C recommendations for adults and 13 level V studies in children.[148,149,154–163,167]

2. Levels of oral anticoagulation therapy that prolong the INR to 2.5–3.5 are recommended based on recommendations in adults.[198]

3. Children with mechanical prosthetic heart valves who suffer systemic embolism despite adequate therapy with oral anticoagulation therapy might benefit from the addition of aspirin, 6–20 mg/kg/day (adult level I study).[199] Dipyridamole, 2–5 mg/kg/day, in addition to oral anticoagulation therapy, is an alternative option (adult level I study).[200,201]

4. When full-dose oral anticoagulation therapy is contraindicated, long-term therapy with oral anticoagulation therapy sufficient to increase the INR to 2.0–3.0 in combination with aspirin, 6–20 mg/kg/day, and dipyridamole, 2–5 mg/kg/day, can be used. This recommendation is an extrapolation of a level I study in adults.[199] There is one level V study in children.[156]

Biologic Prosthetic Heart Valves in Children

Children rarely have biologic prosthetic heart valves. Further clinical investigation is needed before definitive recommendations can be made. One option is to treat children who have biologic prosthetic valves according to adult recommendations.

Treatment of Kawasaki's Disease in Children

In addition to intravenous gamma globulin (400 mg/kg for 4 consecutive days), children with Kawasaki's disease should receive 80–100 mg/kg/day during the acute phase (up to 14 days) as an anti-inflammatory agent, then aspirin, 3–5 mg/kg/day to prevent the formation of coronary aneurysm thrombosis. This grade C recommendation is based on two level III studies.[30,31]

Fontan Operations

Further clinical investigation is needed before definitive recommendations can be made. One option is to initially treat patients with Fontan procedures with therapeutic amounts of heparin followed by oral anticoagulation therapy to achieve an INR of 2.0–3.0 for three months. Patients with fenestrations might benefit from treatment until closure.

Blalock-Taussig Shunts

Further clinical investigation is needed before definitive recommendations can be made. One option is initially to treat patients who have Blalock-Taussig shunts with therapeutic amounts of heparin, followed by aspirin at doses of 3–5 mg/kg/day indefinitely.

Homozygous Protein C– and S–Deficient Patients

1. It is recommended that newborns with purpura fulminans caused by a homozygous deficiency of protein C or S should be treated initially with replacement therapy (either fresh-frozen plasma or protein C concentrate) for approximately six to eight weeks until the skin lesions have healed.
2. Following resolution of the skin lesions and under cover of replacement therapy, oral anticoagulation therapy can be introduced with target INR values of approximately 3.0–4.5. Treatment duration with oral anticoagulants is indefinite. Recurrent skin lesions should be treated with replacement therapy of protein C or S.
3. For patients with homozygous protein C and S deficiency but with measurable plasma concentrations, LMWH is a therapeutic option.[119]

CONCLUSION

Childhood thrombophilia programs do not necessarily have to be hospital based. They can be provided by hospital-based pediatric hematologists linked to a national program. This strategy has been successfully used in Canada, where a free consultative service is readily accessible to physicians 24 hours a day through a 1-800-NO-CLOTS telephone hotline. The program is sponsored for Canadian physicians by the Canadian Children's Thrombophilia Program.

REFERENCES

1. Massicotte P, Marzinotto V, Vegh P, Adams M, Andrew M. Home monitoring of warfarin therapy in children with a whole blood prothrombin time monitor. *J Pediatr.* 1995;127:389–394.
2. Andrew M, Marzinotto V, Brooker L, et al. Oral anticoagulant therapy in pediatric patients: a prospective study. *Thromb Haemost.* 1994;71:265–269.
3. Michelson AD, Bovill E, Andrew M. Antithrombotic therapy in children. *Chest.* 1995;108(suppl 4):506S–522S.
4. Andrew M. Developmental hemostasis: relevance to newborns and infants. In: Nathan DG, Oski FA, eds. *Hematology of Infancy and Childhood.* 5th ed. Philadelphia: WB Saunders; 1998:114–157.
5. Andrew M. Acquired disorders of hemostasis. In: Nathan DG, Oski FA, eds. *Hematology of Infancy and Childhood.* 5th ed. Philadelphia: WB Saunders; 1998:114–157.
6. Massicotte MP, Brooker L, Marzinotto V. Oral anticoagulation therapy in children. In: Poller L, Hirsh J, eds. *Oral Anticoagulants.* London: Arnold; 1996:216–227.
7. Castaman G, Rodeghiero F, Dini E. Thrombotic complications during L-asparaginase treatment for acute lymphocytic leukemia. *Haematologica (Pavia).* 1990;75:567–569.

8. Wise RC, Todd JK. Spontaneous, lower-extremity venous thrombosis in children. *Am J Dis Child.* 1973;126:766–769.
9. Bernstein D, Coupey S, Schonberg S. Pulmonary embolism in adolescents. *Am J Dis Child.* 1986;140:667–671.
10. Coon W, Willis P, Keller J. Venous thromboembolism and other venous disease in the Tecumseh Community Health Study. *Circulation.* 1973;48:839–846.
11. Gjores J. The incidence of venous thrombosis and its sequelae in certain districts in Sweden. *Acta Chir Scand.* 1956;206(suppl):1–10.
12. Carter C, Gent M. The epidemiology of venous thrombosis. In: Coleman R, Hirsh J, Marder V, Salzman E, eds. *Hemostasis and Thrombosis: Basic Principles and Clinical Practice.* Philadelphia: JB Lippincott; 1982:805–819.
13. Andrew M, David M, Adams M, et al. Venous thromboembolic complications (VTE) in children: first analyses of the Canadian Registry of VTE. *Blood.* 1994;83:1251–1257.
14. Berube C, David M, Laxer R, et al. The relationship of antiphospholipid antibodies to thromboembolic disease in systemic lupus erythematosus in children: a cross-sectional study. *Lupus.* 1994;3:360.

15. Montes de Oca MA, Babron MC, Bletry O, et al. Thrombosis in systemic lupus erythematosus: a French collaborative study. *Arch Dis Child.* 1991;66:713–717.

16. David M, Andrew M. Venous thromboembolism complications in children: a critical review of the literature. *J Pediatr.* 1993;123:337–346.

17. Schmidt B, Andrew A. A prospective international registry of neonatal thrombotic diseases. *Pediatr Res.* 1994;35(pt 2):170a. Abstract.

18. Andrew M, Marzinotto V, Pencharz P, et al. A cross-sectional study of catheter-related thrombosis in children receiving total parenteral nutrition at home. *J Pediatr.* 1995;126:358–363.

19. Green R, Meyer T, Dunn M, Glassroth J. Pulmonary embolism in younger adults. *Chest.* 1992;101:1507–1511.

20. Greengard JS, Eichinger S, Griffin JH, Bauer KA. Brief report: variability of thrombosis among homozygous siblings with resistance to activated protein C due to an Arg-Gln mutation in the gene for factor V. *N Engl J Med.* 1994;331:1559–1562.

21. Ganeson V, Kelsey H, Cookson J, Osborn A, Kirkham FJ. Activated protein C resistance in childhood stroke. *Lancet.* 1996;347:260.

22. Hong C, Yun Y, Choi J, et al. Takayasu arteritis in Korean children: clinical report of seventy cases. *Heart Vessels.* 1992;7:91–96.

23. Zheng D, Fan D, Liu L. Takayasu arteritis in China: a report of 530 cases. *Heart Vessels.* 1992;7:32–36.

24. Wiggelinkhuizen J, Cremin B, Cywes S. Spontaneous recanalization of renal artery stenosis in childhood Takayasu arteritis: a case report. *S Afr Med J.* 1980;57(3):96–98.

25. Hall T, McDiarmid S, Grant E, Boechat M, Bosulti R. False-negative duplex Doppler studies in children with hepatic artery thrombosis after liver transplantation. *Am J Roentgenol.* 1990;154:573–575.

26. Flint E, Sumkin J, Zajko A, Bowen A. Duplex sonography of hepatic artery thrombosis after liver transplantation. *Am J Roentgenol.* 1988;151:481–483.

27. Lerut J, Gordon R, Tzakis A, Stieber A, Iwatsuki S, Starzl T. The hepatic artery in orthotopic liver transplantation. *Helv Chir Acta.* 1988;55:367–378.

28. LeBlanc J, Culham J, Chan K, Patterson M, Tipple M, Sandor G. Treatment of grafts and major vessel thrombosis with low-dose streptokinase in children. *Ann Thorac Surg.* 1986;41:630–635.

29. Samara E, Voss B, Pederson J. Renal artery thrombosis associated with elevated cyclosporine levels: a case report and review of the literature. *Transplant Proc.* 1988;20:119–123.

30. Koren G, Rose V, Lavi S, Rowe R. Probable efficacy of high-dose salicylates in reducing coronary involvement in Kawasaki disease. *JAMA.* 1985;254:767–769.

31. Daniels S, Specker P, Capannari TE, Schwartz D, Burke M, Kaplan S. Correlates of coronary artery aneurysm formation in patients with Kawasaki disease. *Am J Dis Child.* 1987;141:205–207.

32. Newburger J, Takahashi M, Burns J, et al. The treatment of Kawasaki syndrome with intravenous gamma globulin. *N Engl J Med.* 1986;315:341–347.

33. Freed M, Keane J, Rosenthal A. The use of heparinization to prevent arterial thrombosis after percutaneous cardiac catheterization in children. *Circulation.* 1974;50:565–569.

34. Rajani K, Goetzman B, Wennberg R, Turner E, Abildgaard C. Effect of heparinization of fluids infused through an umbilical artery catheter on catheter patency and frequency of complications. *Pediatrics.* 1979;63:552–556.

35. Jackson J, Truog W, Watchko J, Mack L, Cyr D, Van Belle G. Efficacy of thromboresistant umbilical artery catheters in reducing aortic thrombosis and related complications. *J Pediatr.* 1987;110:102–105.

36. David R, Merten D, Anderson J, Gross S. Prevention of umbilical artery catheter clots with heparinized infusates. *Dev Pharmacol Ther.* 1981;2(2):117–126.

37. Bosque E, Weaver L. Continuous versus intermittent heparin infusion of umbilical artery catheters in the newborn infant. *J Pediatr.* 1986;108:141–143.

38. Horgan M, Bartoletti A, Polonsky S, Peters J, Manning T, Lamont B. Effect of heparin infusates in umbilical arterial catheters on frequency of thrombotic complications. *J Pediatr.* 1987;111:774–778.

39. Ankola P, Atakent Y. Effect of adding heparin in very low concentration to the infusate to prolong the patency of umbilical artery catheters. *Am J Perinatal.* 1993;10:229–232.

40. Andrew M, MacIntyre B, Williams W, et al. Heparin therapy during cardiopulmonary bypass requires ongoing quality control. *Thromb Haemost.* 1993;70:937–941.

41. Babacan MK, Tasdemir O, Yakut C, et al. Heparin need of the patients with cyanotic congenital heart disease during cardiopulmonary bypass. *J Cardiovasc Surg (Torino).* 1989;30:348–350.

42. Akl B, Vargas G, Neal J, Robillard J, Kelly P. Clinical experience with the activated clotting time for the control of heparin and protamine therapy during cardiopulmonary bypass. *J Thorac Cardiovasc Surg.* 1980;79:97–102.

43. Boonstra P, Gu Y, Akkerman C, Haan J, Juyzen R, van Oeveren W. Heparin coating of an extracorporeal circuit partly improves hemostasis after cardiopulmonary bypass. *J Thorac Cardiovasc Surg.* 1994;107:289–292.

44. Whittlesey G, Drucker D, Salley S, et al. ECMO without heparin: laboratory and clinical experience. *J Pediatr Surg.* 1991;26:320–325.

45. Green T, Isham-Schopf B, Irmiter R, Smith C, Uden D, Steinhorn R. Inactivation of heparin during extracorporeal circulation in infants. *Clin Pharmacol Ther.* 1990;48:148–154.

46. Wilson J, Bower L, Fackler J, Beals D, Bergus B, Kevy S. Aminocaproic acid decreases the incidence of intracranial hemorrhage and other hemorrhagic complications of ECMO. *J Pediatr Surg.* 1993;28:536–541.

47. Bjork V, Olin C, Bjarke B, Thoren C. Right atrial-right ventricular anastomosis for correction of tricuspid atresia. *J Thorac Cardiovasc Surg.* 1979;77:452–458.

48. Breman FJ, Malm J, Hayes C, Gersony W. Physiological approach to surgery for tricuspid atresia. *Circulation.* 1978(suppl 1):I-83.

49. Fontan F, Baudet E. Surgical repair of tricuspid atresia. *Thorax.* 1971;26:240–248.

50. Zahn E, Lima V, Benson L, Freedom R. Use of endovascular stents to increase pulmonary blood flow in pulmonary atresia with ventricular septal defect. *Am J Cardiol.* 1992;70:411–412.

51. Peeters S, Vandenplas Y, Jochmans K, Bougatef A, De Waele M, De Wolf D. Myocardial infarction in a neonate with hereditary antithrombin III deficiency. *Acta Paediatr.* 1993;82:610–613.

52. Zobel G, Trop M, Muntean W, Ring E, Gleispach H. Anticoagulation for continuous arteriovenous hemofiltration in children. *Blood Purif.* 1988;6:90–95.

53. Zobel G, Beitzke A, Stein J, Trop M. Continuous arteriovenous haemofiltration in children with postoperative cardiac failure. *Br Heart J.* 1987;58:473–476.

54. Leone M, Jenkins R, Golper T, Alexander S. Early experience with continuous arteriovenous hemofiltration in critically ill pediatric patients. *Crit Care Med.* 1986;14:1058.

55. Hirsh J. Oral anticoagulant drugs. *N Engl J Med.* 1991;324:1865–1875.

56. Rosenberg RD, Lam L. Correlation between structure and function of heparin. *Proc Natl Acad Sci USA.* 1979;76:1218–1222.

57. Lindahl U, Backstrom G, Hook M, Thunberg L, Fransson L, Linker A. Structure of the antithrombin-binding site of heparin. *Proc Natl Acad Sci USA.* 1979;76:3198–3202.

58. Casu B, Oreste P, Torri G. The structure of heparin oligosaccharide fragments with high anti-(factor Xa) activity containing the minimal antithrombin Ill-binding sequence. *Biochem J.* 1981;197:599–609.

59. Choay J, Lormeau JC, Petitou M, Sinay P, Fareed J. Structural studies on a biologically active hexasaccharide obtained from heparin. *Ann N Y Acad Sci.* 1981;370:644–649.

60. Andrew M, Massicotte MP. Blood: hemostasis. In: Gluckman PD, Heymann MA, eds. *Pediatrics and Perinatology: The Scientific Basis.* 2nd ed. London: Arnold; 1996:877–890.

61. Vieira A, Ofosu F, Andrew M. Heparin sensitivity and resistance in the neonate: an explanation. *Thromb Res.* 1991;63:85–99.

62. Hirsh J. Heparin. *N Engl J Med.* 1991;324:1565–1574.

63. Levine MN, Hirsh J. Hemorrhagic complications of anticoagulant therapy. *Semin Thromb Haemost.* 1986;12:39–57.

64. Nieuwenhuis HK, Albada J, Banga JD, Sixma JJ. Identification of risk factors for bleeding during treatment of acute venous thromboembolism with heparin or low molecular weight heparin. *Blood.* 1991;78:2337–2343.

65. Shojania A, Tetreault J, Turnbull G. The variations between heparin sensitivity of different lots of activated partial thromboplastin time reagent produced by the same manufacturer. *Am J Clin Pathol.* 1988;89:19–23.

66. Refn I, Vestergaard L. The titration of heparin with protamine. *Scand J Clin Lab Invest.* 1954;6:284–287.

67. Teien AN, Lie M. Evaluation of amidolytic heparin assay method. Increased sensitivity by adding purified antithrombin III. *Thromb Res.* 1977;10:399–410.

68. Hirsh J, Dalen J, Warkentin T, Deykin D, Poller L, Raschke R. Heparin: mechanism of action, pharmacokinetics, dosing considerations, monitoring, efficacy and safety. *Chest.* 1995;108 (suppl 4):258S–275S.

69. Andrew M, Marzinotto V, Blanchette V, et al. Heparin therapy in pediatric patients: a prospective cohort study. *Pediatr Res.* 1994;35:78–83.

70. Chiu H, Hirsh J, Yung W, Regoeczi E, Gent M. Relationship between the anticoagulant and antithrombotic effects of heparin in experimental venous thrombosis. *Blood.* 1977;49:171–184.

71. Levine M, Hirsh J, Gent M, et al. A randomized trial comparing the activated thromboplastin time with the heparin assay to monitor heparin therapy in patients with acute venous thromboembolism requiring large daily doses of heparin. *Arch Intern Med.* 1994;154:49–56.

72. Raschke RA, Reilly BM, Guidry JR, et al. The weight-based heparin dosing nomogram compared with a "standard care" nomogram. *Ann Intern Med.* 1993;119:874–881.

73. Andrew M, Ofosu F, Schmidt B, Brooker L, Hirsh J, Buchanan M. Heparin clearance and ex vivo recovery in newborn piglets and adult pigs. *Thromb Res.* 1988;52:517–527.

74. Turner Gomes S, Nitschmann E, Benson L, et al. Heparin is cleared faster in children with congenital heart disease than adults. *J Am Coll Cardiol.* 1993;21(2):59a. Abstract.

75. Gallus A, Jackaman J, Tillett J, Mills W, Wycherley A. Safety and efficacy of warfarin started early after submassive venous thrombosis or pulmonary embolism. *Lancet.* 1986;2:1293–1296.

76. Hull RD, Raskob GE, Rosenbloom D, et al. Heparin for 5 days as compared with 10 days in the initial treatment of proximal venous thrombosis. *N Engl J Med.* 1990;322:1260–1264.

77. Holmgren K, Andersson G, Fagrell B, et al. One-month versus six-month therapy with oral anticoagulants after symptomatic deep vein thrombosis. *Acta Med Scand.* 1985;218:279–284.

78. Cruickshank MK, Levine MN, Hirsh J, Roberts R, Siguenza M. A standard heparin nomogram for the management of heparin therapy. *Arch Intern Med.* 1991;151:333–337.

79. Levine H, Pauker S, Salzman E, Eckman M. Antithrombotic therapy in valvular heart disease. *Chest.* 1992;102(suppl 4):434S–444S.

80. Matzsch T, Bergqvist D, Hedner U, Nilsson B, Ostergaard P. Effects of low molecular weight heparin and unfragmented heparin on induction of osteoporosis in rats. *Thromb Haemost.* 1990;63:505–509.

81. Ginsberg J, Kowalchuk G, Hirsh J, et al. Heparin effect on bone density. *Thromb Haemost.* 1990;64:286–289.

82. Monreal M, Vinas L, Monreal L, Lavin S, Lafoz E, Angles A. Heparin-related osteoporosis in rats. *Haemostasis.* 1990;20:204–207.

83. Monreal M, Olive A, Lafoz E. Heparins, coumarin and bone density. *Lancet.* 1992;338:706.

84. Murdoch I, Beattie R, Silver D. Heparin-induced thrombocytopenia in children. *Acta Paediatr.* 1993;82:495–497.

85. Spadone D, Clark F, James E, Laster J, Hoch J, Silver D. Heparin-induced thrombocytopenia in the newborn. *J Vasc Surg.* 1992;15:306–311.

86. Mocan H, Beattie T, Murphy A. Renal venous thrombosis in infancy: long-term follow-up. *Pediatr Nephrol.* 1991;5:45–49.

87. McDonald MM, Hathaway WE. Anticoagulant therapy by continuous heparinization in newborn and older infants. *J Pediatr.* 1982;101:451–457.

88. Boneu B, Buchanan MR, Caranobe C, et al. The disappearance of a low molecular weight heparin fraction (CY216) differs from standard heparin in rabbits. *Thromb Res.* 1987;46:845–853.

89. Andersson L, Barrowcliffe T, Holmer E, Johnson E, Sims G. Anticoagulant properties of heparin fractionated by affinity chromatography on matrix-bound antithrombin III and by gel filtration. *Thromb Res.* 1976;9:575–583.

90. Johnson E, Kirkwood T, Stirling Y, et al. Four heparin preparations: anti-Xa potentiating effects of heparin after subcutaneous injection. *Thromb Haemost.* 1976;35:586–591.

91. Bergqvist D, Hedner U, Sjorin E, Holmer E. Anticoagulant effects of two types of low molecular weight heparin administered subcutaneously. *Thromb Res.* 1983;32:381–391.

92. Carter C, Kelton J, Hirsh J, Cerksus A, Santos A, Gent M. The relationship between the hemorrhagic and antithrombotic properties of a low molecular weight heparin in rabbits. *Blood.* 1982;59:1239–1245.

93. Ockelford P, Carter C, Cerskus A, Smith C, Hirsh J. Comparison of the in vivo hemorrhagic and antithrombotic effects of a low antithrombin III affinity heparin fraction. *Thromb Res.* 1982;27:679–690.

94. Prandoni P, Vigo M, Cattelan A, Ruol A. Treatment of deep venous thrombosis by fixed doses of a low–molecular-weight heparin (CY216). *Haemostasis.* 1990;20(suppl 1):220–223.

95. Holm H, Ly B, Handeland G, et al. Subcutaneous heparin treatment of deep vein thrombosis: a comparison of unfractionated and low molecular weight heparin. *Haemostasis.* 1986;16(suppl 2):30–37.

96. Lensing A, Prins M, Koopman M, Büller H. Which heparin for proximal deep-vein thrombosis? *Lancet.* 1992;340:311–312.

97. Bratt G, Aberg W, Johansson M, Tornebohm E, Granqvist S, Lockner D. Two daily subcutaneous injections of Fragmin as compared with intravenous standard heparin in the treatment of deep venous thrombosis. *Thromb Haemost.* 1990;64:506–510.

98. Prandoni P, Lensing A, Büller H, et al. A comparison of subcutaneous low–molecular-weight heparin with intravenous standard heparin in proximal deep-vein thrombosis. *Lancet.* 1992,339:441–445.

99. Albada J, Nieuwenhuis H, Sixma J. Treatment of acute venous thromboembolism with low molecular weight heparin (Fragmin). *Circulation.* 1989,80:935–940.

100. Simonneau G, Charbonnier B, Decousus H, et al. Subcutaneous low–molecular-weight heparin compared with continuous intravenous unfractionated heparin in the treatment of proximal deep vein thrombosis. *Arch Intern Mod.* 1993;153:1541–1546.

101. Lockner D, Bratt G, Tornebohm E, Aberg W, Granqvist S. Intravenous and subcutaneous administration of Fragmin in deep venous thrombosis. *Haemostasis.* 1986;16(suppl.):25–29.

102. Duroux P, Ninet J, Bachet P. A randomized trial of subcutaneous low molecular weight heparin (CY216) compared with intravenous unfractionated heparin in the treatment of deep vein thrombosis. A collaborative European multicentre study. *Thromb Haemost.* 1991;65:251–256.

103. Ofosu FA. Mechanisms of action of low molecular weight heparins and heparinoids. *Antithrombotic Therapy.* London: Baillière Tindall; 1990:505–521.

104. Ofosu FA. In vitro and ex-vivo activities of CY216: comparison with other low molecular weight heparins. *Haemostasis.* 1990;20(suppl 1):180.

105. Massicotte P, Adams M, Marzinotto V, Brooker L, Andrew M. Low molecular weight heparin in pediatric patients with thrombotic disease: a dose finding study. *J Pediatr.* 1996;128:313–318.

106. Lane D, MacGregor I, Ivan R, Cella G, Kakkar V. Molecular weight dependence of the anticoagulant properties of heparin. Intravenous and subcutaneous administration of fractionated heparins to man. *Thromb Res.* 1979;16:651–662.

107. Palm M, Mattsson C. Pharmacokinetics of Fragmin. A comparative study in the rabbit of its high and low affinity forms for antithrombin. *Thromb Res.* 1987;48:51–62.

108. Green D, Hirsh J, Heit J, Prins M, Davidson B, Lensing AWA. Low molecular weight heparin: a critical analysis of clinical trials. *Pharmacol Rev.* 1994;46:89–109.

109. Murray WJG, Lindo VS, Kakkar VV, Melissari E. Long-term administration of heparin and heparin fractions and osteoporosis in experimental animals. *Blood Coag Fibrinolysis.* 1995;6:113–118.

110. Muir JM, Andrew M, Hirsh J, et al. Histomorphometric analysis of the effects of standard heparin on trabecular bone in vivo. *Blood.* 1996;88:1314–1320.

111. Shibata Y, Abiko Y, Goto K, Morlya Y, Takiguchi H. Heparin stimulates the collagen synthesis in mineralized cultures of the osteoblast-like cell line, MC3T3–E1. *Biochem Int.* 1992;28:335.

112. Goldhaber P. Heparin enhancement of factors stimulating bone resorption in tissue culture. *Science.* 1965;147:407.

113. Fuller K, Chambers TJ, Gallagher AC. Heparin augments osteoclast resorption-stimulating activity in serum. *J Cell Physiol.* 1991;147:208.

114. Chowdhury MH, Hamada C, Dempster DW. Effects of heparin on osteoclast activity. *J Bone Miner Res.* 1992;7:771.

115. McSheedy PMJ, Chambers TJ. Osteoblastic cells mediate osteoclastic responsiveness to parathyroid hormone. *Endocrinology.* 1986;118:824.

116. Dahlman TC, Sjöberg HE, Ringertz H. Bone mineral density during long-term prophylaxis with heparin in pregnancy. *Am J Obstet Gynecol.* 1994;170:1315–1320.

117. Barbour LA, Kick SD, Steiner JF, et al. A prospective study of heparin-induced osteoporosis in pregnancy using bone densitometry. *Am J Obstet Gynecol.* 1994;170:862–869.

118. Zimran A, Shilo S, Fisher D, Bab I. Histomorphometric evaluation of reversible heparin-induced osteoporosis in pregnancy. *Arch Intern Med.* 1986;146:386.

119. Andrew M, Halton J, Massicotte M. Treatment of homozygous protein C deficiency in two children with low molecular weight heparin (LMWH) therapy. *Thromb Haemost.* 1995;73:939.

120. Ramakrishna R. Heparin-induced thrombocytopenia: cross-reactivity between standard heparin, low molecular weight heparin. *Br J Haematol.* 1995;91:736–738.

121. Warkentin TE. Heparin-induced thrombocytopenia in patients treated with low molecular weight or unfractionated heparin. *N Engl J Med.* 1995;332:1330–1335.

122. Altes A. Heparin-induced thrombocytopenia and heart operation: management with tedelparin. *Ann Thorac Surg.* 1995;59:508–509.

123. Kalangos A, Relland JY, Massonet-Castel S, Acar C, Carpentier A. Heparin-induced thrombocytopenia and thrombosis following open heart surgery. *Eur J Cardiothorac Surg.* 1994;8(4):199–203.

124. Boshkov L, Warkentin T, Hayward C, et al. Heparin-induced thrombocytopenia and thrombosis: clinical and laboratory studies. *Blood.* 1990;76:447a. Abstract.

125. Keeling DM. Platelet aggregation in response to four low molecular weight heparins and the heparinoid ORG 10172. *Br J Haematol.* 1994;86:425–426.

126. Patrassi GM, Luzatto G. Heparin-induced thrombocytopenia with thrombosis of the aorta, iliac arteries and right axillary vein successfully treated by low molecular weight heparin. *Acta Haematol.* 1994;91:55–56.

127. Kikta MJ, Keller MP, Humphrey PW, Silver D. Can low molecular weight heparins and heparinoids be safely given to patients with heparin-induced thrombocytopenia syndrome? *Surgery.* 1993;114:705–710.

128. Andrew M. Developmental hemostasis: relevance to thromboembolic complications in pediatric patients. *Thromb Haemost.* 1995;74(suppl): 415–425.

129. Massicotte M, Marzinotto V, Adams M, et al. Coumarin suppresses thrombin regulation to a greater extent in children compared to adults. *Thromb Haemost.* 1995;73:1117. Abstract.

130. Francis J, Todd P. Congenital factor XIII deficiency in a neonate. *BMJ.* 1978;2:1532.

131. Quick AJ, Grossman AM. Prothrombin concentration in newborns. *Proc Soc Exp Biol Med.* 1939;41:227.

132. Loeliger E, van den Besselaar A, Lewis S. Reliability and clinical impact of the normalization of the prothrombin times in oral anticoagulant control. *Thromb Haemost.* 1985;53:148–154.

133. Roy A, Jaffe N, Djerassi, I. Prophylactic platelet transfusions in children with acute leukemia: a dose response study. *Transfusion.* 1973;13:283.

134. Poller L. Progress in standardization anticoagulation control. *Hematol Rev.* 1987;1:225–241.

135. Poller L. Laboratory control of oral anticoagulants. *BMJ.* 1987;294:1184.

136. International Committee for Standardization in Haematology, International Committee on Thrombosis and Haemostasis. ICSH/ICTH recommendations for reporting prothrombin time in oral anticoagulant control. *Thromb Haemost.* 1985;53:155–156.

137. Aballi A, de Lamerens S. Coagulation changes in the neonatal period and in early infancy. *Pediatr Clin North Am.* 1962,9:785–817.

138. Shearer MJ, Barkhan P, Rahim S, Stimmler L. Plasma vitamin K$_1$ in mothers and their newborn babies. *Lancet.* 1982;2:460–463.

139. Greer FR, Mummah-Schendel LL, Marshall S, Suttie JW. Vitamin K$_1$ (phylloquinone) and Vitamin K$_2$ (menaquinone) status in newborns during the first week of life. *Pediatrics.* 1988;81:137–140.

140. Barnard D, Hathaway W. Neonatal thrombosis. *Am J Pediatr Hematol Oncol.* 1979;1:235–244.

141. Von Kries R, Shearer MJ, McCarthy PT, Haug M, Hanzer G, Gobel U. Vitamin K$_1$ content of maternal milk: influence of the stage of lactation, lipid composition, and vitamin K$_1$ supplements given to the mother. *Pediatr Res.* 1987;22:513–517.

142. Andrew M. The hemostatic system in the infant. In: Nathan DG, Oski FA, eds. *Hematology of Infancy and Childhood.* Philadelphia: WB Saunders; 1993:115–153.

143. Widdershoven J, Kollee L, van Munster P, Bosman AM, Monnens L. Biochemical vitamin K deficiency in early infancy: diagnostic limitation of conventional coagulation tests. *Helv Paediatr Acta.* 1986;41:195–201.

144. Haroon Y, Shearer MJ, Rahim S, Gunn WG, McEnery G, Barkhan P. The content of phylloquinone (vitamin K$_1$) in human milk, cow's milk and infant formula foods determined by high-performance liquid chromatography. *J Nutr.* 1982;112:1105–1117.

145. Von Kries R, Stannigel H, Gobel U. Anticoagulant therapy by continuous heparin-antithrombin III infusion in newborns with disseminated intravascular coagulation. *Eur J Pediatr.* 1985;114:191–194.

146. Evans D, Rowlands M, Poller L. Survey of oral anticoagulant treatment in children. *J Clin Pathol.* 1992;45:707–708.

147. Kumar S, Haigh J, Rhodes L, et al. Poor compliance is a major factor in unstable outpatient control of anticoagulant therapy. *Thromb Haemost.* 1989;62:729–732.

148. Stewart S, Cianciotta D, Alexson C, Manning J. The long-term risk of warfarin sodium therapy and the incidence of thromboembolism in children after prosthetic cardiac valves. *J Thorac Cardiovasc Surg.* 1987;93:551–554.

149. El Makhlouf A, Friedli B, Oberhansli I, et al. Prosthetic heart valve replacement in children. *J Thorac Cardiovasc Surg.* 1987;93:80–85.

150. Sade R, Crawford FJ, Fyfe D, Stroud M. Valve protheses in children: A reassessment of anticoagulation. *J Thorac Cardiovasc Surg.* 1988;95(4):553–561.

151. Rao S, Solymar L, Mardini M, Fawzy M, Guinn G. Anticoagulant therapy in children with prosthetic valves. *Ann Thorac Surg.* 1989;47:589–592.

152. Serra A, McNicholas K, Olivier HJ, Boe S, Lemole G. The choice of anticoagulation in pediatric patients with the St. Jude Medical valve prostheses. *J Cardiovasc Surg.* 1987;28:588–591.

153. McGrath L, Gonzalez-Lavin L, Edlredge W, Colombi M, Restrepo D. Thromboembolic and other events following valve replacement in a pediatric population treated with antiplatelet agents. *Ann Thorac Surg.* 1987;43:285–287.

154. Spevak P, Freed M, Castaneda A, et al. Valve replacement in children less than 5 years of age. *J Am Cardiol.* 1986;8:901–908.

155. Harada Y, Imai Y, Kurosawa H, et al. Ten-year follow-up after valve replacement with the St. Jude Medical prosthesis in children. *J Thorac Cardiovasc Surg.* 1990;100:175–180.

156. Woods A, Vargas J, Berri G, Kreutzer G, Meschengieser S, Lazzari MA. Antithrombotic therapy in children and adolescents. *Thromb Res.* 1986;42:289–301.

157. Bradley LM, Midgley FM, Watson DC, et al. Anticoagulation therapy in children with mechanical prosthetic cardiac valves. *Am J Cardiol.* 1985;56:533–535.

158. Milano A, Vouhe PR, Baillot-Vernant F, et al. Late results after left-sided cardiac valve replacement in children. *J Thorac Cardiovasc Surg.* 1986;92:218–225.

159. Schaffer MS, Clarke DR, Campbell DN, Madigan CK, Wiggins JW Jr, Wolfe RR. The St. Jude Medical cardiac valve and children: role of anticoagulant therapy. *J Am Coll Cardiol.* 1987;9:235–239.

160. Schaff H, Danielson G, DiDonato R, Puga F, Mair D, McGoon D. Late results after Starr-Edwards valve replacement in children. *J Thorac Cardiovasc Surg.* 1984;88:583–589.

161. Borkon AM, Soule L, Reitz BA, Gott VL, Gardner TJ. Five year follow-up after valve replacement with the St. Jude Medical valve in infants and children. *Circulation.* 1986;74(suppl 1):I-110–I-115.

162. Human DG, Joffe HS, Fraser CB, Barnard CN. Mitral valve replacement in children. *J Thorac Cardiovasc Surg.* 1982;83:873–877.

163. Antunes MJ, Vanderdonck KM, Sussman MJ. Mechanical valve replacement in children and teenagers. *Eur J Cardiothorac Surg.* 1989;3:222–228.

164. Hooshang T, Capitanio M. Tracheobronchial calcification: an observation in three children after mitral valve replacement and warfarin sodium therapy. *Radiology.* 1990;176:728–730.

165. Piro L, Whyte M, Murphy W, Birge S. Normal cortical bone mass in patients after long term Coumadin therapy. *J Clin Endocrinol Metab.* 1982;54:470–473.

166. Rosen H, Maitland L, Suttie J, Manning W, Glynn R, Greenspan S. Vitamin K and maintenance of skeletal integrity in adults. *Am J Med.* 1993;94:62–68.

167. Solymar L, Rao PS, Mardini MK, Fawzy ME, Guinn G. Prosthetic valves in children and adolescents. *Am Heart J.* 1991;121:557–568.

168. LeBlanc J, Sett S, Vince D. Antiplatelet therapy in children with left-sided mechanical prostheses. *Eur J Cardiothorac Surg.* 1993;7:211–215.

169. Starko K, Ray C, Dominguez L, Stromberg W, Woodall D. Reye's syndrome and salicylate use. *Pediatrics.* 1980;66:859–864.

170. Arrowsmith JB, Kennedy DL, Kuritsky JN, Faich GA. National patterns of aspirin use and Reye syndrome reporting. United States, 1980 to 1985. *Pediatrics.* 1987;79:858–863.

171. Tonsgard JH, Huttenlocher PR. Salicylates and Reye's syndrome. *Pediatrics.* 1981;68:747–748.

172. Remington P, Shabino C, McGee H, Preston G, Sarniak A, Hall W. Reye syndrome and juvenile rheumatoid arthritis in Michigan. *Am J Dis Child.* 1985;139:870–872.

173. Porter J, Robinson P, Glasgow J, Banks J, Hall S. Trends in the incidence of Reye's syndrome and the use of aspirin. *Arch Dis Child.* 1990;65:826–829.

174. Jorda M, Rodriguez MM, Reik RA. Thrombotic thrombocytopenic purpura as the cause of death in an HIV positive child. *Pediatr Pathol.* 1994;14:919–925.

175. Halpin T, Holtzhauer F, Campbell R, et al. Reye's syndrome and medication use. *JAMA.* 1982;248:687–691.

176. Hurwitz ES, Barrett MJ, Bregman D, et al. Public health service study of Reye's syndrome and medications: report of a main study. *JAMA.* 1987;257:1905–1911.

177. Partin JS, Partin JC, Schubert WK, Hammond JG. Serum salicylate concentrations in Reye's disease. *Lancet.* 1982;1.

178. Prescott LF. Effects of non-narcotic analgesics on the liver. *Drugs.* 1986;32(suppl 4):129–147.

179. Makela A, Lang H, Korpela P. Toxic encephalopathy with hyperammonaemia during high-dose salicylate therapy. *Acta Neurol Scand.* 1980;61:146–151.

180. Andrew M, Vegh P, Johnston M, Bowker J, Ofosu F, Mitchell L. Maturation of the hemostatic system during childhood. *Blood.* 1992;80:1998–2005.

181. Leaker M, Massicotte MP, Brooker L, Andrew M. Thrombolytic therapy in pediatric patients: a comprehensive review of the literature. *Thromb Haemost.* 1996;76:132–134.

182. Corrigan J, Sluth J, Jeter M, Lox C. Newborn's fibrinolytic mechanism: components and plasmin generation. *Am J Hematol.* 1989;32:273–278.

183. Andrew M, Brooker L, Paes B, Weitz J. Fibrin clot lysis by thrombolytic agents is impaired in newborns due to a low plasminogen concentration. *Thromb Haemost.* 1992;68:325–330.

184. Leaker M, Brooker L, Ofosu K, Paes B, Weitz J, Andrew M. Anisoylated streptokinase-plasminogen activator complex offers no advantage over streptokinase for fibrin clot lysis in cord plasma. *Pediatric Research.* 1995;37:283a.

185. Leaker M, Superina R, Andrew M. Fibrin clot lysis by tissue plasminogen activator (tPA) is impaired in plasma from pediatric liver transplant patients. *Transplantation.* 1995;60:144–147.

186. Leaker M, Massicotte M, Brooker L, Andrew M. Thrombolytic therapy in pediatric patients: a comprehensive review of the literature. *Thromb Haemost.* 1996;76:132–134.

187. Kellam B, Fraze D, Kanarek K. Clot lysis for thrombosed central venous catheters in pediatric patients. *J Perinatal.* 19;7:242–244.

188. Mirro JJ, Rao BN, Stokes DC, et al. A prospective study of Hickman/Broviac catheters and implantable ports in pediatric oncology patients. *J Clin Oncol.* 1989;7:214–222.

189. Morris J, Occhionero M, Gauderer M, et al. Totally implantable vascular access devices in cystic fibrosis: a four-year experience with fifty-eight patients. *J Pediatr.* 1990;117:82–85.

190. Winthrop AL, Wesson DE. Urokinase in the treatment of occluded central venous catheters in children. *J Pediatr Surg.* 1984;19:536–583.

191. Deeg K, Wolfel D, Rupprecht T. Diagnosis of neonatal aortic thrombosis by colour coded Doppler sonography. *Pediatr Radiol.* 1992;22:62–63.

192. Cook DJ, Guyatt GH, Laupacis A, Sackett DL, Goldberg RJ. Clinical recommendations using levels of evidence for antithrombotic agents. *Chest.* 1995:108(suppl):227S–230S.

193. Carpentieri U, Nghiem QX, Harris LC. Clinical experience with an oral anticoagulant in children. *Arch Dis Child.* 1976;51:445–448.

194. Doyle JJ, Koren G, Chen MY, Blanchette VS. Anticoagulation with sodium warfarin in children: effect of a loading regimen. *J Pediatr.* 1988;113:1095–1097.

195. Hathaway WE. Use of antiplatelet agents in pediatric hypercoagulable states. *Am J Dis Child.* 1984;138:301–304.

196. Schmidt B, Andrew M. Report of scientific and standardization subcommittee on neonatal hemostasis diagnosis and treatment of neonatal thrombosis. *Thromb Haemost.* 1992;67:381–382.

197. Freed M, Rosenthal A, Fyler D. Attempts to reduce arterial thrombosis after cardiac catheterization in children: use of percutaneous technique and aspirin. *Am Heart J.* 1974;87:283–286.

198. Stein P, Grandison D, Hua T, et al. Therapeutic levels of oral anticoagulation with warfarin in patients with mechanical prosthetic heart valves: Review of literature and recommendations based on International Normalized Ratio. *Postgrad Med J.* 1994;70(suppl 1):S72–S83.

199. Turpie AGC, Gent M, Laupacis A, et al. A comparison of aspirin with placebo in patients treated with warfarin after heart-valve replacement. *N Engl J Med.* 1993;329:524–529.

200. Rajah S, Sreeharan N, Joseph A, et al. Prospective trial of dipyridamole and warfarin in heart valve patients. *Acta Ther (Brussels).* 1980;6:54. Abstract.

201. Turpie AGC, Gunstensen J, Hirsh J, Nelson H, Gent M. Randomised comparison of two intensities of oral anticoagulant therapy after tissue heart valve replacement. *Lancet.* 1988;1:1242–1245.

Chapter 22

Anticoagulation in the Antiphospholipid Syndrome

Barbara M. Alving

One of the most intriguing thrombotic conditions is the antiphospholipid syndrome, which was first described as the *anticardiolipin syndrome* by several rheumatologists in England in 1986.[1] The syndrome includes a wide constellation of clinical manifestations combined with laboratory findings of autoantibodies that are directed against phospholipid-binding proteins such as prothrombin and β2-glycoprotein I (β2-GPI) and not against phospholipids, as was originally described.[2] The clinical manifestations, criteria for diagnosis, and treatment of this condition, which is largely empiric, will be described in the present chapter.

The term *antiphospholipid-protein antibodies (APA)* (formerly *antiphospholipid antibodies*), used in this chapter, refers to antibodies of the IgG, IgM, or IgA isotope directed against phospholipid-binding proteins such as prothrombin or β2-glycoprotein I (β2-GPI). When measured by an enzyme-linked immunosorbent assay (ELISA), the antibodies are called *anticardiolipin antibodies (ACAs)* because assays contain the phospholipid cardiolipin (the phospholipid to which β2-GPI binds). When detected by a phospholipid-dependent clotting assay, they are described as *lupus anticoagulants (LAs)*. The term *antiphospholipid syndrome* is used to refer to a condition characterized by venous or arterial thrombosis, thrombocytopenia, and recurrent fetal loss in association with APA.

ANTIPHOSPHOLIPID SYNDROME: OVERVIEW OF CLINICAL MANIFESTATIONS

The antiphospholipid syndrome should be considered in patients who present with one or more of the following clinical conditions: venous thrombosis, arterial thrombosis (stroke, transient ischemic attack, or myocardial infarction, especially in persons younger than age 55), recurrent pregnancy loss, or thrombocytopenia.[2,3] Associated conditions are vasculitic rashes, arthralgias, necrosis of digits, pulmonary hypertension, and cutaneous skin necrosis.[4] The diagnosis is confirmed if the patient also tests positive for autoantibodies that are detected as LA in phospholipid-dependent clotting assays or as ACA in ELISAs that contain cardiolipin along with β2-GPI. The tests should be positive for LA or for moderate to high levels of ACA (IgG or IgM) on two occasions at least 12 weeks apart.[2] The requirement for sustained positivity for APA is given because results may be only transiently positive and unrelated to clinical symptoms.[5] In the absence of systemic lupus erythematosus (SLE) or other autoimmune connective tissue disorders, the syndrome is considered a primary antiphospholipid syndrome. It is twice as common in women as in men.

The syndrome is considered as a secondary antiphospholipid syndrome if it occurs in patients who have another autoimmune connective tissue disorder. An initial study in patients with SLE indicated that 61% had elevated levels of ACA antibodies of at least one isotope and that 49% had detectable LA.[6] The overlap between LA and ACA was quite

Source: Reprinted from Division of Blood Diseases and Resources, National Heart, Lung and Blood Institute, National Institutes of Health, Bethesda, Maryland.

significant, since ACA levels were increased in 91% of the patients who tested positive for LA. Subsequent prospective[7] and retrospective[8] analyses have confirmed that LA and ACA antibodies are detectable in approximately 50% of patients with SLE. Patients with SLE who have a persistent elevation of ACA will have a significantly increased odds ratio (5.4) for a peripheral thromboembolic event compared to those who test positive for antiphospholipid antibodies on only one occasion.[7]

Neurologic manifestations of the antiphospholipid syndrome include single or recurrent cerebral infarcts, severe vascular headaches, transient ischemic attacks, and visual disturbances.[9] Recurrent strokes are more likely in patients with the antiphospholipid syndrome who also have hypertension or other risk factors for cerebrovascular disease, such as cigarette smoking and hyperlipidemia.[9] As many as 80% of patients with the primary antiphospholipid syndrome have at least one of these additional risk factors. Cerebral angiography performed on such patients shows large-vessel occlusion or stenosis without evidence of vasculitis. Approximately 80% will have only IgG ACA.

In one prospective study, 18% of young adults (ages 15–44 years) who had sustained ischemic stroke or transient ischemic attacks tested positive for ACA.[10] The patients with ACA had a higher probability of recurrent events than those who did not have the antibody. For patients who have transient ischemic attacks at a young age or for those who have these events in association with other features of the antiphospholipid syndrome, testing for ACA and LA appears to be warranted. However, indiscriminate testing of a general patient population with cerebrovascular events is probably not cost-effective.

ELISA FOR APA

The assay measures the level of APA in patient sera in a quantitative fashion, using microtiter plates coated with cardiolipin or another negatively charged phospholipid.[6,11] Most test procedures now involve using a known concentration of β2-GPI. After an incubation period, the plates are washed and the antiphospholipid antibodies are detected by labeled anti-human IgG or IgM.

Test results are expressed in units of MPL or GPL. One MPL is equal to 1 μg of IgM APA, and 1 GPL is equal to 1 μg of IgG APA. The current recommendation is that assay results be described as "high positive" (> 80 GPL U/mL or > 60 MPL U/mL), "moderately positive" (20–80 GPL U/mL, 20–60 MPL U/mL), or "low positive" (< 20 GPL or MPL U/mL). Samples with less than 10 GPL or less than 10 MPL U/mL are considered negative.[12]

TESTING FOR LA

LA are APA that prolong the clotting time of phospholipid dependent coagulation assays by blocking the binding of coagulation factors to the acidic phospholipid surfaces or by enhancing the binding of β2-GPI to the procoagulant phospholipid surface.[13,14] The following are indications for testing for LA:

- *Patients suspected of having APA.* Perform at least two different assays for LA even if screening activated partial thromboplastin time (aPTT) is normal. (LA assays are based on phospholipid dilution and can therefore be positive in the presence of a normal aPTT.)
- *Patients having prolonged aPTT as an incidental finding.* Presence of LA is one of the most common reasons for a prolonged aPTT and is usually due to underlying infection or use of drugs such as phenothiazines or procainamide. Confirm presence of LA if mixing studies suggest inhibitor, and perform appropriate coagulation factor assays to establish factor levels (no further evaluation is necessary if patient has no history suggestive of APA).

The tests for LA are phospholipid-dependent assays in which the phospholipid is either diluted to increase the ability to detect the antibody or increased to "normalize" the test result and to provide confirmation of LA.

An international standardization committee has recommended that more than one study be performed to verify the presence of LA.[15] In one study, the detection of LA increased from 73% with one test to 90% with two tests.[16] Phospholipid dilution assays are currently used for the detection of LA, especially in patients with an aPTT that is normal or only minimally prolonged. Perhaps the most sensitive test for LA is the kaolin clotting time, which relies only on the phospholipid in the plasma. Assays that are performed with addition of dilute phospholipid include the dilute Russell viper venom time (dRVVT)[17,18] and the dilute phospholipid aPTT,[19] both of which use only a single dilution of phospholipid. The dRVVT is a phospholipid dilution assay in which Russell viper venom, an activator of factor X, is used to initiate coagulation in the presence of dilute phospholipid and calcium.[17] One laboratory reported a sensitivity and specificity of 97% and 100%, respectively, in detecting LA when two tests were used (the dRVVT and the dilute aPTT-LA [American Bioproducts]).[18]

In the general medical population, a prolonged aPTT is most frequently due to the presence of LA.[20] Correction studies are frequently not helpful in determining the presence of LA, since they can be normal. LA usually do not cause increasing prolongation of the aPTT with time, since the antibodies are directed against the phospholipid that is added to the assay. Although LA may appear to be the cause of a prolonged aPTT, factor levels are measured in order to exclude a true factor deficiency or the presence of another inhibitor. Patients who have LA or ACA in association with underlying infections or with use of medications are usually not at risk for thrombosis and do not require anticoagulation.

ASSOCIATION OF LA WITH PROTHROMBIN DEFICIENCY

In one study of patients with LA and SLE or other autoimmune connective tissue disorders, the majority had IgG antibodies to prothrombin, although only 30% of patients with antibodies had a detectable prothrombin deficiency.[21] Prothrombin deficiency, when it does occur in patients with LA, appears to be due to the binding of the antibody to prothrombin in vivo, which results in increased clearance.

The antibody production can usually be easily suppressed by administration of corticosteroids and azathioprine, as was demonstrated in one patient in whom the prothrombin time (PT) was normal 7 days after initiation of treatment.[22] In another study, the use of corticosteroids alone increased the prothrombin level even while the prothrombin-antibody complexes were still detectable.[23] If a patient is actively bleeding, treatment with fresh frozen plasma or prothrombin complex concentrates is required.

Antibodies to prothrombin can also be detected in patients who have infections and LA. At least eight cases of LA and clinically significant hypoprothrombinemia have occurred in children under the age of 17 years in association with a viral illness.[24] In these cases, the diagnosis is made because of clinical symptomatology, and the patients improve as the antibody disappears spontaneously. One patient with severe hypoprothrombinemia and gastrointestinal hemorrhage was treated successfully with intravenous methylprednisolone followed by prednisone.[25]

ANTICOAGULATION OF PATIENTS WHO HAVE THE ANTIPHOSPHOLIPID SYNDROME OR LABORATORY MANIFESTATIONS OF APA (LA OR ACA)

Major issues in the management of patients with the antiphospholipid syndrome and thrombosis are the intensity of anticoagulation that should be given, the duration of anticoagulation, and the appropriate monitoring. The following are treatment issues for patients with venous thrombosis and APA:

- *Intensity of anticoagulation.* Anticoagulation with warfarin to maintain an International Normalized Ratio (INR) of 2 to 3, with an attempt to target the INR of 3, may be the best option (with or without aspirin daily at a dose of 75–325 mg/day). (Recurrent thrombotic events per year of follow-up range from 0.07 to 0.23.)[26,27]
- *Duration of anticoagulation.* Anticoagulation should be continued indefinitely after the first thrombotic event. There is a high rate of recurrence if anticoagulation is discontinued 3 months after initiation.
- *Issues with respect to monitoring.* INR has been reported to be falsely increased in patients with LA and initial prolongation of PT. The test appears to be reliable in these patients if PT reagent containing recombinant tissue factor is not used. Some authors have also increased reliability of the test by using plasmas with a calibrated INR as a standard for calculating the patient's INR instead of using the international sensitivity index measured by the manufacturer.

One goal is to reduce other risk factors for thrombosis, such as uncontrolled hypertension, smoking, and use of oral contraceptives.[28] Treatment of asymptomatic patients with LA or with moderate or high titers of ACA is controversial. Some physicians will prescribe low-dose aspirin (75 mg/day) and then use anticoagulation with warfarin or heparin at times of increased risk for thrombosis.[28]

Patients with the antiphospholipid syndrome and venous thromboembolism are at high risk for recurrence if anticoagulation is discontinued after a first episode of venous thrombosis.[26,27,29] In a retrospective study of 19 patients with secondary antiphospholipid syndrome who had 34 episodes of thromboembolism, the discontinuation of warfarin resulted in a 50% probability of recurrent episodes at 2 years, which increased to 78% at 8 years.[27] The rate of recurrence was highest (1.30 per patient-year) in the first 6 months after discontinuation of anticoagulation.[27] In contrast, continuation of warfarin (INR 2.5–4.0) resulted in 100% freedom from thrombosis at the 8-year follow-up.

The appropriate intensity of anticoagulation has not been carefully studied. However, one international trial that is in progress (Warfarin in the Antiphospholipid Syndrome Study) randomizes patients to high-intensity treatment (INR 3–4.5) or to standard treatment.[30] The study should be completed at the end of the year 2000. In a prospective study comparing the clinical manifestations of patients with the primary and secondary antiphospholipid syndrome during a 2-year period, eight persons developed recurrent thrombosis, seven of whom had INR values of less than 3.[31] In a prospective study of the clinical relevance of antiphospholipid antibodies in patients who had venous thromboembolism but not SLE, the authors found no recurrence in patients receiving warfarin at INR intensities of 2 to 2.9 and no difference in the rate of recurrence in patients with and without APA.[32] In a third prospective study, patients with an episode of venous thrombosis who had LA and were randomized to warfarin during a 4-year period had no recurrences when the INR was maintained between 2 and 3. The intensity of anticoagulation required may depend on whether the patient has underlying SLE; however, this issue has also not been resolved. In the meantime, for patients with antiphospholipid syndrome and thrombosis who are receiving warfarin, an INR of 2 to 3, with an attempt to maintain the INR nearer to 3, is recommended if there are no contraindications; furthermore, anticoagulation should be continued on an indefinite basis as long as the risks of bleeding are less than the risk of thrombosis. Low-dose aspirin may be added, depending on whether thrombotic manifestations such as superficial thrombophlebitis persist.

One report has described variability in measuring the INR in patients with LA who also had an increased baseline PT.[33] Such a phenomenon could result in the underutilization of warfarin. However, two other studies have shown that there does not appear to be false prolongation of the INR in such patients,[34,35] although in one study variability in the INR was greatly increased when a recombinant tissue factor was used as the PT reagent.[34] The authors also found increased reliability in measuring the INR when they calibrated patient plasmas against plasma standards that had three different levels of the INR. This was done instead of using the international sensitivity index provided by the manufacturer to determine the INRs of the patient plasmas.

The role of corticosteroids or plasmapheresis has not been documented for patients with the antiphospholipid syndrome. These treatments are reserved for patients with a "catastrophic antiphospholipid syndrome," defined as acute multiorgan failure in patients with antiphospholipid antibodies.[36] In this rare syndrome, mortality is 60%; plasmapheresis may be beneficial in patients who have not responded to heparin, corticosteroids, or immunosuppressive agents.[36]

CONCLUSION

Although the pathophysiology of the antiphospholipid syndrome has not been well established, the specificity of the autoantibodies is now becoming more well defined, and the diagnostic testing as well as the criteria for establishing the diagnosis have been greatly refined.[2,37] A major issue is that of treatment[38]; the type, duration, and intensity of anticoagulation still have not been resolved, but with the development of cooperative international clinical trials, some of these issues may soon be clarified. The antiphospholipid syndrome is a disorder that encompasses many specialties: hematology, neurology, obstetrics, and rheumatology. Thus, the approach to patients with this disorder must be truly interdisciplinary.

REFERENCES

1. Hughes GRV, Harris EN, Gharavi AE. The anticardiolipin syndrome. *J Rheumatol.* 1986;13:486–489.

2. Greaves M. Antiphospholipid antibodies and thrombosis. *Lancet.* 1999,353:1348–1353.

3. Mackworth-Young CG, Loizou S, Walport MJ. Primary antiphospholipid syndrome: features of patients with raised anticardiolipin antibodies and no other disorder. *Ann Rheum Dis.* 1989;48:362–367.

4. Asherson RA. Anti-phospholipid antibodies: clinical complications reported in medical literature. In: Harris EN, Exner T, Hughes GRV, Asherson RA, eds. *Phospholipid-Binding Antibodies.* Boston, Mass: CRC Press, Inc.; 1991:388–402.

5. Vila P, Hernández MC, Lopez-Hernández MF, Batalle J. Prevalence, follow-up and clinical significance of the anticardiolipin antibodies in normal subjects. *Thromb Haemost.* 1994;72:209–213.

6. Harris EN, Gharavi EA, Boey ML, et al. Anticardiolipin antibodies: detection by radioimmunoassay and association with thrombosis in systemic lupus erythematosus. *Lancet.* 1983;2:1211–1214.

7. Long AA, Ginsberg JS, Brill-Edwards P, et al. The relationship of anti-phospholipid antibodies to thromboembolic disease in systemic lupus erythematosus: a cross-sectional study. *Thromb Haemost.* 1991:66:520–524.

8. Love PE, Santoro SA. Antiphospholipid antibodies: anticardiolipin and the lupus anticoagulant in systemic lupus erythematosus (SLE) and in non-SLE disorders. *Ann Intern Med.* 1990;112:682–698.

9. Levine SR, Deegan MJ, Futrell N, Welch KMA. Cerebrovascular and neurologic disease associated with antiphospholipid antibodies: 48 cases. *Neurology.* 1990;40:1181–1189.

10. Nencini P, Baruffi MC, Abbate R, Massai G, Amaducci L, Inzitari D. Lupus anticoagulant and anticardiolipin antibodies in young adults with cerebral ischemia. *Stroke.* 1992;23:189–193.

11. Harris EN. Annotation: antiphospholipid antibodies. *Br J Haematol.* 1990;74:1–9.

12. Harris EN. The Second International Anti-Cardiolipin Standardization Workshop/the Kingston Anti-Phospholipid Antibody Study (KAPS) Group. *Am J Clin Pathol.* 1990;94:476–484.

13. Galli M, Finazzi G, Bevers EM, Barbui T. Kaolin clotting time and dilute Russell's venom time distinguish between prothrombin-dependent and β2-glycoprotein I-dependent antiphospholipid antibodies. *Blood.* 1995;86:617–623.

14. Pengo V, Thiagarajan P, Shapiro SS, Heine MJ. Immunological specificity and mechanism of action of IgG lupus anticoagulants. *Blood.* 1987;70:69–76.

15. Brandt JT, Triplett DA, Alving B, Scharrer I. Criteria for the diagnosis of lupus anticoagulants: an update on behalf of the Subcommittee on Lupus Anticoagulant/Antiphospholipid Antibody of the Scientific and Standardisation Committee of the ISTH. *Thromb Haemost.* 1995;74:1185–1190.

16. Comparison of a standardized procedure with current laboratory practices for the detection of lupus anticoagulant in France: Working Group on Hemostasis of the Société Française Biologie Clinique. *Thromb Haemost.* 1993;70:781–786.

17. Thiagarajan P, Pengo V, Shapiro SS. The use of the dilute Russell viper venom time for the diagnosis of lupus anticoagulants. *Blood.* 1986;68:869–874.

18. Schjetlein R, Wisloff F. An evaluation of two commercial test procedures for the detection of lupus anticoagulant. *Coag Transf Med.* 1995;103:108–111.

19. Alving BM, Barr CF, Johansen LE, Tang DB. Comparison between a one-point dilute phospholipid aPTT and the dilute Russell viper venom time for verification of lupus anticoagulants. *Thromb Haemost.* 1992;67:672–678.

20. Kitchens CS. Prolonged activated partial thromboplastin time of unknown etiology: a prospective study of 100 consecutive cases referred for consultation. *Am J Hematol.* 1988;27:38–45.

21. Eson JR, Vogt JM, Hasegawa DK. Abnormal prothrombin crossed-immunoelectrophoresis in patients with lupus inhibitors. *Blood.* 1984;64:807–816.

22. Bajaj SP, Rapaport SI, Fierer DS, Herbst KD, Schwartz DB. A mechanism for the hypoprothrombinemia of the acquired hypoprothrombinemia-lupus anticoagulant syndrome. *Blood.* 1983;61:684–692.

23. Bajaj SP, Rapaport SI, Barclay S, Herbst KD. Acquired hypoprothrombinemia due to nonneutralizing antibodies to prothrombin: mechanism and management. *Blood.* 1985;65:1538–1543.

24. Lee MT, Nardi MA, Hu G, Hadzi-Nesis J, Karpatkin M. Transient hemorrhagic diathesis associated with an inhibitor of prothrombin with lupus anticoagulant in a 1½-year-old girl: report of a case and review of the literature. *Am J Hematol.* 1996;51:307–314.

25. Bernini JC, Buchanan GR, Ashcroft J. Hypoprothrombinemia and severe hemorrhage associated with a lupus anticoagulant. *J Pediatr.* 1993;123:937–939.

26. Rosove MH, Brewer PMC. Antiphospholipid thrombosis: clinical course after the first thrombotic event in 70 patients. *Ann Intern Med.* 1992;117:303–308.

27. Khamashta MA, Cuadrado MJ, Mujic F, Taub NA, Hunt BJ, Hughes GRV. The management of thrombosis in the antiphospholipid-antibody syndrome. *N Engl J Med.* 1995;332:993–997.

28. Khamashta MA. Management of thrombosis in the antiphospholipid syndrome. *Lupus.* 1996;5:463–466.

29. Kearon C, Gent M, Hirsh J, et al. A comparison of three months of anticoagulation with extended anticoagulation for a first episode of idiopathic venous thromboembolism. *N Engl J Med.* 1999;340:901–907.

30. Galli M, Barbui T. Antiprothrombin antibodies: detection and clinical significance in the antiphospholipid syndrome. *Blood.* 1999;93:2149–2157.

31. Vianna JL, Khamashta MA, Ordi-Ros J, et al. Comparison of the primary and secondary antiphospholipid syndrome: a European multicenter study of 114 patients. *Am J Med.* 1994;96:3–9.

32. Ginsberg JS, Wells PS, Brill-Edwards P, et al. Antiphospholipid antibodies and venous thromboembolism. *Blood.* 1995;86:3685–3691.

33. Moll S, Ortel TL. Monitoring warfarin therapy in patients with lupus anticoagulants. *Ann Intern Med.* 1997;127:177–185.

34. Robert A, Le Querrec A, Delahousse B, et al. Control of oral anticoagulation in patients with the antiphospholipid syndrome: influence of the lupus anticoagulant on International Normalized Ratio. *Thromb Haemost.* 1998;80:99–103.

35. Lawrie AS, Purdy G, Mackie IJ, Machin SJ. Monitoring of oral anticoagulant therapy in lupus anticoagulant positive patients with the anti-phospholipid syndrome. *Br J Haematol.* 1997;98:887–892.

36. Asherson RA, Piette J-C. The catastrophic antiphospholipid syndrome 1996: acute multi-organ failure associated with antiphospholipid antibodies: a review of 31 patients. *Lupus.* 1996;5:414–417.

37. Alving B. Antiphospholipid syndrome, lupus anticoagulants, and anticardiolipin antibodies. In: Loscalzo J, Schafer AI, eds. *Thrombosis and Hemorrhage.* 2nd ed. Baltimore: Williams and Wilkins; 1998:817–833.

38. Schulman S, Svenungsson E, Granqvist S. Duration of Anticoagulation Study Group. Anticardiolipin antibodies predict early recurrence of thromboembolism and death among patients with venous thromboembolism following anticoagulant therapy. *Am J Med.* 1998;104:332–338.

Chapter 23

Anticoagulation in Pregnancy

Shannon M. Bates and Jeffrey S. Ginsberg

Indications for anticoagulation during pregnancy include treatment and prophylaxis of acute venous thromboembolism, prevention of systemic embolism in patients with prosthetic heart valves or native valvular heart disease, and prevention of pregnancy loss in selected women with antiphospholipid antibodies. The use of anticoagulants in pregnancy is problematic, however, because they may produce complications in the fetus, as well as in the mother.

PROBLEMS ASSOCIATED WITH THE USE OF COUMARIN DERIVATIVES DURING PREGNANCY

Warfarin, the most commonly used oral anticoagulant, crosses the placenta[1,2] and has been associated with adverse events in the fetus,[3–10] including warfarin embryopathy[3–7,9,10] and central nervous system abnormalities.[7,10] Warfarin embryopathy is characterized by nasal hypoplasia and/or stippled epiphyses and is associated with warfarin exposure between the 6th and 12th weeks of gestation.[7] Although up to 30% of all infants exposed to warfarin during this time period have been reported to be affected,[9] others have suggested that the true incidence of warfarin embryopathy more likely approximates 5%.[7,10] The central nervous system abnormalities associated with maternal oral anticoagulant use include dorsal midline dysplasia with agenesis of the corpus callosum, Dandy-Walker malformations, and midline cerebellar atrophy, as well as ventral midline dysplasia with optic atrophy and blindness.[7] Unlike warfarin embryopathy, which

has been reported only with first-trimester exposure, central nervous system abnormalities can occur after warfarin exposure at any point in gestation.[7] Although the incidence of these anomalies appears to be less than 5%,[7,9,10] their long-term sequelae can be more devastating than those associated with warfarin embryopathy. The rates of spontaneous abortions and stillbirths are reportedly elevated with warfarin use during pregnancy,[7,9] presumably partly on the basis of placental hemorrhage. When warfarin is continued to term, delivery of the anticoagulated fetus can result in neonatal hemorrhage.[2,8] Warfarin appears safe for the breastfeeding infants of women receiving this drug, for two small studies found no warfarin activity in the breast milk of warfarin-treated patients or in their infants' circulation.[11,12]

On the basis of the above information, if warfarin is used during pregnancy, it should be avoided between the 6th and 12th weeks of gestation to avoid embryopathy and near term to prevent delivery of an anticoagulated fetus.[2,8] Two approaches can be safely used in women requiring long-term anticoagulation who wish to become pregnant. In the first, which assumes that warfarin is safe during the first four to six weeks of gestation, warfarin is continued, and weekly pregnancy tests are performed. As soon as pregnancy is diagnosed, and prior to the 6th week of gestation, heparin therapy is substituted. The other approach is to discontinue warfarin and initiate subcutaneous heparin therapy once the decision is made to attempt pregnancy. While this approach avoids fetal warfarin exposure in the first few weeks following conception, prolonged heparin exposure may place the mother at increased risk of a number of complications.

ALTERNATIVES TO ORAL ANTICOAGULANTS DURING PREGNANCY

Unfractionated heparin does not cross the placenta[13] and would therefore not be expected to produce fetal complications. Both a critical review of the literature[10] and a retrospective cohort study of 100 consecutive pregnancies associated with unfractionated heparin therapy[14] concluded that maternal therapy with unfractionated heparin is safe for the fetus. Therefore, for most indications, heparin is the anticoagulant of choice during pregnancy. In the above cohort study,[14] the rate of major bleeding in pregnant patients treated with heparin was 2%, which is similar to the rates of bleeding reported when adjusted-dose subcutaneous heparin therapy[15] or warfarin therapy[16] is used for the treatment of venous thromboembolism in nonpregnant patients. It has been reported that adjusted-dose subcutaneous heparin can cause a persistent anticoagulant effect at the time of delivery and thus presumably increase the risk of bleeding[17] and epidural hematoma. The mechanism of this prolonged anticoagulant effect is unclear, but it appears to be a feature of subcutaneous administration. Because heparin does not cross the placenta, it does not increase the risk of fetal bleeding.

Treatment with unfractionated heparin has other drawbacks, including heparin-induced thrombocytopenia[18,19] and heparin-associated osteoporosis.[20–27] In addition, treatment with therapeutic doses of unfractionated heparin by either continuous infusion or twice-daily subcutaneous injections requires laboratory monitoring and regular dose adjustments.[28]

Low–molecular-weight heparins have a safety and efficacy profile similar to that of unfractionated heparin in the treatment[29] and prophylaxis of venous thromboembolism in non-pregnant patients.[30–32] Like unfractionated heparin, low molecular-weight heparins do not cross the placental barrier.[33] They have a number of advantages over unfractionated heparin,[34] including an increased plasma half-life, which makes them suitable for once-daily dosing,[35,36] and a more predictable anticoagulant response, which obviates the need for routine laboratory monitoring.[34] These agents cause less heparin-induced thrombocytopenia[37] and probably less osteoporosis.[38–40]

Because the evaluation of low–molecular-weight heparins in pregnancy has been limited to small case series, there is uncertainty about their value in pregnant women requiring antithrombotic therapy. In a recent systematic review of the literature, a total of 486 pregnancies from 21 different studies in which low–molecular-weight heparin was administered as the sole anticoagulant were evaluated.[41] Low–molecular-weight heparin therapy did not appear to be associated with an increased incidence of adverse fetal/infant outcomes.[41] Moreover, the long-term use of low–molecular-weight heparin appears to be safe for the mother, since symptomatic

osteoporosis, bleeding, and heparin-induced thrombocytopenia occurred only infrequently. Of note, however, only 5% of women were treated with "therapeutic" doses of low–molecular-weight heparin, and it is likely that higher doses are associated with an increased risk of bleeding, osteoporosis, and probably heparin-induced thrombocytopenia. Although venous thromboembolic complications occurred in only 0.6% of pregnancies, suggesting that these agents provide effective prophylaxis against venous thrombosis, not all women had an increased risk of this complication. Due to the limitations of the study (pooling of case series) and the heterogeneity of the patients included, definitive conclusions cannot be drawn about the effectiveness and safety of low–molecular-weight heparin therapy in pregnancy. However, on the basis of the best available evidence, we believe that their use during pregnancy is reasonable clinical practice.

THERAPEUTIC RECOMMENDATIONS

There are limited data regarding the efficacy of anticoagulants during pregnancy for the prevention and treatment of venous thromboembolism, as well as the prevention of systemic embolism in patients with valvular heart disease. Treatment recommendations, therefore, have largely been extrapolated from data in nonpregnant patients, in addition to case reports and case series of pregnant patients.[42]

Treatment of Venous Thromboembolism

Unfractionated heparin has traditionally been the anticoagulant of choice during pregnancy because of potential fetal side effects associated with coumarin but not heparin use during pregnancy. Like unfractionated heparin, low–molecular-weight heparins also appear to be safe for the fetus.[41] The efficacy of both these agents for the treatment of venous thromboembolism is well established in the nonpregnant population.[29] While unfractionated heparin has been used during pregnancy for many years,[43] there is growing experience with the use of low–molecular-weight heparins in this population, and we believe that pregnant patients with objectively documented venous thromboembolism can be treated with either unfractionated heparin or low–molecular-weight heparin.

There have been no randomized trials evaluating routes of administration or dosages of unfractionated heparin therapy during pregnancy. On the basis of the results of a randomized trial in nonpregnant patients showing that full-dose intravenous heparin, followed by 3 months of adjusted-dose subcutaneous heparin, is safe and effective,[15] a similar approach is recommended for pregnant patients with acute venous thromboembolism. Depending on the severity of the thrombosis and the response to therapy, patients should receive intravenous unfractionated heparin for 5 to 10 days. This has traditionally been initiated with a bolus of 5000 U, followed by a continuous infusion of at least 30,000 U/24 h titrated to prolong the activated partial thromboplastin time (aPTT) into the therapeutic range.[28] A weight-adjusted heparin dosing nomogram has also been shown to be effective in preventing recurrent venous thromboembolism[44] and, accordingly, has been adopted by many hospitals. After the initial intravenous therapy, subcutaneous unfractionated heparin should be given every 12 hours in doses adjusted to prolong the midinterval (6 hours postinjection) aPTT into the therapeutic range for the duration of the pregnancy. The aPTT should be checked regularly (every 1 to 2 weeks) because unfractionated heparin requirements may vary as the pregnancy progresses. To minimize the volume injected, concentrated heparin solutions should be used. Subcutaneous low–molecular-weight heparin is also likely to be effective and safe for the initial and long-term treatment of acute venous thromboembolism during pregnancy, although information about appropriate dosing in this population is lacking. At present, initiation with a weight-adjusted dose that is increased as the patient's weight increases is recommended.[42] The need for measurement of anti-factor Xa concentrations remains controversial. However, given the limited information available regarding appropriate dosing, measurement of anti-factor Xa levels approximately 4 hours after injection with dose adjustment to a level of approximately 0.5 to 1.2 U/mL appears reasonable if these assays are available.[42]

Venous Thromboembolism Prophylaxis during Pregnancy

Although it is commonly believed that women with a previous history of deep vein thrombosis or pulmonary embolism have an increased risk of recurrence during pregnancy and the postpartum period, published data are conflicting, and the magnitude of this risk is unknown.[45–49] Women who developed their initial thrombosis in the presence of a transient risk factor might be expected to have a lower risk of recurrence than those whose event was idiopathic or who have an ongoing risk factor.[42] It is also likely that women with underlying thrombophilic states have an increased risk of venous thromboembolism during pregnancy and the puerperium.[50–53] In those individuals who are receiving long-term warfarin, oral anticoagulants should be replaced by therapeutic doses of heparin. The optimal approach to venous thromboembolic prophylaxis in pregnant women is not known, and the pattern of practice varies widely, from clinical surveillance to aggressive antepartum heparin therapy with postpartum warfarin therapy. There is no consensus among various expert panels, and many different approaches have been recommended (Table 23–1).[42,54,55]

Prevention of Systemic Embolism in Pregnant Women with Valvular Heart Disease

While it is clear that women with mechanical heart valves or bioprosthetic valves with atrial fibrillation or previous systemic embolism require anticoagulation during pregnancy, optimal antithrombotic management of these women is controversial. A dearth of properly designed trials makes it impossible to issue definitive recommendations. Because of this lack of reliable data and concerns about the fetal safety of warfarin, as well as about the efficacy of subcutaneous heparin in the prevention of thromboembolic complications, the decision as to the most appropriate therapy should be made only after inherent risks of the various treatment options are thoroughly reviewed with the expectant woman and her family. In general, three approaches have been advocated. In the first, heparin therapy is administered throughout pregnancy. The second approach is the use of heparin only during those periods considered high risk for the fetus (the 6th to 12th weeks of gestation and near term). The third approach is the use of warfarin throughout pregnancy.

The failure of unfractionated heparin to prevent thromboembolic events has been documented in retrospective studies and case reports.[56,57] It is possible that these failures are the result of inadequate dosing and/or the use of an inadequate therapeutic range. Therefore, if unfractionated heparin is used, it should be initiated at doses of 17,500 to 20,000 U every 12 hours and adjusted to prolong a midinterval aPTT into the therapeutic range (at least twice the control value) or to provide an anti-factor Xa level of 0.35 to 0.70 U/mL.[28] Careful monitoring is essential because unfractionated heparin requirements fluctuate over time. Low–molecular-weight heparin may be a reasonable substitute for unfractionated heparin, but data regarding appropriate dosing are lacking.

If warfarin is used during pregnancy to reduce the risk of maternal thromboembolism, we believe that it should be discontinued and replaced by heparin between the 6th and 12th week of gestation (to avoid embryopathy) and near term (to prevent delivery of an anticoagulated fetus).[42] On the basis of data from nonpregnant patients with mechanical heart valves, an International Normalized Ratio (INR) of 2.5 to 3.5 is recommended for tilting disk valves and bileaflet prosthetic valves in the mitral position.[58] A target INR of 2.0 to 3.0 is likely to be adequate for those with bileaflet mechanical valves in the aortic position, provided that they do not have an enlarged left atrium and are in sinus rhythm, as well as those with bioprosthetic valves and atrial fibrillation.[58] Careful monitoring of the level of anticoagulation is necessary.

Table 23–1 Consensus Panel Recommendations for Venous Thromboembolic Prophylaxis during Pregnancy

Consensus Panel	During Pregnancy	Postpartum
American College of Chest Physicians (1998)[42]	*Prior VTE secondary to transient factor:* Clinical surveillance *Prior idiopathic VTE/thrombophilia with no prior VTE:* Clinical surveillance or low-dose heparin (5000 U/12 h) or adjusted to produce a heparin level of 0.1–0.2 U/mL *Prior VTE and thrombophilia:* Adjusted-dose subcutaneous heparin	*Prior VTE secondary to transient risk factor:* Warfarin for 4–6 weeks *Prior idiopathic VTE/thrombophilia with no prior VTE:* warfarin for 4–6 weeks *Prior VTE and thrombophilia:* Warfarin for 4–6 weeks
British Society for Haematology Guidelines[54]	Unfractionated heparin 5000 U of sc heparin every 12 hours during the 1st and 2nd trimesters, with an increase in dosage sufficient to prolong the midinterval aPTT to 1.5x control in the 3rd trimester or 10,000 U of unfractionated heparin sc every 12 hours throughout pregnancy unless heparin level >0.3 U/mL.	
Maternal and Neonatal Haemostasis Working Party of the Haemostasis and Thrombosis Task[55]	*Prior VTE not associated with pregnancy:* Prophylaxis throughout pregnancy if previous episode severe or during 3rd trimester if not severe (7500 U of unfractionated heparin sc every 12 hours until 36 weeks gestation and 10,000 U every 12 hours from 36 weeks to term) *Prior VTE associated with pregnancy or postpartum:* Unfractionated heparin as above, starting 4–6 weeks before the stage at which thrombosis occurred	*Prior VTE not associated with pregnancy:* Warfarin for at least 6 weeks *Prior VTE associated with pregnancy or postpartum:* Warfarin for at least 6 weeks

Note: VTE, venous thromboembolism; sc, subcutaneously.

In many countries in Europe, warfarin (or a coumarin derivative) is used throughout pregnancy. This approach is based on two considerations. First, the risk of maternal thromboembolism is unacceptable with heparin. Second, the risk of embryopathy has been overstated. This is a difficult position to advocate in North America because of medicolegal concerns and the statement in the manufacturer's package insert that the drug is contraindicated during pregnancy.

Patients at the highest risk of thromboembolism (those with previous embolic events and those with older-generation mechanical valves) may benefit from the addition of low-dose aspirin (80–100 mg/day). This recommendation is based on data in nonpregnant patients in which the addition of low-dose aspirin to warfarin reduced mortality and major systemic embolism, albeit with an increased risk of minor bleeding.[59]

MANAGEMENT OF ANTICOAGULANTS AT DELIVERY

Because of the possibility of persistent elevation of the aPTT at the time of delivery, planned delivery with discontinuation of subcutaneous injections 24 hours before induction has been advocated for women receiving therapeutic doses of subcutaneous unfractionated heparin.[17] An intravenous infusion of unfractionated heparin should be started after discontinuation of subcutaneous heparin in patients considered at high risk for thromboembolic complications.[60] This infusion can then be discontinued 4 to 6 hours before the anticipated time of delivery, with the expectation that the aPTT will be within normal limits at delivery. Women with spontaneous onset of labor should discontinue injections immediately. The aPTT should be checked in all instances to ensure that it has normalized with discontinuation of heparin. If necessary, rapid reversal of heparinization can be accomplished with protamine sulphate. If the patient is receiving prophylactic doses of heparin at term, they can be discontinued at the onset of true labor. No increased bleeding is expected with this approach.[60]

Although there are no well-designed trials, we also recommend elective induction of labor close to term in women who are receiving "therapeutic" doses of low–molecular-weight heparin, with discontinuation of the drug 24 hours before elective induction. If spontaneous labor occurs while a patient is receiving "therapeutic" doses of low–molecular-weight heparin, the approach is dependent upon the dose, the proximity of the last dose to the expected time of delivery, and, if available, the anti-factor Xa level. If there is a reasonable expectation that, at the expected time of delivery, a significant anticoagulant effect will be present, or if anti-factor Xa levels show an anticoagulant effect, several precautions should be taken. First, epidural analgesia should be avoided. Second, judicious use of protamine sulphate should be considered. Finally, the obstetrician should be made aware of the potential for bleeding and make efforts to minimize the risk. For "prophylactic" doses of low–molecular-weight heparin (less than or equal to 5000 U every 24 h), it is probably reasonable to proceed "as usual," provided that 12 hours have elapsed between the last dose and an invasive procedure like delivery or epidural catheter insertion.

Women receiving warfarin during pregnancy should be switched to subcutaneous unfractionated heparin at approximately 36 weeks of gestation in order to prevent delivery of an anticoagulated fetus. If a mother enters labor while still receiving warfarin, intravenous vitamin K should be administered and the baby delivered by Caesarean section to avoid the risk of traumatic hemorrhage associated with vaginal delivery.

MANAGEMENT OF ANTICOAGULANTS AFTER DELIVERY

In women receiving anticoagulants for the treatment of venous thromboembolism or for prevention of systemic embolism associated with valvular heart disease, therapeutic doses of heparin should be reintroduced as soon as adequate hemostasis is achieved following delivery. Warfarin can be started immediately and the heparin discontinued once the INR has been within the therapeutic range for two consecutive days. Oral anticoagulants should be continued for 4 to 6 weeks postpartum or for a minimum of 3 months when the venous thromboembolic event occurs late in pregnancy. Patients with valvular heart disease require long-term anticoagulation.

REFERENCES

1. Quick AJ. Experimentally induced changes in the prothrombin level of the blood. III. Prothrombin concentration of newborn pups of a mother given Dicoumarol before parturition. *J Biol Chem*. 1946;164: 371–376.

2. Kraus AP, Perlow A, Singer K. Danger of Dicoumarol treatment in pregnancy. *JAMA*. 1949;139:758–782.

3. DiSaia PJ. Pregnancy and delivery of a patient with a Starr-Edwards mitral valve prosthesis: report of a case. *Obstet Gynecol*. 1966;28: 469–472.

4. Kerber IJ, Warr OS, Richardson C. Pregnancy in a patient with a prosthetic mitral valve. *JAMA*. 1968;203:223–225.

5. Becker HM, Genieser NB, Finegold M, Miranda D, Spackman T. Chondroplasia punctata: is maternal warfarin a factor? *Am J Dis Child*. 1975;129:356–359.

6. Shaul WL, Hall JG. Multiple congenital anomalies associated with oral anticoagulants. *Am J Obstet Gynecol*. 1977;27:191–198.

7. Hall JAG, Paul RM, Wilson KM. Maternal and fetal sequelae of anticoagulation during pregnancy. *Am J Med*. 1980;68:122–140.

8. Hirsh J, Cade JF, Gallus AS. Fetal effects of Coumadin administered during pregnancy. *Blood*. 1970;36:623–627.

9. Iturbe-Alessio I, del Carmen Fonseca M, Mutchinik O, Santos MA, Zajarias A, Salazar E. Risks of anticoagulant therapy in pregnant women with artificial heart valves. *N Engl J Med*. 1986;315:1390–1393.

10. Ginsberg JS, Hirsh J, Turner C, Levine MN, Burrows R. Risks to the fetus of anticoagulant therapy during pregnancy. *Thromb Haemost*. 1989;61:197–203.

11. L'E Orme M, Lewis M, DeSwiet M, et al. May mothers given warfarin breast-feed their infants? *Br Med J*. 1977;1:1564–1565.

12. McKenna R, Cole ER, Vasan U. Is warfarin sodium contraindicated in the lactating mother? *J Pediatr*. 1983;103:325–327.

13. Flessa HC, Kapstrom AB, Glueck MJ, Will JJ. Placental transport of heparin. *Am J Obstet Gynecol*. 1965;93:570–573.

14. Ginsberg J, Kowalchuk G, Hirsh J, Brill-Edwards P, Burrows R. Heparin therapy during pregnancy: risks to the fetus and mother. *Arch Intern Med*. 1989;149:2233–2236.

15. Hull R, Delmore T, Carter C, et al. Adjusted subcutaneous heparin versus warfarin sodium in the long-term treatment of venous thrombosis. *N Engl J Med*. 1982;306:189–194.

16. Hull R, Hirsh J, Jay R, et al. Different intensities of oral anticoagulant therapy in the treatment of proximal vein thrombosis. *N Engl J Med*. 1982;307:1676–1681.

17. Anderson D, Ginsberg JS, Burrows R, Brill-Edwards P. Subcutaneous heparin therapy during pregnancy: a need for concern at the time of delivery. *Thromb Haemost*. 1991;65:248–250.

18. Kapsch D, Silver D. Heparin-induced thrombocytopenia with thrombosis and hemorrhage. *Arch Surg*. 1981;116:1423–1427.

19. Aster RH. Heparin-induced thrombocytopenia and thrombosis. *N Engl J Med*. 1995;332:1374–1376.

20. Griffith GC, Nichols G, Asher JD, Hanagan B. Heparin osteoporosis. *JAMA*. 1965;193:191–194.

21. Dahlman TC, Sjoberg HE, Rigertz H. Bone mineral density during long-term prophylaxis with heparin in pregnancy. *Am J Obstet Gynecol*. 1994;160:1315–1320.

22. Dahlman TC, Hellgren MS, Blomback M. Thrombosis prophylaxis in pregnancy with use of subcutaneous heparin concentration in plasma. *Am J Obstet Gynecol*. 1993;168:1265–1270.

23. Howell R, Fidler J, Letsky E, DeSwiet M. The risks of antenatal subcutaneous heparin prophylaxis: a controlled trial. *Br J Obstet Gynaecol*. 1983;30:1124–1128.

24. Ginsberg JS, Kowalchuk G, Hirsh J, et al. Heparin effect on bone density. *Thromb Haemost*. 1990;64:286–289.

25. Dahlman T, Lindall N, Helgren M. Osteopenia in pregnancy during long-term heparin treatment: a radiological study postpartum. *Br J Obstet Gynaecol*. 1990;97:221–228.

26. Barbour LA, Kick SC, Steiner JF, LoVerde ME, Heddleston LN, Lear JL. A prospective study of heparin-induced osteoporosis using bone densitometry. *Am J Obstet Gynecol*. 1994;170:862–869.

27. Douketis JD, Ginsberg JS, Burrows RD, Duku EK, Webber CE, Brill-Edwards P. The effect of long-term heparin therapy on bone density: a prospective matched cohort study. *Thromb Haemost*. 1996;75: 254–257.

28. Hirsh J, Fuster V. Guide to anticoagulant therapy. Part 1: heparin. *Circulation*. 1994;89:1449–1468.

29. Dolovich L, Ginsberg JS. Low molecular weight heparins in the treatment of venous thromboembolism: an updated meta-analysis. *Vessels*. 1997;3:4–11.

30. Nurmohamed MT, Rosendaal FIR, Büller HR, et al. Low–molecular-weight heparin versus standard heparin in general and orthopaedic surgery: a metanalysis. *Lancet.* 1992;340:152–156.

31. Leizorovicz A, Haugh MC, Chapuis FR, Samama MM, Boissel JP. Low–molecular-weight heparins in the prevention of perioperative thrombosis. *Br Med J.* 1992;305:913–920.

32. Jorgensen LN, Wille-Jorgensen P, Hauch O. Prophylaxis of postoperative thromboembolism with low molecular weight heparins. *Br J Surg.* 1993;30:689–704.

33. Forestier F, Daffos F, Rainaut M, Toulemonde F. Low–molecular-weight heparin (CY 216) does not cross the placenta during the third trimester of pregnancy. *Thromb Haemost.* 1987;57:234.

34. Weitz J. Low–molecular-weight heparins. *N Engl J Med.* 1997;337:688–698.

35. Bara L, Samama M. Pharmacokinetics of low molecular weight heparins. *Acta Chir Scand.* 1988;543(suppl):65–72.

36. Bara L, Billaud E, Gramond G, Kher A, Samama M. Comparative pharmacokinetics of a low–molecular-weight heparin (PK10169) and unfractionated heparin after intravenous and subcutaneous administration. *Thromb Res.* 1985;39:631–636.

37. Warkentin TE, Levine MN, Hirsh J, et al. Heparin-induced thrombocytopenia in patients treated with low–molecular-weight heparin or unfractionated heparin. *N Engl J Med.* 1995;332:1330–1335.

38. Monreal M, Lafoz E, Olive A, de Rio L, Vedia C. Comparison of subcutaneous unfractionated heparin with a low molecular weight heparin (Fragmin) in patients with venous thromboembolism and contraindications for coumarin. *Thromb Haemost.* 1994;71:7–11.

39. Melissari E, Parker CJ, Wilson NV, et al. Use of low molecular weight heparin in pregnancy. *Thromb Haemost.* 1992;68:652–656.

40. Sefras J, Farquharson RG. Bone density studies in pregnant women receiving heparin. *Eur J Obstet Gynecol Reprod Biol.* 1996;65:171–174.

41. Sanson B, Lensing AWA, Prins MH, et al. The use of low–molecular-weight heparin in pregnancy: a systematic review. *Thromb Haemost.* 1999;81:668–672.

42. Ginsberg JS, Hirsh J. Use of antithrombotic agents during pregnancy. *Chest.* 1998;114:524S–530S.

43. Villasanta U. Thromboembolic disease in pregnancy. *Am J Obstet Gynecol.* 1965;93:142–160.

44. Raschke RA, Reilly BM, Guidry JR, Fontana JR, Srinivas S. The weight-based heparin dosing nomogram compared with a "standard care nomogram." *Ann Intern Med.* 1993;119:874–881.

45. De Swiet M, Floyd E, Letsky E. Low risk of recurrent thromboembolism in pregnancy. *Br J Hosp Med.* 1987;38:264. Letter.

46. Howell R, Fidler J, Letsky E, et al. The risk of antenatal subcutaneous heparin prophylaxis: a controlled trial. *Br J Obstet Gynecol.* 1983;90:1124–1128.

47. Badaracco MA, Vessey M. Recurrent venous thromboembolic disease and use of oral contraceptives. *Br Med J.* 1974;1:215–217.

48. Tengborn L, Bergqvist D, Matzsch T, Bergqvist A, Hedner U. Recurrent thromboembolism in pregnancy and puerperium: is there a need for thromboprophylaxis? *Am J Obstet Gynecol.* 1989;160:90–94.

49. Lao TT, De Swiet M, Letsky E, Walters BNJ. Prophylaxis of thromboembolism in pregnancy: an alternative. *Br J Obstet Gynecol.* 1985;92:202–206.

50. Conard J, Horellou MH, Van Dreden P, Lecompte T, Samama M. Thrombosis and pregnancy in congenital deficiencies in AT III, protein C, protein S: a study of 78 women. *Thromb Haemost.* 1990;63:319–320.

51. Allaart CV, Poort SR, Rosendaal FR, Reitsma PH, Bertina RM, Briet E. Increased risk of venous thrombosis in carriers of hereditary protein C deficiency defect. *Lancet.* 1993;341:134–138.

52. De Stefano V, Leone G, Mastrangelo S, et al. Thrombosis during pregnancy and surgery in patients with congenital deficiency of antithrombin III, protein C, protein S. *Thromb Haemost.* 1994;61:799–800.

53. McColl M, Ramsay JE, Tait RC, et al. Risk factors for pregnancy associated venous thromboembolism. *Thromb Haemost.* 1997;78:1183–1188.

54. Colvin BT, Barrowcliffe TW. The British Society for Haematology Guidelines on the use and monitoring of heparin, 1992: second revision. *J Clin Pathol.* 1993;97–103.

55. Maternal and Neonatal Haemostasis Working Party of the Haemostasis and Thrombosis Task. Guidelines on the prevention, investigation, and management of thrombosis associated with pregnancy. *J Clin Pathol.* 1993;489–496.

56. Salazar E, Izaguirre R, Verdejo J, Mutchinick O. Failure of adjusted doses of subcutaneous heparin to prevent thromboembolic phenomena in pregnant patients with mechanical cardiac valve prostheses. *J Am Coll Cardiol.* 1996;27:1698–1703.

57. Sbarouni E, Oakley CM. Outcome of pregnancy in women with valve prostheses. *Br Heart J.* 1994;71:196–201.

58. Stein PD, Alpert JS, Horstkotte D, Turpie AGG. Antithrombotic therapy in patients with mechanical and biological prosthetic heart valves. *Chest.* 1998;114:602S–610S.

59. Turpie AGG, Gent M, Laupacis A, et al. Comparison of aspirin with placebo in patients treated with warfarin after heart-valve replacement. *N Engl J Med.* 1993;329:524–529.

60. Demers C, Ginsberg JS. Deep vein thrombosis and pulmonary embolism in pregnancy. *Clin Chest Med.* 1992;13:645–656.

Chapter 24

Prothrombin Time

Douglas A. Triplett

HISTORICAL DEVELOPMENT

During the mid-1930s, Dr. Armand Quick was interested in developing a coagulation test to assess liver function.[1,2] Hemorrhagic episodes not infrequently complicate liver disease; consequently, Quick reasoned that a coagulation-based test might be sensitive in predicting clinical bleeding. At that time, the science of coagulation was limited. There were only four recognized components to hemostasis: fibrinogen, prothrombin, thromboplastin, and a requirement for calcium ions. Thromboplastin was prepared by extraction from either human or animal tissues, most commonly brain. In 1935, Quick and colleagues published their paper describing the prothrombin time (PT) in the *American Journal of Medical Science.*[2]

The work of Karl Link and his colleagues at the University of Wisconsin ultimately led to the widespread clinical use of the PT.[3] Link and his associates were working on an intriguing veterinary medical problem of hemorrhagic disease in cattle exposed to spoiled sweet clover. This substance was found to be dicumarol (3,3'methylenebis[4-hydroxy-coumarin]). Utilizing Quick's PT, Link found that cattle suffering from spoiled sweet clover disease had prolonged PTs, which were due to an alteration of vitamin K's metabolic pathway. Vitamin K is necessary for the addition of a carboxy group to form γ-carboxyglutamic acid (gla) (Figure 24–1).

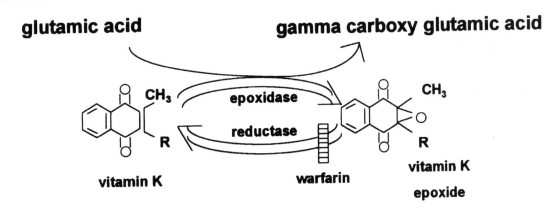

Figure 24–1 Vitamin K epoxide cycle. Vitamin K is a necessary cofactor to convert glutamic acid to γ-carboxyglutamic acid (gla). This reaction is dependent on the epoxidase enzyme. Vitamin K epoxide is no longer functionally able to facilitate production of gla. A reductase enzyme will convert vitamin K epoxide to vitamin K. Warfarin exerts its effect by interfering with the reductase enzyme.

Gla residues are necessary for localization of coagulation factors to phospholipid surfaces. Shortly after Link's description of dicumarol, it was given to patients at the Mayo Clinic to treat postoperative thrombophlebitis. Subsequently, other more easily used oral anticoagulants were introduced.

With the clinical introduction of oral anticoagulation, PT became the most commonly utilized test to monitor oral anticoagulation. Coagulationists also discovered a number of new coagulation factors necessary for the PT test system: factors VII, X, and V. In parallel with the discovery of these coagulation proteins, the concept of intrinsic and extrinsic pathways of coagulation was introduced (Figure 24–2). The PT (tissue factor-induced coagulation time) evaluates the so-called extrinsic system. The activated partial thromboplastin time is a test of the intrinsic pathway of coagulation.[4] Recent studies clearly demonstrate that the concept of discrete intrinsic and extrinsic pathways is erroneous. Nevertheless, it is useful to consider the PT as a test to evaluate the extrinsic pathway (Figure 24–3).

The PT is particularly useful for monitoring oral anticoagulants because three of the four procoagulant vitamin K–dependent proteins are evaluated by the PT: factors VII and X and prothrombin (factor II) (Exhibit 24–1). The PT is also used in screening for vitamin K deficiency from other causes (eg, liver disease, malabsorption, antibiotic therapy). As the popularity of oral anticoagulants increased, a number of additional test systems were introduced to monitor oral anticoagulant therapy. Among these were the thrombotest, prothrombin proconvertin time, and native prothrombin antigen levels.[5–9] Of these, the thrombotest is the only one that has continued significant use (in Scandinavia, The Netherlands, and Japan).[5]

The widespread use of PTs to monitor patients on anticoagulant therapy soon revealed considerable interlaboratory variation among PT results.[10,11] Through collaborative efforts involving many national and international organizations, this issue was addressed by introducing the concept of the International Normalized Ratio (INR).[12–14]

PROTHROMBIN TIME: TECHNICAL AND PROCEDURAL VARIABLES

Although the PT appears to be simple from the standpoint of reagents and technique, a number of important variables can significantly affect PT results. These variables can be conveniently categorized as biologic, preanalytical, analytical, and result reporting.

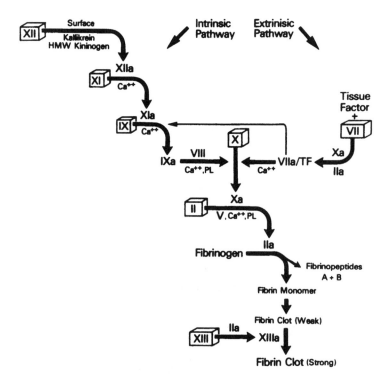

Key: Ca++, calcium ions; HMW, high molecular weight: PL, phospholipid; TF, tissue factor.

Figure 24–2 Coagulation pathways. Coagulation is divided into intrinsic and extrinsic systems. Both systems share the final common pathway beginning with the activation of factor X. It is important to appreciate the amplification aspect of the coagulation process. Source: Reprinted with permission from JE Ansell, *Handbook of Hemostasis and Thrombosis*, p 10, © 1986, Little Brown and Company.

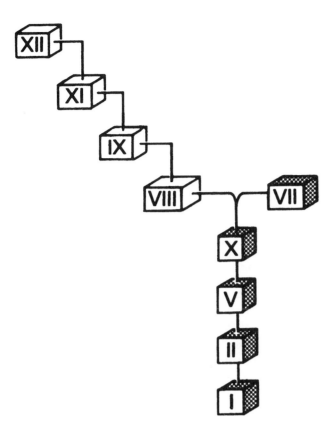

Figure 24–3 The prothrombin time, which evaluates the extrinsic pathway of coagulation (factors VII, X, V, II, and I). In vivo, this pathway is initiated by exposure of blood to tissue factor. Source: Reprinted with permission from JE Ansell, *Handbook of Hemostasis and Thrombosis*, p 20, © 1986, Little Brown & Company.

Biologic Variables

The dietary status of the patient is an important variable. The primary source of vitamin K is dietary (leafy green vegetables). Microorganisms in the gastrointestinal tract also contribute some vitamin K. Vegetarians might require considerably more oral anticoagulants than individuals who eat vegetables infrequently. Seasonal changes in diet often depend on the availability of fresh vegetables. Also, it is important to consider drug-drug interactions that can modify the response to oral anticoagulants. Drugs can alter absorption of the oral anticoagulants from the gastrointestinal tract and also alter their metabolism. Alcohol is a potent suppressor of hepatic microsomal enzyme activity; consequently, alcohol ingestion will prolong the half-life of oral anticoagulants.

Preanalytical Variables

Preanalytical variables are often overlooked in evaluating problems with laboratory procedures. This is also the case

Exhibit 24–1
VITAMIN K–DEPENDENT PROTEINS

PROCOAGULANT	ANTICOAGULANT
• Prothrombin	• Protein C
• Factor VII	• Protein S
• Factor IX	
• Factor X	
OTHER	
• Osteocalcin	
• Protein Z	

with the PT. Appropriate care in acquiring the blood sample from the patient is necessary. The venipuncture should be as atraumatic as possible, and, when feasible, the second tube in a sequence of collection tubes should be used for the PT. Sodium citrate is the anticoagulant of choice. The current recommendations of the National Committee for Clinical Laboratory Standards indicate that sodium citrate (0.129 M) may be used to collect samples for PT testing.[15] Recent evidence, however, suggests there might be significant differences between PT results obtained with 3.2% (109 mM) versus 3.8% (129 mM) citrate concentrations. PT times obtained with 3.8% citrate are typically longer than those obtained with 3.2% citrate.[16] This does have an effect on calculation of the INR. To avoid variability in the INR results, a single citrate concentration should be used within a health care facility. Optimally, 3.2% (109 mM) sodium citrate is recommended. Another important preanalytical variable is potential activation of factor XII (Hageman's factor), which might lead to in vitro activation of factor VII and in shortening of the PT. This phenomenon is seen in plasma stored in glass collection tubes that are not siliconized. It is also enhanced by storage of citrated plasma at 4°C.[17]

Analytical Variables

The analytical variables include choice of thromboplastin and instrumentation and the technical expertise of the person performing the test. It is important to choose a reagent and instrument that are compatible. Typically, manufacturers of reagents and instruments design their products to perform most efficiently when used together. Purchasing an instrument from one manufacturer and a reagent from a second manufacturer might prove to be a less than optimal situation.[18,19] In order to identify performance of instrument/ reagent combinations (systems), the best source of available information is the College of American Pathologists Coagulation Survey Program. These survey results report performance of systems. On an annual basis, oral anticoagulated plasma samples are sent to participating laboratories along with artificially depleted plasma samples (ie, normal plasma that has been adsorbed with barium sulfate to remove vitamin K–dependent proteins—factors II, VII, IX, and X).

Thromboplastins (tissue factor—phospholipids) can be extracted from a variety of human and animal tissues:

- tissue extracts
  - rabbit (brain/lung)
  - human (brain/placenta)
  - bovine (brain)
  - horse
  - monkey (brain)
- recombinant
  - tissue factor
- human tissue factor; cell culture

Brain, lung, and placenta are all rich in thromboplastin. Recently, tissue factor, the protein portion of thromboplastins, has been isolated and sequenced.[20–22] Utilizing recombinant human tissue factor, new thromboplastin reagents have been introduced.[23] With the introduction of recombinant human tissue factor, the biologic variability seen in products prepared from animal or human tissue has been greatly reduced. By utilizing recombinant human tissue factor and carefully controlled lipid preparations, a remarkable degree of homogeneity among lot numbers of thromboplastins can be achieved. Historically, rabbit tissue thromboplastins have been used in the United States. Until recently in the United Kingdom, human brain thromboplastin was the reagent of choice. The thrombotest, which is used in The Netherlands, Norway, and Japan, is prepared from bovine brain thromboplastin.[5] In general, the rabbit brain thromboplastins are less responsive to the oral anticoagulant effect on the PT. Human and bovine thromboplastins are classified as responsive (ie, at a given dose of oral anticoagulant, the PT result will be more prolonged when compared with rabbit brain thromboplastins). The classic concept of a therapeutic range of a PT ratio of 2.0 to 2.5 was based on the use of responsive thromboplastins. When this concept was extrapolated to less responsive thromboplastins, patients were often overanti-

coagulated, with a resulting higher incidence of hemorrhagic complications.[24]

Result Reporting Variables

PT results have been reported in a variety of different formats, including percent activity, PT ratios, index values, and INR. Percent activity is calculated by using a saline or adsorbed plasma dilution of normal plasma, but most laboratories have discontinued using this format. PT ratios are derived by using the patient's PT results in seconds in the numerator and the geometric mean of the normal PT range in the denominator. The PT index is the reciprocal of the ratio reported as a percentage. The INR is discussed in Chapter 25. Until recently, the PT ratio has been the most commonly used means of reporting PT results in the United States. One of the most common errors seen with the PT ratio is the use of a "control" value in the denominator. In many cases, this control value was derived from PT times obtained on control plasmas provided by diagnostic manufacturers. This practice still persists in many laboratories and represents a continuing problem.

DIFFICULTIES WITH PROTHROMBIN TIME AS A THERAPEUTIC GUIDE

Following the introduction of the PT as the principal method for monitoring oral anticoagulant therapy, many modifications of the test were developed.[5,6] To compound the procedural modifications, there was marked diversity of thromboplastins. As noted, various sources of animal tissue were used for thromboplastin preparations. The lack of consistency in PT results led to efforts to standardize reporting of PT values. The INR is recommended for reporting PT results for oral anticoagulant monitoring.[25]

In order to improve the overall performance of PT systems (reagent/instrument combinations), attention must be directed to consistency in the use of 3.2% citrate for collection of samples for PT testing. Also, it is important to recognize the effect of instrumentation on PT results. Laboratories must carefully choose an appropriate reagent/instrument combination.

REFERENCES

1. Quick AJ. The prothrombin time in haemophilia and in obstructive jaundice. *J Biol Chem.* 1935;109:73–74.

2. Quick AJ, Stanley-Brown M, Bancroft FW. A study of the coagulation defect in hemophilia and in jaundice. *Am J Med Sci.* 1935;190: 501–511.

3. Link KP. The anticoagulant from spoiled sweet clover hay. *Harvey Lect.* 1943;39:162.

4. Proctor RR, Rapaport SI. The partial thromboplastin time with kaolin: a simple screening test for first stage plasma clotting factor deficiencies. *Am J Clin Pathol.* 1961;36:212–219.

5. Owren PA. Thrombotest: a new method for controlling anticoagulant therapy. *Lancet.* 1959;2:754–758.

6. Owren PA, Aas K. Control of dicumarol therapy and quantitative determination of prothrombin and proconvertin. *Scand J Clin Lab Invest.* 1951;3:201–208.

7. Furie B, Liebman HA, Blanchard RA, Coleman MS, Kruger SF, Furie BC. Comparison of the native prothrombin antigen and prothrombin time for monitoring oral anticoagulant therapy. *Blood.* 1984;64:445–451.

8. Braun PJ, Szewczyk KM. Relationship between total prothrombin, native prothrombin and the International Normalized Ratio (INR). *Thromb Haemost.* 1992;68:160–164.

9. Le DT, Weibert RT, Sevilla BK, Donnelly KJ, Rapaport SI. The International Normalized Ratio (INR) for monitoring warfarin therapy: reliability and relation to other monitoring methods. *Ann Intern Med.* 1994;120:552–558.

10. Rodman T, Pastor BH, Hoxter BL. Problems encountered in the laboratory control of anticoagulant therapy with the one stage determination of prothrombin complex activity. *Am J Med.* 1961;31:555–563.

11. Quick AJ. Standardization of the one-stage prothrombin time. *Thromb Diathes Haemorrh.* 1972;27:179–180.

12. ICTH/ICSH prothrombin time standardization report of the expert panel on oral anticoagulant control. *Thromb Haemost.* 1979;42:1073–1114.

13. Hermans J, van den Besselaar AMHP, Loeliger EA, van der Velde EA. A collaborative calibration study of reference materials for thromboplastins. *Thromb Haemost.* 1983;50:712–717.

14. Kirkwood TBL. Calibration of reference thromboplastins. *Thromb Haemost.* 1983;49:238–244.

15. National Committee for Clinical Laboratory Standards. *Collection, Transport and Processing of Blood Specimens for Coagulation Testing and Performance of Coagulation Assays.* 2nd ed. Villanova, PA: National Committee for Clinical Laboratory Standards: Approved guideline; 1991: Document H21-A2.

16. Adcock DM, Marlar RA. The effect of sodium citrate concentration on determination of the INR. *Clin Hemost Rev.* 1996;10:18.

17. Gralnick HR. Kessler CR, Palmer R. The prothrombin time: variables affecting results. In: Triplett DA, ed. *Standardization of Coagulation Assays: An Overview.* Skokie. IL: College of American Pathologists; 1982:57–66.

18. Ray MJ, Smith IR. The dependence of the International Sensitivity Index on the coagulometer used to perform the prothrombin time. *Thromb Haemost.* 1990;63:424–429.

19. Thomson JM, Taberner DA, Poller L. Automation and prothrombin time: a United Kingdom field study of two widely used coagulometers. *J Clin Pathol.* 1990;43:679–684.

20. Broze GJ, Leykam JE, Schwartz BD, Miletich JP. Purification of human brain tissue. *J Biol Chem.* 1985;260:10917–10920.

21. Guha A, Bach R, Konigsberg W, Nemerson Y. Affinity purification of human tissue factor: interaction of factor VII and tissue factor in detergent micelles. *Proc Natl Acad Sci USA.* 1986;83:299–302.

22. Morrissey JH, Fair DS, Edgington TS. Structure and properties of the human tissue factor apoprotein. *Thromb Haemost.* 1987;58:257. Abstract.

23. Hoppensteadt DA, Walenga JM, Fareed J, Bermes EG. Comparing r-tissue factor and mammalian tissue reagents for prothrombin time. *Lab Med.* 1995;26:198–203.

24. Hirsh J. Is the dose of warfarin prescribed by American physicians unnecessarily high? *Arch Intern Med.* 1987;147:769–771.

25. Koepke JA, Triplett DA. Standardization of the prothrombin time—finally. *Arch Pathol Lab Med.* 1985;109:800.

Chapter 25

Standardization of the Prothrombin Time

Douglas A. Triplett

VARIABLES AFFECTING PROTHROMBIN TIME

Prothrombin time (PT) results depend on many variables, including appropriate collection of the patient sample, choice of reagent and instrumentation, and reporting of results. When Armand Quick developed the PT, he recommended a carefully described procedure for the preparation and use of rabbit brain thromboplastin in order to ensure consistent results at any time or place.[1] With the introduction of many modifications of the PT, results obtained by different laboratories could not be directly compared.[2] In a Utopian environment, all laboratories would use the same thromboplastin preparation and identical techniques. This is not an achievable objective; consequently, efforts have focused on standardization of PT results by transforming results obtained with various reagents and instruments (systems) into standardized values.[3]

During the 1960s, approaches to standardizing PT results were widely discussed. In 1964, the Manchester comparative reagent (human brain) was introduced in the United Kingdom.[4] Through Dr. Leon Poller's efforts, a remarkable degree of consistency in PT results was achieved in the United Kingdom. Most laboratories utilized the Manchester comparative reagent and also performed PTs with a manual tilt-tube technique. During this same era in the United States, large-scale proficiency testing programs were initiated by the College of American Pathologists.[5] These programs (surveys) subsequently became linked to laboratory accreditation. The early surveys showed significant variability of PT results among samples supplied to laboratories. Utilizing this information, reference plasmas were suggested as a means of standardizing PT results. At meetings of the International Society of Thrombosis and Haemostasis, these two concepts were widely debated.

In 1977, the World Health Organization (WHO) recognized the Manchester comparative reagent as its International Reference Preparation (IRP).[6] In 1983, the International Normalized Ratio (INR) was recommended as the universal scale for reporting PT results from patients receiving oral anticoagulants. By definition, the INR is the PT ratio that would have been obtained on a patient's plasma if the primary IRP had been used to perform the PT with a manual technique. It should be emphasized that the INR was defined only for monitoring oral anticoagulation and not for screening patients with other disorders, such as liver disease or hereditary abnormalities involving coagulation factors of the extrinsic pathway.

INTERNATIONAL NORMALIZED RATIO

The INR is based on the availability of an IRP of thromboplastin and the manual technique for PT determination. Following the introduction of the human brain IRP, various secondary standards, including rabbit brain thromboplastin and a bovine brain preparation were introduced.[7] The availability of secondary standards allows one to calibrate thromboplastins in a like-to-like fashion (ie, rabbit brain thromboplastin used in a given laboratory [working thromboplastin] against the rabbit brain thromboplastin secondary standard).[8]

The secondary standards allow for more consistency (species-species) in thromboplastin calibration.

With widespread automation in modern coagulation laboratories, very few laboratories utilize the manual technique. Initially, it was thought that instrumentation would have little effect on the calculation of INR values. When comparing calibration exercises, however, it soon became evident that different results were obtained on plasma samples evaluated with instrumentation versus those evaluated with the manual technique.[9–11] There is significant instrument variability because of the end-point detection systems used (optical systems, laser detection, electromechanical). Two values, a correctly determined PT ratio and the International Sensitivity Index (ISI) for the thromboplastin being utilized, are needed to calculate the INR:

$$INR = \left[\frac{patient\ PT}{mean\ of\ normal\ PT} \right]^{ISI}$$

The ISI value is dependent on the instrument being used to perform the PT. Commercial thromboplastins must have their ISI values verified on various instruments. Most manufacturers supply ISI values for their optimal instrument and reagent combinations. In many cases, the appropriate instrument is manufactured by the maker of a thromboplastin or by a closely related company that collaborates with the reagent manufacturer.

The ISI value assignment is calculated by the manufacturer. This requires a very detailed protocol utilizing the manufacturer's thromboplastin and RPs provided by the WHO. In order to derive the ISI, it is necessary to test 20 fresh plasma samples from normal individuals and 60 fresh plasma samples obtained from patients who are stabilized on oral anticoagulant therapy. Log PT results for the IRP thromboplastin and working thromboplastin are then plotted, and, by orthogonal regression, the best-fit line is derived (Figure 25–1). The slope of this line is the ISI value. By definition, the IRP has an ISI value of 1.0. The ISI is something of a misnomer because it actually evaluates responsiveness of a thromboplastin to the oral anticoagulant effect. The larger the ISI value, the less responsive is the reagent. When the INR concept began to achieve notoriety in the United States during the early 1990s, the vast majority of thromboplastins had ISI values above 2.0.[12] In many cases, ISI values were greater than 2.5. Thromboplastins with high ISI values result in loss of INR precision, less sensitivity to oral anticoagulants, and a narrow therapeutic range (seconds). Thromboplastins with low ISI values have the advantages of a wider therapeutic window, the ability to monitor low-dose warfarin, a close correlation to the IRP, and more precise monitoring of oral anticoagulation.

With the introduction of the recombinant tissue factor thromboplastins, a marked shift has occurred in the ISI values for thromboplastins used in the United States, and

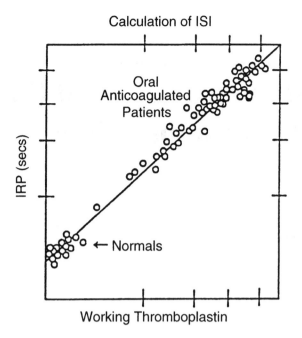

Figure 25–1 Calculation of the International Sensitivity Index (ISI). Samples from 60 stabilized patients on oral anticoagulants and from 20 controls are tested in duplicate with the International Reference Preparation (IRP) and the working thromboplastin. By orthogonal regression, the best-fit line, the slope of which represents the ISI of the working thromboplastin, is derived.

most laboratories now utilize reagents with ISI values of less than 2.0. The ISI values of recombinant tissue factor thromboplastins approach 1.0, which has accelerated the trend for laboratories to use thromboplastins with ISI values of 1.0.[13]

DIFFICULTIES WITH THE INTERNATIONAL NORMALIZED RATIO

The INR is designed to monitor patients who are stabilized on oral anticoagulation therapy. It is not intended to be used for patients who have other clinical conditions (eg, liver disease, malabsorption syndromes, hereditary factor deficiencies), that might affect the PT. Unfortunately, in many institutions, an INR value is now provided on every patient PT result. In some institutions, a PT result is given only as an INR value. This practice has led to significant confusion, particularly for physicians who obtain PTs for reasons other than monitoring oral anticoagulants. For instance, when a gastroenterologist is planning a needle biopsy of the liver, PTs are routinely ordered to assess liver function. Historically, the decision to perform a closed-needle biopsy was based on PT results reported as seconds. Also, these results were obtained using relatively nonresponsive thromboplastins. With the introduction of low ISI thromboplastins, prolonged PTs are more commonly seen, not only for patients with liver disease but also for those with low levels of factor VII resulting from vitamin K deficiency or perhaps for heterozygous patients with hereditary factor VII deficiency. Without a "reference window," a gastroenterologist might be perplexed by the PT or INR results.

The second major problem associated with the INR has been inaccuracy of the ISI values. Although manufacturers carefully calibrate the ISI values on their thromboplastins, they do not, in most cases, provide ISI values that are system specific (thromboplastin/instrument combination).[14] Based on studies of proficiency testing in France and the United States, it appears that the instrument effect might be comparable to the thromboplastin effect on the INR value.[15] One means of overcoming this problem is the use of calibrating plasmas provided by reagent manufacturers. By utilizing plasma samples with carefully calculated INR values, a laboratory can verify the correct ISI value for its system.[16,17] Preliminary trials reported from Europe and the United States are encouraging.

Other circumstances can lead to errors in calculation of the INR. Among these is incorrect determination of the PT ratio (the most common reason for this error is the use of commercial "controls" as the denominator in the PT ratio).[18] Also, the presence of heparin in the sample or the use of the INR value early in the course of oral anticoagulant therapy can yield erroneous results.

The introduction of the INR has greatly advanced the consistency of oral anticoagulant therapy worldwide. Despite these advances, it is important to be aware of the difficulties encountered in maintaining patients within the recommended therapeutic range for the INR (classically, 2.0–3.0).[19] Even in well-controlled patients who are reliable and carefully followed by informed physicians and/or anticoagulant clinics, the best one can hope for in a given individual is to maintain the level of intensity of oral anticoagulation in the therapeutic range approximately 70% of the time.[20,21] During the remaining 30% of the time, because of many complex interactions, the patient will be above or below the appropriate intensity of anticoagulant therapy.

Another interesting problem with respect to the INR has to do with patients with lupus anticoagulants (LAs). LAs are immunoglobulins that prolong phospholipid-dependent coagulation tests (eg, PT, activated partial thromboplastin time, dilute Russell viper time). Paradoxically, LAs are associated with an increased risk of clinical thromboembolic disease. Patients with recurrent venous or arterial thrombi are treated long term (lifelong in some instances) with oral anticoagulants and followed with PTs. In many instances, the intensity of the anticoagulant therapy is greater in these patients than that in patients with isolated thrombotic events. A typical recommendation for an LA patient with recurrent thrombosis is an INR of 3.0–3.5. Recent evidence suggests that LAs have a direct effect on PT results.[22] Thus, in many cases the INR value is erroneously calculated. This can have profound effects resulting in under-anticoagulation of patients with resulting recurrent thrombosis. This phenomenon has been only recently identified; consequently, recommendations concerning the monitoring of these patients have not been rigorously evaluated. It might be necessary to utilize different test systems, such as the prothrombin-proconvertin time or the native prothrombin antigen test.[23,24]

CONCLUSION

The introduction of the INR has improved the monitoring of oral anticoagulant therapy. With the emergence of managed care organizations, the importance of outcome research is emphasized. Preliminary data utilizing INR monitoring suggest that patient outcome is enhanced. The availability of a standardized system of reporting PT results in patients who are orally anticoagulated also allows better interinstitutional studies.

Although problems with the system remain, the use of lyophilized plasma calibrants offers a significant step in ensuring laboratories of correct assignment of ISI values for thromboplastins. Ultimately, practice guidelines will be written for monitoring oral anticoagulant therapy. These guidelines will incorporate the INR as a critical component of optimal patient management.

REFERENCES

1. Quick AJ, Stanley-Brown M, Bancroft FW. A study of the coagulation defect in hemophilia and in jaundice. *Am J Med Sci.* 1935;190: 501–511.

2. Quick AJ. Standardization of the one-stage prothrombin time. *Thromb Diathes Haemorrh.* 1972;27:179–180.

3. Loeliger EA. ICSH/ICTH recommendations for reporting prothrombin time in oral anticoagulant control. *Thromb Haemost.* 1985;54: 155–156.

4. Poller L. The effect of the use of different tissue extracts on one-stage prothrombin time. *Acta Haematol.* 1964;32:292–298.

5. Koepke JA, Gilmer PR, Triplett DA, O'Sullivan MB. The prediction of prothrombin time system performance using secondary standards. *Am J Clin Pathol.* 1977;68:191–194.

6. World Health Organization Expert Committee on Biological Standardization 1977 28th Report. 1977;14–15, 45–51. World Health Organization Technical Report Series 610.

7. Hermans J, van den Besselaar AMHP, Loeliger EA, van der Velde EA. A collaborative calibration study of reference materials for thromboplastins. *Thromb Haemost.* 1983;50:712–717.

8. Thomson JM, Tomenson JA, Poller L. The calibration of the second primary international reference preparation for thromboplastin (thromboplastin human, plain, coded BCT/253). *Thromb Haemost.* 1984;52:336–342.

9. D'Angelo A, Seveso MP, D'Angelo SV, et al. Comparison of two automated coagulometers and the manual tilt tube method for determination of prothrombin time. *Am J Clin Pathol.* 1989;92:321–328.

10. van Rijn JLML, Schmidt NA, Rutten W. Correction of instrument and reagent based differences in determination of the International Normalised Ratio (INR) for monitoring anticoagulant therapy. *Clin Chem.* 1989;355:840–843.

11. Ray MJ, Smith IR. The dependence of the International Sensitivity Index on the coagulometer used to perform the prothrombin time. *Thromb Haemost.* 1990;63:424–429.

12. Triplett DA, Brandt J. International Normalized Ratios: has their time come? *Arch Pathol Lab Med.* 1993;117:590–592.

13. Tripoldi A, Chantarangkul V, Braga M, et al. Results of a multicentre study assessing the status of a recombinant thromboplastin. *Thromb Haemost.* 1994;72:261–267.

14. Hirsch J, Poller L. The International Normalized Ratio. *Arch Intern Med.* 1994;154:282-288.

15. Becker DM, Humphries JE, Walker FB, DeMong LK, Bopp JS, Acker MN. Standardizing the prothrombin time calibrating coagulation instruments as well as thromboplastin. *Arch Pathol Lab Med.* 1993;117:602–605.

16. Clarke K, Taberner DA, Thomson JM, Morris JA, Poller L. Assessment of value of calibrated lyophilized plasmas to determine International Sensitivity Index for coagulometers. *J Clin Pathol.* 1992;45:58–69.

17. Poller L, Triplett DA, Hirsh J, Carroll J, Clarke K. The value of plasma calibrants in correcting coagulometer effects on International Normalized Ratios. *Am J Clin Pathol.* 1995;103:358–365.

18. Critchfield GC, Bennett ST. The influence of the reference mean prothrombin time on the International Normalized Ratio. *Am J Clin Pathol.* 1994;102:806–811.

19. Hirsh J. Oral anticoagulant drugs. *N Engl J Med.* 1991;324:1865–1875.

20. Schulman S. Quality of oral anticoagulant control and treatment in Sweden. *J Intern Med.* 1994;236:143–152.

21. Azar AJ, Deckers JW, Rosendaal FR, et al. Assessment of therapeutic quality control in a long term anticoagulant trial in post-myocardial infarction patients. *Thromb Haemost.* 1994;72:347–351.

22. Della Valle P, Crippa L, Safa O, et al. Potential failure of the International Normalized Ratio (INR) system in the monitoring of oral anticoagulation in patients with lupus anticoagulants. *Ann Med Interne.* 1996;147(suppl 1):10–14.

23. Owren PA, Aas K. Control of dicumarol therapy and quantitative determination of prothrombin and proconvertin. *Scand J Clin Lab Invest.* 1951;3:201–208.

24. Furie B, Liebman HA, Blanchard RA. Coleman MS, Kruger SF, Furie BC. Comparison of the native prothrombin antigen and prothrombin time for monitoring oral anticoagulant therapy. *Blood.* 1984;64:445–451.

Chapter 26

Instrumentation for Prothrombin Times

Linda Barna Cler

INTRODUCTION

Selection of a coagulation instrument requires several considerations. Each of the approximately 10 national manufacturers and distributors typically offers more than one instrument model to accommodate the needs of various laboratory settings (Table 26–1). In addition to the traditional analyzers that utilize plasma samples, several whole blood, point-of-care, or bedside instruments are now on the market or soon will be released (Table 26–2). Small in size, these instruments are designed for monitoring anticoagulant therapy in areas off site from clinical or hospital laboratories.

The initial step in instrument selection is to define the laboratory's present and future needs. What is the expected number of tests per day and what type of testing will be done? Will the efficacy of oral anticoagulant therapy be measured by other tests in addition to the prothrombin time (PT); for example will there be a need to determine the activity levels of vitamin K–dependent factors? Will medications other than warfarin be monitored? Such questions will guide the laboratory personnel in selecting the appropriate instrument.

In addition to the expected test volume and menu, other important factors related to the instrument/reagent system, personnel, and Clinical Laboratory Improvement Amendments of 1988 (CLIA 88) regulations are apart of the selection process:

- number of tests per day
- test menu
- instrument/reagent system
- sample handling
- cost
- CLIA 88 regulations
- service
- bidirectional interface
- bar code
- computer capabilities
- personnel
- safety
- quality control

A PLAN FOR INSTRUMENT SELECTION

Once the design of the anticoagulation management service has been outlined, the selection of an instrument, based on anticipated testing needs, can proceed. Because the choices are numerous, an ample amount of time is needed for a thorough examination of the various instruments. The following list will assist in organizing a plan of action:

- Call the manufacturer: arrange to have a sales representative visit the facility.
- Ask customer service to send literature for review.
- Ask to have the instrument in house for a week to familiarize the staff with its operation.
- Prepare a table of likes and dislikes for each instrument and compare features.
- Network with others who use the instruments that appear favorable.

Table 26–1 Coagulation Analyzers Utilizing Plasma Samples

Instrument	Manufacturer/Distributor
STA ST4	American Bioproducts Company 5 Century Drive Parsippany, NJ 07054 800-ABC-COAG
CoaScreener CoaSystem CoaData	American Labor Corp 8801 Midway West Road Raleigh, NC 27613 800-424-0443
Behring Fibrintimer A	Behring Diagnostics Inc 3403 Yerba Buena Road San Jose, CA 95135 800-227-9948
Microsample Coag Analyzer 210 and 310	Bio/Data Corp 155 Centennial Plaza PO Box 347 Horsham, PA 19044–0347 800-257-3282
Cascade M-4 Cascade 480	Helena Laboratories 1530 Lindbergh Drive PO Box 752 Beaumont, TX 77704–0752 800-231-5663
Electra 750-1600	Hemoliance Medical Laboratory Automation Inc 1001 US Hwy 202 Raritan, NJ 08869 800-697-0099
ACL 100–3000+ ACL Futura	Instrumentation Laboratory/Coulter 113 Hartwell Ave Lexington, MA 02173–3190 800-523-3713
Coag-A-Mate XM Coag-A-Mate RA4 MDA 180	Organon Teknika Corporation 100 Akzo Ave Durham, NC 27704 919-620-2000
KC1–KC40 AMAX CS AMGA CS	Amelung/Sigma 545 S Ewing Ave St. Louis, MO 63103 800-325-3424
CA 1000 CA 5000	Sysmex/Dade Dade International, Inc 1717 Deerfield Road Deerfield, IL 60015 800-242-DADE

Table 26–2 Point-of-Care/Bedside Testing Instruments

Instrument	Manufacturer/Distributor
CoaguChek Plus CoaguChek	Boehringer Mannheim Corp 9115 Hague Rd Indianapolis, IN 46256 800-858-8072
Thrombolytic Assessment System (TAS)	Cardiovascular Diagnostics, Inc 5301 Departure Dr Raleigh, NC 27616 919-954-9871
Hemochron Jr Hemochron 8000 ProTime	International Technidyne Corp 8 Olsen Ave Edison, NJ 08820 800-631-5945
Automated Coagulation Timer II Hepcon Hemostasis Management System	Medtronic Tec, Inc 18501 East Plaza Dr Parker, CO 80134–9061 800-525-7007
Sonodot II	Sienco, Inc 9188 South Turkey Creek Rd Morrison, CO 80465 800-833-7706

product and the names of contact people and telephone numbers. A list of questions (Exhibit 26–1) will standardize information obtained from numerous telephone calls. The manufacturers might also arrange on-site visits to other laboratories for observation of their instruments in operation.

INSTRUMENT CLASSIFICATION BY COST AND INTENDED USAGE

Coagulation analyzers fall into three groups defined by their intended usage: low volume, moderate volume, and high volume. In general, the instrument cost reflects complexity and capabilities (ie, small, low-volume instruments are less costly than the more complex, top-of-the-line models). Smaller instruments, priced at less than $20,000, often serve as backup instruments in large clinical or referral laboratories and might be used for low-volume specialized tests. In small laboratories where coagulation tests are performed infrequently, they can be used for routine PT and/or activated partial thromboplastin time (aPTT) testing. According to operator training manuals and the marketing departments of the various manufacturers, instruments in the price range of $30,000–$55,000 include those typically found in a laboratory of moderate size that performs 25–100 PTs per day (Table 26–3).[1,2] These instruments are often referred to as "workhorses" because they continually turn out results with little personnel intervention. Top-of-the-line models, in the price range of $75,000–$100,000, offer the most flexibil-

Every manufacturer or distributor has a sales and marketing division and is interested in providing assistance. Obtaining literature from several companies in advance provides an opportunity to compare features and narrow down the field. One of the best means to know how the instrument performs is to network with other laboratories. Each manufacturer should be asked for a list of at least five laboratories using its

Exhibit 26–1
QUESTIONS TO ASK OTHER USERS OF A PRODUCT

1. What instrument model are you using?
2. What reagents are you using?
3. What features do you like about the instrument?
4. Have you had any downtime? Did technical service personnel speak to you directly about a problem, or did they ask to call you back? Did they return the call promptly? Were they helpful and courteous?
5. If a service representative was called, did he or she arrive within 24 hours? Was the problem fixed?

6. Is the company helpful and knowledgeable when you call for any kind of assistance?
7. Do you like the computer's features? Is it easy to follow? What do you like most about the computer?
8. Did the company offer a quality control program with your instrument? Do you find it helpful?
9. What do you not like about the instrument or company?
10. Would you recommend this instrument to anyone else?

---

ity (Table 26–4). These are fully automated, multitest, multisample, random-access instruments. The manufacturers of these instruments have already developed or are in the process of placing immunoassays on line. Thus, the instruments are capable of performing tests by three methodologies, clot based, chromogenic, and immunologic, and are suited for the large clinical or referral laboratory.

INSTRUMENT FEATURES

Test Methodologies

Clot-Based or Fibrin-Based Tests

The addition of calcium and a phospholipid source to test plasma initiates the clotting reaction. Subsequent fibrin formation is measured by various mechanisms (eg, photo-optical, mechanical).

Chromogenic Assays

A chromogenic assay is one in which color development is measured from a reaction mixture that includes an enzyme and a synthetic peptide substrate coupled to a dye or chromophore. When the dye is cleaved from the substrate by the specific enzyme, it resumes its native color. The color intensity is measured at a set wavelength, typically 405 nm.

Immunoassays

Antibodies, usually monoclonal antibodies, are bound to a matrix, such as micro latex particles, and mixed with test plasma. The antigen, a coagulation protein, is bound to the antibody to form an immune complex. The resulting turbidity is then measured at 405 nm and compared with a standard curve.

Table 26–3 Automated Instruments for Moderately Sized Laboratories: Price Range, $30,000–$55,000

Instrument	Manufacturer/ Distributor	Cost	Tests/Hour PT/aPTT	Chromogenic Assays	Quality Control Features	Bar Code	Bidirectional Interface
Fibrintimer A	Behring Diagnostics Inc	$54,500	170/120	No	Yes	Yes	Yes
Cascade 480	Helena Laboratories	$29,000	360/144	No	Yes	Yes	Yes
Electra 900C	Hemoliance	$31,000	360/136	Yes	Yes	Yes	No
Electra 1000C	Hemoliance	$49,000	360/136	Yes	Yes	Yes	Yes
Electra 1400C	Hemoliance	$40,000	200/136	Yes	Yes	Yes	Yes
ACL 3000	Instrumentation Laboratory/Coulter	$35,000	175/115	Yes	Yes	Yes	No
CA 1000	Sysmex/Dade	$43,500	160/160	No	Yes	Yes	Yes

Note: List prices effective as of January 1997.

Table 26–4 High-Volume Instruments Capable of Performing Tests by Three Methodologies: Clot Based, Chromogenic, Immunoassays

Instrument	Manufacturer/Distributor	Cost	No. of Reagents on Board at One Time	No. of Analyses Performed Simultaneously
STA	American Bioproducts Company	$100,000	45	12*
BCT	Behring Diagnostics, Inc	$ 85,000	27	20
MDA 180	Organon Teknika	$ 93,000	30	12*
AMAXCS 190	Amelung/Sigma	$ 79,000	24	Not limited
AMGA CS400†		$129,000‡	24	Not limited
CA 6000†	Sysmex/Dade	$ 75,000-$ 80,000	30	20

*Software limitations.

†Pending 510K clearance; not for sale in the United States.

‡Projected cost pending FDA approval.

Note: List prices effective as of January 1997.

Type of Operation

Instruments operate in discrete, batch, or random-access modes.

Discrete

One test type is run on a limited number of samples, typically from one to four. After run completion, the instrument must be completely set up again for the next sample(s). This type of operation is typically found in small, labor-intensive manual instruments used for low-volume testing. Point-of-care instruments are examples of discrete instruments (ie, they run one patient sample at a time).

Batch

The same test is performed on several samples during one run. This type of operation is frequently seen in the clinical laboratory where routine samples for PT and aPTT are run as one group (batch).

Random Access

Several tests can be intermixed in one run; samples are added without regard to test sequence. This is an ideal mode for test profiles in a laboratory performing a large variety of coagulation assays.

The majority of automated instruments today have random access capabilities similar to chemistry analyzers.

End-Point Detection: Clot-Based or Fibrin-Based Tests

Fibrin formation is the end-point determinant for clot-based assays. Three principles, photo-optical, nephelometry, and mechanical, or some modification thereof, describe coagulation analyzers.

Photo-Optical

The majority of instruments are photo-optical. They measure changes in scattered light intensity during fibrin formation. Light from a light-emitting diode shines through the reagent/plasma mixture. Initially, the scatter is low but becomes more intense as coagulation proceeds. The light scatter stabilizes at the end of clotting. A photosensitive detector converts the scattered light into an electrical signal. A microprocessor, in turn, converts the signal to a clotting time in seconds.

Nephelometry

The ACL instruments (Instrumentation Laboratory/Coulter) are microcentrifugal analyzers that determine end point by nephelometry. Nephelometry measures the turbidity of a solution by measuring the amount of light that is scattered at a 90° angle with respect to the incident source.

Mechanical

The ST4 and STA (American Bioproducts Company) determine end point by measuring an increase in plasma viscosity during clotting. This is accomplished by assessing the oscillation rate of an iron ball as it moves in a pendular swing pattern created by an electromagnetic field. When a clot begins to form, the ball oscillation slows down. An algorithm uses variation in oscillation amplitude to determine the clotting time.

Computer

Operations

Software. The software package accompanying an instrument should be user friendly. This is accomplished through a logical menu-driven package that allows the operator to page through the system with ease. The main menu holds the primary functions most frequently used by the operator, such as test selection, instrument preparation, load list, and quality control files. Before purchasing an instrument, one should review the operator's manual and note if there are diagrams and flowcharts for troubleshooting, quality control, and programming.

A busy laboratory welcomes a "walkaway" instrument (ie, one with minimal operator intervention) for routine testing. The instrument selected, however, should be one that allows the operator many programmable capabilities through a wide range of software tools. Software designed for operator interaction enhances an instrument's flexibility. Desirable manipulations include:

- programming setup: incubation and maximum clot detection times, light intensity, reagent and sample volume, and single or duplicate testing
- creating and editing standard curves
- setting parameters for quality control
- selecting calculations, such as the International Normalized Ratio, PT percentage, and PT ratio

Interface. The capability for bidirectional interface is a necessity if a laboratory plans to download patient information from a hospital mainframe system and automatically send out test results from the analyzer. If an instrument has this capability, "output signals" and "RS 232" will be listed on the specification sheet. Interfacing not only shortens turnaround time but also reduces the chance for clerical errors. The favored approach is host query, which further speeds up data handling.

Programming Profiles

Often, laboratories offer profiles to physicians who frequently request a selected test grouping. It is desirable to have software that allows the operator to design such panels or profiles.

Random-access instruments capable of storing several reagents on board can accommodate this approach to laboratory diagnosis.

Upgrades

Manufacturers periodically make software improvements by replacing current programs with updates. These should be provided to the customer at no additional cost. An excellent company welcomes ideas and suggestions and uses this information to improve instrument performance and customer satisfaction.

Reflexive Testing

A relatively new software function is an automatic repeat of samples that exceed the limits of clot detection, which improves turnaround time for the run because there is no delay in repeat testing. This is a favorite feature of laboratories with a high percentage of patients receiving anticoagulant therapy.

Multitasking

Multitasking allows the operator to perform many computer functions while testing is in progress. This enhances turnaround time by permitting the operator to load additional plasma, add tests, retrieve data, or perform other desired functions without waiting for a run to finish.

SAMPLE HANDLING

Automation

A fully automated instrument delivers test plasma, as well as reagents, to the reaction vessel. Customer service refers to this design as a walkaway instrument. Semiautomated instruments require pipetting plasma into cups or cuvettes before testing begins. With some instruments, such as the ST4 (American Bioproducts Company) and the BBL Fibrometer (Becton Dickinson), an operator must pipette both the plasma and reagent. Some refer to these types as *manual* instruments; however, the true manual method is the tilt tube. Even though the ST4 necessitates pipetting both the reagent and test samples, it has a sophisticated computer and a more complex technology than the BBL Fibrometer. The term *semiautomated* thus defines an instrument that requires operator intervention for pipetting the test sample and might or might not be operator dependent for reagent delivery. End-point detection is determined and recorded by the instrument.

Primary Tube Sampling

The advantage of primary tube sampling (from the blood collection tube) is ease of operation as well as safety. Eliminating the step of pipetting test samples into cuvettes prior to testing reduces exposure to bloodborne pathogens. In most instances, the operator must still uncap the tube before placing it on the instrument. Few closed systems are readily available at this time. Exceptions are the MDA 180 (Organon Teknika) and the AMAX CS and AMGA CS (Sigma). Sysmex's soon-to-be-released CA 6000 is also designed as a closed-tube system. Bio/Data's MCA 310 is unique in that it filters plasma from whole blood; the primary tube, unopened and uncentrifuged, is placed onto the instrument.

Another advantage of primary tube sampling is bar-coded patient identification and test ordering. This feature reduces clerical errors and has a large impact on shortening turn-around time.

Tube Size

Most facilities today use evacuated tubes for blood collection. These come in a variety of sizes. A managed care facility might deem that all testing for one analyte or assay take place in a selected laboratory. In this case, samples coming from outside the laboratory might be in tubes of different size or plasma might arrive frozen and necessitate special adapter tubes for automated instruments. The ability of an instrument to accommodate a variety of tube sizes increases its value through flexibility.

QUALITY CONTROL

Control Files

A desired quality control feature is storage of control data. According to CLIA 88, at least two controls, one normal and one abnormal, must be run during each eight hours of daily operation. To determine the number of control files needed, a facility must decide which assays will be performed on the instrument and reserve two files for each. Control files are most useful for tests performed in high volume and for an expected number of controls per month of at least 20. This number will give statistically meaningful data for monthly calculations of mean standard deviation and coefficient of variation. Control data for assays performed infrequently can be recorded in quality control notebooks, rather than in instrument files, if computer memory is limited.

The number of data points the computer can store per file is also a consideration. Monitoring quality control by month is the accepted approach, and the number of data points will depend on how many times a day controls are run. For laboratories operating with two or three shifts, a "sortable" file helps to monitor data by shift. The computer sorts data by time; for example, controls run between 5:30 AM and 2:00 PM are labeled as A (day shift), those run between 2:00 PM and 10:00 PM as B (evening shift), and those run from 10:00 PM to 5:30 AM as C (night shift). This documents that controls for a selected file were run at least once on every shift, a CLIA 88 requirement.

Viewing and Monitoring Quality Control Data

Most instrument quality control programs plot control data, and the operator can access each file to review data for bias, trends, or values outside the acceptable range. A *bias* is 10 consecutive plots of quality control data on one side of the mean. Bias is an indicator of possible systematic error. A *trend* is 5 consecutive plots of quality control values moving in an upward or downward direction. Trends indicate that the analytical system is unstable and failing. The cause may be reagents, standards, calibrators, controls, or a malfunction within the instrument. The technologist performing morning startup must review the control data and confirm that the system is "in control." If it is not, the technologist initiates troubleshooting.

A sophisticated quality control software package offers several ways to view data. One is simply to list the control values and flag those out of range. This gives the reviewer an overall assessment of how well the system is functioning. Another useful tool consists of a variety of control graphs, such as Levey-Jennings plots and frequency bar graphs that visually summarize whether the month's data are clustering around the mean or are trending in a positive or negative direction. (Figures 26–1 and 26–2). Overall, a good program offers several approaches to assist the operator in evaluating the system's performance.

Quality Control Criteria

For reviewing an instrument's quality control program, the Westgard multirules (Table 26–5) are quite helpful in determining whether the system is in control and if patient results can be reported (Figure 26–3). The best program allows the laboratory a choice in selecting which rules to turn on or *enable*. For quality control management, it is also desirable that the operator be able to type in comments and explanations when a rule fails.

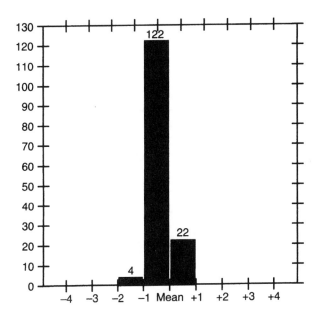

Figure 26–1 Frequency distribution chart

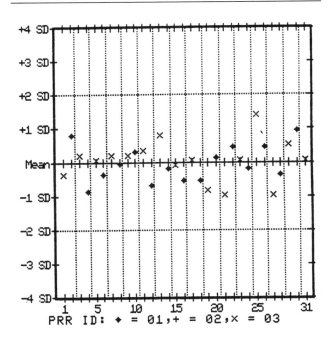

Figure 26–2 Levey-Jennings chart

Table 26–5 Westgard Multirule Quality Control

Rule	Explanation
1 2S	One control value is outside the +/–2 SD range.
1 3S	One control value has exceeded the +/– 3 SD Limit. The patient run should be rejected.
2 2S	One control has exceeded the +/– 2 SD range in two consecutive runs, or two controls in the same run have exceeded the +/– SD range.
4 1S	Control results on four consecutive runs are greater than 1 SD from the mean on the same side of the mean.
10X	The last 10 consecutive runs of one control have fallen on one side of the mean.

Source: Reprinted with permission from J Westgard and T Groth, Design and Evaluation of Statistical Control Procedures: Application of a Computer Quality Control Simulator, *Clinical Chemistry*, Vol 27, No 9, pp 1536–1545, © 1981, American Association of Clinical Chemistry.

SERVICE

One of the most important considerations is service. A full service contract costs approximately 10% of the instrument's list price. Options provided in the contract (eg, full replacement costs for malfunctioning parts, computer updates, 24-hour technical support, biannual preventive maintenance checks) should be reviewed. Networking with other laboratories that have the instrument is an excellent way to know how attentive and responsible a company is to customer needs.

REAGENTS

Each coagulation instrument company either manufactures its own reagents or recommends reagents that work best with its instruments. It is advisable to use the same manufacturer for both the instrument and the reagents. This simplifies operation and offers the best overall performance. Most instruments have open systems (ie, any manufacturers' reagent can be used), but an advantage to using the manufacturer's own reagents is often realized in cost reduction for the entire system.

The national trend for PT reagents is toward the most sensitive preparations, those with a sensitivity index of 1.0. Thromboplastin sources include human placenta, recombinant tissue factor, and rabbit brain preparations.

Liquid reagents offer four advantages over lyophilized products:

1. Lyophilized preparations require reconstitution, usually with water. Historically, water has been a major source of quality control problems in coagulation. According to the National Committee for Clinical Laboratory Standards, coagulation products should be reconstituted with reagent-grade water, type I, as specified in

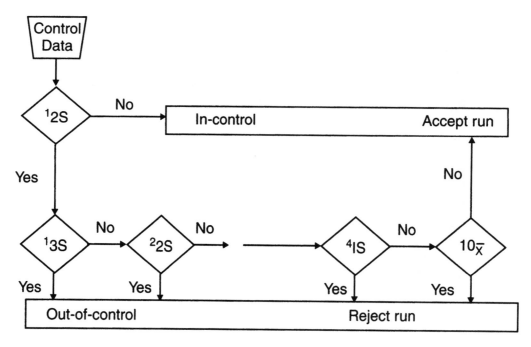

Figure 26–3 Westgaard multiple quality control flowchart. Courtesy of David Risley, Ball Memorial Hospital, Muncie, Indiana.

document C3-A2.[3] This grade of water is nearly impossible to maintain because the grade is lost as soon as the container is opened. Most laboratories purchase high quality water from such sources as Baxter, McGaw Park, IL, product No. B 2F 7113, and Nerl, Providence, RI. Ortho Diagnostics Systems provides a bottled diluent for its PT thromboplastin that standardizes the system and helps to reduce problems.

2. Reconstituting reagents is time-consuming. Once the lyophilized reagent is diluted, it must set for 10–30 minutes before use.

3. There is variation among technologists in reagent preparation, most often in pipetting technique.

4. Pipettes used for reagent reconstitution are a source of expense and frequent problems. Disposable pipettes are costly, and glass pipettes often become contaminated with soap during the cleaning process. The use of glass pipettes is discouraged for this reason.

TOTAL TEST COST

The cost per test varies somewhat among institutions. Manufacturers can give an approximate estimation, but a more accurate figure depends on several considerations. To calculate the cost per test, the cost of every item, from the disposables used by the phlebotomist to reporting results, must be considered. Examples are

- disposables for blood collection
- instrument depreciation
- instrument disposables
- reagents
- labor (technologist's time × salary)

Some instruments are definitely more costly to operate than others. The largest contributing factors are the initial instrument cost and expenses for reagents and disposable supplies.

MEETING CLIA 88 REGULATIONS

CLIA 88 regulations are the minimal requirements for laboratory testing.[4] Thus, compliance with these guidelines forms the bottom-line structure for laboratory operations. CLIA 88 categorizes test complexity by instrument, and test complexity dictates personnel requirements. Therefore, the process of thoroughly investigating instruments and laboratory needs cannot be overemphasized. After September 1, 1997, performing high-complexity testing has required a minimum of an associate's degree or equivalent. The PT is classified as a moderately complex test for the majority of instruments; in contrast, factor assays are highly complex. A minimum of a high school diploma is required for moderate-complexity testing. Another consideration is whether testing personnel work alone. Educational restrictions state that certain levels of testing complexity require oversight by a general supervisor.

CONCLUSION

Several factors must be considered in the choice of an instrument system, in addition to the instrument itself. The best selection is one from a single manufacturer or alliance offering a complete package that includes the instrument, reagents, service, training, and support. Present and future needs should guide the process, and anticipated changes in health care management also must be kept in mind. It is recommended that each laboratory set its own standards because CLIA regulations are minimal. The quality of the laboratory is dependent on its testing personnel and on the accuracy of its instrument and reagent system.

REFERENCES

1. Coagulation product guide, instrument guide. *Clin Hemost Rev.* July 1995:9–16.
2. Coagulation instrumentation. *CAP Today.* February 1996:61–80.
3. National Committee for Clinical Laboratory Standards. *Preparation and Testing of Reagent Water in the Clinical Laboratory.* 2nd ed. Villanova, PA: National Committee for Clinical Laboratory Standards; 1991. Approved guideline. Document C3–A2.
4. Department of Health and Human Services. Clinical Laboratory Improvement Amendments of 1988; Final Rule (42 CFR, Parts 405, et al). *Federal Register.* 1992;57:7001–7288.

Chapter 27

Clinical Laboratories Improvement Act of 1988 Regulations

Linda Barna

HISTORY OF FEDERAL LABORATORY REGULATIONS

Prior to 1977, the Public Health Service (PHS), an agency of the Department of Health and Human Services (DHHS), was the only organization responsible for the administration of federal regulations governing laboratories engaged in interstate testing, in accordance with the Clinical Laboratories Improvement Act of 1967 (CLIA 67). The Health Care Financing Administration (now known as the Centers for Medicare and Medicaid [CMS]) was established in 1977 and assumed inspection and administrative duties for the CLIA and Medicare programs. Currently, PHS and CMS share joint responsibility for the development of federal requirements governing laboratory testing.

In October 1988, CLIA 67 was amended to include all laboratories, not just those engaged in interstate commerce. A laboratory is defined as any testing site that examines materials derived from the human body for the purpose of providing information for the diagnosis, prevention, or treatment of any disease or impairment of, or the assessment of the health of, human beings. The types of testing sites considered as laboratories, either temporary or permanent, are numerous (Exhibit 27–1). The 1988 amendments to CLIA 67 are commonly referred to as CLIA 88. On February 28, 1992, DHHS published regulations in the *Federal Register* to implement CLIA 88.[1] The rules went into effect on September 1, 1992; however, to date, major revisions continue and the final version has yet to be released.

Exhibit 27–1
TESTING SITES RECOGNIZED BY CMS AS LABORATORIES

- Physician office laboratories
- Nursing stations
- Skilled care nursing facilities
- Ambulatory surgical centers
- Hospices and home health agencies
- Emergency departments
- Dialysis facilities
- Bedside testing
- Industrial laboratories performing drug testing
- Shopping malls
- Rural laboratories
- Mobile laboratories
- Insurance company laboratories
- Planned Parenthood clinics
- Military laboratories
- Immediate care facilities
- Government laboratories

Exceptions

- Research laboratories
- Forensic laboratories
- State-exempt laboratories
- National Institute on Drug Abuse urine testing

Source: Federal Register, February 28, 1992, § 493.3.

COMPLIANCE WITH CLIA 88

CLIA 88 addresses seven issues (Table 27–1) requiring laboratory compliance. These requirements are based on test complexity; therefore, applicable regulations differ among laboratories. Those performing moderate- and/or high-complexity tests share the same rules for five of the seven requirements[2]:

1. patient test management
2. quality control
3. quality assurance
4. proficiency testing
5. inspections

The three levels of testing complexity are waived, moderate complexity, and high complexity. The seven determinants for test complexity are listed below:

1. knowledge
2. training and experience
3. reagents and materials preparation
4. characteristics of operational steps
5. calibration, quality control, and proficiency in testing materials
6. test system troubleshooting and instrument maintenance
7. interpretation and judgment

Each determinant is given a score of 1 to 3—1 indicating the lowest level of complexity and 3 the highest. A total score of

---

Table 27–1 CLIA 88 Subparts of Laboratory Requirements

Category	Subpart(s)
1. Certification	B,C,D
2. Proficiency testing for laboratories performing tests of moderate and/or high complexity	H,I
3. Patient test management for laboratories performing tests of moderate and/or high complexity	J
4. Quality control for tests of moderate and/or high complexity	K
5. Personnel for moderate- and high-complexity testing	M
6. Quality assurance for moderate- and/or high-complexity testing	P
7. Inspections	Q

Source: Reprinted from Part 493 of the Federal Register, February 28, 1992.

---

12 or less for all seven determinants indicates that a test is moderately complex; a test scoring above 12 is highly complex. Because all coagulation tests are classified as either moderate complexity or high complexity, discussion of waived tests are not addressed in this chapter.

The seven issues of laboratory compliance are summarized as follows:

1. *Certification or licensure.* A laboratory must do one of two things: obtain a state license in a state with a licensure program *or* obtain one of five licenses issued by a CLIA or CLIA-approved agency:
   - certificate of waiver
   - certificate of registration
   - certificate of accreditation
   - certificate of compliance
   - certificate for provider-performed microscopy (PPM)

   A laboratory in a state with a licensure program must comply with state regulations and is considered "CLIA exempt."

2. *Proficiency testing.* Every laboratory performing tests of moderate and/or high complexity must be enrolled in an approved proficiency-testing program for each specialty, subspecialty, analyte, or test for which it is certified. Tests not included in the proficiency-testing program require a means to establish their accuracy and reliability.

3. *Patient test management.* A system must be in place that ensures optimal integrity and identification of patient specimens throughout the testing process, including accurate reporting of results.

4. *Quality control.* Each laboratory performing moderate- and/or high-complexity testing is required to establish and follow written quality control procedures for monitoring and evaluating the quality of the analytical testing process. The quality control procedures must also ensure the accuracy and reliability of patient test results and reports.

5. *Personnel.* The staff must be qualified to perform tests of each complexity level offered in the laboratory. Qualifications include formal education and training, as well as experience. CLIA 88 also mandates that competency is maintained by individuals performing the tests.

6. *Quality assurance.* Quality assurance encompasses the entire laboratory's operation, including communications, testing, quality control, and personnel. CLIA requires that written policies and procedures be established to maintain a comprehensive quality assurance program.

7. *Inspections.* Every laboratory is required to undergo an on-site CLIA inspection at least once every two years. There are two exceptions: a laboratory that operates in a state with an approved licensure program (CLIA

exempt) *or* a laboratory that qualifies for a "paper survey." This recent ruling allows a laboratory that has performed exceptionally well on a prior inspection for compliance the opportunity to fill out a performance-based assessment form in lieu of an on-site visit. This paper survey is called the Alternate Quality Assessment Survey. No laboratory, however, will go beyond four years without an on-site inspection.

CERTIFICATION

Registration

Before engaging in in vitro testing, a laboratory must first register with CMS (unless it is state exempt). To register, the laboratory contacts its regional CMS office or state agency and requests the CMS-116 application. A certificate of registration is issued to a laboratory that performs moderate-and/or high-complexity tests when registration fees are paid. A laboratory that performs only waived tests does not need to apply for a certificate of registration but will be issued a certificate of waiver instead.

After a laboratory acquires its certificate of registration, it will receive an application that will be used to determine its testing classification by complexity. The laboratory then will be on a schedule for inspection sometime during the following two years. Certificates are valid for two years after each biennial inspection.

Types of Certificates

Certificate of Waiver

A certificate of waiver is issued to a laboratory that performs only waived tests.

Certificate of Registration

A certificate of registration enables a laboratory to conduct moderate- or high-complexity testing, or both, until the laboratory is determined to be in compliance through an on-site survey by CMS or its agent, or it is accredited by an approved accreditation organization.

Certificate of Accreditation

A certificate of accreditation is issued on the basis of a laboratory's accreditation by any of the following accreditation organizations approved by CMS:

- American Association of Blood Banks
- American Osteopathic Association
- American Society of Histocompatibility and Immunogenetics
- College of American Pathologists
- Commission on Office Laboratory Accreditation
- Joint Commission on Accreditation of Healthcare Organizations

Certification by one of these agents indicates that the laboratory meets CLIA requirements.

Certificate of Compliance

A certificate of compliance is issued to a laboratory that performs moderate- and/or high-complexity testing after an inspection by DHHS, rather than by the above-mentioned CMS-approved accreditation agencies.

Certificate for Provider-Performed Microscopy

A certificate for PPM[3] is issued to a laboratory in which a physician, mid-level practitioner, or dentist performs no tests other than PPM procedures and, if desired, waived tests. A mid-level practitioner is defined as a nurse-midwife, nurse-practitioner, or a physician assistant licensed by the state within which the individual practices, if such licensing is required in the state in which the laboratory is located.

PROFICIENCY TESTING

Several organizations qualify as CLIA providers of proficiency testing programs (Table 27–2). To qualify, the programs are required to:

Table 27–2 Organizations Providing Proficiency Testing Programs

Organization	Telephone
American Academy of Family Physicians	800-274-2237
American Proficiency Institute	800-333-0958
American Society for Clinical Chemistry	800-892-1400
American Society of Internal Medicine	800-338-2746
American Thoracic Society	212-315-8808
College of American Pathologists	800-323-4040
New Jersey Department of Health	609-530-6172
New York State Department of Health	518-474-8739

- send samples three times a year to each registered laboratory
- provide five samples for each analyte tested
- ensure that samples provide a full range of values that would be expected in patient specimens
- send an electronic or hard copy of results and all scores within 60 days after the date by which the laboratory must report proficiency testing results to the program
- furnish DHHS with cumulative reports on each individual laboratory
- keep a laboratory's records for a period of five years

CLIA states that proficiency testing samples must be tested along with the patient workload by personnel who routinely perform the assay, and the test method used must be that routinely performed for patients. The minimum overall passing score for coagulation is 80%. The tolerance limits for the prothrombin time (PT) and the activated partial thromboplastin time (aPTT) are +/–15% *or* +/–3 standard deviations (SDs), whichever is greater. For fibrinogen, the tolerance limit is +/–20% *or* +/–3 SDs, whichever is greater.

CLIA defines "unsatisfactory performance" as:

- failure to attain a score of at least 80% of acceptable responses for each analyte
- failure to attain an overall testing event score of at least 80% of all the results for all the analytes tested
- failure to participate in a testing event
- failure to return proficiency testing results to the proficiency testing program within the time frame specified

Failure requires corrective action and documentation of that action. Sanctions are applied only if the laboratory fails an analyte during two consecutive events or during two of three attempted events. In either case, the laboratory's certificate for that specialty, subspecialty, analyte, or test and/or its Medicare approval could be canceled. A laboratory can voluntarily choose to withdraw from certification of an analyte. Certification will be reinstated after a six-month period of satisfactory performance demonstrated during two consecutive proficiency testing events.

PATIENT TEST MANAGEMENT FOR MODERATE- AND HIGH-COMPLEXITY TESTING OR BOTH

This standard states that a laboratory must employ and maintain a system for proper patient preparation, specimen collection, and identification. Policies must be in place as to how the sample is preserved once drawn and how it is transported to the laboratory and processed. The system must ensure a means to maintain specimen integrity and positive identification throughout the preanalytic, analytic, and

postanalytic processes, as well as an accurate reporting protocol. The standards in this subpart are as follows:

- procedures for specimen submission and handling
- test requisition
- test records
- test report
- referral of specimens

QUALITY CONTROL FOR TESTS OF MODERATE AND HIGH COMPLEXITY

Quality control is one aspect of a quality assurance program. Each laboratory must have a written quality control plan that describes procedures designed to provide and ensure accurate, reliable, and valid test results that meet CLIA standards. Quality control monitors the preanalytic, analytic, and postanalytic steps in patient testing, as well as all conditions that affect these steps. Subpart K of Part 493, "Laboratory Requirements," published in the *Federal Register*, addresses the quality control standards. These standards, effective after September 1, 1994, are as follows:

- facilities
- test methods, equipment, instrumentation, reagents, materials, and supplies
- procedure manual
- establishment and verification of method performance specifications
- equipment maintenance and function checks
- calibration and calibration verification
- control procedures
- remedial actions
- quality control records
- quality control specialty: hematology/coagulation

Facilities

The laboratory must be constructed, arranged, and maintained to ensure space, ventilation, and essential utilities for performing and reporting tests. A stable electrical source is necessary to guard against power outages that adversely affect patient results. Safety precautions must be established, posted, and adhered to for protection against physical hazards and biohazardous materials.

Test Methods, Equipment, Instrumentation, Reagents, Materials, and Supplies

All components of this standard must provide accurate and reliable test results and reports. The laboratory is required to have appropriate instruments, equipment, reagents, materials, and supplies for the type and volume of testing performed. Quality is maintained throughout all phases of testing; preanalytic, analytic, and postanalytic. The instruments must be capable of providing test results within the test's stated performance characteristics, which include accuracy, precision, sensitivity, specificity, reportable range, and reference range (normal value). Effective September 1, 1992, a laboratory introducing a new procedure that has been cleared by the Food and Drug Administration (FDA) as meeting the CLIA requirements must demonstrate, prior to reporting patient results, that it can obtain the performance specifications for accuracy, precision, and reportable range. The laboratory must also verify the manufacturer's reference range (normal range) for the local population.

Temperature and humidity must be maintained and monitored to ensure reagent stability. Another concern, especially for coagulation, is water quality. Storage conditions to protect against pH changes or contamination sources are imperative.

Reagents must be labeled to indicate

- identity
- recommended storage requirements
- preparation date and expiration date
- safety warnings

The laboratory cannot use materials that are past their expiration date, are of substandard reactivity, or show signs of deterioration. Reagents cannot be interchanged between test kits of different lot numbers without the manufacturer's approval.

Standard Operating Procedure Manual

Every laboratory must have a written procedure manual for the performance of all tests. It must be readily available and followed by all testing personnel. The procedure manual must include the following components:

- requirements for specimen collection and processing, and criteria for specimen rejection
- step-by-step performance of the procedure, including test calculations and interpretation of results
- reagent preparation
- calibration and calibration verification procedures
- reportable range
- control procedures
- remedial action to be taken
- limitations (interfering substances)
- reference range (normal values)
- imminent life-threatening results (panic values)
- pertinent literature references
- specimen storage criteria

- reporting results
- action to take if the system becomes inoperable
- criteria for referral specimens

Procedures must be initially signed and dated by the laboratory director. If a procedure is discontinued, it must be maintained in the laboratory for two years. A manufacturer's package insert can be used temporarily until a procedure is written.

Verification of Method Performance Specifications

Effective September 1, 1992, a laboratory must verify *or* establish all of the following test performance specifications (except sensitivity and specificity for unmodified FDA-approved kits) before patient results are reported:

- accuracy
- precision (reproducibility)
- sensitivity
- specificity
- reportable range
- reference range (normal range)

CLIA does not require this process for tests established prior to this date. These specifications are determined only once, at the time of initial test setup. Thereafter, controls, calibration checks, and proficiency testing are performed as required. The laboratory must document the verification or establishment of all applicable test performance specifications.

If the new procedure for patient testing is a kit or test system approved by the FDA and the laboratory follows the manufacturer's procedure without modification, CLIA requires the laboratory to verify the accuracy, precision, and reportable range stated by the manufacturer. The laboratory must also establish its own normal reference interval.

If the new procedure is an in-house method, a modification of the manufacturer's procedure, or a method not yet approved by the FDA, the laboratory must establish values for all of the test performance specifications listed above, as applicable.

Accuracy

Results of the new method must be correlated to a method previously validated in the laboratory. For example, if a clot-based test is being replaced by a chromogenic assay, at least 20 specimens are compared by the old and new methods and the results statistically evaluated. This is usually accomplished by regression analysis and the paired Student's t-test. Acceptable criteria must be defined and the new method accepted or rejected on the basis of statistical outcome.

Precision (Reproducibility)

Two controls, normal and abnormal, are run at least 20 times and the mean, SD, and coefficient of variation (CV) calculated. To perform this function, the controls are run for several days, with no more than three runs per day. The CV should be 5% or less.

Sensitivity

Sensitivity is the smallest detectable result obtainable within the linearity of the procedure. To determine this, a reference sample having a known assayed value is diluted until the results are no longer detected by the method and instrument/reagent system.

Specificity

Specificity is the ability of a test to identify those who do not have a disease or abnormality. Some substances or situations, including hemolysis, lipemia, bilirubin, and turbidity, can interfere with this process and invalidate test results by interfering with the end-point detection.

Manufacturers supply specificity and sensitivity data for FDA-approved tests. This information can be obtained from the package insert or by calling the company directly. For in-house methods or those altered from a manufacturer's procedure, specificity is determined by challenging the system with several types of abnormal samples and determining the specificity using truth tables (ie, true negatives divided by the sum of true negatives and false positives).

Reportable Range

The method for determining a reportable range depends on whether the test is a quantitative or qualitative assay. For quantitative assays, a range is established by creating a standard curve and validating linearity. Calibrators or assayed reference materials are used. The reportable range lies between the lowest point and the highest point on the curve.

Linearity is determined by following a four-step procedure:

1. Make several dilutions with mixtures of the highest and lowest calibrators for the assay (eg, 100, 50, 25, 12.5). Run each dilution four times and take the average.
2. Plot the results: observed concentration on the y-axis and expected value on the x-axis.
3. Draw the best straight line through as many data points as possible.
4. Visually accept the linearity if it meets the need; alternatively, analyze the data by computer using a statistical package with regression analysis. Determine acceptable criteria. An r value >0.8 is usually considered acceptable, although values >0.9 are desirable.

Calibrators and/or assayed reference materials are used to create a standard curve from which patient values are interpolated. Once established, the curve is revalidated every six months with another assayed reference preparation.

For nonquantitative tests, the reportable range can be determined by one of several means, depending on the assay in question. Linearity cannot be determined for the PT and aPTT tests because they are not quantitative assays but screening tests that measure several reactions required for fibrin formation. For these coagulation tests, the reportable range is a function of the instrument's limitations, that is, the lower range is determined by the lag time, or guard time, and the upper range is the longest time that the instrument can remain stationary in one position without affecting subsequent samples. Lag time is the short waiting period before the initiation of clot detection. It allows time for turbulence created by reagent delivery to clear. For the PT, the lag time is approximately 7 seconds. Therefore, the lower reportable (detectable) range for the PT is 8 seconds. The upper limit is usually around 100 or 150 seconds, which is the maximum incubation time a cuvette remains in the heating station. Values in these ranges exceed the therapeutic range and are usually due to heparin contamination, overanticoagulation, improper preanalytic steps, instrument out of control, or some other underlying problem. The instrument will indicate that a result is out of range. Appropriate follow-up steps must be documented. In coagulation, there are reference intervals (normal ranges), therapeutic ranges, and reportable ranges. Reportable ranges are those within the instrument's testing limitations.

Reference Range (Normal Range)

To establish a normal reference interval for the local or testing population, the assay is performed on a minimum of 20 normal individuals. These should be healthy adults, 10 females and 10 males, who have no known disorders and are medication free. The mean and one SD are determined and a range established that is +/−2 SDs from the mean.

Equipment Maintenance and Function Checks

The laboratory must establish policies and procedures for the maintenance of equipment, instruments, and test systems and organize a preventive maintenance schedule by creating written tables and charts to assist in documenting the timely performance of these functions. It is recommended that laboratories follow manufacturers' guidelines for scheduling preventive maintenance.

Calibration and Calibration Verification

Calibration verification is required to substantiate the continued accuracy of the test method throughout the reportable range of patient test results. If a calibration curve is linear and at least two levels of an assayed reference material are within range, calibration is acceptable. Calibration verification for each procedure must be performed at least once every six months. Other situations requiring calibration verification include a change in reagent lot number, major maintenance on the instrument, and controls that begin to drift from the mean.

Control Procedures

Control procedures are performed on a routine basis to monitor the stability of the test system. For qualitative tests, the laboratory must include a positive and negative control with each patient run; for quantitative tests, at least two controls of different concentrations are included in the patient run. See the section Quality Control by Specialty: Hematology/Coagulation, below, for tests that are performed several times per day. The controls should challenge both normal and abnormal ranges expected in the patient population. If calibration or control samples are not available, the laboratory must have an alternative method to ensure the quality, accuracy, and precision of test results. All control samples must be tested in the same manner as patient specimens. Prior to reporting patient results, the controls must meet laboratory criteria for acceptability.

Repetitive testing of control data must be monitored over time. Periodic statistical analyses are performed, typically on a monthly basis, that include the mean, SD, and CV. For a new lot number of unassayed control material, such parameters as control ranges are determined concurrently with the present control material. This overlap of old and new lot numbers allows the establishment of an effective control range for the new lot number. For assayed controls, the package insert provides a target value that must be verified by the laboratory.

Remedial Actions

Remedial action policies must be established and applied as necessary to ensure accurate and reliable patient test results and reports. Remedial actions are documented when test systems do not meet the established performance specifications. The following situations apply:

- Equipment or tests do not perform within the established operating parameters.
- Patient test values are outside reportable ranges.

- Control results are outside the established range.
- Turnaround times cannot be met because of either testing difficulties or reporting problems (computer downtime).
- An error was made in reporting results.

When a reporting error is made, the following procedure must be followed:

- promptly notifying the authorized person who ordered or utilized the test results
- issuing corrected reports to the authorized person ordering the test
- maintaining copies of the original report, as well as the corrected report, for two years

Quality Control Records

The laboratory must document all quality control, as discussed in this section, and maintain all records for at least two years.

Quality Control by Specialty: Hematology/Coagulation

Automated Coagulation Testing Systems

The laboratory must include two levels of controls during each eight hours of operation and each time a change in reagents occurs.

Manual Coagulation Tests

Each individual performing tests must assay two levels of controls before testing patient samples and each time a change in reagents occurs. Patient and control samples must be tested in duplicate.

PERSONNEL

Personnel modifications to CLIA 88 were published as a final rule on April 24, 1995. Because of the differences in qualifications between test complexity levels, the following discussion addresses each separately. The regulations do not differentiate between medical technologists and medical technicians but address everyone as "testing personnel."

Moderate-Complexity Testing

The staffing of a laboratory that performs tests of moderate complexity and perhaps waived tests, but not high-complexity tests, include a laboratory director, a technical consultant, a clinical consultant, and testing personnel.

The minimum requirements for testing personnel are high school graduation or equivalent *and* completion of an official military laboratory procedures course of at least 50 weeks *or* documentation of training appropriate for testing performed prior to analyzing specimens. Training requirements must ensure several skills defined in Section 493.1423 of the *Federal Register*, February 28, 1992. Individuals with higher educational qualifications can perform laboratory tests of moderate complexity. All testing personnel must possess a current license issued by the state in which the laboratory is located if such licensing is required.

High-Complexity Testing

The staff of a laboratory that performs one or more tests of high complexity but that might or might not perform waived tests and tests of moderate complexity include a laboratory director, a technical supervisor, a clinical consultant, a general supervisor, and testing personnel. Minimal qualifications for testing personnel of high-complexity testing until September 1, 1997, are high school graduation or equivalent on or before April 24, 1995 and graduation from a medical laboratory or clinical laboratory training program approved by DHHS *or* completion of an official US military medical laboratory procedures training course of 50 weeks. High school graduates who have appropriate training can continue to perform high-complexity tests with supervisory oversight after September 1, 1997, if they were performing such tests on or before April 24, 1995.

Since September 1, 1997, the minimum requirement for testing personnel is an associate degree or equivalent. As with other levels of test complexity, individuals with higher educational levels may perform all laboratory tests. Equivalency requirements for an associate degree are:

- 60 semester hours that include either 24 semester hours of medical laboratory technology courses or 24 hours of science courses
- included in the science courses, 6 semester hours of chemistry; 6 semester hours of biology; 12 semester hours of courses in chemistry, biology, medical laboratory technology, or any combination of the three
- completion of either an accredited clinical laboratory or medical laboratory training program or three months of documented training in each specialty in which the individual performs high-complexity testing

Competency Requirements

The laboratory must have an ongoing mechanism to evaluate the effectiveness of its policies and procedures for ensuring employee competency. Prior to testing patient samples, an individual must have appropriate training, with documentation that he or she is competent to perform preanalytic, analytic, and postanalytic phases of testing. Written documentation is required to show assessment of continued competency twice yearly for each new employee and annually thereafter. The procedures for evaluating competency must include the following:

- direct observation of performance
- monitoring of the recording and reporting of test results
- review of quality control records, proficiency testing results, and preventive maintenance records
- direct observation during operation of an instrument
- assessment of test performance through testing of previously analyzed samples
- assessment of problem-solving skills

QUALITY ASSURANCE FOR MODERATE- OR HIGH-COMPLEXITY TESTING OR BOTH

Quality assurance encompasses all of the above rules and regulations and includes the continued assessment of their effectiveness. As indicated, the laboratory will revise policies and procedures based on the results of ongoing evaluations. All quality assurance activities must be documented. The standards for quality assurance are:

- *Patient Test Management Assessment.* The laboratory must monitor and evaluate the systems described in "Patient Test Management," subpart J of CLIA 88.
- *Quality Control Assessment.* The laboratory must review remedial actions and correct ineffective policies and procedures.
- *Proficiency Testing Assessment.* Corrective action must be taken if any unacceptable and unsatisfactory results in proficiency testing are found.
- *Comparison of Test Methods.* If a laboratory performs the same test (eg, PT) on another instrument other than the main instrument, it must conduct comparison studies twice a year. The relationship between the two instruments or methodologies is statistically evaluated to determine if the two correlate. This application is most often utilized to ensure that a backup method or instrument is within defined specifications.
- *Relationship of Patient Information to Patient Test Results.* The laboratory must have a mechanism to

determine if patient test results are consistent with those expected for age, sex, diagnosis, medications, and relationship to other test parameters.

- *Personnel Assessment.* The laboratory must have a means to evaluate employee competency.
- *Communications.* Documentation must be in place that describes what to do in the event of communication breakdowns, such as those occurring during computer downtime. Corrective actions must be documented to minimize breakdowns.
- *Complaint Investigations.* The laboratory must have a means to receive complaints. Documentation of these complaints and how they are assessed and investigated must be established. In addition, documentation of any corrective action is required.
- *Quality Assurance Review with Staff.* Problems must be addressed with the staff and corrective action taken to prevent recurrences.
- *Quality Assurance Records.* All quality assurance actions must be documented and available to DHHS.

INSPECTIONS

DHHS or its designee will conduct announced and unannounced random validation inspections during hours of laboratory operation. The DHHS inspectors might ask laboratory personnel to perform procedures so that they can observe the testing process. The staff also might be interviewed about all of the standards discussed in this chapter. In addition, test reports and quality assurance documentation might be reviewed. Generally, an inspection is conducted to observe for compliance or to investigate a complaint against a laboratory.

CMS can impose sanctions against laboratories that fail to comply with CLIA 88 requirements. Sanctions include a directed plan of corrective action; civil monetary penalties of up to $10,000 per violation or per day of noncompliance; payment for the costs of on-site monitoring; suspension from the Medicare or Medicaid program; and suspension, limitation, or revocation of the CLIA certificate.

CONCLUSION

CLIA 88 regulations represent the minimal standards for laboratory operations. Although the amendments are relatively brief, the document for implementing them is lengthy and often without clear guidelines. In addition, several revisions have already taken place since 1992 and more are expected. Following all of the changes requires the diligence of one person to retrieve, analyze, and implement the new information. In the author's opinion, it is much easier to register with a CLIA-approved accrediting agency. This removes the burden of daily review of the *Federal Register* from the laboratory and places it with the accrediting agency, which will update information and forward it to the laboratory prior to the inspection. The accrediting agency issues the certificate of accreditation when the laboratory passes the inspection.

Copies of the *Federal Register* are often available in community and hospital libraries. They are also available through the American Society of Clinical Pathologists by one of the following means:

- Via telephone: 202-783-3238
- Via mail: New Orders
             Superintendent of Documents
             PO Box 371954
             Pittsburgh, PA 15250-7954
- Via the Internet: www.archives.gov

REFERENCES

1. Department of Health and Human Services. Clinical Laboratory Improvement Amendments of 1988; Final Rule Part II. (42 CFR, parts 405, 410, 416, 417, 418, 440, 482, 484, 485, 488, 491, 493, 494). *Federal Register.* February 28, 1992:7002–7186.

2. Department of Health and Human Services. Clinical Laboratory Improvement Amendments of 1988; Final Rule Part III. (42 CFR, Part 493). *Federal Register.* February 28, 1992:7187–7288.

3. Department of Health and Human Services. CLIA Program; Categorization of Tests and Personnel Modifications; Final Rule with Comment Period (42 CFR, Part 493). *Federal Register.* April 24, 1995.

Chapter 28

Capillary Whole Blood Prothrombin Time Monitoring: Instrumentation and Methodologies

Jack E. Ansell and Katharine E. Leaning

INTRODUCTION

Prothrombin time (PT) monitoring technologies that allow for capillary whole blood testing or point-of-care testing are a welcome development in the monitoring of patients requiring long-term oral anticoagulation. This chapter reviews the development of capillary whole blood PT monitoring with a focus on the instrumentation and methodologies of each instrument. These new monitors, along with innovative strategies for patient education and training, promise to improve the efficacy and safety of oral anticoagulation, as well as simplify the monitoring process for patients and health care providers. Ultimately, they may provide incentives for more widespread use of oral anticoagulants and better health outcomes for patients requiring long-term oral anticoagulation.

POINT-OF-CARE TESTING

The term *point-of-care testing*, also known as near-patient testing, on-site monitoring, and decentralized testing, describes an analytic process that does not take place in a centralized clinical laboratory but rather where the patient receives care (eg, at the bedside, in a clinic, or in a physician's office). Capillary whole blood PT monitors are used at the site of care delivery to quantify the degree of disruption of the extrinsic coagulation pathway. Currently, several types of capillary whole blood monitors are available (see Table 28–1). Although differences exist in the methodologies of the indi-

vidual monitors, the principal outcome is the same. Each monitor measures the time to clotting, induced by thromboplastin, which is then converted to a plasma PT equivalent by a microprocessor and expressed as PT or International Normalized Ratio (INR). The following discussion outlines the instrumentation and methodologies of these capillary whole blood monitors and summarizes the current literature on their accuracy and precision.

INSTRUMENTATION AND METHODOLOGY

The original capillary whole blood PT monitor was developed by Biotrack and marketed under different names and licensing rights. These instruments are similar to later models having added capabilities.

The first group of monitors includes Protime Monitor 1000 (Biotrack, Inc), Coumatrak (DuPont Pharma), Ciba Corning 512 Coagulation Monitor (Ciba Corning Diagnostics), CoaguChek Plus and CoaguChek Pro (Roche Diagnostics). Each monitor functions according to the same methodology. A cuvette containing dry rabbit brain thromboplastin (ISI [International Sensitivity Index] approximately 2.0) is inserted into the machine at the prompt. A microsample of fresh whole blood (approximately 25 μL, or a large drop) is applied to the target on the cuvette and then drawn by capillary action into the reagent chamber within the cuve[tte]. Mixing of the blood and thromboplastin initiates coa[gula]tion. A coherent laser light focuses through the samp[le]

Table 28–1 Capillary Whole Blood (Point-of-Care) PT Instruments

Instrument	Clot Detection Methodology	Type of Sample	Home Use Approval
Protime Monitor 1000 Coumatrak[1] Ciba Corning 512 Coagulation Monitor[1] CoaguChek Plus[1] CoaguChek Pro[1] CoaguChek Pro/DM[1]	Clot initiation: Thromboplastin Clot detection: Cessation of blood flow through capillary channel	Capillary WB Venous WB	No
CoaguChek CoaguChek Thrombolytic Assessment System Rapidpoint Coag	Clot initiation: Thromboplastin Clot detection: Cessation of movement of iron particles	Capillary WB Venous WB Plasma	Yes[2] (CoaguChek only)
ProTIME Monitor Hemochron Jr[3] GEM PCL[3]	Clot initiation: Thromboplastin Clot detection: Cessation of blood flow through capillary channel	Capillary WB Venous WB	Yes
Avosure Pro+[4] Avosure Pro[4] Avosure PT[4]	Clot initiation: Thromboplastin Clot detection: Thrombin generations detected by fluorescent thrombin probe	Capillary WB Venous WB Plasma	Yes
Harmony	Clot initiation: Thromboplastin Clot detection: Cessation of blood flow through capillary channel	Capillary WB Venous WB	Yes
INRatio[5]	Clot initiation: Thromboplastin Clot detection: Change in impedance in sample	Capillary WB Venous WB	Pending

[1]All instruments in this category are based on the original Biotrack model (Protime Monitor 1000) and licensed under different names. The latest versions available are the CoaguChek Pro and Pro/DM (as models evolved they acquired added capabilities); earlier models no longer available.

[2]CoaguChek not actively marketed for home use at the time of this writing. Thrombolytic Assessment System not available for home use.

[3]Hemochron Jr and GEM PCL are simplified versions of the ProTIME Monitor.

[4]Avosure instruments removed from market when manufacturer (Avocet, Inc.) ceased operations (2001). Technology has since been purchased by Beckman Coulter, Inc.

[5]INRange system manufactured by Hemosense, Inc. has recently been FDA approved for professional use.

Source: Adapted with permission from the *Journal of Thrombosis Thrombolysis*, Vol. 3, pp. 377–384, © 1996, Kluwer Academic Publishers.

chamber of the test cartridge and determines clot formation by the cessation of blood flow. The specimen creates an interference pattern, which is measured by a photodetector. This photodetector then converts the optical signal into an electrical signal, which the microprocessor converts into a quantitative result to be shown on the liquid crystal display as PT, PT ratio, or INR.

This methodology was initially validated in 1987 by Lucas ~1 1 Using 858 samples from 732 subjects (controls, war- ated patients, and heparin-treated patients), the inves- und correlation coefficients of 0.96 between refer- a PTs and capillary whole blood PTs. Results for capillary and venous whole blood measured ent. Within-day precision using two different 's revealed coefficients of variation of 4.9% d 2.9% (level II control). Replicate capil- 's from two different fingersticks and two revealed a correlation coefficient of

0.99. Finally, hematocrits from 23% to 54% did not compromise the accuracy of the instrument. Overall, the investigators found the monitor comparable to the standard laboratory methods.

Numerous subsequent studies confirmed the accuracy of the instrument compared with reference laboratory methods and found correlation coefficients of 0.95[2] and 0.91.[3] The latter investigators, who found a correlation coefficient of 0.91, reasoned that use of the INR (rather than the PT ratio) might have resulted in a higher correlation coefficient. At the time of the study, both participating hospital laboratories reported values as the PT ratio. As a result, corrections were not made for interlot differences in the ISI between the thromboplastin preparations as they would have been if the hospitals had reported results as the INR.

Other investigators have published more qualified support of this instrument's accuracy. A study of the Ciba Corning 512 Coagulation Monitor by Jennings et al[4] examined 104 patients on warfarin and 20 healthy subjects with the capillary PT and compared it with two standard laboratory methods. They found the best INR correlation with the Manchester Reagent, which had a lower thromboplastin ISI, and the worst with the capillary thrombotest INR. The investigators suggest that the relatively high ISI of the capillary instrument's thromboplastin (approximately 2.0) and an inability to determine a local geometric mean normal PT resulted in poor comparability with some thromboplastins, especially the thrombotest.

McCurdy and White,[5] rather than using the correlation coefficient (which measures adherence to a regression line that does not necessarily conform to X = Y), characterize the performance of the portable monitor by focusing on the differences between the monitor and reference laboratory measurements (ISIs approximately 2.4–2.6) in standardized units. In 143 paired specimens, they note that the capillary method yielded the most accurate results in an INR range of 2.0 to 3.0. As the INR increased, the discrepancy between methods increased: the capillary PT was up to 0.5 units lower for INRs of 3.0 to 4.5. The best correlation was found when the INR was approximately 3.0. They also assessed precision of two repeated measurements in 54 patients and found a within-patient standard deviation of 0.23 INR units for the capillary whole blood PT and 0.19 INR units for paired clinical laboratory measurements. Their conclusions are consistent with those of Tripodi et al,[6] who, using the Ciba Corning 512 Coagulation Monitor, recalibrated the ISI of the instrument's thromboplastin against the secondary international reference preparation for rabbit thromboplastin to assess the precision of the INR specifically. The ISI calculated in the study was systematically higher (ISI 2.715) than that reported by the manufacturer (ISI 2.036). They found that the between-assay reproducibility of the monitors was acceptable when results were expressed as PT (coefficient of variation [CV] = 9.7%) but became unacceptable when results were expressed as INR (CV = 18.8%). Like McCurdy and White,[5] they found that the monitor underestimated the result as the INR increased (INR > 4.0). This error did not occur if they calculated the INR by using their recalibrated ISI. The investigators concluded that the monitor might be suitable for oral anticoagulation monitoring if the manufacturers used a more sensitive thromboplastin in the cartridges.

A second type of PT monitor is the CoaguChek. The test cartridge contains dry reagent thromboplastin (ISI approximately 1.0) and paramagnetic iron oxide particles. A microsample of fresh whole blood (approximately 25 µl) is applied to the test strip and drawn into the reagent chamber by capillary action, where it reconstitutes the test reagents. An oscillating magnetic field in the analyzer initiates a particle waving motion that is read optically. Particle movement slows until coagulation stops the particles completely. The time from application of the blood sample to cessation of particle movement represents the time to clotting, which is measured by a microprocessor and displayed on the screen as the PT or INR.

Oberhardt et al[7] initially described this technology and its ability to measure prothrombin times from capillary whole blood, citrated and nonanticoagulated venous whole blood, and citrated plasma. They reported a correlation coefficient of 0.96 in 271 samples of citrated plasma tested on the instrument versus standard laboratory methodology. They also found no effect of hematocrit (from 0% [ie, plasma] to 57%) or of platelet concentration on their results. Rose et al[8] further tested this instrumentation in a clinical setting. Within-day precision for normal and abnormal control plasmas in 20 tests each yielded CVs of 3.7% and 3.6%, respectively. A correlation coefficient of 0.86 was obtained when capillary whole blood PTs were obtained from 50 outpatients and were compared to reference plasma PTs. Somewhat poorer correlations were obtained on inpatients in the coronary and surgical intensive care units, but after outliers were removed, results were similar (r = 0.87 in 37 paired samples and r = 0.86 in 117 paired samples, respectively). Given that this study involved different users, multiple locations (inpatients and outpatients), two lots of thromboplastin, and a number of different instruments over an extended period of time, the investigators found the correlation coefficients acceptable and judged the monitor to be clinically useful.

Fabbrini et al[9] compared this technology with standard laboratory methods by using an MLA 1000 instrument with two different thromboplastins (ISI = 2.46 and 1.01) for two groups of anticoagulated patients (N = 100 and 96, respectively). With the use of citrated blood, reasonable precision was demonstrated (CV = 6% and 4%) with excellent correlation coefficients of 0.92 and 0.91 compared with reference plasma PTs. They concluded that this system was satisfactory for PT monitoring in a point-of-care setting. Kapiotis et al[10] compared results of capillary blood testing on the Coaguchek with results obtained by using the thrombotest reagent on the KC-1 coagulometer. They found a correlation coefficient of r = 0.914 (p < 0.0001) when the INR values were compared for 76 patients on phenprocoumon therapy. Precision was tested using three separate blood drops from the same puncture site on three separate CoaguChek instruments (using test strips from one lot), and correlation coefficients between r = 0.984 and r = 0.990 were found. The investigators also found excellent comparability of different test strip lots and different instruments. Tripodi et al[11] evaluated the calibration of the ISI in this system based on an international reference preparation (IRP) and found that it was extremely close to that adopted by the manufacturer for both whole blood and plasma. Although the CVs of the slopes of the regression lines comparing the system with an international reference were excellent (CV of 2.2 for both whole blood and plasma on the instrument compared with the IRP), the instrument reported significantly higher INRs (3.20 and 3.41 in whole blood and plasma vs 2.92 for plasma in the reference system) using the manufacturer's calibration. The differences were due to a lower mean normal PT adopted by the manufacturer.

Most recently, van den Besselaar[12] evaluated the CoaguChek with two international reference preparations for thromboplastin in 56 coumarin-treated patients. Although capillary whole blood results differed significantly from citrated plasma samples, the mean relative deviation of the INR was not greater than 0.104, and it was felt that the instrument provided a clinically acceptable level of accuracy. van den Besselaar et al[13] also found statistically significant differences in INR results from capillary compared to venous whole blood on the CoaguChek instrument, but once again, the magnitude of the differences was small and was felt to be clinically acceptable.

This instrumentation is marketed as the CoaguCheck instrument. Results of Roche Diagnostics in-house studies on accuracy and precision show correlation coefficients between the instrument and different laboratory thromboplastins, including an IRP (CRM 149R) between 0.88 and 0.92 for more than 1,000 samples tested. Neither hematocrit (approximately 35%–55%) nor fibrinogen (approximately 200 mg/dL–600 mg/dL) significantly affected results.

A recent and important study by Kaatz et al[14] evaluated these two classes of monitors, CoaguChek and Coumatrak, as well as clinical laboratory determinations against the criterion standard established by the World Health Organization (WHO). The criterion standard INR was determined using an international reference thromboplastin and the manual tilt-tube technique. Determinations of INR from four laboratories (using four different thromboplastins and three different instruments) were compared to INR determinations of both monitors. Investigators avoided the correlation coefficient and regression analysis and, instead, evaluated agreement defined as "the proportion of samples that agreed with the criterion standard as being above, within, or below the American College of Chest Physicians' recommended therapeutic ranges." Table 28–2 summarizes important findings from this study. Kaatz et al[14] found that laboratories 1 and 2, which used a more sensitive thromboplastin (ISI = 1.99 and 2.0, respectively) showed close agreement with the criterion standard, whereas laboratories 3 and 4, which used an insensitive thromboplastin (ISI = 2.84 and 2.98, respectively) showed poor agreement. The two monitors fell between these two extremes. As in the study by McCurdy and White,[5] the Coumatrak underestimated the INR at values above 2.5, whereas the CoaguChek simply showed more scatter at INR values above 2.75. Investigators concluded that the accuracy of the portable monitors and laboratories 1 and 2 were clinically acceptable. Interestingly, the determinations of laboratories 3 and 4 were deemed unacceptable. Consistent with the growing evidence that lower ISI reagents yield more accurate results and because the two laboratories that reported inaccurate INR determinations both used an insensitive thrombo-plastin (high ISI), the investigators recommend universal use of more sensitive thromboplastins. INR determinations of the Coumatrak monitor and the CoaguChek were only slightly less accurate than those of the best clinical laboratories.

Table 28–2 Agreement between Criterion Standard INR and Laboratory or Monitor INR Determination

	Laboratory				Monitor	
	1	2	3	4	1	2
International Sensitivity Index	1.99	2.00	2.84	2.98	2.04	2.64
Prothrombin time control (seconds)	11.5	12.5	11.5	11.2	12.0	12.6
ACCP recommended target range:						
Agreement (%)	89	85	69	73	77	78
(95% CI)	(82–93)	(78–90)	(61–76)	(65–80)	(69–83)	(70–84)
Mean absolute relative error (%)	7.8	9.4	22.0[*†§]	25.6[*†§]	12.9[*†]	14.3[*†]
(97.7% CI)	(7–9)	(8–11)	(19–26)	(22–29)	(11–15)	(13–16)

[*] P<0.003 versus laboratory 1

[†] P<0.003 versus laboratory 2

[‡] P<0.003 versus monitor 1

[§] P<0.003 versus monitor 2

Key: ACCP, American College of Chest Physicians; CI, confidence interval; INR, International Normalized Ratio.

Source: Reprinted with permission from *Journal Thrombosis Thrombolysis*, Vol 3, pp 377–384, © 1996, Kluwer Academic Publishers.

The review of the CoaguChek and Coumatrak monitors in the March 1995 *Medical Letter on Drugs and Therapeutics*[15] cites several studies discussed above and presents the two instruments as viable PT monitoring options.

A third type of point-of-care capillary whole blood PT instrumentation has been recently developed by International Technidyne Corporation and approved by the FDA for commercial use. The PT determination is based on capillary whole blood mixing with dry thromboplastin in a capillary channel, but this instrument differs from the previously described instruments in that it performs a PT in triplicate (three capillary channels), as well as internal level 1 and level 2 controls in two additional capillary channels (the previously described monitors both require an external control). The two control channels contain normal and abnormal control material. These channels run concurrently with the PT test and identify sample collection error as well as reagent error. The PT test is run in triplicate (50 µl of capillary whole blood required) and the median value is used in calculating the plasma-equivalent PT result or the INR. The instrument uses recombinant human thromboplastin (Ortho Recomboplastin, ISI = 1.0). The device, known as the ProTIME Monitor, uses an optical detection system (infrared LED light source and detector) and contains computer capabilities to record and compute data.

In a recently completed multi-institutional trial,[16] simultaneous capillary whole blood and venous sample results from 304 warfarin-treated patients and 82 controls were compared with results obtained using standard laboratory methodology at each institution, as well as with results from a reference laboratory. The study also analyzed the ability and accuracy of patients in performing their own measurements compared with the health care provider's ability and accuracy. The ProTIME INR correlated significantly to the reference laboratory for both the health care provider (venous sample, r = 0.92) and the patient (capillary sample, 4 = 0.90). Monitor INR results for fingersticks performed by both the patient and the health care provider were also equivalent and correlated highly (r = 0.92).

Assessment of results from a Bland-Altman analysis of data indicated that the mean difference between the ProTIME venous result with the reference laboratory result was 0.03 INR units. The analysis did show a tendency for the ProTIME result to be slightly less than the reference laboratory result with an increased scatter of results at INR values of 3.0 or greater. In findings similar to those of the previously cited study by Kaatz et al,[14] when the investigators compared the hospital laboratory INR results with the reference laboratory results, they found no significant differences from the ProTIME results compared to the reference laboratory INRs.[16] Nearly 80% of the ProTIME results and hospital laboratory results were within 0.4 INR units of the reference laboratory results.

The same group of investigators compared results from 82 patients who performed self-testing at home and then immediately (within 3 hours) came to the clinic for venous samples tested both in the hospital laboratory and in a reference laboratory.[17] Once again, there was a high correlation between patient self-test (PST) at home and tests at the hospital laboratory (r = 0.92 from 479 comparisons) and reference laboratory (r = 0.86). The average mean difference between the PST and hospital laboratory was 0.03 INR units and there was no evidence of bias in results or systematic error. As before, a Bland-Altman analysis demonstrated a tendency for the PST to be slightly higher than the reference laboratory result.

Other investigators have confirmed the suitability of the ProTIME device in a less structured and more typical environment of real-time patient care. Comparisons were similar to those reported above.[18]

In a separate report on children, Andrew et al[19] reported on the instrument's accuracy and precision in 76 warfarin-treated children and 9 healthy controls. Venous and capillary whole blood tested on the instrument yielded a correlation of r = 0.89. Both results, compared with venous blood tested in a reference laboratory (ISI = 1.0), revealed correlation coefficients of 0.90 and 0.92, respectively. Both reports concluded that the ProTIME Monitor can accurately measure the PT (INR) compared with a plasma PT (INR) assay.

A fourth type of instrument, known as the Avocet$_{PT}$® prothrombin time test system (Avocet, Inc), uses a different technology for clot detection. The reagent test strips contain an ultrathin, sponge-like, asymmetric polysulfone membrane. When whole blood from a fingerstick is applied to the membrane (plasma can also be used), the red blood cells are separated from the plasma. The membrane contains thromboplastin (ISI approximately 1.5), which when hydrated by the blood sample, activates coagulation. As thrombin is generated, it comes in contact with a Rhodamine-110 based fluorescent thrombin substrate. The reaction liberates free rhodamine, an intense fluorophore, and fluorescence is monitored. The time from the initial application of the sample, detected by a resistance drop between two electrodes, to the onset of fluorescence is proportional to the PT. Preclinical studies established the mathematical correlation relationship.

The technology of the Avocet$_{PT}$® monitor was originally described by Zweig et al[20] and its accuracy and precision only recently reported.[21] Within-day precision was assessed by measuring 30 repeat tests each from citrated whole blood and citrated plasma on the instrument, resulting in CVs of 4.8% and 5.5%. Level 1 and level 2 controls were run daily for between-day precision producing CVs of 11.2% (n = 72) and 7.1% (n = 72), respectively. Accuracy was evaluated with capillary whole blood and citrated venous blood tested on the monitor compared to citrated plasma in the reference laboratory using an MLA Electra 800® with Innovin® (ISI ~ 1.0). In samples from 160 patients from three medical centers, a correlation of 0.97 was noted for both capillary blood and citrated venous blood (n = 153 and 157, respectively).

In another study, investigators compared point-of-care tests from 58 patients and 5 normals with tests from a local reference laboratory.[22] The correlation was excellent (r = 0.92 from 125 samples). In an attempt to determine the impact on clinical dosing, the investigators noted that in 82% of the results, the therapeutic dose decision would have been the same. In 18% a different dosing decision would have been indicated, but in no case did the device result endanger the patient by indicating a dosage change opposite to that of the reference.

Most recently, the LifeScan INR monitor (Harmony) was approved for professional and home use. This instrument, like the others, initiates coagulation with thromboplastin (recombinant human with an ISI ~ 1.15) and detects clot formation by cessation of blood flow in a capillary channel. The instrument has two onboard quality control channels such that external controls are not needed. The test requires ~ 20 μl of capillary whole blood from a fingerstick or venous blood. In a correlation study,[23] the LifeScan instrument showed excellent agreement with a local laboratory reference (r = 0.98 for 401 samples). Precision analysis of 199 paired monitor tests yielded a CV of 6.0% for all meters, test strip lots, and samples. When analyzed for clinically relevant agreement, there was a 99% agreement in results between the instrument and the local laboratory results. Finally, when the LifeScan instrument was compared with a WHO reference recombinant thromboplastin (WHO rTF/95), 98% of LifeScan results were in clinical agreement with the WHO rTF/95 results.[24]

In a clinical study, investigators assessed the ability of patients to perform their own INR on the LifeScan instrument after approximately one hour of training.[25] PST results were compared to fingerstick results obtained by study investigators, and all results were compared to those of a local reference laboratory. Results were collected over a 12-week period of time from 278 subjects. Paired results were in agreement 95% and 97% of the time between PST and reference laboratory and investigator-obtained fingerstick and reference laboratory, respectively.

INSTRUMENT COMPARABILITY

With more than a half dozen point-of-care instruments on the market, investigators have attempted to compare instruments to see if one outperforms the others. Unfortunately, these studies are difficult to interpret and conclusions cannot be drawn. Jacobson et al[26] compared eight different instruments and found significant differences between INR results that were large enough to have clinical impact. However, as they caution, one must be careful comparing INR results, not only from different point-of-care instruments, but from different laboratories as well. As McGlasson[27] points out, there are approximately 300 reagent/instrument combinations for PT testing. In his study comparing laboratory INRs, there was up to a 20% difference in INRs using 12 different reagent/instrument combinations. Gosselin et al[28] completed a study on nine point-of-care instruments comparing results to laboratory INRs using three different thromboplastins. Their findings were similar to those of Jacobson et al,[26] with 7 of 9 instruments showing significant differences in INR values.

CONCLUSION

Portable PT monitors, a welcome development, have the potential to lower the risk/benefit ratio and encourage the use of warfarin by physicians. Although these instruments are not yet approved for patient self-testing in the United States, patient self-monitoring of therapy is not far off, given the theoretical potential for improved patient outcomes and overall cost reduction. Although these encouraging results need further confirmation by large randomized prospective trials, they do suggest that the future management of anticoagulation should include patient self-monitoring of therapy.

REFERENCES

1. Lucas FV, Duncan A, Jay R, et al. A novel whole blood capillary technique for measuring the prothrombin time. *Am J Clin Pathol.* 1987;8:442–446.

2. Yano Y, Kambayashi J, Murata K, et al. Bedside monitoring of warfarin therapy by a whole blood capillary coagulation monitor. *Thromb Res.* 1992;66:583–590.

3. Weibert RT, Adler DS. Evaluation of a capillary whole blood prothrombin time measurement system. *Clin Pharm.* 1989;8:864–867.

4. Jennings I, Luddington RJ, Baglin T. Evaluation of the Ciba Corning Biotrack 512 coagulation monitor for the control of oral anticoagulation. *J Clin Pathol.* 1991;44:950–953.

5. McCurdy SA, White RH. Accuracy and precision of a portable anticoagulation monitor in a clinical setting. *Arch Intern Med.* 1992; 152:589–592.

6. Tripodi A, Arbini AA, Chantarangkul V, et al. Are capillary whole blood coagulation monitors suitable for the control of oral anticoagulant treatment by the International Normalized Ratio? *Thromb Hemost.* 1993;70:921–924.

7. Oberhardt BJ, Dermott SC, Taylor M, Alkadi ZY, Abruzzini AF, Gresalfi NJ. Dry reagent technology for rapid, convenient measurements of blood coagulation and fibrinolysis. *Clin Chem.* 1991;37: 520–526.

8. Rose VL, Dermott SC, Murray BF, et al. Decentralized testing for prothrombin time and activated partial thromboplastin time using a dry chemistry portable analyzer. *Arch Pathol Lab Med.* 1993;117:611–617.

9. Fabbrini N, Messmore H, Balbale S, et al. Pilot study to determine use of a TAS analyzer in an anticoagulation clinic setting. *Blood.* 1995;86(suppl l):869a.

10. Kapiotis S, Quehenberger P, Speiser W. Evaluation of the new method Coaguchek® for the determination of prothrombin time from capillary blood: comparison with Thrombotest on KC-1. *Thromb Res.* 1995;77:563–567.

11. Tripodi A, Chantarangkul V, Clerici M, et al. Determination of the international sensitivity index of a new near-patient testing device to monitor oral anticoagulant therapy. *Thromb Haemost.* 1997;78:855–858.

12. van den Besselaar AM. A comparison of INRs determined with a whole blood prothrombin time device and two international reference preparations for thromboplastin. *Thromb Haemost.* 2000;84:410–412.

13. van den Besselaar AM, Meeuwisse-Braun J, Schaefer-van Mansfeld H, van Rijn C, Witteveen E. A comparison between capillary and venous blood international normalized ratio determinations in a portable prothrombin time device. *Blood Coagulation Fibrinolysis.* 2000;11:559–562.

14. Kaatz AA, White RH, Hill J, et al. Accuracy of laboratory and portable monitor International Normalized Ratio determinations. *Arch Intern Med.* 1995;155:1861–1867.

15. Portable prothrombin time monitors. *Med Lett Drugs Ther.* 1995;37:24.

16. Oral Anticoagulation Monitoring Study Group. Point-of-care prothrombin time measurement for professional and patient self-testing use. *Am J Clin Pathol.* 2001;115:288–296.

17. Oral Anticoagulation Monitoring Study Group. Prothrombin measurement using a patient self-testing system. *Am J Clin Pathol.* 2001;115:280–287.

18. Pierce MT, Crain L, Smith J, Mehta V. Point-of-care versus laboratory measurement of the International Normalized Ratio. *Am J Health-Sys Pharm.* 2000;57:2271–2274.

19. Andrew M. Marzinotto V, Adams M, Cimini C, Triplett D, LaDuca F. Monitoring of oral anticoagulant therapy in pediatric patients using a new microsample PT device. *Blood.* 1995;86(suppl 1):863a.

20. Zweig SE, Meyer BG, Sharma S, Min C, Krakower JM, Shohet SB. Membrane-based, dry-reagent prothrombin time tests. *Biomed Instrum Technol.* 1996;30:245–256.

21. Ansell JE, Zweig S, Meyer B, Zehnder J, Lewis J. Performance of the Avocet$_{PT}$ prothrombin time system. *Blood.* 1998;92(suppl 1):112b.

22. Spink BM, Schreiner K, Buschmann DJ, Taborski U. Comparison of a new point-of-care whole blood prothrombin time system to a laboratory reference instrument. *Blood.* 2000;96(Suppl Part 2):102b.

23. Earp B, Chow H, Sharma A. LifeScan INR monitor: system description and calibration traceability. *J Thromb Thrombolys.* 2001;12:110.

24. Earp B, Hambleton J, Spencer F, Jacobson A. Accuracy and precision of the LifeScan INR monitor in anticoagulation clinics. *J Thromb Thrombolys.* 2001;12:109.

25. Earp B, Hambleton J, Spencer F, Jacobson A. Patient self-testing with the LifeScan INR monitor. *Thromb Thrombolys.* 2001;12:109.

26. Jacobson A, Peterson M, Gunnemann T, Westengard J, Ruybalid L. Magnitude of INR variation attributable to differences between point-of-care testing devices. *Thromb Haemost.* 2001;86(Suppl):abstract p802.

27. McGlasson DL. A comparison of INRs after local calibration of thromboplastin international sensitivity indexes. *Clin Lab Sci.* 2002;15:91–95.

28. Gosselin R, Owings JR, White RH, et al. A comparison of point-of-care instruments designed for monitoring oral anticoagulation with standard laboratory methods. *Thromb Haemost.* 2000;83:698–703.

Chapter 29

Pharmacology of Warfarin and Related Anticoagulants

Ann K. Wittkowsky

HISTORY

The history of the development and clinical use of warfarin began in the 1920s when a hemorrhagic disease of cattle appeared in the midwestern United States and western Canada. The source of bleeding was traced to ingestion of improperly cured sweet clover and was associated with a reduction in plasma prothrombin.[1] In 1939, the hemorrhagic agent was isolated at the University of Wisconsin and identified as bishydroxycoumarin (dicumarol), a derivative of 4-hydroxycoumarin.[2,3] While dicumarol was being studied as an anticoagulant in animal models and in humans, a similar compound was synthesized and initially marketed as a rodenticide (Figure 29–1).[4] This agent was given the name warfarin, an acronym derived from the first letters of the Wisconsin Alumni Research Foundation. By 1955, it was available commercially as an anticoagulant for the treatment of thromboembolic disease.

STRUCTURE

The anticoagulant effect of warfarin and related compounds requires the presence of a 4-hydroxycoumarin nucleus with a substituent in the 3 position (Figure 29–2).[5] Several derivatives of 4-hydroxycoumarin (coumarins) are available commercially. Warfarin is the most frequently used coumarin anticoagulant in North America; in Europe, both acenocoumarol and phenprocoumon are widely available. Although they are not commonly used as anticoagulants because of erratic and incomplete absorption, bishydroxycoumarin and ethylbiscoumacetate remain in the pharmacopoeias of several countries. Structural differences among these compounds influence their pharmacokinetic and pharmacodynamic characteristics, as well as dosing requirements, but do not influence their mechanism of anticoagulant effect.[6]

Warfarin, like other coumarins, exists as a racemic mixture of two optical isomers because of the presence of an asymmetric carbon in the substituent group at the 3 position (Figure 29–3).[7] The R and S enantiomers of warfarin are distinguished by their spatial arrangement around the chiral atom. The enantiomers differ with respect to pharmacokinetic and pharmacodynamic characteristics, but their mechanisms of anticoagulant effect are similar.[8,9]

Several derivatives of indan-1,3-dione (indandiones), including phenindione and anisindione, also exhibit an anticoagulant effect similar to that of the coumarins.[5] Because of toxicities, however, these compounds are not used routinely in clinical practice.

MECHANISM OF ACTION

Warfarin and other coumarins and indandiones exert their anticoagulant effect by interfering with the hepatic synthesis of vitamin K–dependent clotting factors, including factors II, VII, IX, and X and proteins C and S (Figure 29–4). In the presence of oxygen, carbon dioxide, and vitamin KH_2 (hydroquinone, reduced vitamin K), glutamic acid (glu) residues

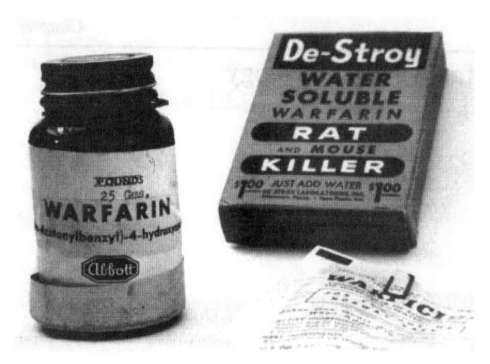

Figure 29–1 Original packaging of warfarin. Courtesy of Wisconsin Alumni Research Foundation, Madison, Wisconsin.

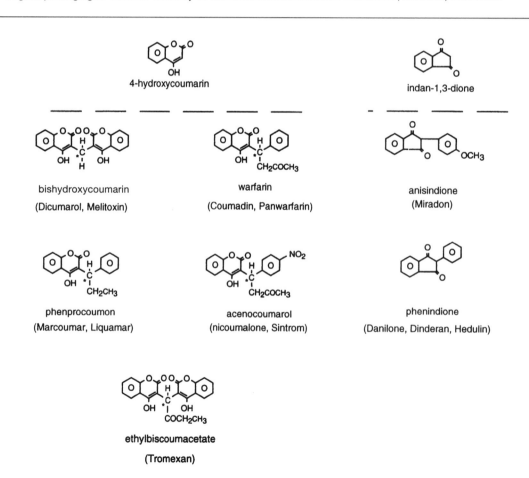

Figure 29–2 Chemical structures of the coumarins and indandiones, including generic and trade names, and identification of asymmetric carbons

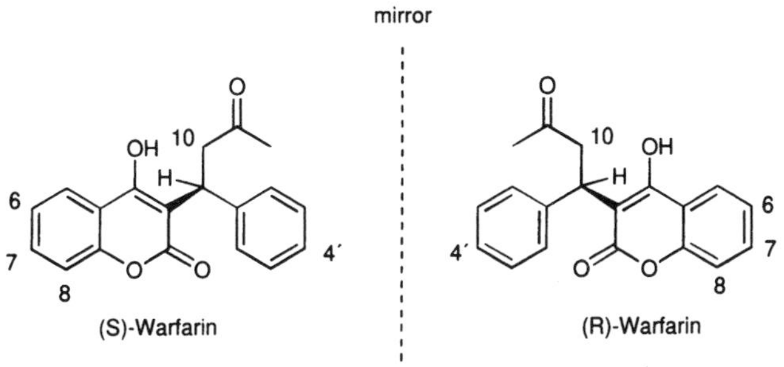

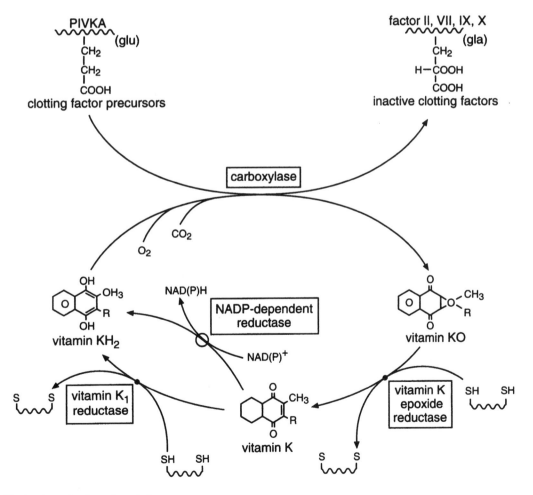

Figure 29–3 Stereoisomerism of warfarin, including sites of oxidative metabolism

found at the NH$_2$-terminal region of precursors to vitamin K–dependent clotting factors undergo γ-carboxylation via a specific carboxylase enzyme to form γ-carboxyglutamic acid (gla) residues.[10,11,12] The presence of gla residues is necessary for the interaction of these proteins with calcium, which confers a conformational change necessary for com-

plexation of these proteins with negatively charged phospholipids found on platelets and endothelial cells.[13,14] These reactions are essential components of the activation of the clotting cascade.

γ-carboxylation also results in oxidation of vitamin KH$_2$ to vitamin K$_{2,2}$-epoxide (Vitamin KO), a form of vitamin K without biologic activity.[15] In order to replenish adequate stores of active vitamin KH$_2$, an hepatic recycling process involving two reductase enzymes converts vitamin KO to vitamin KH$_2$. Vitamin KO is reduced to vitamin K (quinone) by vitamin K epoxide reductase and is further reduced by vitamin K reductase to vitamin KH$_2$. Both enzymes are dithiol dependent.[16,17] The reduction of vitamin K also occurs via an NADPH-dependent reductase enzyme. Each molecule of vitamin K is likely recycled many hundreds of times before it is catabolized to inactive degradation products.[17]

Warfarin interferes with the hepatic recycling of vitamin K by inhibiting the activity of the two diothiol-dependent reductase enzymes (see Figure 29–4).[18] An accumulation of vitamin KO and depletion of vitamin KH$_2$ occurs, which

Figure 29–4 Mechanism of action of warfarin

limits the γ-carboxylation of the glu residues of clotting factor precursors. The result is an accumulation of partially carboxylated or noncarboxylated clotting factor precursors (proteins induced by vitamin K antagonism [PIVKAs]) with markedly reduced ability to contribute to thrombin generation.[19] A reduction in the number of gia residues of prothrombin (factor II) from the normal of 10 to 9, 8, 7, or 6 residues is shown to reduce thrombin-generating activity to 78%, 20%, 7%, and 2% of normal, respectively.[20]

EFFECT ON VITAMIN K–DEPENDENT PROTEINS

Warfarin-induced depletion of vitamin KH_2 results in a reduction in the availability of vitamin K–dependent proteins. Ongoing synthesis of these proteins is inhibited, and previously formed vitamin K–dependent proteins are depleted at rates commensurate with their elimination half-lives (see Table 29–1).[21] In an evaluation of rates of decline of vitamin K–dependent proteins during initiation of warfarin therapy, a 40-mg loading dose of warfarin caused a rapid and substantial decline in factor VII during the first 48 hours (Figure 29–5), but a gradual decline in activity of factors II, IX, and X and proteins C and S over 72 hours (Figure 29–6).[22] In comparison, an initial 10-mg dose of warfarin, followed by two days of warfarin in which dosing was adjusted according to the rate of increase in prothrombin time, lessened the extent but not the rate of initial reduction in factor VII, while other vitamin K–dependent proteins declined gradually (Figures 29–5 and 29–6). Unlike selective suppression of factor II or factor X, suppression of factor VII or factor IX has not been shown to provide adequate protection against tissue factor–induced intravascular coagulation in an experimental animal model.[23] These observations suggest that the initial reduction in factor VII induced by warfarin does not represent adequate anticoagulation despite an increase in International Normalized Ratio (INR).[24]

During long-term warfarin therapy, individual vitamin K–dependent clotting factors are suppressed to different extents. An investigation in stable, anticoagulated patients, in

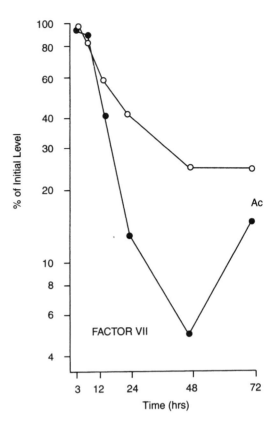

Figure 29–5 Mean factor VII activity following warfarin 40-mg (●) and adjusted warfarin doses (○). Source: Reprinted from *Thrombosis Research*, Vol 45, Weiss et al, pp 783–790, Copyright 1987, with kind permission from Elsevier Science Ltd, The Boulevard, Langford Lane, Kidlington 0X5 1GB, UK.

whom compliance was verified, found a greater degree of suppression of factor II (mean activity, 19%; range, 95–54%) and factor X (mean activity, 18%; range, 9%–45%) than of factor VII (mean activity, 33%; range, 16%–57%) or factor IX (mean activity, 48%; range 26%–94%) (Figure 29–7).[25] Despite considerable variability among patients and in individual patients over time, mean levels of activity of all clotting factors were correlated with intensity of anticoagulation and could be used to predict the INR according to a linear regression model (Figure 29–8).

PHARMACOKINETICS

Absorption

Following oral administration, warfarin is rapidly and extensively absorbed from the stomach and small intestine.[26] Peak concentrations occur between 0.3 and 4 hours.[27] Warfarin is nearly 100% bioavailable, and both oral and intravenous formulations display similar pharmacokinetic characteristics.[28,29] No differences in absorption characteristics or

Table 29–1 Elimination Half-Lives of Vitamin K–Dependent Coagulation Proteins

Protein	Half-Life
Factor II	42–72 hours
Factor VII	4–6 hours
Factor IX	21–30 hours
Factor X	27–48 hours
Protein C	9 hours
Protein S	60 hours

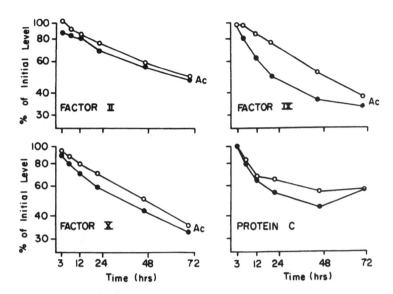

Figure 29–6 Mean factor II, IX, and X activity and protein C antigenicity following warfarin 40-mg (•) and adjusted warfarin doses (○). Source: Reprinted from *Thrombosis Research*, Vol 45, Weiss et al, pp 783–790, Copyright 1987, with kind permission from Elsevier Science Ltd, The Boulevard, Langford Lane, Kidlington 0X5 1GB, UK.

bioavailability of the R and S enantiomers of warfarin have been reported.

The rate but not the extent of absorption of warfarin is reported to be reduced by the presence of food.[30] Small bowel resection (short bowel syndrome) does not appear to alter warfarin absorption; such patients have been adequately anticoagulated with warfarin at normal doses.[31] A single case of acquired warfarin resistance, however, that was due to malabsorption, as verified by pharmacokinetic determination of reduced bioavailability of an oral dosage form, has been reported.[32]

Limited information regarding the comparative bioavailability of various brands of warfarin is available. A comparison of Coumadin (Endo), Warfilone (Frosst), Warnerin (Warner/Chilcott), and Athrombin-K (Purdue Frederick) found that the area under the serum concentration versus time curve (AUC) varied from 87% to 101% of that of the reference product.[33] Differences were also observed in the maximum serum concentration (78%–100% of that of the reference product) and in time to peak concentration (1.8–3.7 hours). Coumadin (Endo), Athrombin-K (Purdue Frederick) and Panwarfarin (Abbott) were compared in a pharmacoki-

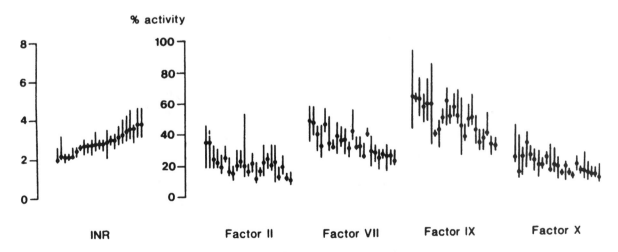

Figure 29–7 Median and range of activity of factors II, VII, IX, and X and corresponding INR values in 23 stable, compliant warfarin-treated patients at four visits over a period of three to six months. Source: Reprinted with permission from Kumar et al, *British Journal of Haemology*, Vol 74, pp 82–85. © 1990, Blackwell Science Ltd.

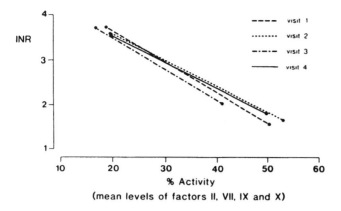

Figure 29–8 Regression of INR on mean of activity levels of factors II, VII, IX, and X at each of four return visits. Source: Reprinted with permission from Kumar et al, *British Journal of Haematology*, Vol 74, pp 82–85, © 1990, Blackwell Science Ltd.

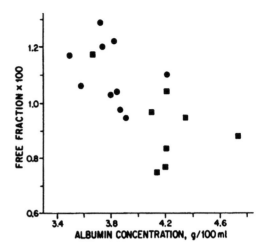

Figure 29–9 Relationship between free fraction of warfarin at 37°C and concentration of albumin in 10 female (c) and 8 male (n) normal human subjects. Source: Reproduced with kind permission from PJD Publications Limited, Westbury, NY 11590, USA, from *Research Communications in Chemical Pathology Pharmacology*, Vol 14, pp 743–746, 1976. Copyright © by PJD Publications Ltd.

netic analysis, in which differences in absorption rate constant, time to peak serum concentration, and AUC were observed among brands.[34] These differences were not considered statistically significant, but their clinical significance could be considerable given the narrow therapeutic index of the anticoagulant effect of warfarin.

Distribution

The average volume of distribution of racemic warfarin is reported to range from 0.11 L/kg to 0.18 L/kg, similar to that of albumin.[35–37] (S)-warfarin and (R)-warfarin appear to exhibit a similar volume of distribution, with an average value of 0.15 L/kg reported for each enantiomer and ranges of 0.11–0.19 L/kg for (S)-warfarin and 0.12–0.22 L/kg for (R)-warfarin.[38,39] These volumes of distribution are reported to correlate with 9.3–26.6% and 7.9–27.4% of total body weight for (S)-warfarin and (R)-warfarin, respectively.[40,41]

Warfarin is extensively bound to plasma proteins, and primarily to albumin.[42] More than 98% of warfarin is protein bound, and only the remaining free, unbound drug is pharmacologically active. The free fraction of warfarin is highly variable among patients and is independent of total warfarin plasma concentrations.[43] The free fraction of warfarin, however, increases proportionately with decreasing albumin concentrations, as demonstrated in normal subjects (Figure 29–9).[44] Similarly, an increase in free fraction and reduction in protein binding has been observed in experimental conditions in patients with disease states associated with decreased serum albumin concentrations, including idiopathic hypoalbuminemia and nephrotic syndrome.[37,45] This increase in free fraction, however, was accompanied by a significant increase in the plasma clearance of warfarin. The relationship between

increasing free fraction and increasing clearance also has been demonstrated in patients treated chronically with warfarin (Figure 29–10).[46] Thus, protein binding is a major determinant of warfarin elimination kinetics. Accordingly,

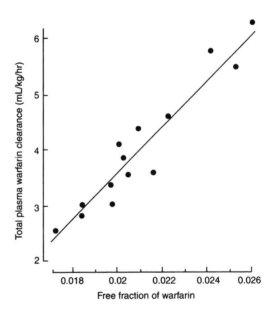

Figure 29–10 Relationships between total plasma warfarin clearance and free fraction of warfarin in 14 patients taking chronic warfarin therapy. Source: Reprinted with permission from Routledge et al, *British Journal of Clinical Pharmacology*, Vol 6, pp 243–247, © 1979, Blackwell Science Ltd.

the significant variability in pharmacokinetic characteristics of warfarin demonstrated among subjects and among patients is the result of differences in extent of protein binding.

Warfarin protein binding displays stereoselective characteristics, with (S)-warfarin binding reported as greater than (R)-warfarin despite significant intersubject and interpatient variability.[47,48] With the use of assay methodology appropriately sensitive to detect small enantiomer concentrations, (S)-warfarin binding was calculated at 99.67% (range, 98.84%–99.98%) compared with 99.44% (range, 98.69%–99.92%) for (R)-warfarin, as determined in a group of patients taking stable doses of warfarin.[49] Significant variability in enantiomer protein binding among patients also has been demonstrated in stable, anticoagulated patients taking racemic warfarin doses of 2.5–12 mg daily (mean 6.1 mg) to reach a similar therapeutic end point. Free concentrations of (S)-warfarin varied from 0.29% to 0.82% and of (R)-warfarin from 0.26% to 0.96%.[50]

Metabolism

Warfarin is metabolized by hepatic microsomal enzymes of the p450 system in the endoplasmic recticulum of the liver parenchyma. Differences in metabolism of (S)-warfarin and (R)-warfarin have been identified by determination of formation clearances of stereospecific oxidative and reductive metabolites (Figure 29–11). (S)-warfarin is approximately 90% oxidized, primarily to 7-hydroxywarfarin and to a lesser extent to 6-hydroxywarfarin, which are formed in roughly a 3:1 ratio.[51–54] In addition, smaller quantities of 10- and

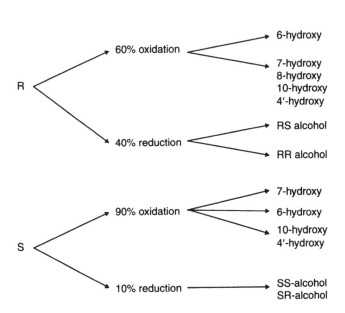

Figure 29–11 Stereoselective metabolism of warfarin

4'-hydroxywarfarin are also formed. Reduction yields diasteriomeric alcohols (SS and SR) that appear to exhibit minor pharmacologic activity.[55] In contrast, (R)-warfarin undergoes approximately 60% reduction, primarily to 6-hydroxywarfarin and to a lesser extent to 4'-, 7-, 8-, and 10-hydroxywarfarin. Additionally, approximately 40% of (R)-warfarin is reduced, primarily to RS alcohol with small quantities of RR alcohol also formed. Significant variability in formation rates of individual oxidative metabolites has been demonstrated between subjects and likely influences the observed differences in warfarin dosing requirements between patients.[56]

Approximately 30 individual enzymes in the cytochrome p450 superfamily have been identified in humans.[57] Each enzyme appears to be responsible for certain, distinct oxidative reactions involved in the metabolism of drug compounds, including warfarin (Figure 29–12). (S)-warfarin is metabolized by the enzyme p450-2C9 to 6- and 7-hydroxywarfarin, and by p450-3A4 to 4'- and 10-hydroxywarfarin.[53] In comparison, (R)-warfarin is oxidized to 6- and 7-hydroxywarfarin by p450-1A2, to 4'- and 10-hydroxywarfarin by p450-3A4, and to 8-hydroxywarfarin by p450-2C19.

Elimination

The hepatic metabolites of warfarin are eliminated by urinary excretion. In a single-dose study, 50% of racemic warfarin administered orally was recovered in the urine over a nine-day period (see Table 29–2).[54] Stereochemical analysis revealed recovery of 31% of (S)-warfarin and 19% of (R)-warfarin, primarily as oxidative and reductive metabolites, with only trace excretion of unchanged drug.

The overall clearance of warfarin is stereospecific, with (S)-warfarin eliminated approximately twice as quickly as (R)-warfarin. Single-dose studies report (S)-warfarin clearance rates of 0.015–0.132 mL/min/kg and (R)-warfarin clearance rates of 0.009–0.121 mL/min/kg.[40,58] Comparatively, multiple dose studies report (S)-warfarin clearance rates of 0.025–0.219 mL/min/kg and (R)-warfarin clearance rates of 0.016–0.087 mL/min/kg.[40,50] Significant intersubject and interpatient variability in clearance has been observed and likely reflects significant differences in protein binding related to subtle differences in plasma albumin concentrations among patients. Accelerated clearance of (S)-warfarin has been associated with relative warfarin resistance.[59]

Differences in clearance of the enantiomers of warfarin are reflected in their elimination half-lives. In single-dose studies, the half-life of (S)-warfarin is reported to range from 18 hours to 52 hours, with an average reported value of 29 hours.[8,40,41,60] In comparison, the average half-life of (R)-warfarin is 45 hours, with a range of 20–70 hours reported in single-dose evaluations.[8,40,41,60]

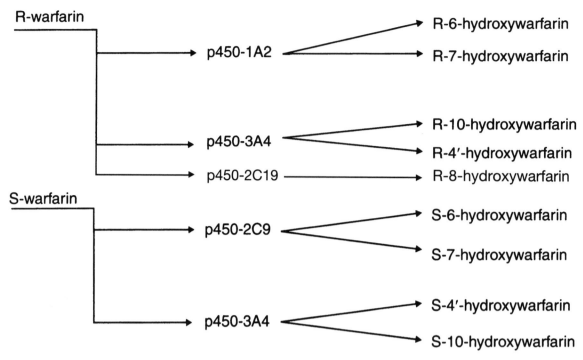

Figure 29–12 Regioselective oxidative metabolism of warfarin enantiomers

PHARMACODYNAMICS

Potency

In humans, stereospecific potency of warfarin is consistently reported. In separate single-dose studies using a Simplastin reagent for monitoring prothrombin time, 1.5 mg/kg racemic warfarin, (S)-warfarin, and (R)-warfarin increased the prothrombin time to a peak of 29, 34, and 21 seconds, respectively, at 48 hours (Figure 29–13).[8] Other investiga-

Table 29–2 Mean Percentage of Warfarin Dose Excreted as Metabolites or as Unchanged Drug over Nine Days Following a Single 1.5-mg/kg Dose in Six Subjects

	R-Warfarin	S-Warfarin
Unchanged drug	1.33%	1.05%
6-Hydroxywarfarin	8.91%	6.31%
7-Hydroxywarfarin	3.26%	21.71%
Warfarin alcohol 1	5.79%	0.06%
Warfarin alcohol 2	0.22%	1.95%
Total	19.51%	31.08%

Source: Reprinted with permission from O'Reilly et al, *Clinical Pharmacology and Therapeutics*, Vol 16, pp 348–354, © 1974, Mosby-Year Book, Inc.

tions, using a variety of experimental designs, have determined that (S)-warfarin is 2.7 to 3.8 times more potent than (R)-warfarin.[40,58] The greater potency and faster elimination clearance of (S)-warfarin suggest a lesser degree of protein binding than (R)-warfarin based on pharmacokinetic principles. (S)-warfarin, however, is more protein bound than (R)-warfarin. Therefore, differential potency of the R and S enantiomers is likely reflective of differences in receptor affinity to vitamin K reductase enzymes, rather than to differences in pharmacokinetic characteristics, including protein binding, volume of distribution, and clearance rates. Despite its lower plasma concentrations, S-warfarin results in a greater accumulation of vitamin $K_{2,3}$ epoxide, thus suggesting a greater degree of vitamin K epoxide reductase inhibition.[61]

Dose/Concentration/Response Relationships

Significant variability in the pharmacokinetic characteristics of warfarin has been observed among subjects and among anticoagulated patients, as described above. In addition, considerable variability in plasma concentrations of warfarin required to maintain a desired intensity of anticoagulation also has been observed. In a group of 36 anticoagulated patients in whom racemic warfarin doses were titrated in order to maintain a prothrombin time index of 30%–50%, total concentrations of warfarin enantiomers were highly variable.[50] (S)-warfarin concentrations ranged from 0.11

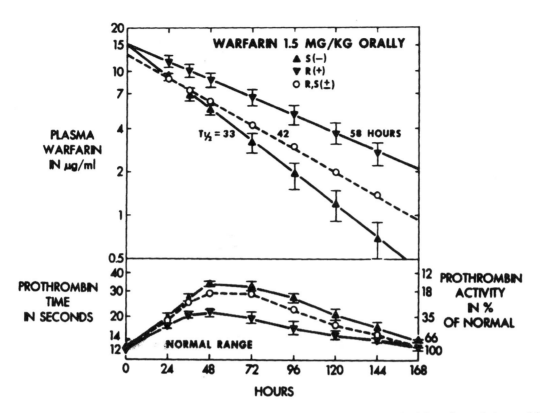

Figure 29–13 Means of warfarin concentrations in plasma and of prothrombin times after single 1.5-mg/kg oral doses of (S)-warfarin, (R)-warfarin, and racemic warfarin in 10 normal subjects. Source: Reprinted with permission from Toon et al, *Clinical Pharmacology and Therapeutics*, Vol 39, pp 15–24, © 1986, Mosby-Year Book, Inc.

μg/mL to 1.02 μg/mL (mean 0.48 μg/mL), and (R)-warfarin concentrations varied from 0.29 μg/mL to 1.82 μg/mL (mean 0.87 μg/mL). Doses of warfarin required to maintain this level of anticoagulation also demonstrated considerable variability (mean, 6.1 mg; range 2.5–12 mg). Significant correlations were observed between each of the following:

- total (S)-warfarin and dose
- total (R)-warfarin and dose
- free (S)-warfarin and dose
- free (R)-warfarin and dose

Similar positive correlations also have been observed between dose and total racemic warfarin concentrations and between dose and unbound racemic warfarin concentrations.[43,62] In these studies of stable anticoagulated patients, however, no correlation between dose and prothrombin time, total warfarin concentration and prothrombin time, or free warfarin concentration and prothrombin time was evident. In an evaluation of anticoagulated patients in whom warfarin was discontinued, a linear relationship between total plasma warfarin concentration and prothrombin time ratio was observed in each individual patient, but there was no similarity between individuals in the warfarin concentration required for a specific response (Figure 29–14).[46]

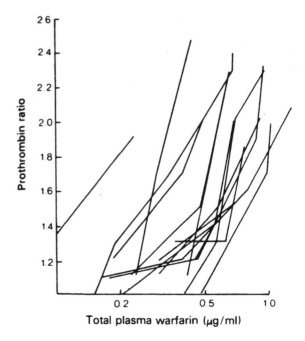

Figure 29–14 Relationship between the logarithm of the total plasma warfarin concentration and the prothrombin time ratio of 15 patients. Source: Reprinted with permission from Routledge et al, *British Journal of Clinical Pharmacology*, Vol 8, pp 243–247, © 1979, Blackwell Science Ltd.

In individual patients, dose/response to warfarin is influenced by pharmacokinetic factors, including the absorption and bioavailability of warfarin, its distribution and extent of protein binding, and the availability and efficiency of metabolizing enzymes. Pharmacodynamic factors, including availability of vitamin K, the efficiency and integrity of clotting factor synthesis and vitamin K recycling, and reductase enzyme receptor affinity and integrity, also impact dose/response. These pharmacokinetic and pharmacodynamic factors are also influenced by a variety of patient-specific factors, including age, diet, disease states, and drug interactions. As a result, dose/response to warfarin is relatively unpredictable and individualization of dosing is required to ensure the safe and effective use of warfarin.

PHARMACOGENOMICS

Cytochrome P4502C9 is the principal hepatic microsomal enzyme responsible for the metabolism of warfarin. While the wild-type allele (CYP2C9*1) predominates in humans, several polymorphisms have been identified (Table 29–3).[63] The frequency of these mutations differs among various ethnic populations, with Caucasians having a higher allelic frequency than African Americans or Asians. The presentation of any polymorphism may be heterozygous (eg, CYP2C9*1/*2) or homozygous (eg, CYP2C9*2/*2). Each variant represents a single nucleotide polymorphism that results in a single amino acid change at a particular locus.

The presence of CYP2C9 mutations has been associated with a reduction in the metabolism of warfarin. The ability of CYP2C9*2 to metabolize S-warfarin to S-7-hydroxywarfarin is only 12% of that of CYP2C9*1.[64] Comparatively, CYP2C9*3 is less than 5% as efficient as CYP2C9*1 in the metabolism of S-warfarin.[65] In addition, the oral clearance of S-warfarin is 66% lower in CYP2C9*3 heterozygotes and 90% lower in CYP2C9*3 homozygotes than in those with the wild-type allele.[66] Clinically, the reduced oxidative capacity of CYP2C9 polymorphisms appears to influence therapeutic response to warfarin.

Cytochrome P4502C9 genotype is independently associated with the warfarin maintenance dosing requirement.[67] In a clinical investigation, 81% of patients with a warfarin maintenance dosing requirement of <1.5 mg per day had a genetic mutation of CYP2C9, whereas mutant alleles were found in only 40% of patients whose mean warfarin dosing requirements were widely varied.[68] Among patients with CYP2C9 polymorphism, both average daily dose (3.5 mg/day vs. 4.6 mg/day) and weight-based total weekly dose (0.397 mg/kg/week vs. 0.307 mg/kg/week) were lower than in patients with the wild-type allele.[69] Other observations have determined that warfarin maintenance dosing requirements are lower in patients with various genetic mutations of CYP2C9 (Table 29–4).[66,70–74] Overall, these data suggest that warfarin dosing requirements are reduced by the presence of CYP2C9*2 polymorphisms and further reduced in patients with CYP2C9*3 variants. These findings are in agreement with previous observations suggesting a greater inhibition of S-warfarin metabolism by CYP2C9*3 than by CYP2C9*2. Additionally, patients with homozygous presentation of CYP2C9 appear to have a greater reduction in dosing requirement than do heterozygotes.

Several investigations have suggested that in addition to increased sensitivity to the effects of warfarin, CYP2C9 mutations are associated with adverse clinical outcomes. In an evaluation of 561 patients during the maintenance period of warfarin therapy, the presence of CYP2C9 mutation did not increase the theoretical risk of bleeding (measured by frequency of INRs > 8.0), or the frequency of overanticoagulation (defined as an INR > 0.5 units above upper limit of the therapeutic range.[73] However, in an evaluation of initiation therapy, 18 of 34 patients with a CYP2C9 mutation experienced an INR greater than 4.0 compared to only 5 of 52 control patients without polymorphisms. Overanticoagulation resulted in an increased length of hospital stay to reach optimal anticoagulation in 9 of 20 patients with mutant alleles compared to no patients in the control group.[71] During the maintenance phase of therapy, major (8.28% vs. 2.25% per patient year; p = 0.007) and minor (5.27% vs. 1.93% per

Table 29–3 Observed Frequency of CYP2C9 Variants among Various Ethnic Groups

	CYP2C9*1	CYP2C9*2	CYP2C9*3	CYP2C9*4	CYP2C9*5
Point mutation	Arg_{144}/Ilc_{359}	Cys_{144}/Ilc_{359}	Arg_{144}/Leu_{351}	Arg_{144}/Thr_{359}	Arg_{144}/Glu_{360}
Caucasians	79%–86%	8%–19.1%	6%–10%	nd	nd
Indigenous Canadians	91%	3%	6%	nd	nd
African Americans	98.5%	1%–3.6%	0.5%–1.5%	nd	2.3%
Asians	95%–98.3%	0	1.7%–5%	0–1.6%	0

nd: not determined.

Table 29–4 Effect of CYP2C9 Genotype on Mean Warfarin Maintenance Dosing Requirement (mg per day) and Percentage Dosage Reduction in Comparison to the Wild-Type Allele

Population	N	*1/*1	*1/*2	*1/*3	*2/*2	*2/*3	*3/*3
Causasian (ref 70)	94	4.7mg	3.8mg (19% ↓)	nd	nd	nd	nd
Caucasian (ref 71)	52	4.25mg	3.5mg (18% ↓)	2.5 (41% ↓)	3.5mg (18% ↓)		nd
Caucasian (ref 72)	180	6.7mg	5.2mg (22% ↓)	3.8mg (43% ↓)	5.2mg (22% ↓)	1.8 (73% ↓)	nd
Caucasian (ref 73)	561	5.01mg	4.31mg (14% ↓)	3.97mg (21% ↓)	3.04mg (39% ↓)	4.09mg (18% ↓)	0
Caucasian (ref 74)	185	5.6mg	4.9mg (13% ↓)	3.3mg (41% ↓)	4.07mg (27% ↓)	2.3mg (59% ↓)	1.6mg (71% ↓)
Asian (ref 66)	47	3.0mg	nd	1.75mg (42% ↓)	nd	nd	0.4mg (87% ↓)

nd: not determined.

patient year) bleeding events were higher in patients with CYP2C9 polymorphisms.

Eighty-eight patients with CYP2C9*1, 62 patients with CYP2C9*2, and 28 patients with CYP2C9*3 were followed over 1.4–1.9 years, including initiation and maintenance of warfarin therapy.[72] Major and minor bleeding events occurred at a rate of 10.7% per patient year in patients with the wild-type allele, compared to 22.5% per patient year in *2 carriers and 37.2% in *3 carriers. Median INR at the time of bleeding episodes was not statistically different in patients with and without CYP2C9 mutations (3.26 vs. 3.5; p = 0.495). Genetic variation of CYP2C9 was an independent risk factor for warfarin-related bleeding complications (OR 2.24; CI 1.04–4.81).

In a recent retrospective evaluation of 185 patients followed over a mean of 2.3 years, the incidence of serious (10.92% vs. 4.89% per patient year) and life-threatening (1.56% vs. 0.7% per patient year) bleeding was higher in patients with CYP2C9 polymorphisms than in those with the wild-type allele.[74] In addition, patients with genetic mutations had an increased risk of above-range INRs (hazard ratio 1.4) and took more time to achieve a stable warfarin dose (mean difference: 95 days; p < 0.004). Polymorphisms were also associated with an increased risk of bleeding during initiation therapy (hazard ratio 3.94) or at any time during treatment (hazard ratio 2.39), and bleeding events occurred sooner after initiation of therapy (p = 0.013).

In summary, patients with CYP2C9 polymorphisms appear to have lower warfarin dosing requirements, a higher risk of bleeding, and higher variability of anticoagulant response. They may also be more susceptible to drug interactions involving inhibition of CYP2C9. Pharmacogenetic screening may one day play a role in identifying patients who are candidates for lower initiation and maintenance dosing and who are at risk for certain drug interactions. However, its cost-effectiveness is yet to be determined.

OTHER ORAL ANTICOAGULANTS

Few details are available regarding the pharmacokinetics and pharmacodynamics of oral anticoagulants other than warfarin, with the exception of phenprocoumon and acenocoumarol. These agents are widely available outside the United States and are used clinically throughout Europe. The most significant differences between these agents and warfarin are their comparative elimination half lives, stereochemistry, and manner of hepatic metabolism (Table 29–5).[75–79] As a result, each of these oral anticoagulants differs with respect to time required to reach steady state, time to reversal of therapeutic effect when the drug is discontinued, and susceptibility to drug interactions involving induction or inhibition of various cytochrome P450 isozymes. Phenprocoumon appears to be less susceptible than warfarin to P450-based drug interactions due to its long elimination half life and significant degree of clearance of unchanged drug.[80] While acenocoumarol might be expected to be more susceptible than warfarin to P450-based interactions, this is not supported in documented case reports or studies, primarily due to a comparatively lower rate of use and drug interaction evaluation.

Early studies suggested that longer acting coumarins provided more stable anticoagulation than coumarins with short elimination half lives.[81,82] Two more recent clinical studies have compared the quality of oral anticoagulation with warfarin in comparison to acenocoumarol. A retrospective evaluation compared 142 patients treated with warfarin to 142 patients treated with acenocoumarol matched for age, gender, disease state, and duration of anticoagulation.[83] Cases and controls had all been anticoagulated for > 100 days. Over a 22-month period, warfarin therapy was associated with a statistically higher rate of therapeutic INRs during the course of treatment (72.5% vs. 67%; p < 0.001) and greater stability of therapy as measured both by the frequency of required

Table 29–5 Comparative Pharmacokinetics of Coumarin Anticoagulants

	Warfarin	Acenocoumarol	Phenprocoumon
Elimination half life	R: 29 hrs S: 45 hrs	R: 9 hrs S: 0.5 hrs	R: 5.5 days S: 5.5 days
Stereochemical potency	S 2.7–3.8 × more potent than R	R more active due to faster clearance of S	S 1.5–2.5 × more potent than R
Primary cytochrome P450 enzymes responsible for metabolism	R: 1A2>3A4>2C19 S: 2C9>3A4	R: 2C9>2C19 S: 2C9	R: 2C9 S: 2C9 1/3 eliminated unchanged

INR measurements (24 vs. 26 INRs per patient; p < 0.001) and the percentage of INR results leading to an anticoagulant dosing adjustment (58% vs. 64%; p < 0.001). Minor bleeding complications occurred at a similar rate in both groups.

In another clinical trial, 103 patients who had been anticoagulated with acenocoumarol were switched to warfarin therapy.[84] After a 2-month period of restabilization, monitoring outcomes during the last 6 months of acenocoumarol treatment were compared to the next 6-month period of warfarin treatment. No differences were found in the frequency of required INR measurements (12 vs. 11 INRs per patient), or the number of INRs within the therapeutic range (59% vs. 62%). Clinical outcomes were not evaluated. However, in a prospective inception-cohort study, bleeding events in patients treated with warfarin and acenocoumarol were found to be similar.[85] The quality of oral anticoagulation with acenocoumarol compared to phenprocoumon was evaluated in a clinical trial involving patients in an anticoagulation clinic setting.[86] Two hundred twenty-eight patients taking acenocoumarol were matched for age, gender, and indication for anticoagulation with 228 patients taking phenoprocoumon. Over a combined duration of 230 treatment years, phenoprocoumon therapy was associated with a higher rate of INRs in the therapeutic rate (42.7% vs. 36.5%), a higher percentage of time spent in the therapeutic range (46.6% vs. 41.6%) compared to acenocoumarol therapy. Although the incidence of minor bleeding complications was slightly higher in patients treated with phenprocoumon, major bleeding events were similar for both drug therapies. The longer half life of phenprocoumon led to more stable anticoagulation in comparison to acenocoumarol.

GENERIC WARFARIN: THERAPEUTIC CONSIDERATIONS

Generic warfarin products, like other generic drugs, must meet US Food and Drug Administration (FDA) criteria for bioequivalence.[87] *Bioavailability* is the rate and extent of absorption of active drug that reaches the site of action.

Bioavailability studies define mean parameters for area under the serum concentration vs. time curve, maximum concentration (C_{max}), time to maximum serum concentration (T_{max}) in healthy volunteers exposed to single doses of brand and generic formulations in a two crossover design with washout period. According to FDA specifications, a generic product is considered bioequivalent if the 90% confidence intervals of its rate and extent of absorption fall within 80% to 125% of that of the innovator product.

As previously described, there is significant variability among patients in the concentration of warfarin obtained with a certain dose. More important, there is significant variability among patients in the concentration of warfarin required to reach a specific INR, as well as the dose of warfarin required to reach the goal INR or target therapeutic range. Clinical response, as measured by INR, is a much more significant parameter than serum concentrations of warfarin. Bioequivalence, however, is based on serum concentrations of drug rather than on therapeutic response to those serum concentrations.

In addition to meeting FDA bioequivalence criteria, generic drug products must meet tablet content uniformity specifications outlined by the United States Pharmacopeia (USP).[88] Stage 1 testing requires that 10 tablets from any batch of drug contain 85% to 115% of the labeled drug strength with a relative standard deviation of less than 6%. If one tablet falls outside this range but within 75% to 125%, then 20 additional tablets must be tested. Stage 2 testing requires that all 30 tablets contain 75% to 125% of the labeled strength and no more than one tablet is outside of 85% to 115%, with a standard deviation of less than 7.8%.

When Coumadin was manufactured by DuPont Pharma, a stricter content uniformity specification was used than was required by the USP.[89] Dupont's stage 1 testing required that 10 tablets from any batch of drug contain 92.5% to 107.5% of the labeled drug strength with a relative standard deviation of less than 3%. If one tablet fell outside this range, but within 87.5% to 112.5%, then 20 additional tablets were tested. Stage 2 testing required that all 30 tablets contain 87.5% to 112.5% of the labeled strength and no more than one tablet be outside the 92.5% to 107.5% range, with a standard deviation of less than 3.9%.

Batch-to-batch and tablet-to-tablet variability in tablet contents for DuPont's Coumadin was not a concern, but it is a potential problem for generic warfarin products. To maintain patients within the appropriate INR range, warfarin dosage adjustments of 5% to 15% of the total daily dose are made and response to therapy is reevaluated within 1 to 2 weeks. USP tablet content uniformity standards allow for greater variation in tablet contents than is used for dosage adjustments (Table 29–6). Patients using generic warfarin may inadvertently receive a significant change in drug dose each time a prescription is refilled. Patients switching from brand to generic warfarin or from one generic to another, as well as patients in whom therapy is initiated with a generic form of the drug, are at risk for complications of over- or under-anticoagulation unless additional therapeutic monitoring is instituted to ensure consistent therapeutic response. Bristol Myers Squibb, the current manufacturer of warfarin, has not released its tablet content uniformity specifications.

Despite these concerns, trials that have compared patients exposed to brand versus generic warfarin have not found clinically or statistically significant differences in clinical or monitoring outcomes.[90–93] Product source should be considered one of many possible explanations for variability in anticoagulant response, particularly when warfarin prescriptions are refilled.

Table 29–6 Possible Variation in Tablet Contents According to DuPont Pharma and USP Tablet Content Uniformity Criteria

	1 mg	2 mg	2.5 mg	4 mg	5 mg	7.5 mg	10 mg
DuPont							
Stage 1 (mg)	0.93–1.08	1.85–2.15	2.31–2.69	3.70–4.30	4.63–5.38	6.94–8.06	9.25–10.75
Stage 2 (mg)	0.88–1.23	1.75–2.25	2.19–2.81	3.50–4.50	4.38–5.63	6.56–8.44	8.75–11.25
USP							
Stage 1 (mg)	0.85–1.15	1.70–2.30	2.13–2.88	3.40–4.60	4.20–5.75	6.38–8.63	8.50–11.50
Stage 2 (mg)	0.75–1.25	1.50–2.50	1.88–3.13	3.00–5.00	3.75–6.25	5.63–9.38	7.50–12.50

REFERENCES

1. Roderick LM. A problem in the coagulation of blood: sweet clover disease of cattle. *Am J Physiol.* 1931;96:413–425.

2. Campbell HA, Link KP. Studies on the hemorrhagic sweet clover disease. IV: The isolation and crystallization of the hemorrhagic agent. *J Biol Chem.* 1941:138:21–33.

3. Stahman MA, Huebner CF, Link KP. Studies on the hemorrhagic sweet clover disease. V: Identification and synthesis of the hemorrhagic agent. *J Biol Chem.* 1941;138:513–527.

4. Link KP. The discovery of dicoumarol and its sequels. *Circ.* 1959; 19:97–107.

5. Majerus PW, Broze GJ, Miletich JP, Tollefsen DM. Anticoagulant, thrombolytic, and antiplatelet agents. In: Goodman Oilman A, et al, eds. *The Pharmacologic Basis of Therapeutics.* New York: Pergamon Press; 1990.

6. Thijssen HHW, Hamulyak K, Willigers H. 4-hydroxycoumarin oral anticoagulants: pharmacokinetics-response relationship. *Thromb Haemost.* 1988;60:35–38.

7. Lam YWF. Stereoselectivity: an issue of significant importance in clinical pharmacology. *Pharmacother.* 1988;8:147–157.

8. O'Reilly RA. Studies on the optical enantiomorphs of warfarin in man. *Clin Pharmacol Ther.* 1974;16:348–354.

9. Thijssen HHW, Baars LGM, Vervoort HTM. Vitamin 2,3-epoxide reductase: the basis for the stereoselectivity of 4-hydroxycoumarin anticoagulant activity. *Br J Pharmacol.* 1988;95:675–682.

10. Bovill EG, Mann KG. Warfarin and the biochemistry of vitamin K dependent proteins. *Adv Exp Med Biol.* 1987;214:17–46.

11. Stenflo J, Fernlund P, Egan W, Roepstorff P. Vitamin K dependent modifications of glutamic acid residues in prothrombin. *Proc Natl Acad Sci USA.* 1974;71:2730–2733.

12. Nelsestuen GL, Zytkovicz TH, Howard JB. The mode of action of vitamin K. Identification of gamma-carboxyglutamic acid as a component of prothrombin. *J Biol Chem.* 1974;249:6347–6350.

13. Nelsestuen GL. Role of gamma-carboxy glutamic acid. An unusual protein transition required for calcium-dependent binding of prothrombin to phospholipid. *J Biol Chem.* 1976;251:5648–5656.

14. Borowski M, Furie BC, Bauminger S, Furie B. Prothrombin requires two sequential metal-dependent conformational transitions to bind phospholipids. *J Biol Chem.* 1986;261:14969–14975.

15. Suttie JW. Vitamin K dependent carboxylation of glutanyl residues of proteins. *Biofactors.* 1988;1:55–60.

16. Whitlon DS, Sadowski JA, Suttie JW. Mechanism of coumarin action: significance of vitamin K epoxide reductase inhibition. *Biochemistry.* 1978;17:1371–1377.

17. Vermeer C, Hamulyak K. Pathophysiology of vitamin K deficiency and oral anticoagulants. *Thromb Haemost.* 1991;66:153–159.

18. Fasco MJ, Hildebrandt EF, Suttie JW. Evidence that warfarin anticoagulant action involves two distinct reductase activities. *J Biol Chem.* 1982;257:11210–11212.

19. Malhotra OP, Nesheim ME, Mann KG. The kinetics of activation of normal and gamma-carboxyglutamic acid-deficient prothrombins. *J Biol Chem.* 1985;260:279–287.

20. Malhotra OP. Dicoumarol induced 9-gamma-carboxyglutamic acid prothrombin: isolation and comparison with 6-, 7-, 8-, and 10-gamma-carboxyglutamic acid isomers. *Biochem Cell Biol.* 1990;68:705–715.

21. Stirling Y. Warfarin-induced changes in procoagulant and anticoagulant proteins. *Blood Coag Fibrinolysis.* 1995;6:361–373.

22. Weiss P, Soff GA, Halkin H, Seligsohn U. Decline of proteins C and S and factors II, VII, IX and X during the initiation of warfarin therapy. *Thromb Res.* 1987;45:783–790.

23. Zevelin A, Roa LVM, Rapaport SI. Mechanism of the anticoagulant effect of warfarin as evaluated in rabbits by selective depression of individual procoagulant vitamin K–dependent clotting factors. *J Clin Invest.* 1993;92:2131–2140.

24. Blanchard RA, Furie BC, Jorgensen M, et al. Acquired vitamin K carboxylation deficiency in liver disease. *N Engl J Med.* 1981;305:242–248.

25. Kumar S, Haight JRM, Tate G, et al. Effect of warfarin on plasma concentrations of vitamin K dependent coagulation factors in patients with stable control and monitored compliance. *Br J Haematol.* 1990;74:82–85.

26. Pyoralak K, Jussila J, Mustala O, Siurala M. Absorption of warfarin from stomach and small intestine. *Scand J Gastroenterol.* 1971;6(suppl 9):95–103.

27. Stirling Y, Howarth DJ, Stockley R, et al. Comparison of the bioavailabilities and anticoagulant activities of two warfarin formulations. *Br J Haematol.* 1982;51:37–45.

28. Breckenridge A, Orme M. Kinetics of warfarin absorption in man. *Clin Pharmacol Ther.* 1973;14:955–961.

29. Andreasen PB, Vesell ES. Comparison of plasma levels of antipyrine, tolbutamide and warfarin after oral and intravenous administration. *Clin Pharmacol Ther.* 1974;16:1059–1065.

30. Musa MN, Lyons LL. Absorption and disposition of warfarin: effects of food and liquids. *Curr Ther Res.* 1976;20:630–633.

31. Lutomski DM, LaFrance RJ, Bower RH, Fischer JE. Warfarin absorption after massive bowel resection. *Am J Gastroenterol.* 1985;80:99–102.

32. Talstad I, Gamst ON. Warfarin resistance due to malabsorption. *J Intern Med.* 1994;236:465–467.

33. Reudy J, Davies RO, Gagnon MA, et al. Drug bioavailability. *Can Med Assoc J.* 1976;115:105.

34. Wagner JG, Welling PG, Lee KP, Walker JE. In vivo and in vitro availability of commercial warfarin tablets. *J Pharm Sci.* 1971;60:666–677.

35. O'Reilly RA, Welling PG, Wagner JG. Pharmacokinetics of warfarin following intravenous administration in man. *Thromb Haemost.* 1971;25:178–186.

36. O'Reilly RA, Trager WF, Motley CH, Howald W. Stereoselective interaction of phenylbutazone with [12C/13C] warfarin pseudo-racemates in man. *J Clin Invest.* 1980;65:746–753.

37. Piroli RB, Passanati T, Shively CA, Vesell ES. Antipyrine and warfarin disposition in a patient with idiopathic hypoalbuminemia. *Clin Pharmacol Ther.* 1981;30:810–816.

38. Choondara IA, Cholerton S, Haynes BP, et al. Stereoselective interaction between the R enantiomer of warfarin and cimetidine. *Br J Clin Pharmacol.* 1986;21:271–277.

39. Banfield C, O'Reilly R, Chan E, Rowland M. Phenylbutazone-warfarin interaction in man: further stereochemical and metabolic considerations. *Br J Clin Pharmacol.* 1983;16:669–675.

40. Breckenridge A, Orme M, Wesseling H, et al. Pharmacokinetics and pharmacodynamics of the enantiomers of warfarin in man. *Clin Pharmacol Ther.* 1973;15:424–430.

41. Hewick DS, McEwen J. Plasma half-lives, plasma metabolites, and anticoagulant efficacies of the enantiomers of warfarin in man. *J Pharm Pharmacol.* 1973;25:458–465.

42. O'Reilly R. Interaction of the anticoagulant drug warfarin and its metabolites with human plasma albumin. *J Clin Invest.* 1969;48:193–202.

43. Yacobi A, Udall JA, Levy G. Serum protein binding as a determinant of warfarin body clearance and anticoagulant effect. *Clin Pharmacol Ther.* 1976;19:552–558.

44. Yacobi A, Stoll RG, DiSanto R, Levy G. Intersubject variation of warfarin binding in serum of normal subjects. *Res Commun Chem Pathol Pharmacol.* 1976;14:743–746.

45. Ganeval D, Fischer AM, Barre J, et al. Pharmacokinetics of warfarin in the nephrotic syndrome and effect on vitamin K dependent clotting factors. *Clin Nephrol.* 1986;25:75–80.

46. Routledge PA, Chapman PH, Davies DM, Rawlins MD. Pharmacokinetics and pharmacodynamics of warfarin at steady state. *Br J Clin Pharmacol.* 1979;8:243–247.

47. Yacobi A, Levy G. Protein binding of warfarin enantiomers in serum of humans and rats. *J Pharmacokinet Biopharm.* 1977;5:123–131.

48. Sellars EM, Koch-Weser J. Interaction of warfarin stereoisomers with human albumin. *Pharm Res Comm.* 1975;7:331–336.

49. Cai WM, Pettigrew LC, Dempsey RJ, Chandler MHH. A simplified high performance liquid chromatographic method for direct determination of warfarin enantiomers and their protein binding in stroke patients. *Ther Drug Monit.* 1994;16:509–512.

50. Chan E, McLachlan AJ, Pegg M, et al. Disposition of warfarin enantiomers and metabolism in patients during multiple dosing with rac-warfarin. *Br J Clin Pharmacol.* 1994;37:563–569.

51. Lewis RJ, Trager WF. Warfarin metabolism in man: identification of metabolites in urine. *J Clin Invest.* 1970;49:907–913.

52. Lewis RJ, Trager WF, Chan KK, et al. Warfarin: stereochemical aspects of its metabolism and the interaction with phenylbutazone. *J Clin Invest.* 1974;53:1607–1617.

53. Rettie AE, Korzekwa KR, Kunze KL, et al. Hydroxylation of warfarin by human cDNA—expressed cytochrome p450: a role for p450-2C9 in the etiology of (S)-warfarin drug interactions. *Chem Res Toxicol.* 1992;5:54–59.

54. Toon S, Low LK, Gibaldi M, et al. The warfarin-sulfinpyrazone interaction: stereochemical considerations. *Clin Pharmacol Ther.* 1986;39:15–24.

55. Lewis RJ, Trager WF, Robinson AJ, Chan KK. Warfarin metabolites: the anticoagulant activity and pharmacology of warfarin alcohols. *J Lab Clin Med.* 1973;81:925–931.

56. Kaminsky LS, Dunbar DA, Wang PP, et al. Human hepatic cytochrome p450 composition as probed by in vivo microsomal metabolism of warfarin. *Drug Metab Disp.* 1984;12:470–477.

57. Nelson DR, Kamataki T, Waxman DJ, et al. The p450 superfamily: update on the new sequences, gene mapping, accession numbers, early trivial names of enzymes and nomenclature. *DNA Cell Biol.* 1993;12:1–51.

58. Wingard LB, O'Reilly RA, Levy G. Pharmacokinetics of warfarin enantiomers: a search for intrasubject correlations. *Clin Pharmacol Ther*. 1973;15:424–430.

59. Hallak HO, Wedlund PJ, Modi MW, et al. High clearance of (S)-warfarin in a warfarin-resistant subject. *Br J Clin Pharmacol*. 1993;35:327–330.

60. Hignite C, Uetrecht J, Tschanz C, Azaroff D. Kinetics of the R and S warfarin enantiomers. *Clin Pharmacol Ther*. 1980;28:99–105.

61. Choondara IA, Haynes BP, Cholerton S, et al. Enantiomers of warfarin and vitamin K1 metabolism. *Br J Clin Pharmacol*. 1986;22:729–732.

62. Hotraphinyo K, Triggs EJ, Maybloom B, Maclaine-Cross A. Warfarin sodium: steady state plasma levels and patient age. *Clin Exp Pharmacol Physiol*. 1978;5:143–149.

63. Takahashi H, Echizen H. Pharmacogenetics of warfarin elimination and its clinical implications. *Clin Pharmacokinetics*. 2001;40(8):587–603.

64. Rettie AE, Wienkers LC, Gonzales FJ, et al. Impaired S-warfarin metabolism catalyzed by R144C allelic varient of CYP2C9. *Pharmacogenetics*. 1994;4:39–42.

65. Haining RL, Hunter AP, Veronese ME, et al. Allelic variants of human cytochrome P4502C9:bacilovirus-mediated expression, purification, structural characterization, substrate stereoselectivity and prochiral selectivity of the wild-type and I359L mutant forms. *Arch Biochem Biophys*. 1996;333:447–458.

66. Takahashi H, Kashima T, Nomoto S, et al. Comparison between in vitro and in vivo metabolism of S-warfarin: catalytic activities of cDNA-expressed CYP2C9, its Leu359 variant, and their mixture versus unbound clearance in patients with the corresponding CYP2C9 genotypes. *Pharmacogenetics*. 1998;8:365–373.

67. Loebstein R, Yonath H, Peleg D, et al. Individual variability in sensitivity to warfarin. Nature or nurture. *Clin Pharmacol Ther*. 2001;70:159–164.

68. Aithal GP, Day CP, Kesteven PJL, Daly AK. Association between polymorphisms of cytochrome P450 CYP2C9 with warfarin dose requirements and risk of bleeding complications. *Lancet*. 1999;353:717–719.

69. Freeman BD, Zehnbauer BA, McGrath S, et al. Cytochrome P450 polymorphisms are associated with a reduced warfarin dose. *Surgery*. 2000;128:281–285.

70. Furuya H, Fernandez-Salguero P, Gregory W, et al. Genetic polymorphisms of CYP2C9 and its effect on warfarin maintenance dose requirement in patients undergoing anticoagulation therapy. *Pharmacogenetics*. 1995;5:389–392.

71. Aithal GP, Day CP, Kesteven PJL, Daly AK. Warfarin dose requirement and CYP2C9 polymorphisms. *Lancet*. 1999;353:1972–1973.

72. Margaglione M, Colaizzo D, D'Andrea G, et al. Genetic modulation of oral anticoagulation with warfarin. *Thromb Haemost*. 2000;84:775–778.

73. Taube J, Halshall D, Baglin T. Influence of cytochrome P450 CYP2C9 polymorphisms on warfarin sensitivity and risk of overanticoagulation in patients on long term treatment. *Blood*. 2000;96:1816–1819.

74. Higashi M, Veenstra DL, Wittkowsky AK, et al. Influence of CYP2C9 genetic variants on the risk of overanticoagulation and of bleeding events during warfarin therapy. *JAMA*. 2002;287:1690–1698.

75. Godbillon J, Richard J, Gerardin A, et al. Pharmacokinetics of the enantiomers of acenocoumarol in man. *Br J Clin Pharmacol*. 1981;12:621–629.

76. Thijssen HK, Flinois JP, Beaune PH. Cytochrome P4502C9 is the principal catalyst of racemic acenocoumarol hydroxylation reactions in human liver microsomes. *Drug Metabolism Disposition*. 2000;28:1284–1290.

77. Jahnchen E, Mienertz T, Gilfrich HJ, et al. The enantiomers of phenoprocoumon: pharmacodynamic and pharmacokinetic studies. *Clin Pharmacol Ther*. 1976;20:342–349.

78. Toon S, Heimark LD, Trager WF, O'Reilly RA. Metabolic fate of phenoprocoumon in humans. *J Pharm Sci*. 1985;74:1037–1040.

79. Haustein KO. Pharmacokinetic and pharmacodynamic properties of oral anticoagulants, especially phenprocoumon. *Semin Thromb Haemost*. 1999;25:5–11.

80. Trager WF. Oral Anticoagulants. In: Levy RH, Thummel KE, Trager WF, et al. *Metabolic Drug Interactions*. Lippincott Williams & Wilkins, Philadelphia, 2000.

81. Breed WPM, can Hoof JP, Haanen C. A comparative study concerning the stability of the anticoagulant effect of acenocoumarol and phenprocoumon. *Acta Med Scand*. 1969;186:283–288.

82. Rodman T, Pastor BH, Resnick ME. Phenprocoumon, diphenadione, warfarin and bishydroxycoumarin: a comparative study. *Am J Med Sci*. 1964;247:655–664.

83. Pattacini C, Manotti C, Pini M, et al. A comparative study on the quality of oral anticoagulant therapy (warfarin vs. acenocoumarol). *Throm Haemost*. 1994;71:188–191.

84. Barcellona D, Vannini ML, Fenu L, et al. Warfarin or acenocoumarol: which is better in the management of oral anticoagulants? *Thromb Haemost*. 1998;80:899–902.

85. Palareti G, Leili N, Coccheri S, et al. On behalf of the Italian Study on Complications of Oral Anticoagulant Therapy. Bleeding complications of oral anticoagulant treatment: an inception cohort prospective collaborative study (ISCOAT). *Lancet*. 1996;348:423–428.

86. Gadisseru APA, vanderMeer FJM, Andriaansen HJM, Fihn SD. Therapeutic quality control of oral anticoagulant therapy comparing the short acting acenocoumarol and the long-acting phenprocoumon. *Br J Haematol*. 2002;117:940–946.

87. Benet LZ, Goyan JE. Bioequivalence and narrow therapeutic index drugs. *Pharmacotherapy*. 1995;15:433–440.

88. United States Pharmacopeia. *Uniformity of Dosage Units*. Rockville, MD: USP-23 Convention, Inc; 1995.

89. Wittkowsky AK. Generic warfarin: implications for patient care. *Pharmacotherapy*. 1997;17:640–643.

90. Neutel JM, Smith DHG. A randomized crossover study to compare the efficacy and tolerability of Barr warfarin sodium to the currently available Coumadin. *Cardiovasc Rev Rep*. 1998;2:49–59.

91. Handler J, Nguyen TT, Rush S, Pham NT. A blinded, randomized crossover study comparing the efficacy and safety of generic warfarin sodium to Coumadin. *Prev Cardiol*. 1998;4:13–20.

92. Swenson CN, Fundak G. Observational cohort study of switching warfarin sodium products in a managed care organization. *Am J Health Syst Pharm*. 2000;57:452–455.

93. Weibert RT, Yeager BF, Wittkowsky AK, et al. A randomized crossover comparison of warfarin products in the treatment of chronic atrial fibrillation. *Ann Pharmacother*. 2000;34:981–988.

Chapter 30

Initiation of Therapy and Estimation of Maintenance Dose

Kari A. Wieland and Ann K. Wittkowsky

INTRODUCTION

Once the need for oral anticoagulation therapy has been determined, the clinician must decide how the therapy will be initiated. A number of factors that might alter the patient's response to therapy must be considered so that appropriate dosing can be selected. Initiation dosing protocols can be utilized, but they must be used in conjunction with individual patient considerations and practical patient management guidelines.

PATIENT CONSIDERATIONS IN INITIAL DOSING

Age

A number of studies conclude that advanced age increases sensitivity to warfarin, which leads to a reduced warfarin dosage requirement. In one study,[1] patients who were 35 years old and younger required an average dose of warfarin of 8.1 mg ±0.7 mg per day, whereas patients who were 75 years of age and older required 3.7 mg ± 0.7 mg per day. There were no statistically significant differences in their prothrombin ratios, which indicate that the levels of anticoagulation were similar. Another study[2] concludes that warfarin dosing requirements decreased by an average of 10.9% per decade of age, corresponding to an average decrease of about 0.5 mg per 10 years. This correlated with a geometric mean dose of about 6 mg for 30-year-old patients, which

decreased to about 3.5 mg for 80-year-old patients. In another study,[3] the mean daily dose of warfarin for various age groups decreased with increasing age:

Age	Warfarin Dose
<50 years	6.4 mg
50–59 years	5.1 mg
60–69 years	4.2 mg
>70 years	3.6 mg

Other researchers found that dosing requirements dropped by one-fourth to one-third for 70-year-old patients compared with a 30-year-old patient.[4]

One study did not demonstrate differences in warfarin pharmacokinetics in younger versus older subjects but hypothesized that the increased effect of warfarin in the elderly might result from an increased intrinsic sensitivity to warfarin.[5] This altered sensitivity is believed to be either a decreased affinity for vitamin K or an increased affinity for warfarin in the elderly, or it might be due to inherent vitamin K deficiency (eg, reduced intake, defective absorption, or altered pharmacokinetics of vitamin K). The age of the patient should be considered in light of other patient-specific factors (eg, other medications, liver and kidney function, diet, activity level) when selecting an initial dose of warfarin.

Weight

The weight of the patient can be a consideration during initiation of anticoagulation therapy. One study[6] shows a significant relationship when age and weight are considered together for the maintenance dose of warfarin, rather than either factor alone. The researchers found that patients who were younger and weighed more required more warfarin for a therapeutic response than patients who were older and weighed less.

Race or Ethnic Background

In anecdotal professional experience, Asian patients often require smaller doses of warfarin than patients of other ethnic backgrounds. Although no published reports confirm this observation, it should be considered in caring for patients of Asian descent.

Liver Function

Because oral anticoagulants are almost entirely metabolized in the liver, impaired hepatic function can potentiate their effects.[7] This is probably due to an inability to synthesize vitamin K–dependent clotting factors.[8] Patients with severe liver disease are also subject to impaired coagulation because of decreased synthesis of the vitamin K–dependent coagulation factors. In these patients bleeding becomes a significant concern, as these patients are usually unable to respond to vitamin K. No data are available regarding warfarin metabolism in patients who have chronic liver disease.

Congestive heart failure (CHF) has been shown to lead to an increased response to oral anticoagulants.[9] Anecdotal reports by anticoagulation practitioners suggest that worsening CHF can lead to unexpected elevations in prothrombin time (PT), possibly because of increased passive congestion of the liver. Patients with cancer who develop, or who have worsening, metastatic disease to the liver are also more sensitive to the effects of oral anticoagulants and might warrant closer monitoring than individuals who do not have cancer.

Renal Disease

Metabolites of warfarin excreted by the kidneys have minimal anticoagulant effects; thus impaired renal function is unlikely to alter warfarin dosing requirements significantly.[7] In patients with end-stage renal disease, however, these metabolites can potentiate uremic bleeding.[10] Patients with significant renal impairment might require lower doses of oral anticoagulants. Clinicians need to titrate warfarin dosing to a therapeutic level based on patient characteristics and individual response.

Hyperthyroidism

The rate of decay of vitamin K–dependent clotting factors is noted to be increased up to threefold in patients with hyperthyroidism.[7,8] No differences in distribution or metabolism of warfarin have been observed. This physiologic response usually becomes clinically significant only when a patient has acute hyperthyroid symptoms or when patients with hypothyroidism begin thyroid replacement therapy. Management of the clinically significant drug interaction between warfarin and thyroid hormones is discussed in more detail in Chapter 35.

Fever

Patients who have prolonged elevated temperature or fever appear to have an increased rate of decay of vitamin K–dependent clotting factors, sometimes as high as three or four times the normal rate.[8] No changes in the rate of metabolism or distribution of warfarin have been observed. The clinical significance of this interaction in patients is largely unknown. Patients must be aware that they might need to be evaluated if they develop an illness with a prolonged fever, and caregivers might need to modify doses based on individual patient response.

Vitamin K

Dietary vitamin K content can impact anticoagulation control if significant changes in intake occur (see Chapter 36 for further details). According to DA Triplett (personal communication), chewing tobacco has the highest vitamin K content per gram of any source of vitamin K that can be ingested. This factor can be important in patients who stop or start chewing tobacco, and it has been anecdotally reported to affect anticoagulation control when patients switch brands of chewing tobacco.

Medications

When patients are started on oral anticoagulants, it is important to obtain a thorough history of medication use, including prescription medications, nonprescription medications, and herbal and home remedies. Drug interactions are common reasons for alterations in intensity of anticoagulation (see Chapter 35 for further details).

Hereditary Warfarin Resistance

Several cases of hereditary warfarin resistance have been reported.[11–13] This rare phenomenon has been attributed to tissue resistance at the site of warfarin action. A group of investigators developed an algorithm to determine if this condition is the cause of warfarin resistance in patients.[13] The daily dose of warfarin, the plasma warfarin level, and the plasma clearance of warfarin first need to be determined and then the algorithm is followed to determine if the resistance is due to kinetic resistance (poor compliance) or tissue resistance (Figure 30–1).

Diarrhea

According to anecdotal reports, patients with severe diarrhea (five or six loose to watery stools per day) for several days have developed elevations in PT. This effect is believed to be due either to impaired absorption of vitamin K_1 from food sources or to the altered ability of gut bacteria to synthesize vitamin K_2.[8] Patients who have recurrent diarrhea (eg, irritable bowel disease) can have difficulty with the stabilization of warfarin therapy.

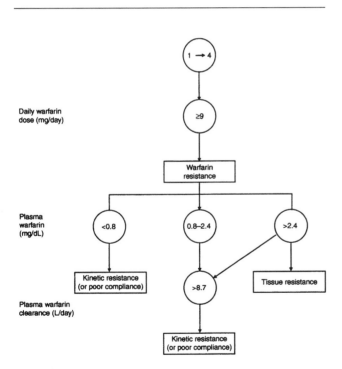

Figure 30–1 Algorithm to determine cause to warfarin resistance. Source: Reprinted with permission from DP Bentley et al, *British Journal of Clinical Pharmacology*, Vol 22, p 39, © 1986, Blackwell Science Ltd.

Alcohol

Although chronic alcohol use appears to cause induction of warfarin metabolism (Coumadin package insert), acute alcohol ingestion results in inhibition of warfarin metabolism. Patients who binge-drink tend to have higher International Normalized Ratio (INR) readings and are at greater risk for hemorrhage because of both overanticoagulation and an increased risk of falling than are patients who do not binge-drink. Complete abstinence from alcohol would be the safest advice to patients on oral anticoagulation in order for them to avoid bleeding risks. An occasional alcoholic drink or light to moderate drinking, however, does not appear to be detrimental to a patient's coagulation status.[14]

INITIATION DOSING

Initiation dosing of warfarin therapy may be accomplished by a number of methods. Selection of a particular method is dependent on whether the patient is hospitalized, whether it is necessary to reach the therapeutic INR range within a short period of time, and the comfort and experience of practitioners with available methods.

Average Daily Dosing Method

In an evaluation of over 2000 patients taking stable doses of warfarin for a number of indications, the daily warfarin dose ranged from 1 mg to 24 mg.[2] The geometric mean dose was 4.57 mg and the arithmetic mean dose was 5.13 mg. These results are used in the warfarin initiation dosing strategy known as the average daily dosing method. This method is frequently used in outpatients who begin therapy without concurrent heparinization, but it also can be used successfully in inpatients and in ambulatory patients who are using subcutaneous unfractionated heparin or low–molecular-weight heparin at home.

Patients who do not meet specific criteria that indicate sensitivity to the effects of warfarin are initiated at 4 to 5 mg daily, with INR values checked within 3 to 5 days. Dosing adjustments are made based on response to initiation therapy, and response is reevaluated in another week. Patients who may be particularly sensitive to the effects of warfarin can also begin warfarin therapy using this initiation strategy, but at doses of 1 to 3 mg daily. The following are factors that increase sensitivity to warfarin:

- greater than 70 years of age
- elevated baseline INR
- fever

- diarrhea
- malignancy
- malnutrition, decreased oral intake, nothing by mouth for more than 3 days
- clinical CHF
- clinical hyperthyroidism
- end-stage renal failure
- concurrent use of drugs known to decrease warfarin dosing requirements

Flexible Initiation Dosing Method

Flexible dosing takes into account individual patient response to warfarin by adjusting the daily dose of warfarin according to the daily rate of increase in INR. Flexible dosing protocols are a common method for initiating warfarin in hospitalized patients, and many institutions have developed internal initiation protocols based on a flexible approach to dosing.

A well-established flexible dosing protocol, developed by Fennerty et al,[15] considers patient-specific responses to initial doses of warfarin in order to determine daily doses and eventual maintenance dose requirements. The loading dose schedule was calculated from data provided by Routledge et al.[16] The Fennerty study[15] evaluated 50 consecutive patients who had venous thromboembolic disorders and were receiving heparin. The study included three patients with CHF and two with chronic liver disease. The average patient age was 52 years. Each patient received 10 mg of warfarin at 5 PM on the third day of the heparin infusion (warfarin day 1). The following morning at approximately 9 AM, the INR was measured. The INR was evaluated and the 5 PM dose of warfarin (warfarin day 2) was determined (Table 30–1). This procedure was repeated on warfarin days 3 and 4. The final maintenance dose of warfarin was based on the INR results for warfarin day 4. All 50 patients were within the therapeutic range by day 6, and prediction and actual maintenance doses were significantly related (p < 0.001).[15] Patients were followed for a median of 21 days. At this time, 44 of the patients were in the therapeutic range and their actual doses were within 1 mg of their predicted maintenance doses.

Cosh et al[17] applied the flexible dosing protocol by Fennerty et al[15] to elderly patients. Consecutive patients beginning warfarin for any reason were enrolled. Patients with a baseline INR greater than 1.3 were excluded, as were patients who had received warfarin or vitamin K within the last 10 days. Warfarin doses were administered at 4 PM and laboratory results were obtained between 7 AM and 9 AM. Of the 141 eligible patients, 100 completed the study, including 15 patients with heart failure and 2 patients with a diagnosis of alcoholism.[17] Patients were reevaluated on day 10 (follow-up point A), day 18 (follow-up point B), and day 34 (follow-up point C). During this period, warfarin doses were adjusted empirically to maintain a therapeutic INR. At follow-up point A, 76% of patients were in therapeutic range and were taking a maintenance dose that was ± 1 mg of the predicted maintenance dose. At follow-up point B, 69% were within therapeutic range, and at follow-up point C, 63% were within therapeutic range. Bleeding occurred in three patients (two patients with hematuria and one patient with epistaxis), but it was not attributable to excessive anticoagulation.

Table 30–1 Tailored Loading Dose Schedule for Warfarin Administration According to the INR

Day	INR	Warfarin dose (mg)
1	<1.4	10.0
2 (16 hours after first 10 mg dose)	<1.8	10.0
	1.8	1.0
	>1.8	0.5
3 (16 hours after second dose)	<2.0	10.0
	2.0–2.1	5.0
	2.2–2.3	4.5
	2.4–2.5	4.0
	2.6–2.7	3.5
	2.8–2.9	3.0
	3.0–3.1	2.5
	3.2–3.3	2.0
	3.4	1.5
	3.5	1.0
	3.6–4.0	0.5
	>4.0	nil
4 (16 hours after third dose)		Predicted maintenance dose:
	<1.4	<8.0
	1.4	8.0
	1.5	7.5
	1.6–1.7	7.0
	1.8	6.5
	1.9	6.0
	2.0–2.1	5.5
	2.2–2.3	5.0
	2.4–2.6	4.5
	2.7–3.0	4.0
	3.1–3.5	3.5
	3.6–4.0	3.0
	4.1–4.5	Miss next day's dose, then give 2 mg
	>4.5	Miss 2 days' doses, then give 1 mg

Source: Reprinted with permission from Fennerty et al, *British Medical Journal*, Vol 288, p 1269, 1984, BMJ Publishing Group.

Special Considerations for Flexible Initiation

Risk of Overanticoagulation

Despite the relative success with flexible initiation, practitioners should be aware of the potential for overanticoagulation when using dosing nomograms, which may lead to bleeding complications. In the Fennerty et al study,[15] 3 patients on day 4 were above the therapeutic range despite holding doses. Hemorrhagic complications were not addressed in the study. The authors suggest if a patient has a baseline ratio of more than 1.4 (and this is not because of anticoagulation resulting from the use of heparin), lower initial induction doses should be administered.

In a comparison of initial dosing using the Fennerty nomogram[15] versus empiric initiation, Doeck et al[18] found that the presence of any one of three complicating factors (interfering medications, heart failure, or chronic alcohol abuse) increased the likelihood of overanticoagulation, defined as an INR greater than 4 on days 4 through 9. Of 84 patients initiated according to the nomogram, 18% were overanticoagulated, including 27% of 22 patients with complicating factors and 14.5% of patients with no complicating factors. Empiric dosing was used to initiate therapy in 88 patients; of these, 26% were overanticoagulated, including 48% of 25 patients with complicating factors and 17% of 63 patients with no complicating factors. However, overanticoagulation was not associated with bleeding in any patient. The authors conclude that the nomogram was safer to use than empiric initiation, especially in patients with risk factors for excessive anticoagulation.

Wilkinson et al[19] compared 3 initiation dosing regimens in 202 patients with a variety of indications for anticoagulation. Patients received either 10 mg daily for 2 days, 10 mg on day 1 and 5 mg on day 2, or 5 mg daily for 2 days. Subsequent dosing was based on INR results. Overanticoagulation was defined as an INR greater than 4 at any time during the first 7 days of therapy. Significant predictors of overanticoagulation included:

- baseline INR greater than 1.3
- receiving more than 3 mg of warfarin on day 2 if day 2 INR is greater than 1.5 after 1 10-mg dose
- receiving more than 2 mg of warfarin on day 3 if day 3 INR is greater than 2.0 after 2 10-mg doses

Practitioners may want to compare these results with the details of the Fennerty nomogram[15] in order to develop more precise guidelines for initiation dosing.

Anticoagulant versus Antithrombotic Effects

Following initial doses of warfarin, early elevations in the prothrombin time reflect depletion of factor VII, the vitamin K dependent clotting factor with the shortest elimination half life. This anticoagulant effect must be differentiated from the eventual antithrombotic effect of warfarin, associated with depletion of factors II and X, each with significantly longer elimination half lives.[20] Patients being treated for acute thromboembolic episodes must continue unfractionated heparin or low–molecular-weight heparin for a minimum of 4 to 5 days even if the INR appears to be within the therapeutic range on day 2 or 3. An appropriate duration of heparin therapy in the setting of acute thromboembolism is required to prevent recurrent thromboembolism.[21]

Hypercoagulability from Protein C Depletion

Historically, loading doses of 20 mg and higher were used for initiation of warfarin therapy. One of the first studies that compared doses of 1.5 mg/kg (range 60 to 153 mg) to smaller loading doses of 10 to 15 mg per day found no significant differences between the two methods of administration in the amount of reduction of any of the four clotting factors.[22] However, these doses were associated with warfarin-induced skin necrosis and increased hemorrhagic rates.[23,24] The authors suggest the avoidance of what were considered customary doses at that time and the use of lower initiation doses, especially in patients with enhanced sensitivity to the effects of the drug.

Warfarin-induced skin necrosis has been associated with rapid reductions in protein C (a vitamin K–dependent anticoagulant with a short elimination half life) and the development of a hypercoagulable state due to a greater degree of protein C depletion than factor II depletion.[23,24] The potential for hypercoagulability has been suggested as a reason to avoid initial 10 mg doses of warfarin. Harrison et al[25] compared warfarin initiation with a 10 mg starting dose versus a 5 mg starting dose in 49 patients with acute thromboembolism who were receiving concurrent heparin therapy. Subsequent dosing was adjusted according to a dosing nomogram published separately.[26] Slow decline of factors II and X was no different between the two groups, but factor VII and protein C declined more quickly and were significantly lower in patients initially dosed with 10 mg than in those initially dosed with 5 mg.

The clinical significance of these findings is questionable. The authors suggest that the initial decline of protein C with near-normal levels of factors II and X might result in a hypercoagulable state that could lead to thrombus extension, recurrent thromboembolism, or warfarin-induced skin necrosis.[25] However, this response is more likely to occur in patients with protein C deficiency; a population in whom warfarin use without concurrent heparinization has been associated with warfarin-induced skin necrosis.[23,24] Patients with protein C deficiency are typically diagnosed with this hypercoagulable state in the process of evaluation for idiopathic thromboembolism. Because a presentation of acute thrombosis requires heparin therapy while warfarin is initiated, such patients are protected from potential hypercoagu-lability associated with rapid declines in protein C. The concerns expressed by the authors may be valid if patients begin warfarin therapy without concurrent heparinization, particularly in patients with unrecognized protein C deficiency.

Appropriate Use

The flexible dosing guidelines may be particularly useful for patients who are hospitalized, because daily dosing determination depends on daily PT evaluation. Concurrent heparinization can avoid the possibility of hypercoagulability, especially in protein C deficient patients. Follow-up outpatient visits can then determine actual dosage needs based on diet, activity level, social habits (eg, alcohol intake), and compliance.

Other Initiation Dosing Methods

Computerized Dosing Schedules

Several computer dosing programs for estimating initial warfarin doses have been studied (see Chapter 9). Some studies found that computer-assisted dosing improved the accuracy of dosing and shortened the time to achieve stable therapeutic doses when used by physicians who did not routinely manage warfarin therapy.[27] Warfarin dosage adjustments using computer modeling can be comparable to the skill of a professional with anticoagulation dosing experience.[28]

Prediction Methods

A number of dosing methods have been reported that use a patient's initial response to warfarin to predict warfarin dosing requirements.[16,29–33] Some studies limit patient selection by not enrolling patients who take medications known to interact with warfarin [16,30,31] or by not enrolling patients with disease states known to influence warfarin therapy.[16,31] Many studies developed regression equations but were limited to predicting values because prothrombin time ratio rather than INR was used.[16,29–31]

A multicenter evaluation of six methods for predicting warfarin maintenance doses from initial responses shows that one method predicted doses that were significantly lower than actual dosing requirements, and three methods predicted doses that were significantly higher than actual requirements.[33] Only one method was able to be used in 23 of 45 patients because of the number of PT measurements needed, and the correlation was not found to be significant. Only one method was useful in determining that the actual maintenance dose and a therapeutic response was predicted in 83% of the cases. The authors noted that these techniques do not represent all sources of patient variability (eg, patient sensitivity and compliance), and more careful titration of doses is preferred in certain patients.

Bayesian pharmacokinetic and pharmacodynamic forecasting were also evaluated in patients taking warfarin.[34] The investigators found that the population parameters need to be refined because Bayesian forecasting is largely dependent on this factor for accurate application.

PRACTICAL CONSIDERATIONS FOR INITIATION DOSING

Start of Initial Dosing

The timing of initial warfarin doses in heparinized patients has been debated. One group studied the early (within 48 hours of starting heparin) versus late (96 hours or later) initiation of warfarin.[35] Early initiation of warfarin during heparin therapy decreased the length of hospitalization and hospital costs, reduced the incidence of heparin-induced thrombocytopenia, and was as effective as late initiation of warfarin.

In patients receiving concurrent heparin and warfarin, the effect of heparin on PT/INR must be considered. Reductions in PT following discontinuation of heparin have been observed. In a study of 25 warfarin-treated patients, in whom PT was evaluated four to six hours after heparin infusion was stopped, a mean reduction of 1.6 seconds was noted, which did not correlate with heparin dose or activated partial thromboplastin time.[36] Because patients are not usually at steady state with respect to warfarin therapy when they are discharged from the hospital, early outpatient follow-up is warranted.

Time of Day for Dosing

The time of day at which patients take their oral anticoagulants should be addressed with individual patients. Many practitioners recommend that patients take warfarin in the late afternoon or early evening. In the event a patient needs a dose change (eg, holding a dose), it may still be accomplished after the patient's clinic visit and before the daily dose is taken. One small study found that there may be significant variations in PT results over a 24-hour period in patients treated with warfarin.[37] The PT results had a mean change of 9.3% ± 3.7%, and the INRs had a mean change of 10.6% ± 6.5%. In this study, warfarin administration occurred at 6 PM, with peak PT results occurring between 4 AM and 8 AM and troughs between 6 PM and midnight. Whether a reverse trend would have been seen in patients taking warfarin in the morning was not evaluated. Regardless of the time of day selected for warfarin administration, consistency is important and should be stressed.

Frequency of Prothrombin Time Evaluation and Patient Assessment

When patients are started on oral anticoagulant therapy, a number of factors should be considered to ensure desired patient outcomes. Following initial dosing, patients should be evaluated at intervals depending on the dosing method used and the duration of therapy (Exhibit 30–1). Therapeutic response and risk factors for hemorrhage will influence these guidelines, and laboratory monitoring and patient assessment may need to be performed more frequently if a patient has an unexpected response or medical instability. Many practitioners advocate the routine monitoring of complete blood counts, urinalysis, and occult blood to ensure that toxicity is avoided, but the cost-effectiveness of this approach is unknown.

CONCLUSION

Many factors need to be considered in patients before starting oral anticoagulation therapy (Figure 30–2). Once oral anticoagulation is determined to be the therapeutic option of choice, a number of patient factors need to be considered because of their effects on response to therapy. Initiation dosing protocols may be helpful, but one must be aware of their limitations. Experience in the dosing of warfarin is an important element of successful patient management.

Exhibit 30–1
FREQUENCY OF INR MONITORING AND PATIENT ASSESSMENT DURING INITIATION THERAPY

• Flexible initiation method	Daily through day 4, then within 3–5 days
• Average daily dosing method	First within 3–5 days, then within 1 week
• After hospital discharge	If stable, within 3–5 days; if unstable, within 1–3 days
• First month of therapy	Weekly
• After first month	Use maintenance therapy guidelines

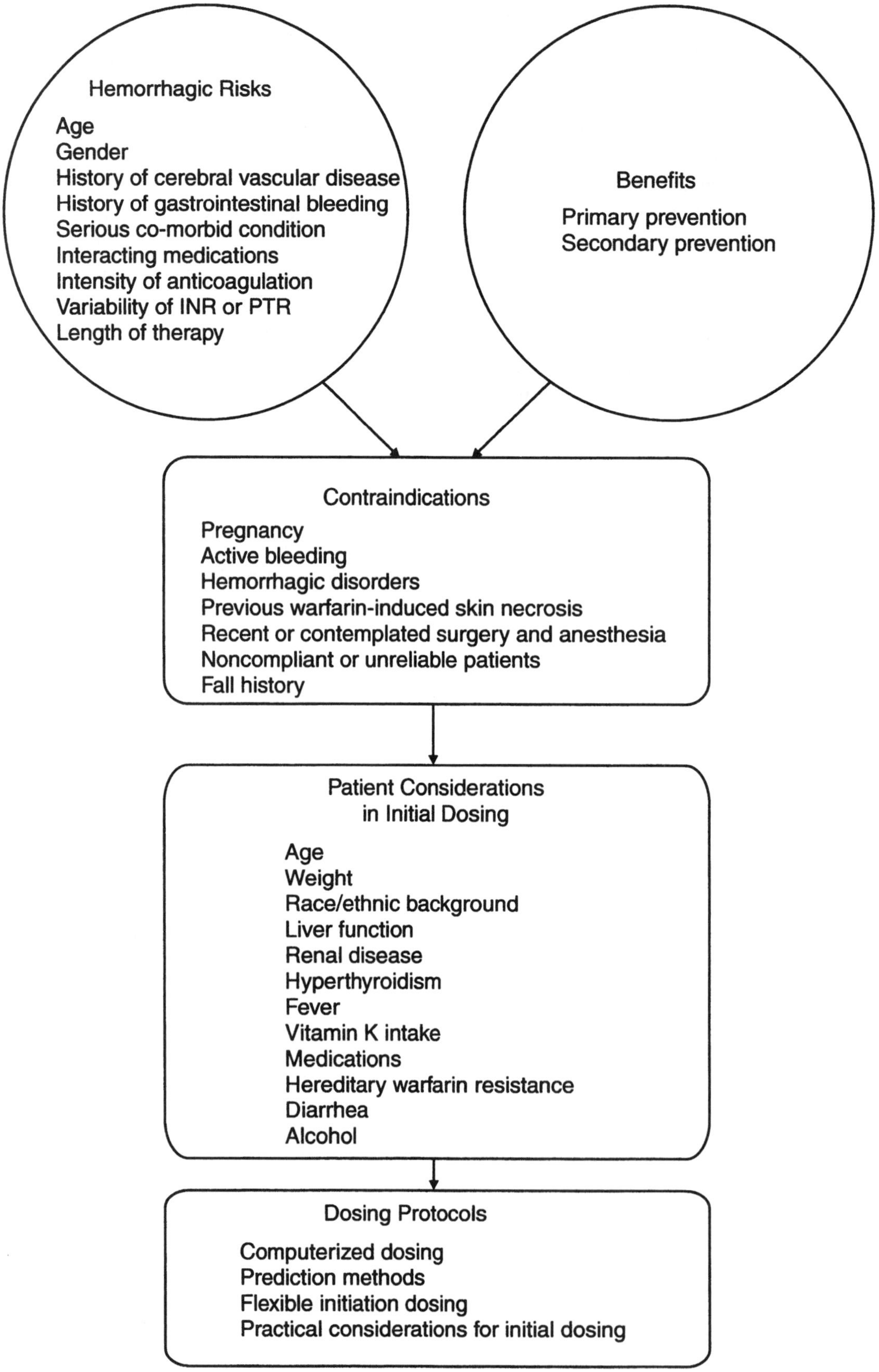

Hemorrhagic Risks

Age
Gender
History of cerebral vascular disease
History of gastrointestinal bleeding
Serious co-morbid condition
Interacting medications
Intensity of anticoagulation
Variability of INR or PTR
Length of therapy

Benefits

Primary prevention
Secondary prevention

Contraindications

Pregnancy
Active bleeding
Hemorrhagic disorders
Previous warfarin-induced skin necrosis
Recent or contemplated surgery and anesthesia
Noncompliant or unreliable patients
Fall history

**Patient Considerations
in Initial Dosing**

Age
Weight
Race/ethnic background
Liver function
Renal disease
Hyperthyroidism
Fever
Vitamin K intake
Medications
Hereditary warfarin resistance
Diarrhea
Alcohol

Dosing Protocols

Computerized dosing
Prediction methods
Flexible initiation dosing
Practical considerations for initial dosing

Figure 30–2 Summary of factors to be considered for the initiation of oral anticoagulation

REFERENCES

1. Routledge PA, Chapman PH, Davies DM, Rawlins MD. Factors affecting warfarin requirements: a prospective population study. *Eur J Clin Pharmacol.* 1979;15:319–322.

2. James AH, Britt RP, Raskino CL, Thompson SG. Factors affecting the maintenance dose of warfarin. *J Clin Pathol.* 1992;45:704–706.

3. Gurwitz JH, Avorn J, Ross-Degnan D, Choodnovsky I, Ansell J. Aging and the anticoagulant response. *Ann Intern Med.* 1992;116: 901–904.

4. Redwood M, Taylor C, Bain BJ, Matthews JH. The association of age with dosage requirement for warfarin. *Age Aging.* 1991;20:217–220.

5. Shepherd AMM, Hewick DS, Moreland TA, Stevenson IH. Age as a determinant of sensitivity to warfarin. *Br J Clin Pharmacol.* 1977;4: 315–320.

6. Dobrzanski S, Duncan SE, Harkiss A, Wardlaw A. Age and weight as determinants of warfarin requirements. *J Clin Hosp Pharm.* 1983;8: 75–77.

7. Shetty HGM, Fennerty AG, Routledge PA. Clinical pharmacokinetic considerations in the control of oral anticoagulant therapy. *Clin Pharmacokinet.* 1989;16:238–253.

8. Breckenridge A. Oral anticoagulant drugs: pharmacokinetic aspects. *Semin Hematol.* 1978;15:19–26.

9. Killip T, Payne MA. High serum transaminase activity in heart disease. *Circulation.* 1960;21:646–660.

10. Kelly JG, O'Malley K. Clinical pharmacokinetics of oral anticoagulants. *Clin Pharmacokinet.* 1979;4:1–15.

11. Alving BM, Strickler MP, Knight RD, Barr CF, Berenberg JL, Peck CL. Hereditary warfarin resistance: investigation of a rare phenomenon. *Arch Intern Med.* 1985;145:499–501.

12. Diab F, Feffer S. Hereditary warfarin resistance. *South Med J.* 1994; 87:407–409.

13. Bentley DP, Backhouse G, Hutchings A, Haddon RL, Spragg B, Routledge PA. Investigation of patients with abnormal responses to warfarin. *Br J Clin Pharmacol.* 1986;22:37–41.

14. Harris JE. Interaction of dietary factors with oral anticoagulants: review and applications. *J Am Diet Assoc.* 1995;95:580–584.

15. Fennerty A, Dolben J, Thomas P, et al. Flexible induction dose regimen for warfarin and prediction of maintenance dose. *Br Med J.* 1984;288:1268–1270.

16. Routledge PA, Davies DM, Bell SM, Cavanagh JS, Rawlins MD. Predicting patients' warfarin requirements. *Lancet.* 1977;2:854–855.

17. Cosh DG, Dally RJ, Moritz CK, Gallus AS, Ashman KJ. Prospective evaluation of a flexible protocol for starting treatment with warfarin and predicting its maintenance dose. *Aust NZ J Med.* 1989;19: 191–197.

18. Doeck CJ, Cosh DG, Gallus AS. Standardized initial warfarin treatment: evaluation of initial treatment response and maintenance dose prediction by randomised trial, and risk factors for an excessive warfarin response. *Aust NZ J Med.* 1991;21:319–324.

19. Wilkinson TJ, Sainsbury R, Heaton DC, Gilchrist NL. Initial warfarin treatment in hospital: room for less caution? A twelve month prospective audit. *NZ Med J.* 1992;105:478–479.

20. Hirsh J, Dalen JE, Deykin D, Poller L, Bussey H. Oral anticoagulants: mechanism of action, clinical effectiveness and optimal therapeutic range. *Chest.* 1995;180(suppl 4):231–246.

21. Hyers TM, Hull RD, Weg JG. Antithrombotic therapy for venous thromboembolic disease. *Chest.* 1995;180(suppl 4):335–351.

22. O'Reilly RA, Aggeler PM. Studies on Coumarin anticoagulant drugs: initiation of warfarin therapy without a loading dose. *Circulation.* 1968;38:169–177.

23. Horn JL, Danziger LH, Davis RJ. Warfarin-induced skin necrosis: report of four cases. *Am J Hosp Pharm.* 1981;38:1763–1768.

24. Comp PC, Elrod JP, Karzenski S. Warfarin-induced skin necrosis. *Semin Thromb Hemostas.* 1990;16(4):293–298.

25. Harrison L, Johnston M, Massicotte MP, Crowther M, Moffat K, Hirsh J. Comparison of 5 mg and 10 mg loading doses in initiation of warfarin therapy. *Ann Intern Med.* 1997;126:133–135.

26. Crowther MA, Harrison L, Hirsh J. Warfarin: less may be better. *Ann Intern Med.* 1997;127:332–333.

27. White RH, Hong R, Venook AP, et al. Initiation of warfarin therapy: comparison of physician dosing with computer-assisted dosing. *J Gen Intern Med.* 1987;2:141–148.

28. White RH, Mungall D. Outpatient management of warfarin therapy: comparison of computer-predicted dosage adjustment to skilled professional care. *Ther Drug Monitor.* 1991;13:46–50.

29. Miller DR, Murray MA. Predicting warfarin maintenance dosage based on initial response. *Am J Hosp Pharm.* 1979;36:1351–1355.

30. Williams DB, Karl RC. A simple technique for predicting daily maintenance dose of warfarin. *Am J Surgery.* 1979;137:572–576.

31. Sharma NK, Routledge PA, Rawlins MD, Davies DM. Predicting the dose of warfarin for therapeutic anticoagulation. *Thromb Hemostas.* 1982;47(3):230–231.

32. Carter BL, Reiders TP, Hamilton RA. Prediction of maintenance warfarin dosage from initial patient response. *Drug Intell Clin Pharm.* 1983;17:23–26.

33. Sawyer WT, Poe TE, Canady BR, et al. Multicenter evaluation of six methods for predicting warfarin maintenance-dose requirements from initial response. *Clin Pharm.* 1985;4:440–446.

34. Svec JM, Coleman RW, Mungall DR, Ludden TM. Bayesian pharmacokinetic/pharmacodynamic forecasting of prothrombin response to warfarin therapy: preliminary evaluation. *Ther Drug Monitor.* 1985;7:174–180.

35. Mohiuddin SM, Hilleman DE, Destache CJ, Stoysich AM, Gannon JM, Sletch MH. Efficacy and safety versus late initiation of warfarin during heparin therapy in acute thromboembolism. *Am Heart J.* 1992;123(3):729–732.

36. Lutomski DM, Djuric PE, Draeger RW. Warfarin therapy: the effect of heparin on prothrombin times. *Arch Intern Med.* 1987;147:432–433.

37. Bleske BE, Welage LS, Warren EW, Brown MB, Shea MJ. Variations in prothrombin time and international normalized ratio over 24 hours in warfarin-treated patients. *Pharmacother.* 1995;15(6):709–712.

Chapter 31

Managing Maintenance Therapy

Lynn B. Oertel

INTRODUCTION

Continued safe and effective management for patients who take oral anticoagulants requires timely and diligent assessment of their responses to therapy and factors that might increase the potential for bleeding and thromboembolic complications. This chapter focuses on the importance of developing an organized approach within a practice setting to improve patient management and monitoring.

Goldhaber[1] describes a closed claim case in which a 45-year-old woman was admitted to the hospital, diagnosed with pulmonary embolism, and promptly treated with heparin and warfarin. Within a month after hospital discharge, a fatal pulmonary embolism occurred. During the course of review, it was learned that the patient had not received effective anticoagulation for 13 days. Terrible tragedies such as this can be avoided if a system is in place to

- identify clearly the responsible party for anticoagulation management
- identify persistent nontherapeutic results
- implement a tracking method that alerts clinicians to tardy patients or missing International Normalized Ratio (INR) values (especially after a recent hospitalization)

MANAGEMENT STRATEGIES

When monitoring warfarin therapy, three important assumptions affecting patient management should be kept in mind:

1. Patients require individualized warfarin doses to achieve therapeutic levels of anticoagulation.
2. The indication for therapy determines the intensity, as well as duration, of therapy.
3. Periodic blood tests are critical to monitor the therapeutic effects.

During the induction or initiation phase of therapy, the goal is to achieve a therapeutic response as soon as possible. Warfarin, with its relatively narrow therapeutic index, requires diligent surveillance because a patient's response to therapy can change over time. Frequent monitoring is necessary to promote safety and to observe effects of treatment throughout the maintenance phase, although complications occasionally occur in patients with therapeutic INRs. Monitoring response to therapy via an INR is not the only task at hand during day-to-day management. Assessment of potential side effects of therapy and clinical symptoms suggestive of treatment failure is crucial throughout the entire course of therapy, as well as assessment of factors causing fluctuations in the INR. Reinforcement of the educational plan also should be incorporated into the maintenance phase for successful management.

If the planned duration of therapy is brief, the anticipated ending date should be clearly documented in the patient's record and the patient's referring physician should be contacted before warfarin therapy is terminated. For each patient on long-term therapy, the anniversary date of the patient's care by the anticoagulation management service (AMS) is an ideal time to complete an annual retrospective review of his or her anticoagulation history and performance and to notify the patient's referring physician of the results.

Dose Adjustments

The response to treatment fluctuates over time and is influenced by numerous factors. Among these factors are the following:

- changes in medications, including deletions or additions of prescribed and over-the-counter drugs and dose adjustments of existing medications
- intercurrent illnesses
- dietary habits and any changes in nutritional status
- lifestyle habits, such as alcohol use, exercise regimens, and travel
- inaccuracies in laboratory processing or point-of-care device
- issues related to patient compliance

Generally, the first month of therapy requires greater scrutiny of each patient's response to therapy. INR monitoring during the first week of therapy is generally more frequent, perhaps daily, until the INR falls within therapeutic range. The frequency interval can be expanded to several days for the next week or two, depending on the INR results. Loading doses of warfarin are generally not implemented, and initial starting doses of 4 or 5 mg per day usually generate

a therapeutic INR within 4 or 5 days.[2] Of course, exceptions based on patient-specific factors are possible. An increased incidence in adverse events is more likely to occur early in treatment.[3] This time period is also crucial for assessing patient adherence to the prescribed regimen and reinforcement of patient education.

During the maintenance phase, the intervals between INR testing can be expanded up to four weeks, provided the INR response remains close to the INR therapeutic target. Dose adjustments during this phase may require more frequent INR testing to assess the response to the new dose adjustment. Practical dose adjustments are easily achieved by calculating the total milligrams per week and using approximately 10% of that figure to make incremental or decremental changes in dose. Slight variations in the amount of daily doses are forgiven by the relatively long half-life of warfarin. The simplicity of dosing strategies using single-strength tablets minimizes the opportunity for dosing errors and is generally the favored approach. A great deal of flexibility can be achieved by using multiples or fractions of single-strength tables and basing dose instructions accordingly. Table 31–1 illustrates an example of such variation achieved by using a 5-mg tablet.

In contrast, several successful anticoagulation clinics have promoted the use of "same-daily-dose" strategies, meaning

Table 31–1 Flexible Weekly Dosing Patterns Using a 5-mg Tablet

	Sun	Mon	Tues	Wed	Thurs	Fri	Sat	Total mg/week
Mg/day	2.5	2.5	2.5	2.5	2.5	2.5	2.5	17.5
Tablets/day	½	½	½	½	½	½	½	
Mg/day	2.5	2.5	2.5	5	2.5	2.5	2.5	20.0
Tablets/day	½	½	½	1	½	½	½	
Mg/day	2.5	5	2.5	5	2.5	5	2.5	25.0
Tablets/day	½	1	½	1	½	1	½	
Mg/day	5	5	5	5	5	5	5	35.0
Tablets/day	1	1	1	1	1	1	1	
Mg/day	5	7.5	5	5	7.5	5	5	40.0
Tablets/day	1	1½	1	1	1½	1	1	
Mg/day	5	7.5	5	7.5	5	7.5	5	42.5
Tablets/day	1	1½	1	1½	1	1½	1	
Mg/day	7.5	7.5	7.5	7.5	7.5	7.5	7.5	52.5
Tablets/day	1½	1½	1½	1½	1½	1½	1½	
Mg/day	10	10	10	10	10	10	10	70.0
Tablets/day	2	2	2	2	2	2	2	

patients receiving the same mg dose every day. This often requires that patients have available several different strengths of warfarin. Concerns are raised regarding the potential for patient confusion resulting in dose errors. Unfortunately, very few studies have addressed the issue between same-daily-dosing versus alternate-day-dosing strategies. A single study reported lower rates of confusion and dosing errors in patients taking same-daily dose when compared to patients receiving alternate-day-dose regimens.[4] The authors conclude, however, that whenever selecting a warfarin dosing regimen, clinicians need to make a careful assessment of patient-specific risks for confusion and dose errors, associated costs, practicality of dose adjustment, and patient preference.

An average maintenance dose approximates 4.5 mg/day (31.5 mg/week), but the range can vary widely from less than 1 mg/day to 20 mg/day or more among patients in the same therapeutic range. Older patients might have a more pronounced response to warfarin and require closer surveillance.[5–9]

Common sense prevails when applying the 10% rule of thumb for dose adjustments. For example, in an elderly patient using a 1-mg tablet daily (total weekly dose, 7 mg), 10% of this relatively small weekly total might be too sharp a change and an approximate 5% adjustment makes more clinical sense. To effect a change to 6.5 mg/week, a suggested dose instruction (using 1-mg tablets) is ½ tablet on Wednesday and 1 tablet on the remaining days of the week. On the other hand, a 50-year-old man with persistent subtherapeutic INRs, who is using a 10-mg tablet daily, might require a 20% increment in weekly dose, rather than 10%. Dose instructions (using a 10-mg tablet) in this case would be 1½ tablets on Monday, Wednesday, and Friday and 1 tablet on the remaining days of the week, for a new weekly total of 85 mg.

In general, once a dose has been adjusted, allow two weeks before scheduling the next prothrombin time (PT). For a patient with an INR slightly above or below the intended therapeutic range, the dose should not be adjusted based on this single, isolated occurrence. Better success at maintaining a stable dose can be achieved by repeating the INR in another week, and, if it is still nontherapeutic, a dose adjustment at this point would be prudent. Mildly elevated INRs generally respond to withholding warfarin for 1 or 2 days, repeating the INR, and resuming at the same or slightly lower dose. Again, the next INR should be rescheduled in two weeks whenever a mild dose adjustment has been implemented.

Instructions to patients must be clear, concise, and simple. Written instructions following oral or telephone instructions can help to ensure accurate dose administration. Several anticoagulation programs use a reminder card at the time of a visit or mail a postcard to the patient's home with dose instructions. Examples of dosing algorithms and other management aids are located in Appendix 31A.

INR Monitoring

The frequency of INR monitoring changes over time, as dictated by dose response and current clinical information. The INR is usually performed daily until the therapeutic INR range is achieved and maintained for at least two consecutive days. Weekly testing is usually required during the next 2–3 weeks; even more frequent testing is warranted if a stable dose is not evident. Increased monitoring is required when factors known to alter anticoagulation response occur or if nontherapeutic INRs are received. Caution is recommended against frequently adjusting warfarin doses for patients with slightly out-of-range results. Repeating the INR within a week will often provide information on whether or not to initiate a dose change.

Performing PT tests at intervals of four weeks is recommended for a patient who achieves a stable dose and response. Clinical experience, however, shows that the mean interval for PT testing in many AMSs is between two and three weeks. The American Heart Association recommends a maximum duration between testing for safe monitoring at four-week intervals,[10] which is consistent with the recommendations of the American College of Chest Physicians in its most recent consensus report.[11]

Other Factors To Optimize Management

Clinicians are often challenged as they strive to manage their patients' anticoagulation therapy and achieve good outcomes. Additional factors from those discussed above (physiologic, pharmacologic, and social) also affect the attainment of this goal.[12] Interventions designed to provide an organized, consistent approach to patient management ultimately lead to successful outcomes.[13] The formation of anticoagulation management services or clinics, as a model of care delivery, has made a positive impact on cost-effectiveness and the quality of patient care and outcomes.[14–16]

The development and testing of computerized programs aids clinicians in many aspects of clinic management. Some programs attempt to extend the testing interval,[17–19] whereas others support more frequent INR testing.[20] Fihn et al[18] describe the collective experience of five anticoagulation clinics in which patients were randomly assigned to a computer-guided intervention or traditional management group. The interval between PT tests for the control group was 3.5 weeks as compared to 4.4 weeks for patients in the computer-driven intervention group. Clinically important bleeding rates were not significantly different between groups; however, the intensity of therapy was better managed in the computerized group. Only 15% of the bleeding episodes in the intervention group had PT ratios greater than 2.0, whereas nearly 50% of patients with bleeding episodes in the control group had PT ratios over 2.0. Skordis and Whitehead[19] implemented a computerized management system in an anticoagulation clinic and also found a significant increase in the time interval between blood tests from 2.6 to 3.6 weeks after the computer program was begun. Although the computerized management system did not significantly impact the INR performance, improvement in other aspects of patient management in the clinic were reported.

In contrast to these data, recent work has suggested that more frequent INR testing is the key to maintaining maximum control on the patient's response to therapy and will lead to better outcomes. The underlying premise is that if more time is spent in therapeutic range, then the opportunity for adverse events is minimized. A report in which patients performed self-testing every 2–4 days seemed to achieve great success by reportedly being in range 89% of the observed time.[20] Patient self-testing and self-management are potential factors to significantly improve warfarin management.

An important, but often time-consuming function of an AMS is tracking patient compliance with monitoring. For example, the determination of whether or not a patient obtained a PT test on the date scheduled is essential and must be part of the overall monitoring plan. Computerized applications assist clinicians by organizing, and perhaps automating, time-consuming patient tracking and follow-up procedures. Computer applications can also aid patient surveillance strategies and monitor patient progress over time. Computerized automation of patient information greatly impacts the efficiency and organization of management, thereby resulting in improved quality of care.

Communicating critical information to patients in a timely fashion is another important factor to optimize management. Clinicians may have difficulty reaching patients within a relatively short time period to notify them of either dangerously elevated or low INRs. At the same time, they need to make an assessment of the patient's status and elicit information that may help to explain the current INR value. Maintaining an up-to-date list of emergency contact names and telephone numbers is essential for efficient operations and patient safety.

Results from several studies[21–24] demonstrate increased adverse events when the INR drifts out of therapeutic range. Dosing algorithms and protocols have been used for many years and the superiority of these dosing applications has been documented in clinical trials.[25–27]

PATIENT INVOLVEMENT FOR SUCCESSFUL THERAPY

Implementing a system of periodic checks and periodic quality control indicators will not guarantee success unless the patient is involved and actively participates in the prescribed therapy. Open dialogue between the patient and health care provider is vital to the program's success. The patient should clearly understand the importance of the anticoagulation program, and other health care providers should encourage and foster the development of communication among the anticoagulation monitoring team. The anticoagulation monitor should be clearly identified, and the significance of this role emphasized to the patient in order to enhance communication with other providers involved in the patient's care. Written guidelines are useful, but they can never replace individual case-by-case assessment.

Interventions designed to help patients remember daily doses will enhance the opportunity for success. For example, patients are traditionally taught to take their warfarin in the evening. Although this arrangement allows time for the clinician to telephone and implement dose changes during the same day of the INR test, with some patients it provides the opportunity for potential errors in terms of missed or forgotten doses at that late time of day. In some cases, instructions to take warfarin in the morning might be a better alternative. Therefore, exceptions to the traditional routine are warranted to improve patient adherence to medication instructions.

Challenging Patient Situations—The Noncompliant Patient

Another aspect of management is the issue of managing difficult or challenging patients. In some cases, these patients may exhaust all available options and the difficult decision to terminate them from the AMS is made. To avoid future litigation, a complete record of patient/provider interactions must be thoroughly documented. This documentation should include:

- the patient's indication for therapy and therapeutic plan
- a summary of the patient's understanding of the treatment plan, risks, and benefits
- an assessment of educational needs, teaching plan, and reinforcement of same
- interventions and techniques attempted thus far
- attempts and methods to communicate with patient
- contact with primary care provider apprising of situation and requesting assistance

Searching out a family member or significant other for aid may also be of help. In the end, patients bear responsibility for their own care, and if the risks of therapy now outweigh the potential benefits, then the difficult situation to withdraw therapy is considered.

Many clinics utilize a tiered-cascade of written reminders or warning letters to communicate with the patient during this process. Each tier of the cascade contains more strongly worded warnings and consequences. With persistent absence or no positive action, a final termination-from-clinic letter is warranted. The structure of each letter needs to be individualized and should capitalize on the opportunity to further educate the patient about his or her medical condition and the potential dangerous consequences of his or her actions.

Many clinics follow the general parameters listed below to suspect a patient from services:

1. AMS director informed of the "challenging" patient, including clinical history, anticoagulation history, initial interventions by AMS staff
2. Patient contacted in writing of failure to comply with clinic standards (may opt to repeat, verify address, or use alternate address)
3. primary care provider contacted for additional assistance
4. patient contacted, in writing, via certified, guaranteed delivery service with request for receipt
5. final termination letter sent, via certified, guaranteed delivery service with request for receipt
6. documentation in patient's medical record of above actions.

All supporting documents should remain with the patient's AMS records and a detailed note should be placed in the patient's medical record. The multifaceted issues relative to patient compliance are further discussed in Chapter 39, The Challenges and Opportunities of Anticoagulation Compliance.

CONCLUSION

Experienced managers of warfarin therapy agree that patients for whom stable maintenance doses cannot be easily reached present real challenges. A detailed assessment of factors known to affect the pharmacodynamics and pharmacokinetics of warfarin often uncover the cause of instability or lead to further exploration. Because of warfarin's narrow therapeutic margin, the potential consequences of nontherapeutic INRs can be serious. Chronic anticoagulation requires persistent surveillance and high levels of organization for effective patient monitoring throughout the course of therapy. Utilizing computer technology can help in patient management and further improve safety, utilization, and clinical outcomes. Continued efforts in research will determine future refinements for anticoagulant-related protocols for dosing strategies and PT scheduling. AMSs are continually developing and providing improved monitoring systems to optimize patient care.

REFERENCES

1. Goldhaber SZ. Outpatient monitoring of anticoagulation. *Forum.* 1994;15:14–15.

2. Harrison L, Johnston M, Massicotte MP, et al. Comparison of 5 mg and 10 mg loading doses in initiation of warfarin therapy. *Ann Intern Med.* 1997;126:133–136.

3. Landefeld CS, Rosenblatt MW, Goldman L. Bleeding in outpatients treated with warfarin: relation to the prothrombin time and important remediable lesions. *Am J Med.* 1989;87:153–159.

4. Wong W, Wilson Norton J, Wittkowsky AK. Influence of warfarin regimen type on clinical and monitoring outcomes in stable patients in an anticoagulation management service. *Pharmacother.* 1999;19 (12):1385–1391.

5. Gurwitz JH, Avorn J, Ross-Degnan D, Choodnovsky I, Ansell J. Aging and the anticoagulant response to warfarin therapy. *Ann Intern Med.* 1992;116:901–904.

6. Fihn SD, Callahan CM, Martin DC, McDonell MB, Henikoff JG, White RH. The risk for and severity of bleeding complications in elderly patients treated with warfarin. *Ann Intern Med.* 1996;124: 970–979.

7. Mungall D, White R. Aging and warfarin therapy. *Ann Intern Med.* 1992;117:878–879.

8. McCormick D, Gurwitz JH, Goldberg J, et al. Long-term anticoagulation therapy for atrial fibrillation in elderly patients: efficacy, risk and current patterns of use. *J Thromb Thrombolysis.* 1999;7: 157–163.

9. James AH, Britt RP, Raskino CL, et al. Factors affecting the maintenance dose of warfarin. *J Clin Pathol.* 1992;45:704–706.

10. Hirsh J, Fuster V. Guide to anticoagulant therapy, II: oral anticoagulants. *Circulation.* 1994;89:1469–1480.

11. Hirsh J, Dalen JE, Anderson DR, et al. Oral anticoagulants: mechanism of action, clinical effectiveness, and optimal therapeutic range. *Chest.* 2001;119(suppl):8S–21S.

12. Ansell J, Hirsh J, Dalen J, et al. Managing oral anticoagulant therapy. *Chest.* 2001;119(suppl):22S–38S.

13. Landefeld CS, Anderson PA. Guideline-based consultation to prevent anticoagulant-related bleeding: a randomized, controlled trial in a teaching hospital. *Ann Intern Med.* 1992;116:829–837.

14. Cortelazzo S, Finazzi G, Viero P, et al. Thrombotic and hemorrhagic complications in patients with mechanical heart valve prosthesis attending an anticoagulation clinic. *Thromb Haemost.* 1993;69: 316–320.

15. Wilt VM, Gums JG, Ahmed OT, et al. Pharmacy operated anticoagulation service: improved outcomes in patient on warfarin. *Pharmacother.* 1995;15:732–779.

16. Chiquette E, Amato MG, Bussey HI. Comparison of an anticoagulation clinic and usual medical care: anticoagulation control. Patient outcomes, and health care costs. *Arch Intern Med.* 1998;158:1641–1647.

17. Kent DL, Vermes D, McDonell MB, et al. A model for planning optimal follow-up for outpatients on warfarin anticoagulation. *Med Decis Making.* 1992;12:132–141.

18. Fihn SD, McDonell MB, Vermes D, et al. A computerized intervention to improve timing of outpatient follow-up: a multicenter randomized trial in patients treated with warfarin. *J Gen Intern Med.* 1994;9: 131–139.

19. Skordis CM, Whitehead S. Computerized management of an oral anticoagulant clinic. *Aust NZ J Med.* 1992;22:496–497.

20. Horstkotte D, Piper C, Wiemer M. Optimal frequency of patient monitoring and intensity of oral anticoagulation therapy in valvular heart disease. *J Thromb Thrombolysis.* 1998;5:S19–S24.

21. Hylek EM, Singer DE. Risk factors for intracranial hemorrhage in outpatients taking warfarin. *Ann Intern Med.* 1994;120:897–902.

22. Cannegieter SC, Rosendaal FR, Wintzen AR, et al. The optimal intensity of oral anticoagulant therapy in patients with mechanical heart valve prostheses: the Leiden artificial valve and anticoagulation study. *N Engl J Med.* 1995;333:11–17.

23. ASPECT Research Group. Effect of long-term oral anticoagulant treatment on mortality and cardiovascular morbidity after myocardial infarction. *Lancet.* 1994;343:499–503.

24. Stroke Prevention in Reversible Ischemia Trial (SPIRIT) study group. A randomized trial of anticoagulants versus aspirin after cerebral ischemia of presumed arterial origin. *Ann Neurol.* 1997;42:857–865.

25. Poller L, Wright D, Rowlands M. Prospective comparative study of computer programs used for management of warfarin. *J Clin Pathol.* 1993;46:299–303.

26. Poller L, Chiach CR, MacCallum P, et al. The European concerted action on anticoagulation (ECAA): multicentre randomized study of computerized anticoagulant dosage. *Lancet.* 1998;352:1505–1509.

27. Geno W, Turpie AGG. A randomized comparison of a computer-based dosing program with a manual system to monitor oral anticoagulant therapy. *J Thromb Thrombolysis.* 1998;5(suppl):S69.

Management Tools for the Clinician (Suggested Therapeutic Guidelines, Decision-Making Nomograms, Sample Letters/Postcards To Assist Patient Management)

General Guidelines for INR Intensity Range, Dose Adjustments, and PT Scheduling

INR

A. 1. INR 2.0–3.0: most thromboembolic situations or prophylaxis.
   2. INR 2.5–3.5: mechanical prosthetic value and recurrent systemic embolism.

DOSE GUIDELINES

B. 1. 5 mg/day if patient is <75 years old and >110 lb; otherwise, begin 2.5 mg/day.
   2. If dose needs adjustment, increase or decrease by 10% of weekly dose.
   3. If first PT is slightly out of range, no change in dose and recheck in one week.
   4. Unless INR is very high, do not hold warfarin for more than two days.

PROTIME SCHEDULING

C. 1. PT weekly for stent patients. PT weekly for first month.
   2. Maximum length of time between tests: six to eight weeks for stable patients in range.
   3. Allow two weeks before next PT when making dose adjustments.
   4. Check PT frequently with changes in medications (eg, antibiotics, pain medication, and digoxin).
   5. For patients discharged from hospital or patients new on warfarin schedule, protime one week from discharge.
   6. Hemoglobin and hematocrit every six months.

D. 1. Whenever there's a question, call physician.

E. 1. _____ will be contact physician if patient's physician is not available.

Anticoagulation Clinic Guidelines

GENERAL INSTRUCTIONS

- Use 5-mg tablets when possible (occasionally, 2-mg tablets).
- When twice weekly, use on Wednesdays and Saturdays.
- When once weekly, use on Saturdays.
- Check PT once weekly for 4 weeks; then, if stable, every 10–14 days for three months. Then, if stable, check every two to four weeks. When a dose change is made, the PT should be rechecked in one week.
- If the INR is >6.0, notify the primary physician and the anticoagulation clinic physician. It might be advantageous to give a small dose of vitamin K subcutaneously. Hold for 2 days and recheck the PT. The patient needs to be informed about the significant risk of bleeding until the PT returns to the therapeutic range and to call at once or go to the emergency room if any significant bleeding occurs. These instructions should be documented in the chart.

STARTING WARFARIN AS AN OUTPATIENT

If the patient is under age 70 and over 60 kg, give 5 mg daily and check the PT in 4–6 days. If over age 70 or under 60 kg, start with 2 mg tablets, giving 4 mg for 2 days followed by 2 mg daily and check the PT in 4–6 days.

ADJUSTMENT PROTOCOL: INR 2.0–3.0

INR	Adjustment
1.00–1.70	Extra dose 4–5 mg and increase by 2.0–2.5 mg twice weekly
1.71–2.00	Extra dose 2.0–2.5 mg and increase by 2.0–2.5 mg weekly
2.10–2.50	Continue same dose
2.51–3.00	Continue same dose or decrease by 2.0–2.5 mg weekly
3.10–4.50	Decrease by 2.0–2.5 mg weekly
4.51–6.00	Hold today and decrease by 2.0–2.5 mg twice weekly
>6.00	Hold 2 days, check patient and decrease by 2.0–2.5 mg three times weekly

ADJUSTMENT PROTOCOL: INR 2.5–3.5

INR	Adjustment
1.00–1.70	Extra dose 4.0–5.0 mg and increase by 2.0–2.5 mg three times weekly
1.71–2.00	Extra dose 4.0–5.0 mg and increase by 2.0–2.5 mg twice weekly
2.10–2.50	Extra dose 4.0–5.0 mg and increase by 2.0–2.5 mg weekly
2.51–3.00	Continue same dose
3.10–3.50	Continue same dose or decrease by 2.0–2.5 mg weekly
3.51–4.50	Decrease dose by 2.0–2.5 mg weekly
4.51–6.00	Hold today and decrease by 2.0–2.5 mg once weekly
>6.00	Hold 2 days, check PT and decrease by 2.0–2.5 mg twice weekly

Patients on warfarin doses of 10 mg or more or 2 mg or less per day will need more or less, respectively, of a change in dose than per protocol.

Warfarin Dosage Guidelines

1. If the International Normalized Ratio (INR) is less than 1.5, may increase warfarin dosage by up to 5.0 mg daily.

2. If the INR is greater than 1.5 but falling, may increase warfarin dosage up to 2.5 mg daily.

3. If the INR is less than 4.0 but rising, may decrease the warfarin dosage by up to 2.5 mg daily.

4. If the INR is greater than 4.0 but less than 5.0, may stop warfarin for up to two days and then reduce dose.

5. If the INR is greater than 5.0 with no evidence of bleeding, stop warfarin, monitor the INF, and proceed as above. If the INR is greater than 6.0 or if there is a question of bleeding, consultation with attending physician.

Courtesy of Coumadin Clinic, Veterans Affairs Medical Center, Albuquerque, NM.

Protocol for Regulating Warfarin

INTRODUCTION

This protocol allows a nurse-practitioner (NP) to adjust warfarin dosage within the protocol guidelines. The NP may write prescriptions to renew warfarin through the hospital pharmacy. The protocol does not allow NPs to initiate warfarin therapy.

RECOMMENDED THERAPEUTIC RANGE FOR ORAL ANTICOAGULANT THERAPY

Indication	INR
Prophylaxis of venous thrombosis (high-risk surgery)	
Treatment of venous thrombosis	
Treatment of pulmonary embolism	
Prevention of systemic embolism	
– tissue heart valves	
– biosynthetic prosthetic heart valves	2.0–3.0
– acute myocardial infarction (to prevent systemic embolism)	
– valvular heart disease	
– atrial fibrillation	
– recurrent systemic embolism	
Mechanical prosthetic valves (high risk)	2.5–3.5

FREQUENCY OF PROTHROMBIN TIME

The PT will be checked about once every month by the hospital laboratory. The interval between PT laboratory checks can be extended to longer intervals of six to eight weeks for selected patients with stable control. Other local laboratory arrangements can be made on an individual basis.

A patient with frequent recurrent courses of antibiotics (other than trimethoprim and sulfamethoxazole, metronidazole, and erythromycin) and previously documented lack of INR change with same antibiotic and no other health status or medication changes need *not* have PT rechecked sooner than routinely scheduled follow-up.

After discharge from hospitalizations longer than two days, PT will be checked within one to two weeks, regardless of whether medications were adjusted while inpatient.

CHANGE DOSE

1. Low-intensity anticoagulation
   - INR <2: do approximately 10% increase in total weekly warfarin intake.
   - INR >3: do approximately 10% decrease in total weekly warfarin intake.
   - INR >3.0 <6.0: patients may be individually evaluated for need to hold warfarin for one or two doses in addition to the 10% or greater decrease.
2. High-intensity anticoagulation
   - INR <2.5: do approximately 10% increase in total weekly warfarin intake.
   - INR >3.5: do approximately 10% decrease in total weekly warfarin intake.
   - INR >3.5 and <6.0: the patient can be individually evaluated for need to hold warfarin for one or two doses in addition to the 10% dose decrease.

continues

Protocol for Regulating Warfarin continued

3. For INRs >6.0, a physician will be consulted as soon as possible and within 24 hours. The following recommendations will be evaluated by the physician:
   - If the INR is above 6.0 but below 10.0 and the patient is not bleeding, or more rapid reversal is required because the patient requires elective surgery, then vitamin K_1 intravenously in a dose of 0.5–1 mg can be given with the expectation that a demonstrable reduction of the INR will occur at 8 hours, and many patients will be in the therapeutic range of 2.0–3.0 in 24 hours. If the INR is still too high at 24 hours, the dose of 0.5 mg can be repeated. Warfarin treatment then can be resumed at a lower dose. In patients with low risk of bleeding and INR between 6.0–8.0, oral or subcutaneous vitamin K, 1–2 mg, and withholding warfarin dose(s) can be used at physician's discretion.
   - If the INR is above 10.0 but below 20.0 and the patient is not bleeding, a higher dose of vitamin K of 3–5 mg intravenously should be given with the expectation that INR will be reduced substantially at 6 hours. The INR should be checked every 6–12 hours, and vitamin K then can be repeated if necessary. Consideration will be given to hospitalization of these patients.
   - If a rapid reversal of an anticoagulant effect is required because of serious bleeding or major warfarin overdose (eg, INR >20.0), vitamin K in a dose of 10 mg should be given by intravenous injection and the INR checked every 6 hours. Vitamin K might have to be repeated every 12 hours and supplemented with plasma transfusion or factor concentrate, depending on the urgency of the situation.
   - In case of life-threatening bleeding or serious warfarin overdose, replacement with factor concentrates is indicated, supplemented with intravenously given vitamin K, 10 mg, to be repeated as necessary depending on the INR.
   - If continued warfarin therapy is indicated after high doses of vitamin K administration, then heparin can be given until the effects of vitamin K have been reversed and the patient becomes responsive to warfarin.

The decision to recheck a questionable PT/INR prior to dosage adjustments can be made on an individual basis. For dose adjustments within the 10% change limit, the PT will be rechecked in 3–14 days. Once the INR is within the target range on two consecutive laboratory tests, the monthly surveillance schedule will be resumed.

MEDICATION INTERACTIONS

A physician is consulted prior to initiating or changing use of NSAIDs, trimethoprim and sulfamethoxazole, cholesterol-lowering agents, and other medications that have high potential for interactions. PT is rechecked in 5–14 days.

LABORATORY FOLLOW-UP

- PT level is checked every month.
- Urinalysis and serial stool guaiacs are checked once a year.
- Evaluation for melena, bruising, hematuria, or abnormalities in any of these laboratory tests will be brought to the physician's attention as soon as possible.
- Duration of anticoagulation will be determined in collaboration with the patient's physician.

continues

Protocol for Regulating Warfarin continued

PATIENT EDUCATION

Patient education is essential to assist in medication compliance and effectiveness. Each patient or caregiver

- will receive the warfarin patient education handouts
- will be able to report dosage to the nurse verbally
- will be able to state symptoms that might indicate dosage of warfarin that is too high
- will be informed of the need for the patient to wear medical alert identification
- will know how and whom to contact if there is a problem or questions regarding anticoagulation medication
- will be offered the opportunity to view a film on the use of warfarin in the hospital library
- will be offered a pillbox

Physician signature: _____

Key: INR, International Normalized Ratio; PT, prothrombin time.

Courtesy of Red Primary Care Team, Veterans Affairs Medical Center, Salt Lake City, UT.

Patient Assessment Nomogram Guidelines for Warfarin

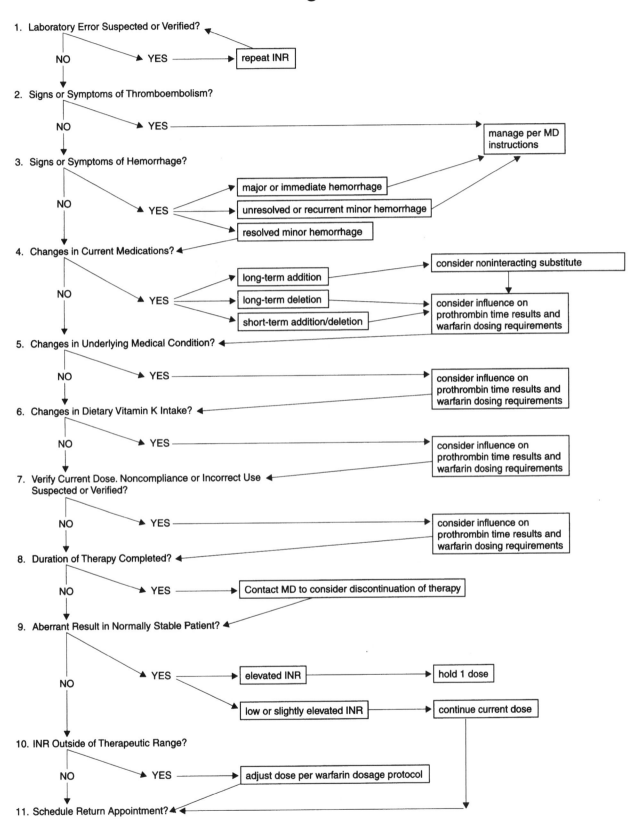

Courtesy of University of Washington, Seattle, WA.

Warfarin Dosage Protocol

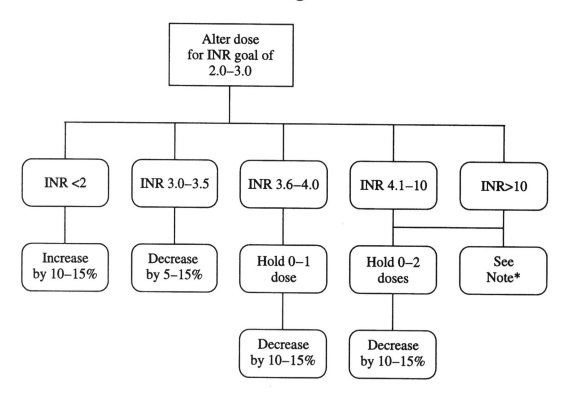

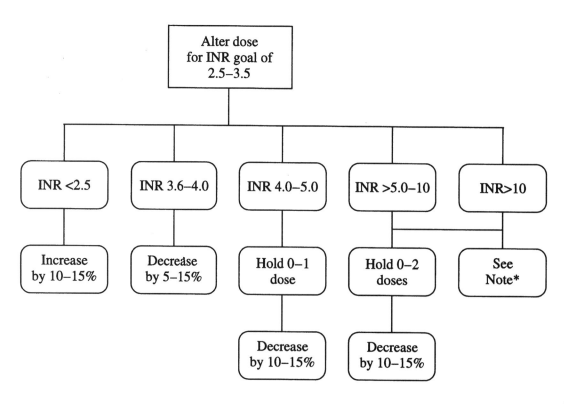

continues

Warfarin Dosage Protocol continued

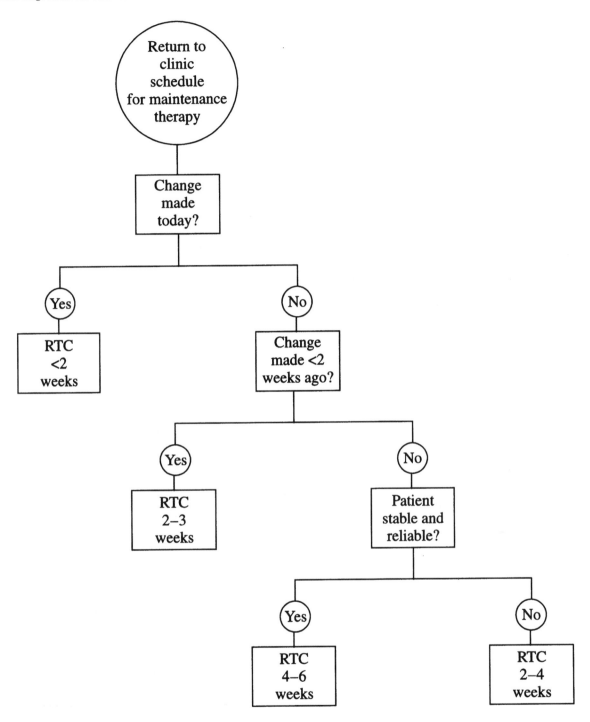

continues

Warfarin Dosage Protocol continued

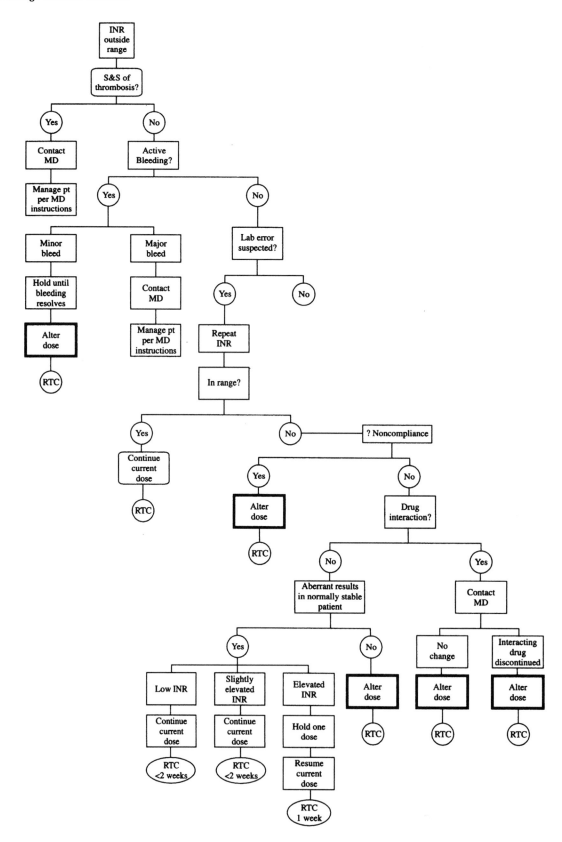

continues

Warfarin Dosage Protocol continued

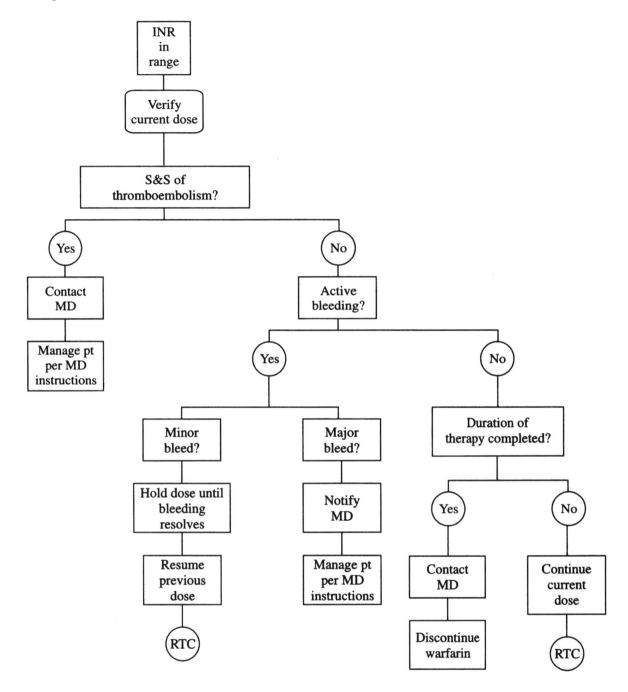

Key: INR, International Normalized Ratio; pt, patient; RTC, return to clinic; S&S, signs and symptoms.

*Note: See **Managing Excessive Prolongation of the International Normalized Ratio in the Outpatient Setting** in this Appendix.

Courtesy of Anticoagulation Clinic, University of Washington Medical Center, Seattle, WA.

Optimal Therapeutic Range and Duration of Warfarin Therapy

Indication	Target INR Range	Duration	Comment
ATRIAL FIBRILLATION (AF)			
Age < 65/no risk factors	None	Chronic	Use aspirin alone
Age < 65 years with risk factors for stroke	2.5 (2.0–3.0)	Chronic	
[hx TIA/stroke/TE; HTN, CHF, ↓ LV fxn; rheumatic mitral valve dz; valve replacement, diabetes, CAD; thyrotoxicosis]			
Age 65–75/no risk factors	2.5 (2.0–3.0)	Chronic	or aspirin
Age 65–75 with risk factors	2.5 (2.0–3.0)	Chronic	
Age > 75	2.5 (2.0–3.0)	Chronic	
precardioversion (AF or flutter > 48 hours in duration)	2.5 (2.0–3.0)	3 weeks	
postcardioversion (in NSR)	2.5 (2.0–3.0)	4 weeks	
CARDIOEMBOLIC STROKE			
With risk factors for stroke	2.5 (2.0–3.0)	Chronic	
[AF, CHF, LV dysfxn; mural thrombus, hx TIA/stroke/TE]			
Following embolic event despite anticoagulation	2.5 (2.0–3.0)	Chronic	Add antiplatelet therapy
LEFT VENTRICULAR DYSFUNCTION (LV DSYFXN)			
Ejection fraction < 30%	2.5 (2.0–3.0)	Chronic	
Transient, following myocardial infarction	2.5 (2.0–3.0)	3 months	
Following embolic event despite anticoagulation	2.5 (2.0–3.0)	Chronic	Add antiplatelet therapy
MYOCARDIAL INFARCTION (MI)			
Following anterior MI	2.5 (2.0–3.0)	3 months	
Following inferior MI with transient risk(s)	2.5 (2.0–3.0)	3 months	
[AF; CHF, LV dysfxn, mural thrombus, hx TE]			
Following initial tx with persistent risks	2.5 (2.0–3.0)	Chronic	
THROMBOEMBOLISM (DVT, PE)			
Treatment/prevention of recurrence			
Transient risk factors	2.5 (2.0–3.0)	3–6 months	
Idiopathic	2.5 (2.0–3.0)	6 months	
Persistent risk factors	2.5 (2.0–3.0)	Chronic	
[AT-III, protein C, protein S deficiencies; factor V Leiden; malignancy]			
Antiphospholipid antibody syndrome	3.0 [2.5–3.5]	Chronic	higher range may be required
Following recurrent DVT/PE	2.5 (2.0–3.0)	Chronic	
VALVULAR DISEASE			
Aortic valve disease	2.5 (2.0–3.0)	Chronic	
with mitral valve disease, AF, or hx systemic embolization			
Mitral annular calcification	2.5 (2.0–3.0)	Chronic	
with AF or hx systemic embolization			
Mitral valve prolapse:			
With AF or hx systemic embolization	2.5 (2.0–3.0)	Chronic	
With history of TIA despite ASA therapy	2.5 (2.0–3.0)	Chronic	
S/p embolic event despite anticoagulation	2.5 (2.0–3.0)	Chronic	Add antiplatelet tx
Rheumatic mitral valve disease:			
With AF, hx systemic embolization, LA > 5.5cm	2.5 (2.0–3.0)	Chronic	
S/p embolic event despite anticoagulation	2.5 (2.0–3.0)	Chronic	Add antiplatelet tx
VALVE REPLACEMENT—BIOPROSTHETIC			
Aortic or mitral	2.5 [2.0–3.0]	3 months	Followed by aspirin
with LA thrombus	2.5 [2.0–3.0]	> 3 months	Followed by aspirin
With history systemic embolism	2.5 [2.0–3.0]	3–12 months	Followed by aspirin
With AF	2.5 [2.0–3.0]	Chronic	
Following systemic embolism	2.5 [2.0–3.0]	Chronic	Add aspirin
VALVE REPLACEMENT—MECHANICAL			
Aortic			
Bileaflet			
In NSR, nl EF, nl LA size	2.5 (2.0–3.0)	Chronic	
All others	3.0 (2.5–3.5)	Chronic	*Or 2.0–3.0 plus aspirin 81 mg*
Tilting disk	3.0 (2.5–3.5)	Chronic	*Or 2.0–3.0 plus aspirin 81 mg*
Ball and cage	3.0 (2.5–3.5)	Chronic	With aspirin
Mitral	3.0 (2.5–3.5)	Chronic	
Bileaflet	3.0 (2.5–3.5)	Chronic	*Or 2.0–3.0 plus aspirin 81 mg*
Tilting disk	3.0 (2.5–3.5)	Chronic	*Or 2.0–3.0 plus aspirin 81 mg*
Ball and cage	3.0 (2.5–3.5)	Chronic	With aspirin
With additional risk factors or following TE	3.0 (2.5–3.5)	Chronic	Add aspirin

Note: hx, history; TIA, transient ischemic attack; TE, thromboembolism; HTN, hypertension; CHF, congestive heart failure; ↓, lowered; LV, left ventricular; fxn, function; dz, disease; CAD, coronary artery disease; AF, atrial fibrillation; NSR, normal sinus rhythm; MI, myocardial infarction; dysfxn, dysfunction; tx, treatment; DVT, deep venous thrombosis; PE, pulmonary embolism; ASA, aspirin; s/p, status post; LA, left atrium; nl, normal; EF, ejection fraction.

*In patients with risks for hemorrhage.

Courtesy of University of Washington Medical Center, Seattle, WA.

Patient Treatment Guidelines from the Thrombosis Interest Group

WARFARIN AND VITAMIN K–DEPENDENT FACTORS

The molecular structures of clotting factors VII, IX, X, and II are modified by an enzymatic system in the presence of vitamin K. This is an essential step in the activation of these factors.

The activation of the coagulation factors will ultimately lead to the formation of thrombin—the key enzyme that produces fibrin, an essential component in thrombus formation.

Warfarin will inhibit thrombin formation by interfering with vitamin K metabolism. The degree of inhibition will depend on the treatment intensity.

MONITORING

The prothrombin time (PT) is the most commonly used test to monitor oral anticoagulant therapy.

The PT should be reported using the International Normalized Ratio (INR). By using the INR, monitoring of warfarin is simplified and its safety is improved by the standardization of the therapeutic range irrespective of the thromboplastin reagent used. Many laboratories now report INRs.

The INR is calculated from the observed PT using the formula:

$$INR = \left(\frac{Patient's\,PT}{Mean\,of\,PT\,of\,normal\,range\,in\,seconds} \right)^{ISI}$$

The ISI is the International Sensitivity Index for a given reagent. The mean of the normal range should be calculated by obtaining the mean of a minimum of 20 patients' PTs, with the PT determined with the laboratory's individual thromboplastin. This calculation is done by the laboratory.

PRACTICAL TIPS

- Obtain baseline INR, PTT.
- Initiate warfarin with expected maintenance, dose, 4 or 5 mg/day.
- Check INR.
- Monitor potential side effects.

The occasional patient might show extreme sensitivity.

If the results are marginally above or below the range and the patient is not bleeding, do not overreact. Repeat PT test in three days. Then, if results are still outside the range, adjust dosage accordingly:

- If no bleeding—INR above 6.0
  - withhold warfarin for one day
  - consider small doses of vitamin K (eg, 1 mg)
  - monitor patient's INR closely

continues

Patient Treatment Guidelines continued

- If rapid reversal is required because of serious bleeding or INR > 20.0
  - administer IV vitamin K, 10 mg
  - check patient's INR every 6 hours
  - vitamin K might have to be repeated every 12 hours and supplemented with plasma transfusion depending on the urgency of reversal

THERAPEUTIC RANGE

Once a stable anticoagulation level is reached, patients should be maintained within an INR range of 2.0–3.0 except for mechanical prosthetic valve replacement, where an INR range of 2.5–3.5 is recommended.

Because the half-lives of coagulation factors vary from 6 to 72 hours and the half-life of warfarin is 2.5 days, changes made to the dosage will not be reflected in the INR value completely until day 3 or 4. Order tests accordingly.

The initiation/stopping of concomitant therapies should result in more frequent monitoring of the PT, especially in regard to antibiotic therapy. Follow Practical Tips.

WARNING TO PATIENTS

- No IM injections.
- No ASA, NSAIDs without consultation.
- No contact sports—but otherwise normal activities.
- Moderate alcohol intake is not harmful but excessive alcohol intake (bingeing) is.
- Significant changes in diet should be reported and PT monitored.
- Consult physician or pharmacist before taking any over-the-counter medication.

PREGNANCY

If anticoagulation is necessary during pregnancy, heparin is the treatment of choice. Warfarin should not be used. It crosses the placenta and causes embryopathy, CNS abnormalities, and fetal bleeding. Women planning to become pregnant should avoid warfarin therapy. Women who become pregnant while on warfarin therapy should notify the physician immediately.

THE PRODUCTS

Warfarin is available as Coumadin and Warfilone. They are not interchangeable. Coumadin is available in six dosage forms: 1-, 2-, 2.5-, 4-, 5-, and 10-mg tablets, each having a different color.
Warfilone is available in 5-mg tablets.

continues

ADVERSE EFFECTS

Bleeding is the most important complication of anticoagulant therapy. The intensity of anticoagulation, the concomitant use of ASA and NSAIDs, and the underlying clinical disorder are factors influencing the risk of bleeding.

Skin rash and alopecia are uncommon adverse effects and can be managed by changing oral anticoagulants.

Skin necrosis is a rare complication and usually appears within a few days of the start of oral anticoagulation therapy.

DRUG INTERACTIONS

There are many factors, alone or in combination, that can affect the anticoagulant response. In some instances, the net effect of warfarin on anticoagulant response might be unpredictable. For these reasons, it is imperative to monitor the patient's response when other medications are initiated or discontinued and to modify the dosage of warfarin accordingly.

THROMBOSIS INTEREST GROUP

The Thrombosis Interest Group (TIG) is dedicated to furthering education and research in the prevention and treatment of thrombosis.

The group consists of Canadian health care professionals from medicine, nursing, and laboratory technology whose primary interest is investigation and management of thromboembolic disease. The TIG is involved in clinical research, various educational activities, has a fellowship program, and represents a source of information for the medical community.

This material is part of a series of practical treatment guidelines developed to help the clinician keep abreast on the newest ways of managing thromboembolic disease. Developed by TIG members, it is based on medical literature and on current Canadian medical practice. The brochure will be revised and reprinted as new clinical information becomes available.

Key: ASA, acetylsalicylic acid; CNS, central nervous system; IM, intramuscular; IV, intravenous; NSAIDs, nonsteroidal anti-inflammatory drugs; PTT, partial thromboplastin time.

Managing Excessive Prolongation of the International Normalized Ratio in the Outpatient Setting

INR	Recommendation
4–6	Omit one or more doses of warfarin; consider reduced dose.
6–10	Hold warfarin until INR is therapeutic, then reinstitute at a reduced dose.
10–20	Consider vitamin K, 0.5–2.0 mg*; check INR in 12–24 hours and repeat vitamin K if necessary; reinstitute warfarin at a reduced dose.
>20	Consider vitamin K, 1.0–5.0 mg*; close observation and consider fresh-frozen plasma depending on degree of INR elevation and specific patient risks for bleeding; reinstitute warfarin at lower dose when INR becomes therapeutic.

Note: Serious bleeding requires the use of fresh-frozen plasma to replace missing factors and parenteral vitamin K*; factor concentrates may be considered in life-threatening or intracranial hemorrhage.

*Because of the potential for hypersensitivity reaction or anaphylaxis to intravenous vitamin K, it should be given slowly (not >1 mg/min); alternatively, it can be given by the subcutaneous route or orally, but response might be delayed if absorption is impaired. Vitamin K can lead to a brief period of relative warfarin resistance and difficulty in reestablishing a therapeutic range; higher doses of warfarin may be needed, but frequent monitoring is imperative.

Courtesy of Boston University Medical Center Anticoagulation Clinic, Boston, MA.

Anticoagulation Center Procedure for Oral Vitamin K Administration

Patients with an INR > 6.0 and < 10.0 who are not actively bleeding may receive oral vitamin K to decrease the INR and lower the risk of bleeding. By administering oral vitamin K and withholding Coumadin, the INR will fall into a safe range in approximately 24 hours. Administration of oral vitamin K in the clinic setting decreases emergency room visits for subcutaneous vitamin K administration. In addition, oral vitamin K does not completely reverse Coumadin and therefore does not make patients Coumadin resistant. Patients with signs and/or symptoms of active bleeding are not candidates for oral vitamin K and should be seen in the emergency department.

1. The patient's physician will be immediately notified by a pharmacist if the INR is > 6.

2. A patient having an INR > 6.0 and < 10.0 without signs and/or symptoms of bleeding is a potential candidate for oral vitamin K administration.

3. A verbal order from the patient's referring physician for oral vitamin K administration will be taken by the pharmacist and recorded on the designated log sheet. Should the referring physician be unable to be contacted, the covering physician or the medical director of the clinic will be contacted.

4. The log sheet data are to include the following information:
   –patient name and medical record number
   –date and time
   –INR result
   –vitamin K dose, lot, and expiration date
   –name of physician authorizing the verbal order
   –name or initials of pharmacist administering the vitamin K
   –follow-up INR and the date follow-up performed

5. The single dose of vitamin K 2.5 mg orally will then be administered to the patient while in clinic.

6. The patient will return to clinic the following business day for a recheck of the INR.

Courtesy of Lutheran General Hospital-Advocate Health Care, Park Ridge, Illinois.

Management of No-Shows

I. The patient is responsible for rescheduling all missed appointments.
II. The first time a patient misses a scheduled appointment:
    A. The patient will be notified by telephone.
    B. Another appointment will be scheduled.
    C. A note will be written in the progress notes of the patient's chart stating that the appointment was missed.
III. The second time a patient misses a scheduled appointment:
    A. The patient will be notified by telephone.
    B. Another appointment will be scheduled.
    C. A letter will be sent to the patient.
    D. A copy of above letter will be placed in the correspondence section of the patient's chart.
    E. A note will be written in the progress notes of the patient's chart stating that the appointment was missed.
IV. The third time a patient misses a scheduled appointment:
    A. The patient will be notified by telephone.
    B. Another appointment will be scheduled. The urgency and importance of this will be stressed.
    C. The program director will be notified.
    D. A letter co-signed by the program director will be sent to the patient's primary physician.
    E. A copy of above letter will be placed in the correspondence section of the patient's chart.
    F. A letter will be sent to the patient.
    G. A copy of above letter will be placed in the correspondence section of the patient's chart.
    H. A note will be written in the progress notes of the patient's chart stating that the appointment was missed, and that the program director and the primary physician were notified.
V. The fourth time a patient misses a scheduled appointment:
    A. The patient will be notified by telephone. The patient will be told that a letter will be sent by certified mail. If the patient fails to respond after letter sent, then patient will be terminated from the anticoagulation program.
    B. A letter signed by the program director outlining alternative forms of care will be sent via certified mail.
    C. A copy of above letter will be placed in the correspondence section of the patient's chart.
    D. A note will be written in the progress notes of the patient's chart stating that the appointment was missed, and that a letter was sent via certified mail.
VI. If the patient has not contacted the office within 10 working days:
    A. The program director will be notified.
    B. A letter will be sent to the patient's primary physician stating that the patient has been terminated from the anticoagulation program.
    C. A termination note will be written in the progress notes of the patient's chart.

Courtesy of Division of Internal Medicine, Anticoagulation Program, Thomas Jefferson University Hospital, Philadelphia, PA.

Initiation of Therapy Letter

Date _____

Dear _____:

Clinic No. _____

Your physician has requested that the _____ Clinic monitor and adjust your warfarin therapy. Please realize that there are potentially serious risks involved in taking warfarin without careful monitoring. To help ensure your safety, you are expected to share in the responsibility by following these four guidelines:

1. Regular blood testing of prothrombin time (PT) is usually done at _____ Clinic. In special circumstances, the testing can be done elsewhere if you agree to obtain the PT results and call us with them that day for warfarin adjustments.

2. Adjust your warfarin as instructed after each test.

3. Return for your regular PT test and clinic visit as directed. If the time is missed, notify us and be sure to come at the next available time.

4. Call us or your physician if any problems or questions arise regarding the warfarin treatment.

Thank you,

_____, RN

_____ CLINIC

Courtesy of Jacksonville Coumadin Clinic, Mayo Clinic, Jacksonville, Florida.

Anticoagulation Program Introduction Letter

Dear _____:

Welcome to the Anticoagulation Program! The Anticoagulation Program is a service directed by Dr _____ and staffed by registered nurses and pharmacists with specific knowledge in anticoagulation therapy. Oral anticoagulant care is managed under the supervision of physicians in the Department of Medicine.

CLINIC HOURS

Tuesday 12:00 PM to 4:00 PM
Friday 9:00 AM to 12:00 noon

Clinic visits are by appointment only. The PT (protime) test will be checked by fingerstick with a special machine that provides the results within a few seconds. Then, you will be seen by the nurse or the pharmacist.

FREQUENCY OF PT TESTING

The PT test will need to be checked one or two times a week until stable. The frequency of testing will be gradually decreased to every two weeks, then to every month. The test must be done at least once a month after therapy is stable. After a change in dose is made, you will be instructed to have the PT checked at least once a week until stable. These are only general guidelines applied to all our patients. The frequency of testing will also depend on other factors, such as your clinical condition and your physician's recommendations.

If you are unable to keep your appointment, please notify the office and reschedule. Failure to keep your appointments or to follow any of the instructions given to you might result in serious health risks and/or termination from the program.

Because we are only authorized to manage the anticoagulation part of your medical care, it is very important that you see your primary physician, as directed, for your medical needs. If you do not have a physician, we will be happy to refer you to a physician from our department.

We are happy to participate in your care, and we look forward to seeing you. Please feel free to call us if you have any questions or problems about your warfarin.

Our telephone number is _____ .

This is a 24-hour number. If you call after the business day, the answering service will answer and notify the physician on call, who will contact you.

Sincerely yours,

_____

Courtesy of Division of Internal Medicine, Anticoagulation Program, Thomas Jefferson University Hospital, Philadelphia, PA.

Monitoring Letter

Date _____

Dear Dr _____:

Your patient, _____, Clinic No. _____, was seen in the _____ Clinic for monitoring his or her warfarin therapy. Instructions were given concerning the potential risks and benefits of this medication and the need for blood testing, adjustment of dosage, and the patient's responsibility for compliance and reporting any possible side effects.

We will adjust the patient's warfarin dose to maintain a goal therapeutic INR range of _____.

The anticipated duration of therapy is _____ months *or* an indefinite period of time.

You will be contacted if there is a question regarding the appropriate level or duration of therapy, if more information is needed, or if there is a significant complication or noncompliance.

Contact us if there is any change in the warfarin orders or other medications, or if there are questions regarding the recommended duration or intensity of treatment.

Sincerely,

_____, MD

_____, RN

Courtesy of Jacksonville Coumadin Clinic, Mayo Clinic, Jacksonville, Florida.

Update Letter to Physician

Date _____

Dear Dr _____:

   Your patient, _____, was seen in the Anticoagulation Program on _____. Prothrombin time (PT) results were as follows:

PT: _____
PT Ratio: _____
INR: _____

   The current dose of warfarin is _____. The patient is due for a prothrombin time again on _____.

   If you require any further information regarding this patient's anticoagulation, please do not hesitate to contact us.

Sincerely,

_____RN

_____PharmD

_____MD

Courtesy of Division of Internal Medicine, Anticoagulation Program, Thomas Jefferson University Hospital, Philadelphia, PA.

Letter to Dentist: Planned Dental Procedure

Date:_____

To whom it may concern:

PT = _____sec   INR = _____

_____ is currently taking warfarin (Coumadin) for
_____(patient name)_____

_____ and is followed by the _____
_____(indication)_____
Anticoagulation Service. The patient has informed us that (s)he may undergo a dental procedure in the near future. Attached are review articles that may assist you in managing this patient.

It is **not necessary to discontinue or alter warfarin therapy** for patients receiving **routine dental cleanings or other low-risk dental procedures** such as restorations, endodontics, prosthetics, and minor periodontal therapy **provided** the patient is stable on warfarin therapy and has been tested within two (2) weeks of the dental procedure.

For procedures with a **moderate risk of hemorrhage,** such as tooth extractions, we recommend the use of local hemostatic agents and altering the warfarin therapy as follows:

- Patients at low to moderate risk for thromboembolism. We recommend discontinuing warfarin for 2 days prior to the procedure and reinstituting therapy the night following the procedure.
- Patients at high risk for thromboembolism. We recommend continuing warfarin at a lower level of anticoagulation intensity (INR 2.0–2.5) immediately prior to the procedure. Following the procedure, reinstitute the patient's previous "full-dose" warfarin therapy.

For procedures with a **high risk of hemorrhage,** please call _____ so that we can discuss a strategy for proper patient management.

Please remember that prophylactic antibiotics are recommended to prevent bacterial endocarditis for patients with a prosthetic heart valve, valvular heart disease, or hypertrophic cardiomyopathy.

If you have any questions, contact me directly at _____ or page me at _____.

Most sincerely,

_____
Director, Anticoagulation Service

References: Wahl MJ. *Arch Intern Med.* 1998;158:1610–1616. Beirne OR, et al. *J Oral Maxillofac Surg.* 1996;54:1115–1118. Weibert R. *Clin Pharm.* 1992;11:857–864.

Reminder Card Presented to Patient during Appointment

Name _____ Date _____

Warfarin, _____-mg tablets   Protime _____

                                          INR _____

Number of tablets to take each date:

Monday _____ Friday _____

Tuesday _____ Saturday _____

Wednesday _____ Sunday _____

Thursday _____

Next appointment _____

_____, PharmD

Telephone _____

Courtesy of Anticoagulation Clinic, Royal C Johnson Memorial Hospital/Veterans Affairs, Sioux Falls, South Dakota.

Postcard Mailed to Patient with Dose Instructions

Your blood test from _____
was received.

Please take your warfarin as follows:
Number of pills per day
(using _____-mg size tablet):

Sun	Mon	Tues	Wed	Thurs	Fri	Sat
___	___	___	___	___	___	___

Patient Name _____

Address _____

_____

Your next blood test is on: _____

If you have any questions,
please call _____

Courtesy of Anticoagulant Therapy Unit, Massachusetts General Hospital, Boston, MA.

Postcard Notifying Patient of Test Results

Date _____

Dear _____ :

Your prothrombin time (PT) today resulted in an INR of _____ .

_____ Please continue your current dose of warfarin.

_____ Change your dose of warfarin to _____

using _____-mg tablets.

Thank you.

_____ RN

_____ Clinic

Telephone: _____

Courtesy of Jacksonville Coumadin Clinic, Jacksonville, Florida.

Anticoagulation Service Patient Instruction Form

TODAY's Test Result   DATE:_____

Your INR:_____   Your Goal:_____

Please take your warfarin (Coumadin) as follows:

_____ mg tablets

	SUN	MON	TUES	WED	THUR	FRI	SAT
tablets							

Special Instructions: _____

_____

_____

_____

Your next appointment is _____ at _____ PM. If you are unable to keep this appointment, call _____ to reschedule.

Unless otherwise instructed, we will see you at your next appointment. We will discuss the results of your blood test with you and ask a few questions at the time of your appointment. **You must stay in the clinic to be seen. DO NOT LEAVE THE CLINIC before being seen. Please arrive on time for your appointment. If you are late, we may not be able to see you.** Please bring **all** your medication bottles, including any over-the-counter medication you take regularly, with you.

Your health is our concern. Please follow the directions above carefully. Do not skip doses without our permission to do so. Do not take double doses.

_____

PharmD

_____

RN

Anticoagulation Service
(insert address and phone number)

Courtesy of University of Maryland, School of Pharmacy, Baltimore, MD.

Missing Blood Work Letter

Date _____

Dear _____:

Re: Warfarin therapy

There is a problem with your warfarin therapy. We have not been able to contact you and have not received any blood (prothrombin time) values recently.

We wish to notify you that unless the problem is resolved, we will no longer be able to share with you in the responsibility for your care. Please realize that there are potentially serious risks involved in taking warfarin without careful monitoring.

Please contact us as soon as possible.

Thank you,

_____, MD

_____, RN

Courtesy of Jacksonville Coumadin Clinic, Mayo Clinic, Jacksonville, Florida.

Overdue Reminder Letter

Date _____

Dear _____:

This is a reminder that you are due to have your PT (Protime test) checked. Please call us at _____ to schedule an appointment, or have your blood test checked at your usual laboratory. Thank you very much.

Sincerely,

_____RN

_____PharmD

_____MD

Courtesy of Division of Internal Medicine, Anticoagulation Program, Thomas Jefferson University Hospital, Philadelphia, PA.

Missed Appointment Letter
(Sent after Two or More Missed Appointments)

Date _____

Dear _____:

You had an appointment on _____ in the Anticoagulation (Coumadin) Clinic. You did not keep this appointment. I am concerned that you have missed your last _____ (number of missed appointments) appointments in our clinic. As you know, it is very important to obtain blood tests regularly to determine the effects of your Coumadin therapy. Without regular blood tests, it is impossible for you (or us) to know whether the dose of Coumadin is right for you. The amount of Coumadin that is safe and effective for you may change from time to time. Although it can protect you from getting harmful blood clots, Coumadin can be a dangerous medication if taken incorrectly.

I have scheduled your next appointment in the Anticoagulation Clinic for _____. If you are unable to keep this appointment, please call _____ as soon as possible to reschedule. If you are no longer taking Coumadin or someone else is following your Coumadin therapy, please let us know immediately.

If you do not keep your appointment on _____, I will not reschedule your appointment; it will be your responsibility to call us at _____ to make future appointments in the Anticoagulation Clinic. If you are unable to come to our clinic, it is very important that you obtain follow-up blood tests at a minimum of every 4 to 5 weeks through your primary care physician. If you have any questions or concerns, please call _____. Your good health and well-being is important to me.

Sincerely,

_____
Director, Anticoagulation Clinic

Courtesy of University of Maryland School of Pharmacy, Baltimore, MD.

Final Warning Reminder Letter

Date _____

Dear _____:

Unfortunately, you have not had your protime done as we have requested. We have attempted to contact you _____ times to remind you to have your protime checked.

As you know, warfarin can be a very dangerous medication if used improperly or if your protime is not checked regularly. We are not able to instruct you properly on your warfarin dosage without a recent prothrombin time test.

If your protime is too high, serious bleeding or hemorrhage can occur. If your protime is too low, blood clots can form and lead to heart attack, stroke, or pulmonary embolus (blood clot in the lung).

We are responsible for informing you when your protime should be checked, but it is up to you to follow through. We realize that it might be inconvenient for you to have repeated blood testing, but it is for your own safety.

This will be your last reminder from our clinic until we receive a protime result from your laboratory or you come in to the clinic for an appointment. If, because of unforeseen circumstances, you are unable to have your protime checked, please notify the office at _____.

Sincerely,

_____RN

_____PharmD

_____MD

Courtesy of Division of Internal Medicine, Anticoagulation Program, Thomas Jefferson University Hospital, Philadelphia, PA.

Noncompliance Letter

Date _____

Dear _____:

Re: Warfarin therapy

We regret to advise you that, as a result of your lack of cooperation in having blood work (prothrombin time) drawn for monitoring of your warfarin therapy, we will no longer share with you in the responsibility of management of this therapy. We are, therefore, advising you that we hereby withdraw from further attendance upon you.

Please realize that there are potentially serious risks involved with taking warfarin without careful monitoring. We feel that your warfarin therapy requires further care and monitoring and, accordingly, suggest that you take steps to place yourself under the care of another practitioner. In the event that an emergency arises before you have had the opportunity to engage a new physician, we, of course, will be available to you.

After thirty (30) days following the receipt of this letter, we shall expect that you will have placed yourself under the care of another physician.

Upon your written request and instructions, I should be happy to provide your new physician with the summary of the care and treatment provided to you, together with copies of any records your physician may require.

Sincerely,

_____

_____

cc:_____

Courtesy of Jacksonville Coumadin Clinic, Mayo Clinic, Jacksonville, Florida.

Chapter 32

Assessing Risk Factors for Bleeding

Rebecca J. Beyth

INTRODUCTION

Bleeding is the major complication of oral anticoagulant therapy and it is what limits its more widespread use. Varying criteria for bleeding severity across studies has hampered direct comparison of bleeding rates among studies. The major determinants of oral anticoagulant-related bleeding are the intensity of the anticoagulant effect, patient characteristics, concomitant use of drugs known to affect hemostasis, and the length of therapy. The risk for anticoagulant-related bleeding cannot be considered in isolation, and the potential benefits need to be weighed carefully in each individual patient, regardless of age.

INTENSITY OF ANTICOAGULANT EFFECT

The relationship between the intensity of the anticoagulant effect and the risk of major bleeding has been well established. Clinical trials of patients with venous thromboembolism,[1] tissue heart valves,[2] and mechanical heart valves[3,4] have shown a statistically and clinically significant reduction in the frequency of major and minor bleeding in patients receiving lower intensity therapy (International Normalized Ratio [INR] 2.0–3.0) compared to those randomly assigned to more intense warfarin therapy (INR >3.0). For example, among patients with proximal vein thrombosis, bleeding occurred in 4% of the less intensely treated group (2 major bleeds) compared to 22% of the more intensely anticoagu-

lated group (2 major bleeds, 9 minor bleeds).[1] Similarly, among patients with tissue heart valves,[2] bleeding complications were more frequent in the more intensely anticoagulated groups (5 major bleeds, 10 minor bleeds) compared to the lower intensity groups (6 major bleeds). Lower intensity anticoagulant therapy for mechanical heart valves also was associated with less bleeding. Saour et al[3] noted 0.95 major and 5.2 minor bleeding episodes per 100 patient years in lower intensity patients versus 2.1 major and 10.2 minor bleeding episodes per 100 patient years in the higher intensity patients. Altman et al[4] noted bleeding rates of 3.8% versus 20.8% among patients with mechanical heart valves with lower intensity and higher intensity anticoagulant therapy, respectively.

Similarly, randomized clinical trials of patients with atrial fibrillation have reported very low rates of major bleeding with less intense warfarin therapy. For example, the annual incidence of major bleeding averaged 1.3% in those patients randomly assigned to target INRs of 2.0 to 3.0 compared to 1.0% in those patients randomly assigned to placebo.[5] A target INR of 2.5 (range, 2.0–3.0) has been shown to minimize the risk of both major bleeding and thromboembolism in patients with atrial fibrillation.[6,7]

The intensity of anticoagulant effect is considered the most important risk factor for intracranial hemorrhage.[8] For each 0.5 increase in prothrombin time ratio (PTR), the risk for intracerebral hemorrhage doubled (odds ratio, 2.1; 95% confidence interval, 1.4 to 2.9). For subdural hemorrhage, the risk increased substantially with a PTR of 2.0 (INR = ~4.0). Also, increased variation in the anticoagulant effect, as indicated by variability in the INR, is associated with an increased frequency of bleeding independent of the mean INR.[9,10] Fihn and colleagues[9] noted that variability of the PTR over time was independently associated with the first episode of serious bleeding; relative risk for the highest compared to the lowest tertile, 1.6 (95% confidence interval, 1.2 to 2.7). Similarly, The Stroke Prevention in Atrial Fibrillation Investigators[10] noted in univariate analyses that PTR fluctuation was associated with warfarin-related bleeding. Age (P = .006), increasing the number of prescribed medications (P = .007), and intensity of anticoagulation (P = .02) were independent risks for bleeding at any site during anticoagulant therapy.

PATIENT CHARACTERISTICS

Patient characteristics or co-morbidities that are considered risk factors for anticoagulant-related bleeding are a history of gastrointestinal bleeding, cerebrovascular disease, liver disease, and renal insufficiency.[11-14] Other co-morbidities such as atrial fibrillation, hypertension, and malignancy have been reported as risk factors, but not consistently.[9,11,12,15] Some of the differences in the co-morbid conditions reported may have been influenced by higher intensity of anticoagulant therapy in earlier studies, lower frequency of use of anticoagulant therapy in some co-morbidities (e.g., alcoholism), and inaccurate documentation of co-morbid conditions in the medical record.[14]

Of particular concern is the risk of anticoagulant-related bleeding in patients with a history of ischemic cerebral vascular disease. Oral anticoagulant therapy has been associated with increased bleeding in randomized trials comparing oral anticoagulant therapy with no treatment, very–low dose anticoagulant, or antiplatelet therapy after an acute episode of ischemic cerebrovascular disease;[16-23] major bleeding varied from 2.% to 13%. Higher intensity of the anticoagulant effect (INR > 4), uncontrolled hypertension, initiation of anticoagulant therapy in the setting of an acute cerebral ischemia, and unsuspected initial intracerebral hemorrhage are probable reasons for the higher frequency of bleeding noted in the earlier studies.[24]

Whether age, in and of itself, is a risk factor for anticoagulant-related bleeding remains controversial. Older patients may be at increased risk for anticoagulant-related bleeding for the same reasons that put them at risk for any adverse drug reaction.[25] They are more likely to have more than one chronic disease,[26-28] and they are more likely to be taking more than one type of medication.[29,30] Additionally, the anticoagulant effect is increased in older patients. Older patients require smaller doses of anticoagulants, and the anticoagulant response to warfarin is enhanced with age.[31-34] Last, vascular integrity may become impaired with age.[25-37]

Increased vascular endothelial fragility may make older patients more susceptible to anticoagulant-related bleeding, especially intracranial bleeding.[8] Several studies have found anticoagulant-related bleeding to be more common in older patients,[6,12,15,38-44] whereas some studies[9,45-50] have not. The evidence is conflicting. There are too few data on patients 75 years and older, and few studies report the absolute age-associated risk, which is more pertinent to decision making. The evidence suggests that anticoagulant-related bleeding may be more common in older patients, with a relative risk of bleeding of 2 compared with younger patients.[51] Although this risk may be high enough to avoid anticoagulants in some older patients, it is unlikely that age-related risk alone outweighs the potential benefits.

CONCOMITANT USE OF DRUGS KNOWN TO AFFECT HEMOSTASIS

The concomitant use of drugs in patients taking warfarin can result in either pharmacokinetic or pharmacodynamic interactions. A large number of drugs are known to interact with anticoagulants, and since patients tend to take anticoagulants for several months there is sufficient exposure time for an adverse reaction to occur. Pharmacokinetic interactions can alter the response of warfarin by affecting absorption, distribution, metabolism, or excretion. Pharmacokinetic interactions are seen with drugs that potentiate the anticoagulant effect, resulting in an increased prothrombin time and risk of bleeding. Examples of these drugs include cimetidine,[52-54] metronidazole,[55] phenytoin,[56] and erythromycin.[57-60] Other drugs, such as barbiturates[61-63] and rifampin[64,65] increase hepatic metabolism, which decreases the anticoagulant effect, thereby increasing the dosage requirements. Discontinuation of these latter drugs can lead to an increased prothrombin time and an increased risk of bleeding.

Pharmacodynamic interactions are related to the biochemical and physiologic effects of warfarin. When pharmacodynamic interactions occur, medications have additive effects that cannot be avoided. A common pharmacodynamic interaction occurs between warfarin and aspirin and nonsteroidal anti-inflammatory drugs (NSAIDs) by inhibiting platelet aggregation.[66-68] NSAID use increases the likelihood of hemorrhagic peptic ulcer disease.[66,67] NSAIDs have been shown to increase the risk of peptic ulcer disease in the elderly three to five times.[69,70] The inhibition of cytoprotective prostaglandins in the gastrointestinal tract[71] and inhibition of platelet cyclooxygenase[72] are the putative causes of this increased risk. Shorr et al[66] found that the concurrent use of NSAIDs and oral anticoagulants was associated with a 13-fold increase in the risk of developing hemorrhagic peptic ulcer disease in a retrospective cohort study of Tennessee Medicaid enrollees aged 65 years and older. NSAID exposure was attributable to almost 10% of the hospitalizations for hemorrhagic peptic ulcer disease among users of anticoagulant therapy.

Concomitant use of aspirin has been associated with a higher frequency of bleeding even in patients treated with low-intensity warfarin.[73–75] In a large randomized trial[73] comparing the combination of low-dose warfarin therapy (INR < 2.0) and aspirin (80 mg/day) to aspirin (160 mg/day) in patients with prior myocardial infarction, the frequency of spontaneous major bleeding during the first year of therapy was 1.4% compared to 0.7%, respectively (p = 0.01). Similarly, in a primary prevention trial of ischemic heart disease,[74] the rate of hemorrhagic stroke was 0.09%/year for those treated with low-intensity warfarin (target INR 1.5) and aspirin (75 mg/day), 0.01%/year with low-intensity warfarin alone; 0.02%/year with aspirin; and none with the placebo group.

LENGTH OF THERAPY

The cumulative risk of anticoagulant-related bleeding is directly related to the length of anticoagulant therapy.[24] Higher frequencies of bleeding are seen early in the course of therapy.[9,12,40,76] For example, Landefeld et al[12] reported that the frequency of major bleeding was noted to decrease from 3% during the first month of outpatient warfarin therapy to 0.8%/month during the rest of the first year of therapy to 0.3%/month thereafter.[12] Similarly, Fihn et al[77] noted that the relative risks for serious bleeding during the first three months of therapy, compared with the rest of the first year and the second year and anytime thereafter were 1.9 (95% confidence intervals, 1.2 to 3.0), 3.0 (95% confidence intervals, 1.8 to 4.0), and 5.9 (95% confidence intervals, 3.8 to 9.3), respectively. Other studies[49,78,79] have reported similar observations, though it has not been universal.

SITES OF BLEEDING COMPLICATIONS FROM ORAL ANTICOAGULANTS

The most common sites of anticoagulant-related bleeding are the gastrointestinal tract, the genitourinary tract, and soft tissues, including wounds.[9,11,40,46,80,81] The risk of gastrointestinal bleeding is increased with the concomitant use of NSAIDs, and they should be avoided if at all possible in older patients receiving oral anticoagulant therapy. Intracranial bleeding is the most feared site of anticoagulant-related bleeding, especially in older patients. It is posited to be one of the major deterrents to more widespread use of warfarin therapy in stroke prevention.[29,82–84] Rates of anticoagulant-related intracerebral hemorrhage have been estimated to range from 0.3% to 2.0% per year.[9,12,43,85–90] Hart et al[29] recently reviewed the issue of oral anticoagulant-related intracerebral bleeding and found that most were intracerebral

hematomas, of which 60% were fatal. Predictors of anticoagulant-related intracerebral hematoma were advanced age, prior ischemic stroke, hypertension, and intensity of the anticoagulant effect. Because risk factors for ischemic stroke (advanced age, hypertension, and prior stroke) are similar, the potential reduction in thromboembolism must be weighed against the potential increase in hemorrhage.

HEMORRHAGIC RISK ASSESSMENTS AND PREDICTION MODELS

Prediction models have been developed for estimating the risk of major bleeding during oral anticoagulant therapy. A prediction rule for estimating the risk of major bleeding during long-term warfarin therapy was recently prospectively validated and shown to be more accurate than physicians' predictions.[13] The index included four independent risk factors for major bleeding: (1) age 65 years or greater, (2) history of gastrointestinal bleeding, (3) history of stroke, and (4) one or more of four specific co-morbid conditions (recent myocardial infarction, anemia, renal insufficiency, or diabetes). The cumulative incidence of major bleeding at 48 months was 3%, 12%, and 53% in low-, intermediate-, and high-risk patients, respectively. Kuijer et al[91] also recently developed a prediction model for anticoagulant-related bleeding that included age, gender, and the presence of malignancy. Rates of major bleeding were 7%, 4%, and 1% after three months of therapy for patients classified as high, middle, and low risk, respectively.

These prediction models can be used as an evidence-based starting point for assessing the risks of anticoagulant-related bleeding at the initiation of therapy rather than relying on subjective assessments. They by no means should be the sole criterion for deciding whether to initiate therapy, but should be used in conjunction with other assessments, such as the patient's functional and cognitive status and likelihood of adherence. Such considerations may determine that more frequent monitoring of therapy is needed. These assessments could be easily incorporated into the medical chart, reviewed at the initiation of therapy, and then periodically assessed throughout the course of anticoagulant therapy. Likewise, the risks of anticoagulant-related bleeding may need to be modified to incorporate the effects of new treatments for underlying co-morbidities, such as the treatment of *Helicobacter pylori* for peptic ulcer disease.

SUMMARY

Hemorrhage is the major complication of anticoagulant therapy. The major determinants of oral anticoagulant-related bleeding are the intensity of the anticoagulant effect, patient characteristics, concomitant use of drugs known to affect hemostasis, and the length of therapy. The therapeutic benefits of primary or secondary prophylaxis need to be balanced against the bleeding risks for each individual patient, taking into consideration the relative and absolute contraindications to anticoagulant therapy. Once the decision has been made to initiate long-term anticoagulant therapy, then efforts should be directed toward optimizing the management of therapy to minimize the risks.

REFERENCES

1. Hull R, Hirsh J, Jay R, Carter C, England C, Gent M, et al. Different intensities of oral anticoagulant therapy in the treatment of proximal-vein thrombosis. *N Engl J Med*. 1982;307(27):1676–1681.

2. Turpie AGG, Gunstensen J, Hirsh J, Nelson H, Gent M. Randomised comparison of two intensities of oral anticoagulant therapy after tissue heart valve replacement. *Lancet*. 1988;1(8597):1242–1245.

3. Saour JN, Sieck JO, Mamo LAR, Gallus AS. Trial of different intensities of anticoagulant therapy in patients with prosthetic heart valves. *N Engl J Med*. 1990;322(7):428–432.

4. Altman R, Rouvier J, Gurfinkel E, D'Ortencio O, Manzanel R, de La Fuente L, et al. Comparison of two levels of anticoagulant therapy in patients with substitute heart valves. *J Thorac Cardiovasc Surg*. 1991;101(3):427–431.

5. Atrial Fibrillation Investigators. Risk factors for stroke and efficacy of antithrombotic therapy in atrial fibrillation. Analysis of pooled data from five randomized controlled trials. *Arch Intern Med*. 1994;154:1449–1457.

6. EAFT (European Atrial Fibrillation Trial) Study Group. Secondary prevention in non-rheumatic atrial fibrillation after transient ischaemic attack or minor stroke. *Lancet*. 1993;342:1255–1262.

7. Hylek EM, Skates SJ, Sheehan MA, Singer DE. An analysis of the lowest effective intensity of prophylactic anticoagulation for patients with nonrheumatic atrial fibrillation. *N Engl J Med*. 1996;335:540–546.

8. Hylek EM, Singer DE. Risk factors for intracranial hemorrhage in outpatients taking warfarin. *Ann Intern Med*. 1994;120:897–902.

9. Fihn SD, McDonell M, Martin D, Henikoff J, Vermes D, Kent D, et al. Risk factors for complications of chronic anticoagulation. A multicenter study. *Ann Intern Med*. 1993;118(7):511–520.

10. The Stroke Prevention in Atrial Fibrillation Investigators. Bleeding during antithrombotic therapy in patients with atrial fibrillation. *Arch Intern Med*. 1996;156(Feb 26):409–416.

11. Landefeld CS, Beyth RJ. Anticoagulant-related bleeding: clinical epidemiology, prediction and prevention. *Am J Med*. 1993;95:315–328.

12. Landefeld CS, Goldman L. Major bleeding in outpatients treated with warfarin: incidence and prediction by factors known at the start of outpatient therapy. *Am J Med*. 1989;87:144–152.

13. Beyth RJ, Quinn LM, Landefeld CS. Prospective evaluation of an index for predicting risk of major bleeding in outpatients treated with warfarin. *Am J Med*. 1998;105:91–99.

14. Levine MN, Raskob G, Landefeld CS, Kearon C. Hemorrhagic complications of anticoagulant treatment. *Chest*. 2001;119(Suppl 1):108S–121S.

15. Launbjerg J, Egeblad H, Heaf J, Nielsen NH, Fugleholm AM, Ladefoged K. Bleeding complications to oral anticoagulant therapy: multivariate analysis of 1010 treatment years in 551 outpatients. *J Intern Med*. 1991;229:351–355.

16. Enger E, Boyesen S. Long-term anticoagulant therapy in patients with cerebral infarction. *Acta Med Scand*. 1965;178(Suppl):7–55.

17. McDowell F, MeDevitt E, Wright IS. Anticoagulant therapy: five years experience with the patient with an established cerebrovascular accident. *Arch Neurol*. 1963;8:209–214.

18. Baker RN, Broward JA, Fang HC, et al. Anticoagulant therapy in cerebral infarction: report on cooperative study. *Neurology*. 1962;12:832–835.

19. Fisher CM. Anticoagulant therapy in cerebral thrombosis and cerebral embolism. *Neurology*. 1961;11:119–131.

20. Hill AB, Marshall J, Shaw DA. A controlled clinical trial of long-term anticoagulant therapy in cerebrovascular disease. *Quarterly J Med*. 1960;29:597–609.

21. Hill AG, Marshall J, Shaw DA. Cerebrovascular disease: trial of long-term anticoagulant therapy. *BMJ*. 1962;2:1003–1006.

22. Olsson JE, Brechter C, Backlund H, et al. Anticoagulant vs. antiplatelet therapy as prophylactic against cerebral infarction in transient ischemic attacks. *Stroke*. 1980;11:4–9.

23. The stroke prevention in reversible ischemia trial (SPIRIT) study group. A randomized trial of anticoagulant versus aspirin after cerebral ischemic of presumed arterial origin. *Ann Neurol*. 1997;42:857–865.

24. Levine GN, Ali MN, Schafer AJ. Antithrombotic therapy in patients with acute coronary syndromes. *Arch Intern Med*. 2001;161:937–948.

25. Beyth RJ, Shorr RI. Epidemiology of adverse drug reactions in the elderly by drug class. *Drugs and Aging*. 1999;14(3):231–239.

26. Guralnik JM, LaCroix AZ, Everett DF, Kovar MG. Aging in the eighties: the prevalence of comorbidity and association with disability. In: National Center for Health Statistics, ed. *Advance Data from Vital and Health Statistics* (PHS) 89-1250. 170, 1–8. Hyattsville, MD: U.S. Department of Health and Human Services, May 26-1989.

27. Seeman TE, Guralnik J, Kaplan GA, Knudsen L, Cohen R. The health consequences of multiple morbidity in the elderly. The Alameda County Study. *J Aging Health*. 1989;1:50–66.

28. U.S. Senate Special Committee on Aging (1987–88). *Aging America, 1988: Trends and Projections*. Washington, DC: U.S. Department of Health and Human Services; 1991.

29. Hart RG, Boop BS, Anderson DC. Oral anticoagulants and intracranial hemorrhage. Facts and hypotheses. *Stroke*. 1995;26(8):1471–1477.

30. Nolan L, O'Malley K. Prescribing for the elderly. Part II. Prescribing patterns: difference due to age. *J Am Geriatr Soc*. 1988;36:245–254.

31. Toohey M. Clinical trial of phenylindanedione as an anticoagulant. *BMJ*. 1953;1:650–662.

32. Gurwitz JH, Avorn J, Ross-Degnan D, Choodnovskiy I, Ansell J. Aging and the anticoagulant response to warfarin therapy. *Ann Intern Med*. 1992;116:901–904.

33. O'Malley K, Stevenson IH, Ward CA, Wood AJJ, Crooks J. Determinants of anticoagulant control in patients receiving warfarin. *Br J Clin Pharmacol*. 1977;4:309–314.

34. Shepherd AMM, Hewick DS, Moreland TA, Stevenson IH. Age as a determinant of sensitivity to warfarin. *Br J Clin Pharmacol*. 1977;4:315–320.

35. Friedman SA. Organ systems: cardiovascular disorders. In: Berkow R, Abrams WB, eds. *The Merck Manual of Geriatrics*. Whitehouse Station, New Jersey: Rahway, Merck and Company, Inc.; 1990:408.

36. Masuda J, Tanak K, Ueda K, Omae T. Autopsy study of incidence and distribution of cerebral amyloid angiopathy in Hisayama, Japan. *Stroke*. 1988;19(2):205–210.

37. Vonsattel JP, Myers RH, Hedley-White ET, Ropper AH, Bird ED, Richardson EP Jr. Cerebral amyloid angiopathy without and with cerebral hemorrhages: a comparative histological study. *Ann Neurol*. 1991;30(5):637–649.

38. Coon WW, Willis PWI. Hemorrhagic complications of anticoagulant therapy. *Arch Intern Med*. 1974;133:386–392.

39. Fihn SD, Callahan CM, Martin DC, McDonnell MB, Henikoff JG, White RH. The risk and severity of bleeding complications in elderly patients treated with warfarin. *Ann Intern Med*. 1996;124:970–979.

40. Palareti G, Leali N, Coccheri S, Poggi M, Manotti C, D'Angelo A, et al. Bleeding complications of oral anticoagulant treatment: an inception-cohort, prospective collaborative study (ISCOAT). *Lancet*. 1996;348:423–428.

41. Petitti DB, Strom BL, Melmon KL. Prothrombin time ratio and other factors associated with bleeding in patients treated with warfarin. *J Clin Epidemiol*. 1989;42:759–764.

42. Pollard JW, Hamilton MJ, Christensen NA, Achor RWP. Problems associated with long-term anticoagulant therapy. *Circulation*. 1962;25:311–317.

43. Stroke Prevention in Atrial Fibrillation Investigators. Stroke prevention in atrial fibrillation study. Final results. *Circulation*. 1991;84:527–539.

44. van der Meer FJM, Rosendaal FR, Vandenbroucke JP, Briet E. Bleeding complications in oral anticoagulant therapy: an analysis of risk factors. *Arch Intern Med*. 1993;153:1557–1562.

45. Davis FB, Estruch MT, Samson-Corvera EB, Voigt GC, Tobin JD. Management of anticoagulation in outpatients. Experience with an anticoagulation service in a municipal hospital setting. *Arch Intern Med*. 1977;137:197–202.

46. Forfar JC. A 7-year analysis of hemorrhage in patients on long-term anticoagulant treatment. *Br Heart J*. 1979;42:128–132.

47. Gurwitz JH, Goldberg RJ, Holden A, Knapic N, Ansell J. Age-related risks of long-term oral anticoagulant therapy. *Arch Intern Med*. 1988;148:1733–1736.

48. Lundstrom T, Ryden L. Hemorrhagic and thromboembolic complications in patients with atrial fibrillation on anticoagulant prophylaxis. *J Intern Med*. 1989;225:137–142.

49. McInnes GT, Helenglass G. The performance of clinics for outpatient control of anticoagulation. *J Royal Coll Phys London*. 1987;21:42–45.

50. Peyman MA. The significance of hemorrhage during the treatment of patients with the coumarin anticoagulants. *Acta Med Scand*. 1958;339:1–62.

51. Beyth RJ, Landefeld CS. Anticoagulants in older patients: a safety perspective. *Drugs and Aging*. 1995;6:45–54.

52. Serlin MJ, Sibeon RG, Mossman S, Breckenridge AM, Williams JR, Atwood JL, et al. Cimetidine: interaction with oral anticoagulants in man. *Lancet*. 1979;2(8138):317–319.

53. Silver BA, Bell WR. Cimetidine potentiation of the hypopro-thrombinemic effect of warfarin. *Ann Intern Med*. 1979;90(348):349.

54. Bell WR, Anderson KC, Noe DA, et al. Reduction in the plasma clearance rate of warfarin induced by cimetidine. *Arch Intern Med*. 1986;146:2325–2328.

55. O'Reilly RA. The stereoselective interaction of warfarin and metronidazole in man. *N Engl J Med*. 1976;295:354–357.

56. Nappi JM. Warfarin and phenytoin interaction [letter]. *Ann Intern Med*. 1979;90:852.

57. Bartle WR. Possible warfarin-erythromycin interaction. *Arch Intern Med*. 1980;140:985–987.

58. Schwartz J, Bachmann K, Perrigo E. Interaction between warfarin and erythromycin. *Southern Med J*. 1983;76:91–93.

59. Weibert RT, Adler DS. Evaluation of a capillary whole-blood prothrombin time measurement system. *Clin Pharmacol*. 1989;8:864–867.

60. Sato RI, Gray DR, Brown SE. Warfarin interaction with erythromycin. *Arch Intern Med*. 1984;144:2413–2414.

61. MacDonald MG, Robinson DS. Clinical observations of possible barbiturate interference with anticoagulation. *JAMA*. 1968;204:97–100.

62. Udall JA. Clinical implications of warfarin: interactions with five sedatives. *Am J Cardiol*. 1975;35:67–71.

63. O'Reilly RA, Trager WF, Rettie AE, et al. Interaction of secobarbital with warfarin pseudoracemates. *Clin Pharmacol Ther*. 1980;28:1895–1899.

64. O'Reilly RA. Interaction of sodium warfarin and rifampin: studies in man. *Ann Intern Med*. 1974;81:337–340.

65. O'Reilly RA. Interaction of chronic daily warfarin therapy and rifampin. *Ann Intern Med*. 1975;83:506–508.

66. Shorr RI, Ray WA, Daugherty JR, Griffin MR. Concurrent use of nonsteroidal anti-inflammatory drugs and oral anticoagulants places elderly persons at high risk for hemorrhagic peptic ulcer disease. *Arch Intern Med*. 1993;153:1665–1670.

67. Chan TYK. Adverse interactions between warfarin and nonsteroidal anti-inflammatory drugs: mechanisms, clinical significance, and avoidance. *Ann Pharmacother*. 1995;29:1274–1283.

68. Turpie AGG, Gent M, Laupacia A, et al. A comparison of aspirin with placebo in patients treated with warfarin after heart-valve replacement. *N Engl J Med*. 1993;329:524–529.

69. Gabriel SE, Jaakkimainen L, Bombardier C. Risk for serious gastrointestinal complications related to use of nonsteroidal anti-inflammatory drugs. A meta-analysis. *Ann Intern Med*. 1991;115:787–796.

70. Griffin MR, Piper JM, Daugherty JR, Snowden M, Ray WA. Non-steroidal anti-inflammatory drug use and increased risk for peptic ulcer disease in elderly persons. *Ann Intern Med*. 1991;114:257–263.

71. Brooks PM, Day RO. Nonsteroidal antiinflammatory drugs: differences and similarities. *N Engl J Med*. 1991;324:1716–1725.

72. Ali M, McDonald JWD. Reversible and irreversible inhibition of platelet cyclooxygenase and serotonin release by nonsteroidal antiinflammatory drugs. *Thrombosis Res*. 1978;13:1057–1065.

73. Coumadin Aspirin Reinfarction Study (CARS) Investigators. Randomised double-blind trial of fixed low-dose warfarin with aspirin after myocardial infarction. *Lancet*. 1997;350:389–396.

74. Medical Research Council. The Medical Research Council's general practice research framework. *Lancet*. 1998;351:233–241.

75. Blackshear JL, Kopecky SL, Litin SC, Safford RE, Hammill SC. Management of atrial fibrillation in adults: prevention of thromboembolism and symptomatic treatment. *Mayo Clin Proc*. 1996;71:150–160.

76. Petitti DB, Strom BL, Melmon KL. Duration of warfarin anticoagulant therapy and the probabilities of recurrent thromboembolism and hemorrhage. *Ann Intern Med*. 1986;81:255–259.

77. Fihn SD, McDonell M, Martin D, Henikoff J, Vermes D, Kent D, et al. Risk factors for complications of chronic anticoagulation. A multicenter study. *Ann Intern Med*. 1993;118(7):511–520.

78. Fuller JA, Melb MB. Experiences with long-term anticoagulant treatment. *Lancet*. 1959;2:489–491.

79. Mosley DH, Schatz IJ, Breneman GM, et al. Long-term anticoagulant therapy. *JAMA*. 1963;186:914–916.

80. Gitter MJ, Jaeger TM, Petterson TM, Gersh BJ, Silverstein MD. Bleeding and thromboembolism while receiving anticoagulation therapy: a population-based study in Rochester, Minnesota. *Mayo Clin Proc*. 1995;70:725–733.

81. White RH, McKittrick T, Takakuwa J, Callahan C, McDonell M, Fihn S. Management and prognosis of life-threatening bleeding during warfarin therapy. *Arch Intern Med*. 1996;156:1197–1201.

82. Gustafsson C, Asplund K, Britton M, Norrving B, Olsson B, Marke L. Cost effectiveness of primary stroke prevention in atrial fibrillation: Swedish national perspective. *BMJ*. 1992;305:1457–1460.

83. Man-Son-Hing M, Nichol G, Lau A, Laupacis A. Choosing antithrombotic therapy for elderly patients with atrial fibrillation who are at risk for falls. *Arch Intern Med*. 1999;159:677–685.

84. Monette J, Gurwitz J, Rochon PA, Avorn J. Physician attitudes concerning warfarin for stroke prevention in atrial fibrillation: results of a survey of long-term care practitioners. *J Am Geriatr Soc*. 1997; 45:1060–1065.

85. Boston Area Anticoagulation Trial for Atrial Fibrillation Investigators. The effect of low-dose warfarin on the risk of stroke in patients with nonrheumatic atrial fibrillation. *N Engl J Med*. 1990;323(22): 1505–1511.

86. Connolly SJ, Laupacis A, Gent M, Roberts RS, Cairns JA, Joyner C, et al. Canadian atrial fibrillation anticoagulation (CAFA) study. *J Am Coll Cardiol*. 1991;18:349–355.

87. Ezekowitz MD, Bridgers SL, James KE, Carliner NH, Colling CL, Gornick CC, et al. Warfarin in the prevention of stroke associated with nonrheumatic atrial fibrillation. *N Engl J Med*. 1992;327:1406–1412.

88. Petersen P, Boysen G, Godtfredsen J, Andersen ED, Andersen B. Placebo-controlled, randomized trial of warfarin and aspirin for prevention of thromboembolic complications in chronic atrial fibrillation: the Copenhagen AFASAK study. *Lancet*. 1989;1:175–179.

89. Stroke Prevention in Atrial Fibrillation Study Group Investigators. Warfarin versus aspirin for prevention of thromboembolism in atrial fibrillation: stroke prevention in atrial fibrillation II study. *Lancet*. 1994;343:687–691.

90. Vieweg WVR, Piscatelli RL, Houser JJ, Proulx RA. Complications of intravenous administration of heparin in elderly women. *JAMA*. 1970;213:1303–1306.

91. Kuijer PMM, Hutten BA, Prins MH, Buller HR. Prediction of the risk of bleeding during anticoagulant treatment for venous thromboembolism. *Arch Intern Med*. 1999;159:457–460.

Chapter 33

Evaluation and Management of Excessive Anticoagulation and Bleeding

Jack E. Ansell

INTRODUCTION

The appropriate management of excessive anticoagulation or bleeding during warfarin therapy is an important function of an anticoagulation management service. Although the health care provider who manages the therapy might not make the ultimate therapeutic decisions, it is important to triage patients requiring physician intervention appropriately. The initial evaluation usually occurs in the setting of serious bleeding or markedly elevated International Normalized Ratios (INRs). The health care provider is expected to discuss each patient with the director of the service and contact the primary care or referring physician.

EXCESSIVE ANTICOAGULATION IN THE ABSENCE OF BLEEDING

Managing excessive anticoagulation is fraught with difficulties. One problem relates to managing patients, often by telephone, who are geographically dispersed. When an INR result is received, the patient usually has returned home from the office or laboratory where the test was done. This difficulty can be overcome by the use of point-of-care testing if the patient attends the anticoagulation management service office. Frequently, the question is one of balancing the urgency for corrective action against the inconvenience to the patient to travel to a nearby health center for treatment. The greater use of oral vitamin K (described below) can improve this situation.

Another problem is the stratification of levels of risk with elevated INRs, especially with more sensitive reagents (ie, thromboplastins with an International Sensitivity Index [ISI] of ~1.0). Many laboratories have an upper limit cutoff for reporting elevated INRs of approximately 8.0–10.0. Above these values, the sensitivity of the test becomes extremely poor. This is not the case with the end points achieved when using a less sensitive thromboplastin (ISI >2.0). This difficulty should make no difference in the management of elevated INRs. It simply means that stratification of risk at higher levels is not possible. Further, although the literature strongly points to an increased risk of bleeding with greater intensity of therapy, the risk is certainly time dependent. Thus, an individual with a transient elevation of an INR might be at a considerably different risk than one who presents with bleeding and an elevated INR, the duration of which is generally unknown.

There is increasing evidence that simply holding therapy or using oral vitamin K is a practical way of managing patients with mild to moderate degrees of excessive anticoagulation (INR 5.0–10.0).

Glover and Morrill,[1] in a retrospective review of their experience in treating elevated INRs in 51 patients attending an anticoagulation service, found that 48 of the patients (94%) were successfully managed by simply withholding warfarin and increasing the frequency of monitoring. The INR range of these 48 patients was 6.0–10.0 in 32 subjects, 10.0–20.0 in 10 subjects, and 23.5–80.9 in 6 individuals. The other 3 patients received intravenous vitamin K_1. One of the 48 patients had minor bleeding (hematuria) within 24 hours after the elevated INR was noted. It is not recommended simply to observe patients with such elevated INRs (>10), but this study does indicate that the INR can be very high in some patients without bleeding. The time course for the reduction in the INR by withholding therapy is nicely shown in the study by White et al,[2] who prospectively determined the rate of decline of the INR in 22 patients who were stably anticoagulated (mean INR 2.6) before cessation of treatment. The mean INR following discontinuation of therapy was 1.6 at 2.7 days and 1.1 at 4.7 days.

Looking at predictors of a prolonged delay in INR return to the therapeutic range, Hylek et al[3] found that an individual's steady-state warfarin dose (higher = longer), advanced age, and extreme elevation in the INR were associated with a prolonged delay in INR decline. Decompensated congestive heart failure and an active cancer increased the risk of this slow decline.

The act of withholding vitamin K for INRs greater than 10.0 is one with which many providers will be uncomfortable. The potential consequences are better illustrated in a study by Brophy et al.[4] In a prospective series of patients managed in an anticoagulation program, 23 patients presented with an INR > 10.0. With INRs between 10.0 and 13.0, 6 patients were observed; 2 of them developed spontaneous hemorrhage (epistaxis and gross hematuria). Patients with INRs between 11.00 and 21.00 were treated with escalating doses of intravenous vitamin K_1 (0.1–1.0 mg). The best response in the shortest interval of time was judged to occur following the 1.0-mg dose. These patients did not experience difficulty in reestablishing therapeutic levels. This treatment with intravenous vitamin K supports the earlier work by Shetty et al,[5] which shows that only 1 mg or less of intravenous vitamin K_1 is adequate to reverse elevated INRs without causing subsequent resistance to reestablishing stable anticoagulation.

More recent studies suggest that, in fact, the same clinical outcomes can be achieved with small doses of oral vitamin K, an intervention that would facilitate the treatment of ambulatory patients who live at a distance from or are unable to travel to a health care facility to receive parenteral therapy. Crowther et al[6] prospectively evaluated 62 patients on warfarin with INR values between 4.0 and 10.0. The next warfarin dose was held, and vitamin K_1, 1 mg, was given orally. At 24 hours, the INR was reduced in 59 (95%) of patients, and in 53 (85%) patients it was reduced to less than 4.0. Only 22 (35%) of patients had an INR of less than 1.9. Warfarin resistance did not develop in any of these patients. Weibert et al[7] assessed the outcome of 94 outpatients, with INRs >5.0 or with minor bleeding, who were treated by withholding warfarin and giving 2.5 mg of oral vitamin K_1. For patients with INRs of 5.00–10.00, the INR was reduced to <5.0 within 24–48 hours on 73 of 78 occasions (94%). When the INR was >10, it was reduced to <5 on only 5 of 10 occasions (50%) by 24–48 hours. The INR was overcorrected to 1.6–2.0 on only 17 of these 88 occasions. Minor bleeding was adequately controlled in all patients.

Most recently, Crowther et al,[8] in a randomized controlled trial, showed that giving vitamin K_1 to individuals with INRs between 5 and 10 resulted in fewer bleeding episodes in the following three months compared to those who received placebo. Two of forty-five patients who received 1 mg vitamin and K_1 had bleeding compared to 8/44 who received placebo. All but one of the episodes was minor. Similar to the findings of Crowther et al,[6] more patients who received vitamin K_1 were in therapeutic range the next day, although a greater number in this group were also subtherapeutic.

Based on a compilation of recent studies, as well as the author's personal experience, Exhibit 33–1 lists recommendations for managing excessive anticoagulation and/or bleeding. There is still a need for more clinical investigations to refine these recommendations, especially as they pertain to the use of fresh-frozen plasma and/or prothrombin complex concentrates.

INVESTIGATIVE EVALUATION OF GROSS OR OCCULT BLEEDING

Numerous studies analyze the rate of major or minor bleeding and the source of bleeding in anticoagulated patients, but few studies adequately address two problematic questions:

1. What is the likelihood of bleeding from an unknown gastrointestinal or genitourinary lesion (the two most common sites where important remediable lesions are likely to be found)?
2. What is the value of an extensive investigation when bleeding occurs in the setting of therapeutic or excessive anticoagulation?

The traditional dictum is to investigate thoroughly those individuals who manifest bleeding with a therapeutic level of anticoagulation, whereas the return on evaluation is significantly less if bleeding occurs in the face of excessive anticoagulation. Unfortunately, there are few well-designed prospective studies to ascertain the value of this approach.

As discussed in Chapter 32, there is abundant evidence that the risk of bleeding increases with the intensity of therapy.[9–13] Although soft tissue bleeding is probably the most common site of all bleeding,[14] the gastrointestinal and urinary tracts are not far behind and certainly the most likely sites in which to find important remediable lesions.[9,12,14–16] A comparative analysis of past studies to answer the above questions, however, is difficult because of a number of variables, including the definition of major bleeding, study design (retrospective or prospective), whether bleeding originated from known or unknown conditions, and the unknown intensity of therapy (variable thromboplastins and lack of INR reporting).

Exhibit 33–1
RECOMMENDATIONS FOR THE MANAGEMENT OF EXCESSIVE ORAL ANTICOAGULATION OR BLEEDING

INR above therapeutic but less than 5.0 with no significant bleeding

Lower dose or omit dose and resume at lower dose with INR therapeutic; if only minimally above therapeutic range, no dose reduction may be required.

INR > 5.0 but < 9.0 with no significant bleeding

Omit next one or two doses, monitor more frequently, and resume at lower dose when INR therapeutic. Alternatively, omit dose and give vitamin K_1 (1 to 2.5 mg) orally, particularly if at increased risk of bleeding. If more rapid reversal is required because the patient requires urgent surgery, vitamin K_1 (2 to 4 mg) orally can be given with the expectation that a reduction of the INR will occur in 24 hr. If the INR is still high, additional vitamin K_1 (1 to 2 mg) orally can be given.

INR > 9.0 with no significant bleeding

Hold warfarin and give higher dose of vitamin K_1 (3 to 5 mg) orally with the expectation that the INR will be reduced substantially in 24–48 hrs. Monitor more frequently and use additional vitamin K_1 if necessary. Resume therapy at lower dose when INR therapeutic.

INR therapeutic or elevated with serious or life-threatening bleeding

Hold warfarin and give vitamin K_1 (10 mg) by slow IV infusion and supplemented with fresh plasma or prothrombin complex concentrate depending on the urgency of the situation. Vitamin K_1 can be repeated every 12 hr.

Note: If continuing warfarin therapy is indicated after high doses of vitamin K_1, heparin or in many cases low–molecular-weight heparin can be given until the effects of vitamin K_1 have been reversed and the patient becomes responsive to warfarin therapy.

Source: J Ansell, J Hirsh, J Dalen, et al. Managing oral anticoagulation therapy, *Chest.* 119(Suppl), pp 225–385, © 2001.

Gastrointestinal Blood Loss

One might first ask whether the administration of warfarin leads to an increase in occult blood in the stool. This simple question is not so easy to answer, as reflected in two recent studies where very accurate quantitative occult blood measurements were made detecting blood below the threshold discernible by the usual clinical examination occult blood assays. Blackshear et al[17] reported on three groups from the Stroke Prevention in Atrial Fibrillation II trial; 54 patients on aspirin alone (325 mg daily) had a mean value of 0.8 mg hemoglobin/gm of stool, compared with 32 patients on warfarin (INR 2.0–3.0) who had a mean value of 1.0 mg hemoglobin/gm of stool. In 31 patients on low-dose warfarin (INR <1.5) plus aspirin (325 mg), a mean value of 1.7 mg hemoglobin/gm of stool was found. In the standard group and low-dose warfarin plus aspirin group combined, 11% of individuals had >2 mg of hemoglobin/gm of stool and 8% had >4 mg hemoglobin/gm of stool, which is greater than the normal limit of ~2 mg hemoglobin/gm stool.

In the same year, Greenberg et al[18] reported results from a prospective study showing that 25 warfarin-treated patients (INR 2.0–3.0) excreted a mean of 0.51 mg hemoglobin/gm of stool, compared with 25 control patients who excreted a mean of 0.68 mg hemoglobin/gm stool (p = 0.55). Patients who received aspirin excreted 0.82 mg hemoglobin/gm of stool (81 mg acetylsalicyclic acid [ASA] daily) or 1.04–1.41

mg hemoglobin/gm stool (325 mg ASA daily in the two groups). In the warfarin group, there was no difference in hemoglobin excretion based on the INR, although only a few INRs were above 3.5 and the highest was ~4.5.

Both of these studies benefit from the use of an INR, but the study by Greenberg et al[18] represents a more general population of medical patients than does the study by Blackshear et al.[17] In either case, the amount of hemoglobin in the stool was generally small and, in most cases, below the normal limit of 2 mg hemoglobin/gm of stool except for a small percentage in the latter study. Further, large studies in nonanticoagulated older patients have found that between 4%–6% of older patients will have >2 mg hemoglobin/gm of stool.[19] Based on the Greenberg and Blackshear studies, one should not consider the finding of occult blood in the stool, especially when the INR is within therapeutic range, simply a manifestation of anticoagulation; as in the general population, it might represent an underlying lesion. The significance of occult gastrointestinal bleeding in excessively anticoagulated individuals remains unclear.

With less quantitative screening, older studies provide further insight into the management of occult or gross gastrointestinal bleeding. In 1987, Jaffin et al[20] found a 12% prevalence of positive stool occult blood tests in 175 patients on warfarin or heparin, compared with 3% in 74 controls (p<.005). Most of these patients were inpatients, and they had a significantly higher rate of positivity (17% inpatient versus

3% outpatient). Approximately 30% were on heparin. In the anticoagulated patients, there was no difference in the mean prothrombin or activated partial thromboplastin time between positive and negative patients. In 16 patients who were evaluated, 15 (94%) were found to have lesions not previously suspected; 4 of the 16 (25%) lesions were found to be neoplastic disease. In a report by Wilcox and Truss,[21] 50 patients were retrospectively identified over a 15-year period with gastrointestinal bleeding during warfarin therapy. A source of bleeding was found in 53% of the patients; in 3 of these patients (6% of the total), the bleeding was related to cancer. Finally, the retrospective analysis of Landefeld et al[9] found 14 of 41 patients (34%) with gastrointestinal bleeding to have important remediable lesions. The lesions in 2 patients were malignant (5%). This limited information further supports the need for investigation if occult blood is found in the stool. The chance of finding important remediable lesions is at least 33%, but the likelihood of finding a source is generally greater than 50%. Less than 25% of these lesions are likely to be malignant.

Hematuria

The clinical circumstances pertaining to hematuria are not too different from those found in occult gastrointestinal bleeding. In a prospective controlled study, Culclasure et al[22] identified the incidence and prevalence of hematuria in a large sample of patients attending an anticoagulation clinic over a two-year period. All hematuria was found to be microscopic. Hematuria occurred at a rate of 0.05/100 patient months in the anticoagulated group with a prevalence of 3.2% (243 subjects), compared with a rate of 0.08/100 patient months and a prevalence of 4.8% (258 subjects) in the control group. No significant difference was noted between the groups. Surprisingly, there was no difference in the rate of hematuria in the anticoagulated group for patients with INRs between 1.0 and >5.0, although it is not known how high the INRs went. After a second episode of hematuria, 43 patients

(32 anticoagulated and 11 control) were investigated; 27 (84%) of the anticoagulated and 8 (73%) of the control patients (81% of the total) were found to have significant underlying disease with three cancers found in the combined group (7%). This study is important because of its suggestions that microscopic hematuria is no more frequent in anticoagulated patients than in nonanticoagulated patients, and that excessive anticoagulation does not seem to enhance the frequency of hematuria, although this latter fact is disputed by other studies.[9,14] In an abstract by Caralis et al[23] with limited information, the results of prospectively screening 172 orally anticoagulated patients for hematuria indicate that a surprisingly high 33% of patients had hematuria. It is unclear whether all subjects were within therapeutic range. Of the 49 patients who underwent investigative evaluation, many had multiple causes of hematuria, with a significant finding noted in 96% of patients, including 5 with cancer (10%).

In a retrospective study by Schuster and Lewis,[24] patients were examined who presented with gross (24 patients) or microscopic (5 patients) hematuria; 3 patients were on heparin and 26 on warfarin. All patients were therapeutically anticoagulated. The investigators found a cause of bleeding in 80% of the patients, 58% of whom were judged to have significant urologic conditions. Four cases (14% of patients) of cancer were uncovered. In a series of cases studied by van Savage and Fried,[25] 30 therapeutically anticoagulated patients with gross (24 patients) or microscopic (6 patients) hematuria were evaluated. An underlying lesion was found in 25 patients (83%), and 24 of these lesions were significant findings; 2 patients (7% of the total) had cancer. These studies support the finding that in anticoagulated or even nonanticoagulated individuals with persistent hematuria, there is a high likelihood of finding a significant underlying cause (~80% of the time). The potential to identify a cancer will occur in 5% to 15% of patients. As with gastrointestinal bleeding, additional studies are needed to determine the significance of hematuria in the setting of excessive anticoagulation.

REFERENCES

1. Glover JJ, Morrill GB. Conservative treatment of overanticoagulated patients. *Chest*. 1995;108:987–990.

2. White RH, McKittrick T, Hutchinson R, Twitchell J. Temporary discontinuation of warfarin therapy: changes in the International Normalized Ratio. *Ann Intern Med*. 1995;122:40–42.

3. Hylek EM, Regan S, Go AS, Hughes RA, Singer DE, Skates SJ. Clinical predictors of prolonged delay in return of the International Normalized Ratio to within the therapeutic range after excessive anticoagulation with warfarin. *Ann Intern Med*. 2001;135:460–462.

4. Brophy MT, Fiore LD, Deykin D. Low dose vitamin K therapy in excessively anticoagulated patients: a dose finding study. *J Thromb Thrombolysis*. 1997;4:289–292.

5. Shetty HG, Backhouse G, Bentley OP, et al. Effective reversal of warfarin-induced excessive anticoagulation with low dose vitamin K₁. *Thromb Haemost*. 1992;67:13–15.

6. Crowther MA, Donovan D, Harrison L, et al. Low dose oral vitamin K reliably reverses over-anticoagulation due to warfarin. *Thromb Haemost*. 1998;79:1116–1118.

7. Weibert RT, Le DT, Kayser SR, Donnelly KJ, Sevilla BK, Rapaport SI. Correction of excessive anticoagulation with oral vitamin K₁. *Ann Intern Med*. 1997;125:959–962.

8. Crowther MA, Julian J, McCarty D, et al. Treatment of warfarin-associated coagulopathy with oral vitamin K: a randomized controlled trial. *Lancet*. 2000;356:1551–1553.

9. Landefeld CS, Rosenblatt MW, Goldman L. Bleeding in outpatients treated with warfarin: relation to the prothrombin time and important remediable lesions. *Am J Med.* 1989;87:153–159.

10. Fihn SD, McDonell M, Martin D, et al. Risk factors for complications of chronic anticoagulation: a multicenter study. *Ann Intern Med.* 1993;118:511–520.

11. Saour JN, Sieck JO, Mamo LAR, Gallus AS. Trial of different intensities of anticoagulation in patients with prosthetic heart valves. *N Engl J Med.* 1990;322:428–432.

12. van der Meer FJM, Rosendaal FR, Vandenbroucke JP, Briet E. Bleeding complications in oral anticoagulant therapy: an analysis of risk factors. *Arch Intern Med.* 1993;153:1557–1562.

13. Cannegieter SC, Rosendaal FR, Wintzen AR, van der Meer FJM, Vandenbroucke JP, Briet E. Optimal oral anticoagulant therapy in patients with mechanical heart valves. *N Engl J Med.* 1995;33:11–17.

14. Landefeld CS, Beyth R. Anticoagulant-related bleeding: Clinical epidemiology, prediction, and prevention. *Am J Med.* 1993;95:315–328.

15. Landefeld CS, Goldman L. Major bleeding in outpatients treated with warfarin: incidence and prediction by factors known at the start of outpatient therapy. *Am J Med.* 1989;87:144–152.

16. White RH, McKittrick T, Takakuwa J, et al. Management and prognosis of life-threatening bleeding during warfarin therapy. *Arch Intern Med.* 1996;156:1197–1201.

17. Blackshear JL, Baker VS, Holland A, et al. Fecal hemoglobin excretion in elderly patients with atrial fibrillation. *Arch Intern Med.* 1996;156:658–660.

18. Greenberg PD, Cello JP, Rockey DC. Asymptomatic chronic gastrointestinal blood loss in patients taking aspirin or warfarin for cardiovascular disease. *Am J Med.* 1996;100:598–604.

19. Ahlquist DA, Wiand HS, Moertel GC, et al. Accuracy of fetal occult blood screening for colorectal neoplasia: a prospective study using Hemoccult and HemoQuant. *JAMA.* 1993;269:1262–1267.

20. Jaffin BW, Bliss CM, Lamont JT. Significance of occult gastrointestinal bleeding during anticoagulation therapy. *Am J Med.* 1987;83:269–272.

21. Wilcox CM, Truss CD. Gastrointestinal bleeding in patients receiving long-term anticoagulant therapy. *Am J Med.* 1988;84:683–690.

22. Culclasure TF, Bray VJ, Hasbargen JA. The significance of hematuria in the anticoagulated patient. *Arch Intern Med.* 1994;154:649–652.

23. Caralis P, Gelbard M, Washer J, Rhamy R, Marcial E. Incidence and etiology of hematuria in patients on anticoagulant therapy. *Clin Res.* 1989;37:791A.

24. Schuster GA, Lewis GA. Clinical significance of hematuria in patients on anticoagulant therapy. *J Urol.* 1987;137:923–925.

25. van Savage JG, Fried FA. Anticoagulant associated hematuria: a prospective study. *J Urol.* 1995;153:1594–1596.

Nonhemorrhagic Complications of Warfarin Therapy

Janet Hiatt Dailey

INTRODUCTION

Most adverse reactions associated with warfarin are bleeding-related complications. Nonhemorrhagic adverse reactions of warfarin are rare and therefore not easily recognized by clinicians. When nonhemorrhagic complications induced by warfarin remain unidentified or misinterpreted, their consequences can be as severe, challenging, and unpredictable as hemorrhagic complications.

ADVERSE DERMATOLOGIC EFFECTS

Skin Necrosis

History

Warfarin-induced skin necrosis (WISN) is the most serious nonhemorrhagic complication of oral anticoagulation.[1-3] Although skin necrosis was initially recognized by Flood et al in 1943 as thrombophlebitis migrans disseminate,[4] not until the 1950s did Verhagen, based on his clinical observation of 13 patients,[5] properly identify the causative agent as oral anticoagulants.[3-5]

Incidence

Estimation of the incidence of WISN is difficult because of the rarity of this condition. Incident rates of 1:1000,[6] 1:5000,[1] and 1:10,000[7] have been reported. Although WISN is infrequent, more than 200 cases have been reported.

Clinical Presentation

WISN most commonly occurs in middle-aged (range, 16–93 years) obese females following a thromboembolic event.[8-15] In fact, a compilation of cases by Eby[3] revealed that 82% of WISN cases involved women with a diagnosis of either deep venous thrombosis or pulmonary embolus. In a few reported cases, cerebral vascular accident, coronary thrombosis, and prosthetic valves were the indications for anticoagulation.[16,17]

Areas that WISN can affect include large subcutaneous adipose tissues, such as the breast, thighs, buttocks, and abdomen.[9,18] Cases involving hands, feet, nose, male genitals, the adrenal gland, uterus, and choroid plexus have been reported.[1,7,10,12] The lesions can be single, although it has been reported that 40% of patients present with multiple lesions.[12,19,20] Underlying disease states, previous exposures to warfarin, and intensity of anticoagulation are not associated with WISN.[5,14,21] Patients with either subtherapeutic or supratherapeutic prothrombin times can be affected. In most reported cases, however, the level of anticoagulation is within the therapeutic range at the time of clinical presentation. Skin necrosis usually does not recur with subsequent courses of warfarin, although a few cases of recurrent coumarin-induced necrosis are documented.[11,14,22-24]

The development of necrosis is similar in all patients and begins abruptly with the sensation of pain.[13-15] Dermal manifestations usually become evident between the third and eighth days of therapy,[1,3,5] but the appearance of lesions has been reported to occur from four hours to three years following initiation of therapy.[1,2,10,12] Changes progress quickly; within hours, a regional evanescent flush, petechiae, and, in some patients, edema develop.[2,5,10,11] The petechiae coalesce to form irregular, marginated ecchymoses surrounded by an erythematous halo,[7,11,12] followed by the formation of hemorrhagic bullae, the hallmark of hemorrhagic infarction and irreversible skin necrosis.

Laboratory evaluation is of no value in the diagnosis of WISN. Verhagen[5] notes that erythrocytes, leukocytes, platelet count, bleeding, and coagulation time were similar to pretreatment values in 13 patients. Bone marrow and peripheral smear are typically normal.[25] Schramm et al,[26] however, describe a single patient who presented with thrombocytopenia at the time of onset of skin necrosis.

Etiology and Dermatopathology

The etiology of skin necrosis is not well understood. The most widely accepted theory for this phenomenon is rapidly decreasing levels of factor VII and protein C (see Chapter 17), compared with levels of other vitamin K–dependent factors, following the initiation of warfarin, particularly if large loading doses are administered.[27] The lower level of protein C results in a hypercoagulable state and triggers the development of microthrombi in very small venules. The development of thrombosis of the lower dermal venules leads to gangrenous necrosis that results in the formation of a pigmented eschar. The presence of hemorrhagic bullae is thought to represent the initial damage to the vascular endothelium in the arteriole-capillary junction.[7,10] Subsequently, extensive edema and ulceration, progressing into the subcutaneous tissues, lead to extensive scarring (see Table 34–1).[1,7,11,16] Because the appearance of the lesions rapidly changes and the histopathologic features of skin necrosis and other related conditions associated with dermal vascular thromboses are similar, biopsy is nondiagnostic and not mandatory.[1,6,10] Histologically, however, if a biopsy is performed, the lesions reflect infarcts with occlusion of the dermal capillaries and venules with fibrin and platelet thrombi.[6,28,29] Microvascular thrombosis in the arteries and arterioles is absent, as well as histopathologic evidence of vasculitis, such as inflammation and hemorrhage of the epidermis and endothelium.[1,6,13,16,28,29]

Even relatively minor stimuli, such as venipuncture, local hypoxia, and pressure-induced ischemia, seem to be able to initiate the microvascular thrombosis in predisposed subjects.[1] Patients with congenital or acquired protein C deficiency and, less commonly, protein S deficiency are thought to have a higher susceptibility to WISN.[2] Gallerani et al[1] suggest that 3% of patients with protein C deficiency experience WISN. This complication, however, also has been observed in nondeficient individuals.[23,30,31] Of interest, the

Table 34–1 Correlation of the Pathophysiology and the Clinical Signs of Warfarin-Induced Skin Lesions

Pathophysiology	Clinical Signs
Capillary dilation secondary to endothelial damage in dermovascular loop	Initial flush
Rupture of the capillary walls in the dermis at the junction of precapillary arterioles and capillaries	Petechiae
Coalescence of petechial hemorrhage	Ecchymosis
Thrombosis of vessels	Hemorrhagic infarct (gangrenous necrosis)

protein C deficiency state causing purpura fulminans in infants is thought to be related to WISN because the dermal manifestation of the two conditions is similar, which suggests that the level of protein C, not the drug per se, is responsible for the etiology.[23] In addition, isolated cases of antithrombin III deficiency and the presence of a lupus anticoagulant have been described as predisposing factors for WISN.[32,33] Finally, WISN also has been reported in benign monoclonal gammopathy associated with disseminated intravascular coagulopathy (DIC).[6] Additional predisposing factors that have been associated with coumarin-induced skin necrosis include estrogen deficient states, diabetes mellitus, antibiotics, and analgesics,[32] although the pathophysiologic relationships between these factors and the development of WISN have not been described.

Differential Diagnosis

In addition to distinguishing WISN from other types of dermal vascular thromboses. Cole et al[12] advise that differentiating skin necrosis secondary to warfarin therapy from soft tissue hemorrhage is important because treatments differ substantially (see Table 34–2). The clinical presentation of WISN mimics several other conditions, including purpura fulminans, necrotizing fasciitis, microembolization, early stages of inflammatory breast cancer, and decubitus ulcers.[15] The classification of purpura associated with dermal vascular thrombosis, as in WISN, is[6]

- disseminated intravascular coagulation
- coumarin- and heparin-induced skin necrosis

Table 34–2 Comparison of Hemorrhage and Necrosis in Soft Tissues Associated with Warfarin Therapy

Hemorrhage	Necrosis
Occurs in men and women equally	Occurs mainly in women
Onset unrelated to initiation of therapy	Occurs 3–8 days after initiation of therapy
Corrected with discontinuance of therapy and/or vitamin K	Progressive despite discontinuance of therapy and/or vitamin K
Continuing therapy worsens the situation	Continuing therapy has no effect on the progression of skin lesions
Occurs in arterial and venous disease	Rarely occurs in arterial disease
Tissue necrosis absent	Tissue necrosis present
Surgical treatment usually not indicated	Surgical treatment usually necessary

Source: Adapted with permission from M Cole et al, *Surgery*, Vol 103, No 3, p 274, © 1988, Mosby-Year Book, Inc.

- skin necrosis associated with antiphospholipid antibodies
- purpura fulminans
- idiopathic purpura fulminans
- acute infectious purpura fulminans
- myeloblastemia
- thrombotic thrombocytopenic purpura
- paroxysmal nocturnal hemoglobinuria
- cryoglobulinemia

Much confusion exists in distinguishing skin necrosis from purpura fulminans. Thus, Adcock and Hicks[6] propose a new classification of purpura fulminans that includes systemic manifestations of DIC and protein C deficiency. Therefore, WISN under the new classification would be categorized under the following conditions associated with either decreased protein C levels or impaired functional capacity of the protein C system[6]:

- hereditary or acquired dysfunction of the protein C anticoagulant system (purpura fulminans)
  - hereditary protein C deficiency
  - protein S deficiency
  - coumarin therapy
  - disseminated intravascular coagulopathy
  - cholestasis associated with severe vitamin K deficiency
  - antiphospholipid antibodies
- acute infectious purpura fulminans
- idiopathic purpura fulminans

Prevention and Treatment

The key to treatment of WISN is the early establishment of a correct diagnosis and clinical differentiation. Because the extent and severity of lesions are variable, preventing extension of the necrosis is difficult. Although predicting which patients might develop WISN is not possible, one method of prevention is to avoid initial development of a hypercoagulable state.[15] The warfarin loading dose, once commonly utilized, is not recommended.[11] Instead, initiating oral anticoagulation therapy at lower doses and slowly increasing the dose, combined with therapeutic doses of heparin therapy, are suggested.[13,16,17,34–36] This regimen is especially important in patients with acquired or congenital deficiency of protein C or protein S. Alternative regimens have been used when intravenous heparin and slow progressive doses of oral anticoagulation are not possible. For instance, a homozygous protein C–deficient patient with recurrent episodes of skin necrosis and DIC, when rechallenged with intravenous heparin and incremental dose adjustment of oral anticoagulant, was treated successfully for more than two years with a low–molecular-weight heparin.[23,34] Melissarie and Kakkar[37] used a low–molecular-weight heparin as a long-term prophylactic agent for two years in five protein C–deficient patients, two of whom previously had developed skin necrosis with warfarin.

Fortunately, warfarin-induced skin lesions remain localized.[2] Supportive therapy, with or without continuing warfarin, has not been shown to alter the progression or development of new areas of necrosis. Most authors, however, recommend stopping anticoagulation therapy but not withholding it indefinitely.[9,10,12,15,21,33] Several other treatment modalities have been attempted with minimal success: local hypothermia; topical and systemic therapy, including corticosteroids, vasodilators, vitamin C, sympathetic nerve block, and hyperbaric oxygen; blood transfusion; and vitamin K.[1,2,7,12,14,16] In one patient with protein C deficiency and a history of warfarin necrosis, fresh-frozen plasma and intravenous heparin were used to prevent WISN during the reinitiation of warfarin.[38] However, one case of a life-threatening fluid overload following the administration of fresh-frozen plasma has been reported.[39]

In patients with hereditary protein C or antithrombin III (AT-III) deficiency, purified preparations of protein C or AT-III concentrates, respectively, can be used to treat WISN.[31,40–43] Schramm et al[26] treated skin necrosis in a patient with acquired protein C deficiency by using an initial dose of 1,500 IU of monoclonal antibody-purified protein C concentrate. The patient experienced immediate pain relief and disappearance of skin erythema. A total dose of 21,000 IU of protein C over a period of 45 days was used without any bleeding complications or adverse effects. This therapy also has been used successfully in the treatment of purpura fulminans in a homozygous protein C-deficient newborn.[44] In addition, one report describes the use of subcutaneous heparin and titrated warfarin doses in increments of 1 mg/week in a patient with AT-III deficiency.[41] Finally, cloning of cDNA-encoding protein C is being investigated.[45] Even though protein C, protein S, and AT-III deficiency might predispose patients to warfarin-induced skin necrosis, measuring these factors prior to starting warfarin therapy is often not feasible or practical.[1]

Despite these therapies, more than 50% of patients with WISN require some type of surgical intervention, such as debridement, skin grafting, or amputation.[9,13,15,46–48] It is important to involve a general surgeon and, in some instances, an orthopaedic surgeon early in the treatment care plan. Postoperative recovery in these patients usually is prompt, with no extension of the necrosis.[8]

Purple Toe Syndrome

History and Clinical Characteristics

Purple toe syndrome is a rare, nonhemorrhagic adverse effect of warfarin. It was first described in the literature by Feder and Auerbach in 1961 as "dark, blue-tinged bilateral purple discoloration of feet."[49] A comparison of the clinical features of purple toe syndrome versus warfarin-induced skin necrosis is depicted in Table 34–3.

Etiology

Several mechanisms, including a direct toxic effect of warfarin on the capillary and a vasodilating action on the smooth muscle, have been suggested for the etiology of purple toe syndrome.[49] Most investigators, however, believe that purple toe syndrome is a manifestation of cholesterol microembolization.[50–52] Although the syndrome can occur without anticoagulation therapy, several authors of case reports have observed a causal relationship between warfarin ingestion and the occurrence of purple toes. The proposed mechanism for the syndrome is that anticoagulation therapy can interfere with the healing of ulcerated atheromatous plaques, thus causing or initiating fragments to dislodge.[52] Interestingly, warfarin-related cholesterol embolization without the manifestation of purple toes also has been demonstrated.[53]

Histology

Biopsies reveal widespread cholesterol microembolization and hyperkeratosis. Inflammation or hemorrhage is not seen.[50,52]

Prognosis and Treatment

The sequela from purple toe syndrome depends on the scope of the underlying vascular atherosclerosis and the location and extent of ulcerated plaques. Some patients fare well with the discontinuation of warfarin. If warfarin can cause cholesterol embolization, however, the possible occurrence of potentially life-threatening systemic embolization is a concern.[50] Therefore, it is recommended that anticoagula-

Table 34–3 Comparison of Clinical Characteristics of Purple Toe Syndrome and Warfarin-Induced Skin Necrosis

Purple Toe Syndrome	Warfarin-Induced Skin Necrosis
More common in men	More common in women
Occurs 3–8 weeks after initiation of warfarin	Occurs 3–8 days after initiation of warfarin
Lesions usually bilateral	Bilateral lesions not always present
Digits on extremities involved	Digits on extremities rarely involved
Absence of necrosis and skin loss	Presence of necrosis and skin loss
Symptoms resolved with discontinuation of warfarin	Lesions not resolved with discontinuation of warfarin
Progression of skin blanches, with pressure, that fade with elevation of legs	Absence of skin blanches with pressure and elevation of legs

tion therapy be discontinued, if clinically possible, in patients who develop purple toe syndrome.

Maculopapular, Vesicular, Urticarial, and Pruritic Skin Eruptions

Incidence

Allergic maculopapular eruptions resulting from warfarin therapy have been reported infrequently. In 1959, Sheps and Gifford[54] reported the development of transient urticaria in a 50-year-old man 40 minutes after ingesting 50 mg of warfarin. Adams and Pass[55] describe a patient presenting with pruritic maculopapular eruption, including mouth erosions, after ingesting warfarin for four weeks.

Diagnosis

At clinical presentation, most cases of warfarin-related allergic skin eruptions are diagnosed as dermatitis medicamentosa.[56] Kwong et al[57] report the results of a biopsy, performed six days after a patient had a recurrent episode of pruritus and rash following a rechallenge with warfarin, as minimal nonspecific perivascular chronic inflammation and mild actinic degeneration of the papillary dermal collagen.

Prognosis and Treatment

Urticaria and rash associated with warfarin use are self-limiting and resolve when the medication is discontinued.[58] In some patients, an antihistamine relieves urticarial symptoms. It is possible that the coloring dyes used in compounding warfarin tablets are the causative agents. Among the dosage forms of warfarin, only the 10-mg strength does not contain a dye. Therefore, it might be reasonable to rechallenge patients who develop allergic reactions with the 10-mg dosage form as a means of determining whether the urticaria and/or rash recur in the absence of a coloring agent.

The literature differs as to whether allergic cross-sensitivity occurs among other coumarin derivatives. Substituting warfarin with another anticoagulant agent might result in relief of allergic symptoms.[54,55] Kruis-de Vries et al[59] report that a 24-year-old woman with a four-year history of Crohn's disease developed pruritus and/or rash with acenocoumarol, phenprocoumon, and warfarin. The only one of these coumarin derivatives that contained a dye was acenocoumarol. Several investigators substituted warfarin with bishydroxy-coumarin (not available since 1992), and patients obtained

relief from urticaria.[54,55,57] One case report describes urticaria being successfully avoided when warfarin was substituted with anisindione, an indandione anticoagulant.[60]

ADVERSE NONDERMATOLOGIC EFFECTS

Drug-Induced Hepatitis

Few well-documented cases of coumarin-induced hepatitis have been described. Little is known about the mechanism of warfarin-induced hepatitis.[61] It is unclear whether the metabolism of the drug or the metabolites change the antigenicity of hepatocytes, which results in an immunologic response.[62] Rhenqvist[63] reports two cases of intrahepatic jaundice that were probably due to warfarin therapy. There is some suggestion that cross-reactivity among coumarin derivatives occurs. In one case, a woman with a mitral valve replacement experienced recurrent episodes of hepatitis and jaundice when rechallenged with phenprocoumon. The patient experienced a similar reaction with warfarin. The authors note that phenprocoumon caused a hepatitis-like picture, whereas warfarin resulted in a cholestatic effect. The patient was switched to a low–molecular-weight heparin with no further recurrence.[64]

Tracheobronchial Calcification

Although tracheobronchial ring calcification is a teratogenic side effect of warfarin, several cases suggest a causal association between tracheal calcification or tracheobronchial calcification and long-term prophylactic usage of warfarin in all age groups. Case reports describe radiographic tracheal changes in three children taking warfarin for mitral valve replacement.[65] Moncada et al[66] determined that the prevalence of tracheal and bronchial cartilaginous rings was higher in patients taking warfarin than in a control group aged less than 60 years. The authors present additional information suggesting that a higher prevalence of rings correlated with a longer duration of warfarin therapy.

Alopecia

Rare cases of warfarin-induced alopecia have been reported.[67–69] One case occurred in which alopecia developed 3–20 weeks after the initiation of warfarin.[68] Complete recovery occurred following discontinuation of the medication. In some patients, alopecia occurred more than 10 years after warfarin was started.[69] It is not certain whether the process is the consequence of the drug or occurs as the result of a recent illness or stressful reaction.

Priapism

In a single case report, a 40-year-old man experienced frequent chilling episodes, recurrent intermittent priapism, spermatic cord pain, and testicular swelling thought to be related to warfarin.[60] The patient remained symptom free when warfarin was substituted with anisindione.

CONCLUSION

Nonhemorrhagic complications of warfarin therapy are fortunately uncommon. Recognizing and minimizing warfarin-induced nonhemorrhagic complications are difficult and challenging for even an experienced health care provider. The most serious nonhemorrhagic complication induced by warfarin is skin necrosis. Additional nonhemorrhagic complications have been reported in the literature. Health care providers, especially those involved in the management of anticoagulated patients, need to be mindful that nonhemorrhagic side effects of warfarin, although rare, do exist.

REFERENCES

1. Gallerani M, Manfredini R, Moratelli S. Non-haemorrhagic adverse reactions of oral anticoagulant therapy. *Int J Cardiol.* 1995;49:1–7.

2. Sternberg ML. Warfarin sodium-induced skin necrosis. *Ann Emerg Med.* 1995;26:94–97.

3. Eby CS. Warfarin-induced skin necrosis. *Hematol Oncol Clin North Am.* 1993;7:1291–1300.

4. Flood EP, Redish MH, Bociek SJ. Thrombophlebitis migrans disseminata: report of a case in which gangrene of a breast occurred. *NY State J Med.* 1943;43:1121–1124.

5. Verhagen H. Local haemorrhage and necrosis of the skin and underlying tissues during anticoagulant therapy with dicumarol or dicumacyl. *Acta Med Scand.* 1954;148:453–462.

6. Adcock DM, Hicks MJ. Dermatopathology of skin necrosis associated with purpura fulminans. *Semin Thromb Hemost.* 1990;16:283–292.

7. Horn JR, Danziger LH, Davis RJ. Warfarin-induced skin necrosis: Report of four cases. *Am J Hosp Pharm.* 1981;38:1763–1768.

8. Nudelman HL, Kempson RL. Necrosis of the breast: a rare complication of anticoagulant therapy. *Am J Surg.* 1966;111:728–733.

9. Lacy JP, Goodin RR. Warfarin-induced necrosis of skin. *Ann Intern Med.* 1975;82:381–382. Letter.

10. Nalbandian RM, Mader IJ, Barrett JL, et al. Petechiae, ecchymoses, and necrosis of skin induced by coumarin congeners. *JAMA.* 1965;192:603–608.

11. Teepe RGC, Broekmans AW, Vermeer BJ, et al. Recurrent coumarin-induced skin necrosis in a patient with an acquired functional protein C deficiency. *Arch Dermatol.* 1986;122:1408–1412.

12. Cole MS, Minifee PK, Wolma FJ. Coumadin necrosis. A review of the literature. *Surgery.* 1988;103:271–277.

13. Caldwell EH, Stewart S. Skin necrosis as a consequence of Coumadin therapy. *Plast Reconstr Surg.* 1983;72:231–233.

14. Schleicher SM, Fricker MP. Coumarin necrosis. *Arch Dermatol.* 1980;116:444–445.

15. DeFranzo AJ, Marasco P, Argenta LC. Warfarin-induced necrosis of the skin. *Ann Plast Surg.* 1995;334:203–208.

16. Kahn S, Stern HD, Rhodes GA. Cutaneous and subcutaneous necrosis as a complication of Coumadin-congener therapy. *Plast Reconstr Surg.* 1971;48:160–166.

17. Faraci PA, Deterling RA, Stein AM, et al. Warfarin induced necrosis of the skin. *Surg Gynecol Obstet.* 1978;146:695–700.

18. Kagan RJ, Glassford GH. Coumadin-induced breast necrosis. *Am Surg.* 1981;47:509–510.

19. Comp PC, Eirod JP, Karzenski S. Warfarin-induced skin necrosis. *Semin Thromb Hemost.* 1990;16:293–298.

20. Jillson OF. Coumarin-induced necrosis of the skin. *Arch Dermatol.* 1967;95:87–88.

21. Jones RR, Cunningham J. Warfarin skin necrosis. The role of factor VII. *Br J Dermatol.* 1979;100:561–565.

22. Boss JM, Summerly R. Prevention of warfarin-induced skin necrosis. *Br J Dermatol.* 1979;100:617. Letter.

23. Hofmann V, Frick PG. Repeated occurrence of skin necrosis twice following coumarin intake and subsequently during decrease of vitamin K dependent coagulation factors associated with cholestasis. *Thromb Haemost.* 1982;48:245–246.

24. Pescatore P, Horellou HM, Conrad J, et al. Problems of oral anticoagulation in an adult with homozygous protein C deficiency and late onset of thrombosis. *Thromb Haemost.* 1993;69:311–315.

25. Brooks LW, Blais FX. Coumarin-induced skin necrosis. *J Am Osteopath Assoc.* 1991;91:601–605.

26. Schramm W, Spannagl M, Bauer KA, et al. Treatment of Coumarin-induced skin necrosis with a monoclonal antibody purified protein C concentrate. *Arch Dermatol.* 1993;129:753–756.

27. Broekmans AW, Bertina RM, Loeliger EA, et al. Protein C and the development of skin necrosis during anticoagulant therapy. *Thromb Haemost.* 1984;49:244. Letter.

28. Bhajanjit SB, Gruba DM. Coumadin-induced necrosis of the skin after total knee replacements. *J Bone Joint Surg.* 1991;73–A:129–130.

29. Gold JA, Watters AK, O'Brien E. Coumadin versus heparin necrosis. *J Am Acad Dermatol.* 1987;16:148–149.

30. Humphries JE, Gardner JH, Connelly JE. Warfarin skin necrosis: Recurrence in the absence of anticoagulant therapy. *Am J Hematol.* 1991;37:197–200.

31. Rowbotham B, Clouston W, Kime N, et al. Coumarin skin necrosis without protein C deficiency. *Aust N Z J Med.* 1986;16:513.

32. Kiehl R, Hellstern P, Wenzel E. Hereditary antithrombin III deficiency and atypical localization of a coumarin necrosis. *Thromb Res.* 1987;45:191–193.

33. Moreb J, Kitchens CS. Acquired functional S deficiency, central venous thrombosis, and coumarin skin necrosis in association with antiphospholipid syndrome; report of two cases. *Am J Med.* 1989;87:207–210.

34. Enzenauer RJ, Berenberg JC, Campbell J. Progressive warfarin anticoagulation in protein C deficiency: a therapeutic strategy. *Am J Med.* 1990;88:697–698.

35. Samama M, Horellou MH, Soria J, et al. Successful progressive anticoagulation in a severe protein C deficiency and previous skin necrosis at the initiation of oral anticoagulant therapy. *Thromb Haemost.* 1984;51:132–133.

36. Locht H, Lindström FD. Severe skin necrosis following warfarin therapy in a patient with protein C deficiency. *J Intern Med.* 1993; 233:287–289.

37. Melissarie E, Kakkar VV. Congenital severe protein C deficiency in adults. *Br J Haematol.* 1989;72:222–228.

38. Zauber NP, Stark MW. Successful warfarin anticoagulation despite protein C deficiency and a history of warfarin necrosis. *Ann Inter Med.* 1986;104:659–660.

39. Majer RV, Chisholm M, Hickton MC. Replacement therapy for protein C deficiency using fresh frozen plasma. *Br J Haematol.* 1989;72:475.

40. Bick RL. Hypercoagulability and thrombosis. *Med Clin North Am.* 1994;78:635–665.

41. Colman RW, Rao AK, Rubin RN. Warfarin skin necrosis in a 33-year-old woman. *Am J Hematol.* 1993;43:300–303.

42. Lewandowski K, Zawilska K. Protein C concentrate in the treatment of warfarin-induced skin necrosis in the protein C deficiency. *Thromb Haemost.* 1994;71:395. Letter.

43. Munteah W, Finding K, Gamillscheg A, Schwarz HP. Multiple thromboses and coumarin-induced skin necrosis in a child with anticardiolipin antibodies. Effects of protein C concentrate administration. *Thromb Haemost.* 1991;65:1254.

44. Dreyfus M, Magny JF, Bridey F, et al. Treatment of homozygous protein C deficiency and neonatal purpura fulminans with a purified protein C concentrate. *N Engl J Med.* 1991;325:1565–1568.

45. Tuddenham E, Takase T, Thomas AE, et al. Homozygous protein C deficiency with delayed onset of symptoms at 7 to 10 months. *Thromb Res.* 1989;53:475–484.

46. Kipin CS. Gangrene of the breast—a complication of anticoagulant therapy—report of two cases. *N Engl J Med.* 1961;265:638–640.

47. Bahadir I, James EC, Fedde CW. Soft tissue necrosis and gangrene complicating treatment with the Coumadin derivatives. *Surg Gynecol Obstet.* 1977;145:497–500.

48. Campbell R, Clanton TO, Heckman JD. Necrosis and gangrene as a complication of Coumadin therapy. A case report. *J Bone Joint Surg.* 1980;62(A):1016.

49. Feder W, Auerbach R. "Purple toes": an uncommon sequela of oral coumarin drug therapy. *Ann Intern Med.* 1961;55:911–917.

50. Hyman BT, Landas SK, Ashman RF, et al. Warfarin-related purple toes syndrome and cholesterol microembolization. *Am J Med.* 1987;82:1233–1237.

51. Park S, Schroeter AL, Park YS, et al. Purple toes and livido reticularis in a patient with cardiovascular disease taking Coumadin. *Arch Dermatol.* 1993;129:777, 780.

52. Moldveen Geronimus M, Merriam JC. Cholesterol embolization: from pathological curiosity to clinical entity. *Circulation.* 1967;35: 946–953.

53. Burns FJ, Segel DP, Adler S. Control of cholesterol embolization by discontinuation of anticoagulant therapy. *Am J Med Sci.* 1978;275: 105–108.

54. Sheps SG, Gifford RW. Urticaria after administration of warfarin sodium. *Am J Cardiol.* 1959;3:118–120.

55. Adams CW, Pass BJ. Extensive dermatitis due to warfarin sodium (Coumadin). *Circulation.* 1960;22:947–948.

56. Schiff BL, Pawtucket RI, Kern AB. Cutaneous reactions to anticoagulants. *Arch Dermatol.* 1968;98:136–137.

57. Kwong P, Roberts P, Prescott SM, Tikoff G. Dermatitis induced by warfarin. *JAMA.* 1978;239:1884–1885.

58. Antony SJ, Krick SK, Mehta DM. Unusual cutaneous adverse reaction to warfarin therapy. *South Med J.* 1993;86:1413–1414.

59. Kruis-de Vries MH, Stricker BHC, Coenraads PJ, Nater JP. Maculo-papular rash due to coumarin derivatives. *Dermatologica.* 1989;178: 109–111.

60. Grosset ABM, Allen JE, Rodgers GM. Anticoagulation with anisindione in patients who are intolerant of warfarin. *Am J Hematol.* 1994;46:138–140.

61. Sonnenblick M, Oren A, Jacobsen B. Hypertransaminasaemia with heparin therapy. *Br Med J.* 1975;13:77.

62. De Man RA, Wilson JHP, Schalm SW, et al. Phenprocoumon-induced hepatitis mimicking non-A, non-B hepatitis. *J Hepatol.* 1990;11: 318–321.

63. Rehnqvist N. Intrahepatic jaundice due to warfarin therapy. *Acta Med Scand.* 1978;2044:335–336.

64. Hohler T, Schnutgen M, Helmreich-Becker I, et al. Drug-induced hepatitis: a rare complication of oral anticoagulants. *J Hepatol.* 1994; 21:447–449.

65. Taybi J, Capitanio MA. Tracheobronchial calcification: an observation in three children after mitral valve replacement and warfarin sodium therapy. *Radiology.* 1990;176:728–730.

66. Moncada RM, Venta LA, Venta ER, et al. Tracheal and bronchial cartilaginous rings: warfarin sodium-induced calcification. *Radiology.* 1992;184:437–449.

67. Cornbleet T, Hoit L. Alopecia from coumarin. *AMA Arch Dermatol.* 1957;75:440–441.

68. Baker H, Levein GM. Drug reactions V: cutaneous reactions to anticoagulants. *Br J Dermatol.* 1969;81:236–238.

69. Umlas J, Harken DE. Warfarin-induced alopecia. *Cutis.* 1988;42: 63–64.

Chapter 35

Warfarin Drug Interactions

Philip Hansten and Ann K. Wittkowsky

INTRODUCTION

More is known about the drug interactions of warfarin than perhaps any other drug. Several factors account for this:

- Warfarin has been in clinical use for many years.
- An objective measure of its effect (prothrombin time) is performed in all patients taking the drug.
- The adverse outcomes of the interactions (bleeding or clotting) are usually obvious.
- Warfarin has a number of properties that predispose it to drug interactions.

Accordingly, the responsibility of health care providers for the prevention of adverse drug interactions in patients receiving warfarin is probably greater than their responsibility for most other adverse drug interactions. This is true not only because of the available information but also because the adverse consequences of excessive or inadequate warfarin response can be life threatening. Moreover, for most warfarin drug interactions, a simple method for early detection exists, namely, determination of the prothrombin time expressed as INR (International Normalized Ratio). In addition, patients who receive warfarin along with drugs with which it interacts, possibly incur higher costs as a result of the interactions.[1]

INTERACTIVE PROPERTIES OF WARFARIN

Warfarin exhibits a number of properties that make it susceptible to interactions with other drugs. Interactions that influence the handling of warfarin are termed *pharmacokinetic* interactions, and those that influence the physiology of hemostasis are *pharmacodynamic* interactions.

Most drug interactions involve some alteration in the hypoprothrombinemic response of warfarin, which culminates in a change in prothrombin time (PT). Interactions that result in an increase in warfarin response and elevation in PT are described in Table 35–1; interactions that decrease the PT by reducing response to warfarin are described in Table 35–2. In addition to the determination of interacting agents, interest in warfarin drug interactions has resulted in the identification of drugs that do not appear to influence response to warfarin. These agents are described in Table 35–3.

PHARMACOKINETIC INTERACTIONS

Absorption

Oral warfarin is well absorbed, and only a few agents have been shown to reduce warfarin bioavailability. Thus, interference with absorption is not a common mechanism for warfarin drug interactions. The bile acid sequestrant, cholestyramine, can bind with warfarin and reduce its absorption.[24] This effect can be minimized by separating the doses (eg, giving warfarin two hours before or six hours after cholestyramine). Because warfarin appears to undergo enterohepatic circulation, however, cholestyramine might somewhat reduce warfarin response no matter how far apart the doses of the two drugs are spaced. Colestipol also appears to bind with warfarin in the gastrointestinal tract, but limited

Table 35–1 Drugs That Can Increase Warfarin Response[2-23]

Drug	Comments
Acetaminophen	Usually little or no effect, but large doses for more than a week are reported to increase warfarin effect in some patients.
Alcohol	Alcohol intoxication can substantially increase the hypoprothrombinemic response to warfarin, but smaller amounts appear to have little effect. Chronic excessive alcohol use can enhance warfarin metabolism, resulting in reduced warfarin effect.
Allopurinol	Increased warfarin effect noted in some patients, but incidence is not known.
Aminoglycosides	Oral aminoglycosides can increase warfarin effect in some patients, but the incidence is not known. Aminoglycosides IV have not been shown to do so.
Aminosalicylic acid	Purported increase in warfarin effect in one patient, but a causal relationship is not established.
Amiodarone	Marked increase in warfarin effect; slow onset (weeks) and offset (months) of effect. Magnitude of effect dependent on dose of amiodarone.
Androgens	Large increases in warfarin effect reported; extent of effect can vary with different androgens.
Ascorbic acid	Isolated case reports of reduced warfarin response, but a causal relationship is not established.
Azithromycin	Isolated cases of increased warfarin effect, but a causal relationship is not established.
Capecitabine	Increased hypoprothrombinemic response to warfarin; reduction in warfarin dose likely to be needed.
Cephalosporins	Cefoperazone, cefamandole, cefotetan, cefmetazole, and moxalactam can cause hypoprothrombinemia through effects on vitamin K production and/or activity.
Chloral hydrate	Displaces warfarin from plasma protein binding and produces a transient increase in the hypoprothrombinemic response.
Chloramphenicol	Increases the hypoprothrombinemic response to dicumarol; theoretically, it would also increase warfarin effect, but data are lacking.
Cimetidine	Inhibits the hepatic metabolism of warfarin and increases its hypoprothrombinemic response. The effect is usually modest, but substantial increases in warfarin effect are occasionally seen.
Ciprofloxacin	Several cases of increased hypoprothrombinemic response to warfarin reported, but the incidence and magnitude of this interaction is not established. Isolated cases of increased warfarin effect have also been reported with other fluoroquinolones, but a causal relationship was not established.
Clofibrate	Increases the hypoprothrombinemic response to warfarin; bleeding has occurred.
Corticosteroids	Case reports have suggested both increased and decreased effects of warfarin.
Danazol	Can markedly enhance the hypoprothrombinemic response to warfarin; bleeding has occurred.
Diflunisal	Limited clinical data suggest that discontinuation might increase warfarin requirements.
Digoxin immune Fab	Isolated cases of increased warfarin effect, but a causal relationship is not established.
Disulfiram	Inhibits the hepatic metabolism of warfarin and consistently increases the hypoprothrombinemic response.
Erythromycin	Several case reports of marked increase in hypoprothrombinemic response to warfarin, but studies in healthy subjects suggest smaller interaction. It might occur only in certain predisposed individuals.
Ethacrynic acid	Isolated case reports suggest increased hypoprothrombinemic response to warfarin, but the clinical importance is not established.
Etoposide	Isolated cases of increased warfarin effect, but a causal relationship is not established.
Fenofibrate	Isolated cases of increased warfarin effect; more data needed to establish clinical importance.
Fluconazole	Inhibits the hepatic metabolism of warfarin and increases its hypoprothrombinemic response.
Fluorouracil	Isolated cases of increased hypoprothrombinemic response to warfarin.
Gemfibrozil	Limited clinical evidence indicates that gemfibrozil can increase the hypoprothrombinemic response to warfarin. Gemfibrozil is in the same class as clofibrate, a drug known to enhance warfarin effect.
Glucagon	Can increase the hypoprothrombinemic response to warfarin, but the clinical importance is not established.
Glyburide	A case of increased warfarin effect has been reported, but a causal relationship is not established.
Griseofulvin	Can inhibit the hypoprothrombinemic response to warfarin, possibly by increasing warfarin hepatic metabolism.
Ifosfamide	Isolated cases of increased hypoprothrombinemic response to warfarin, but a causal relationship is not established.
Influenza vaccine	Has been associated with altered hypoprothrombinemic response to warfarin in some patients, but the effect appears to be minimal in most cases.

continues

Table 35–1 continued

Drug	Comments
Interferon	Case reports of increased hypoprothrombinemic response to warfarin; more study is needed.
Isoniazid	Isolated case reports suggest that isoniazid can increase the hypoprothrombinemic response to warfarin, possibly by inhibiting the hepatic metabolism of warfarin.
Ketoconazole	Appears to increase the hypoprothrombinemic response to warfarin probably by inhibiting its hepatic metabolism.
Levamisole	Isolated cases of increased hypoprothrombinemic response to warfarin, but the incidence and magnitude of the effect are not established.
Lovastatin	Appears to increase the hypoprothrombinemic response to warfarin, but the mechanism is not established.
Metronidazole	Inhibits the metabolism of S-warfarin and can markedly increase the hypoprothrombinemic response to warfarin.
Miconazole	Probably inhibits the hepatic metabolism of warfarin and can markedly increase its hypoprothrombinemic effect, even when the miconazole is applied as an oral gel or vaginally.
Nalidixic acid	Isolated cases of increased hypoprothrombinemic response to warfarin, but a causal relationship is not established.
Nonsteroidal anti-inflammatory drugs	Some nonsteroidal anti-inflammatory drugs (NSAIDs) such as azapropazone and phenylbutazone, can markedly increase the hypoprothrombinemic response to warfarin. Other NSAIDs, such as meclofenamate, piroxicam, and sulindac, have more modest effects on warfarin and/or only affect warfarin occasionally. NSAIDs that appear unlikely to affect the hypoprothrombinemic response to warfarin include ibuprofen, naproxen, diclofenac, ketoprofen, and tolmetin.
Omeprazole	Studies in patients and normal subjects suggest only slight increase in hypoprothrombinemic response to warfarin with 20 mg/day of omeprazole.
Phenytoin	Both increased and decreased warfarin effects have been described. Several mechanisms are possible: induction of warfarin metabolism; competition for plasma protein binding sites; both are metabolized by CYP2C9 (competition?).
Propranolol	Propranolol slightly increases warfarin serum concentrations; the clinical importance of this effect is questionable.
Propafenone	Increased hypoprothrombinemic response to warfarin reported in healthy subjects.
Quinidine	Several cases reported of quinidine-induced increase in warfarin hypoprothrombinemic response, but most patients appear minimally affected.
Ropinirole	Isolated cases of increased warfarin effect; more data needed to establish clinical importance.
Simvastatin	Limited clinical evidence suggests that Simvastatin slightly increases the hypoprothrombinemic response to warfarin.
Sulfinpyrazone	Marked increases in warfarin hypoprothrombinemic response reported.
Tamoxifen	Increased hypoprothrombinemic response to warfarin reported in several patients.
Terbinafine	Isolated cases of increased hypoprothrombinemic response to warfarin, but *decreased* warfarin effect also reported.
Tetracycline	Increased hypoprothrombinemic response to warfarin reported in several patients.
Thyroid hormones	Increase catabolism of clotting factors, thus increasing the hypoprothrombinemic response to warfarin.
Tricyclic antidepressants	Increased hypoprothrombinemic response reportedly has occurred, but clinical evidence is minimal.
Trimethoprim-sulfamethoxazole	Inhibits the hepatic metabolism of S-warfarin and substantially increases warfarin's hypoprothrombinemic response.
Vitamin E	Increased hypoprothrombinemic response to warfarin reported in several patients; effect is probably minimal with small supplemental doses found in multivitamins.
Valproic acid	Possible displacement of warfarin from plasma protein binding, resulting in transient increase in hypoprothrombinemic response; more study is needed.
Zafirlukast	Increased hypoprothrombinemic response to warfarin reported, probably due to inhibition of CYP2C9.

Table 35–2 Drugs That Can Reduce the Effect of Warfarin[12,19,24–28]

Drug	Comments
Aminoglutethimide	Reduced warfarin effect; effect is probably large and occurs in most patients.
Antithyroid drugs: methimazole propylthiouracil	Reducing thyroid status reduces warfarin effect; rare cases of hypoprothrombinemia with propylthiouracil alone.
Azathioprine	Isolated case reports of reduced warfarin response, but a causal relationship is not established.
Barbiturates	Well-documented reduction in warfarin effect; bleeding has occurred when barbiturate stopped.
Binding resins: cholestyramine colestipol	Binding of warfarin in gastrointestinal tract, reducing warfarin effect. Spacing doses of binding resin from warfarin can reduce interaction but not eliminate it because warfarin undergoes enterohepatic circulation.
Carbamazepine	Reduced warfarin effect in several case reports; carbamazepine is a known enzyme inducer.
Contraceptives, oral	Although oral contraceptives have been reported to affect the response to some oral anticoagulants, there is little information on warfarin. Patients with thromboembolic disorders, however, generally should avoid oral contraceptives.
Cyclophosphamide	Limited clinical evidence suggests that cyclophosphamide inhibits the hypoprothrombinemic response to warfarin; more study is needed.
Cyclosporine	Isolated case reports suggest a reduction in the effect of both warfarin and cyclosporine, but a causal relationship is not established.
Dicloxacillin	As with nafcillin, decreased warfarin response has been observed, but little is known about other penicillinase-resistant penicillins.
Disopyramide	Limited clinical data suggest that disopyramide inhibits the hypoprothrombinemic response of warfarin, but causal relationship is not established.
Ethchlorvynol	Limited clinical evidence indicates that ethchlorvynol inhibits the hypoprothrombinemic response to warfarin; more study is needed.
Etretinate	Limited clinical evidence suggests that etretinate inhibits the hypoprothrombinemic response to warfarin, but a causal relationship is not established.
Glutethimide	Enhances the hepatic metabolism of warfarin; the hypoprothrombinemic response is substantially reduced in most patients.
Griseofulvin	Limited clinical evidence suggests that griseofulvin inhibits the hypoprothrombinemic response to warfarin, probably by enzyme induction.
Haloperidol	Limited clinical evidence suggests that haloperidol inhibits the hypoprothrombinemic response to phenindione, but its effect on warfarin is not known.
Mercaptopurine	Limited clinical evidence indicates that mercaptopurine inhibits the hypoprothrombinemic response to warfarin.
Mesalamine	Isolated case reports of reduced warfarin effect, but the mechanism is not established.
Mitotane	Isolated cases of decreased hypoprothrombinemic response to warfarin, but a causal relationship is not established.
Nafcillin	Several case reports suggest that nafcillin inhibits the hypoprothrombinemic response to warfarin; dicloxacillin can affect warfarin similarly, but little is known regarding other penicillinase-resistant penicillins.
Phenytoin	Both increased and decreased warfarin effects have been described. Several mechanisms are possible: induction of warfarin metabolism; competition for plasma protein-binding sites; both are metabolized by CYP2C9 (competition?).
Rifampin	Marked reduction in warfarin response; substantial increase in warfarin dose usually required.
Sucralfate	Isolated cases of decreased hypoprothrombinemic response to warfarin reported, but other investigators found little effect.

Table 35-3 Drugs That Appear To Have Minimal Effect on Warfarin[12,19,29–32]

Drug	Comments
Antacids	Magnesium and aluminum hydroxides do not appear to affect warfarin absorption.
Bumetanide	Studies in healthy subjects suggest no alteration in warfarin effect.
Chlordiazepoxide	Several studies suggest no alteration in warfarin effect.
Diazepam	Diazepam does not appear to affect the hypoprothrombinemic response to warfarin.
Famotidine	Available evidence suggests that famotidine does not affect the hypoprothrombinemic response to warfarin.
Felodipine	Available evidence suggests that felodipine does not affect warfarin pharmacokinetics or hypoprothrombinemic response.
Flurazepam	Flurazepam does not appear to affect the hypoprothrombinemic response to warfarin.
Furosemide	Furosemide appears to have little or no effect on the hypoprothrombinemic response to warfarin.
Meprobamate	Meprobamate does not appear to affect the hypoprothrombinemic response to warfarin.
Modafinil	Study in healthy subjects suggests that modafinil does not affect warfarin pharmacokinetics.
Nizatidine	Available evidence suggests that nizatidine does not affect the hypoprothrombinemic response to warfarin.
Pravastatin	Available evidence suggests that pravastatin does not affect the hypoprothrombinemic response to warfarin.
Ranitidine	The bulk of the clinical evidence suggests that ranitidine has little or no effect on the hypoprothrombinemic response to warfarin.
Tacrine	Tacrine has no effect on the hypoprothrombinemic response in patients stabilized on chronic warfarin therapy.

evidence suggests that the effect is less than the effect with cholestyramine. Sucralfate also has been reported to inhibit the gastrointestinal absorption of warfarin, but some of the evidence is conflicting.[25]

Plasma Protein Binding

Warfarin is about 99% bound to plasma proteins, primarily albumin. Thus, one might expect that other highly bound drugs would displace warfarin and increase its hypoprothrombinemic response. In fact, many drugs do appear to displace warfarin from plasma protein–binding sites, but there is little evidence to suggest that this causes much clinical difficulty. When warfarin is displaced from plasma protein–binding sites, the increase in hypoprothrombinemic response is transient. This is because the increased unbound warfarin is available not only to sites of action but also to sites of elimination. Thus, protein–binding displacement drug interactions tend to be self-limited. An example is chloral hydrate, which appears to displace warfarin from plasma protein–binding sites and usually results in a modest increase in the hypoprothrombinemic response to warfarin that lasts a few days.[17] Valproic acid also can displace warfarin from plasma protein binding.[18] Although it is possible that even a transient increase in warfarin effect could increase bleeding risk, the primary risk of warfarin displacement probably

occurs when the patient is also receiving a drug that inhibits warfarin metabolism. In such a situation, the compensatory increase in warfarin elimination that occurs following plasma protein-binding displacement would be prevented.

Induction of Metabolism

Warfarin is extensively metabolized by cytochrome P450 enzymes in the liver. Although several isozymes are involved, the most important is CYP2C9, which metabolizes (S)-warfarin. Thus, agents that enhance CYP2C9 activity (enzyme inducers) reduce the hypoprothrombinemic response to warfarin.

Enzyme inducers can substantially reduce the hypoprothrombinemic response to warfarin, thus reducing the PT and requiring an increase in warfarin dose.[26,27] If the enzyme inducer is subsequently discontinued, the patient is likely to become overanticoagulated; fatal bleeding episodes have occurred. The effect of enzyme inducers on warfarin response is gradual because it requires the synthesis of new drug-metabolizing enzymes. Induction can begin after only a few days, but a period of one to two weeks, or longer, might be required before maximal effects on the hypoprothrombinemic response occurs. The dissipation of enzyme induction is also gradual, being dependent on elimination of the inducer from the body and the decay of the increased drug-metabolizing enzyme stores. Although all inducers result in gradual effects, there can be differences in the time course, depending on the enzyme inducer. For example, enzyme induction that is due to rifampin tends to have a more rapid onset and offset than a drug, such as phenobarbital, that has a long half-life. The following can enhance warfarin metabolism[12,19,26,27]:

- aminoglutethimide
- barbiturates
- carbamazepine
- glutethimide
- griseofulvin
- nafcillin
- phenytoin
- primidone
- rifampin

Inhibition of Metabolism

The number of drugs that have been shown to inhibit warfarin hepatic metabolism far exceeds the number of those that induce warfarin metabolism; however, there is considerable variation in the potency with which inhibitors affect warfarin metabolism. This is probably due to the specific cytochrome P450 isozymes affected by the various inhibitors. Because CYP2C9 is the most important isozyme in the metabolism of (S)-warfarin, potent inhibitors of CYP2C9 can dramatically increase warfarin effect. On the other hand, CYP1A2 and CYP3A4 are the primary isozymes involved in the metabolism of the less active enantiomer (R)-warfarin, which is the less potent of the enantiomers of warfarin. Inhibitors of these latter enzymes tend to have more modest and/or inconsistent effects on the hypoprothrombinemic response to warfarin. For example, in 13 men stabilized on chronic warfarin therapy, ticlopidine increased (R)-warfarin serum concentrations by 25% but had no effect on mean INR values.[33] Nonetheless, occasional predisposed individuals on warfarin might manifest clinically important increases in the hypoprothrombinemic response when given inhibitors of CYP1A2 or CYP3A4. Exhibit 35–1 lists drugs that inhibit specific metabolizing enzymes of warfarin.

Given that the (S) enantiomer of warfarin is considerably more active than the (R) enantiomer, it is important to use warfarin enantiomer concentration data when studying pharmacokinetic drug interactions with warfarin. Often, a drug that inhibits the metabolism of (R)-warfarin but not (S)-warfarin has little or no effect on warfarin's hypoprothrombinemic response. An example would be diltiazem, which decreases the clearance of (R)-warfarin but not (S)-warfarin,

---

Exhibit 35–1
DRUGS KNOWN OR SUSPECTED TO INHIBIT THE CYTOCHROME P450 ENZYMES INVOLVED IN METABOLISM OF (S)- AND (R)-WARFARIN[34–36]

CYP1A2	CYP3A4	CYP2C9
Cimetidine	Clarithromycin	Amiodarone
Ciprofloxacin	Cyclosporine	Disulfiram
Diltiazem	Danazol	Fluconazole
Erythromycin	Diltiazem	Fluvoxamine
Fluvoxamine	Erythromycin	Fluvastatin
Mexiletine	Fluconazole (large doses)	Metronidazole
Norfloxacin	Fluoxetine	Miconazole
Tacrine	Fluvoxamine	Propoxyphene
	Grapefruit juice	Sulfaphenazole
	Itraconazole	Trimethoprim-sulfamethoxazole
	Ketoconazole	
	Miconazole	
	Nefazodone	
	Omeprazole	
	Propoxyphene(?)	
	Quinidine	
	Ritonavir	
	Troleandomycin	
	Verapamil	

Note: CYP1A2 and CYP3A4 are the primary isozymes for the metabolism of (R)-warfarin. CYP2C9 is the primary isozyme in the metabolism of (S)-warfarin.

and does not affect the hypoprothrombinemic response.[29] Thus, it is important to measure the effect of drugs on both warfarin enantiomers in order to avoid faulty conclusions about the nature of the interactions.

Inhibitors of drug metabolism generally begin to interfere with the hepatic metabolism of warfarin as soon as sufficient concentrations of the inhibitor are achieved in the liver (ie, usually within the first 24 hours of therapy). Nonetheless, it may take 7 to 10 days for a new steady-state hypoprothrombinemic response because warfarin has a relatively long half-life and the inhibitor can prolong the warfarin half-life even more.

PHARMACODYNAMIC INTERACTIONS

Clotting Factor Synthesis and Degradation

Some drugs have intrinsic effects on clotting factors or fibrinolysis and thus can increase the bleeding risk without interacting directly with warfarin. For example, drugs that increase circulating levels of thyroid hormones (eg, thyroid replacement) increase the catabolism of clotting factors and increase warfarin response. The opposite is true of drugs that reduce circulating thyroid hormone concentrations. Other drugs, such as quinidine, and large doses of salicylates can reduce the production of clotting factors, thus potentially increasing the hypoprothrombinemic response to warfarin. Table 35–4 describes agents that interact with the pharmacodynamic effect of warfarin by interfering with hemostasis.

Platelet Inhibition

Drugs that impair platelet function also tend to increase the risk of bleeding in patients receiving warfarin. For example, nonsteroidal anti-inflammatory drugs (NSAIDs) inhibit platelet function and appear to increase the risk of severe gastrointestinal bleeding in patients on warfarin.[37] Aspirin also inhibits platelet function, but, unlike NSAIDs, its effects last for the life of the platelet. Nonacetylated salicylates, such as choline salicylate, salsalate, and sodium salicylate, however, have minimal effects on platelet function. They are also less likely than NSAIDs or aspirin to cause gastric erosions. It should be noted that impaired platelet function is not reflected in the INR, so that the increased bleeding risk is not likely to be detected with normal monitoring. Table 35–5 describes agents that increase the risk of bleeding associated with warfarin by inhibiting platelet aggregation without interfering with PT response.[12,19,33,37–42]

INTERACTIONS WITH DIETARY SUPPLEMENTS

The use of herbal medicinals (botanicals), amino acids, and other nonprescription products has increased dramatically in the last decade. A recent survey suggested that approximately 50% of Americans have used dietary supplements for health purposes, with up to 20% reporting regular use.[48] However, up to 60% of patients do not report use of alternative therapies to their health care providers.[49]

Dietary supplements are regulated by the Food and Drug Administration (FDA) Dietary Supplement Health and Education Act of 1994.[50] However, unlike drug products, dietary supplements are not tested prior to marketing for safety, efficacy, dosing requirements, or interactions with other medications. They are not required to meet quality standards for labeling, nor are they required to follow good manufacturing practices or to meet United States Pharmacopeia standards for tablet content uniformity.[51] Without regulation of tablet contents, patients may be exposed to unlisted ingredients and potential contaminants, as well as to varying doses of the active ingredient, whether taking apparently similar

Table 35–4 Pharmacodynamic Interactions with Warfarin: Clotting Factor Synthesis and Degradation[12,19]

Drugs	Comments
Cephalosporins	Some cephalosporins, such as cefamandole, cefoperazone, cefotetan, and moxalactam. can produce hypoprothrombinemia through effects on vitamin K production and/or activity.
Methimazole	Reported to reduce response to warfarin by antithyroid activity.
Propylthiouracil	Several cases of propylthiouracil-induced hypoprothrombinemia have been reported, but incidence appears to be low. Much more common would be the antithyroid effects of propylthiouracil that reduce the hypoprothrombinemic response to warfarin.
Thyroid hormones	Thyroid hormones increase catabolism of clotting factors, thus increasing the hypoprothrombinemic response to warfarin.
Vitamin K	Vitamin K, given as a drug or ingested in foods, can antagonize the hypoprothrombinemic response to warfarin.

Table 35–5 Pharmacodynamic Interactions with Warfarin: Platelet Inhibition[12,19,33,37–47]

Drugs	Comments
Aspirin	Aspirin can produce gastrointestinal bleeding; risk is increased in patients on warfarin. Salicylate-induced inhibition of platelet function can also increase bleeding risk. Benefits of additive anticoagulant effects with warfarin might outweigh risks in many patients. Low-dose aspirin used for platelet inhibition in patients on warfarin appears to increase the risk of minor bleeding but not major bleeding. Note that inhibition of platelet function does not affect the INR. Unlike aspirin, nonacetylated salicylates, such as choline salicylate, magnesium salicylate, and salsalate, have minimal effects on platelets and are unlikely to produce gastrointestinal bleeding.
Nonsteroidal anti-inflammatory drugs	NSAIDs can produce gastrointestinal bleeding, and the risk is increased in patients on warfarin. NSAID-induced inhibition of platelet function would also theoretically increase the bleeding risk (without affecting the INR). There are no comparative studies to determine the relative risk of bleeding for one NSAID versus another in patients on warfarin. Ideally, all NSAIDs should be avoided in patients on warfarin. Nonetheless, when it is necessary to use NSAIDs and warfarin, four general guidelines can be made:[37] 1. avoid (serious risk of interaction): mefenamic acid, and probably piroxicam and ketoprofen 2. use if drugs from 3 and 4 (below) cannot be used (moderate risk of interaction or inadequate data): diflunisal, etodolac, fenbufen, indomethacin, ketoprofen, sulindac, tenoxicam, and tolmetin 3. might be less likely to interact: ibuprofen, nabumetone, and naproxen 4. least likely to interact: nonacetylated salicylates
Selective serotonin reuptake inhibitors	These inhibitors can increase the bleeding risk in some patients on warfarin without affecting hypoprothrombinemic response, which might result from inhibition of platelet function. Some case reports suggest that fluoxetine increases warfarin hypoprothrombinemic response.
Clopidogrel/Ticlopidine	Increased risk of bleeding due to inhibition of platelet function.
Tramadol	Isolated case reports of increased bleeding risk with warfarin; mechanism is not established.
COX-2 Inhibitors	Unlike standard NSAIDs, the cyclooxygenase-2 (COX-2) inhibitors, celecoxib, rofecoxib, and valdecoxib do not affect platelet function and are less likely than NSAIDs to produce gastrointestinal ulceration and bleeding. While several case reports describe increased INR and/or bleeding when COX-2 inhibitors were added to warfarin therapy, results of pharmacokinetic and pharmacodynamic studies suggest that COX-2 inhibitors only slightly increase warfarin effect (rofecoxib, valdecoxib) or have no effect on warfarin (celecoxib). Overall, it seems likely that COX-2 inhibitors are safer than standard NSAIDs in patients receiving warfarin (lack of platelet effect, less gastrointestinal toxicity) but still should be used with caution due to a possible increase in the risk of gastrointestinal bleeding.

products produced by different manufacturers or batches of the same product from a single manufacturer. These limitations influence the risk of adverse effects associated with interactions between dietary supplements and drug products, including warfarin. They also influence the availability and reliability of information regarding potential interactions.

Case reports constitute the majority of information regarding interactions with warfarin and dietary supplements. In addition, limited knowledge of the pharmacodynamic effects of certain herbal medicinals suggests potential interactions with warfarin despite a lack of case reports. Certain products may increase the possibility of warfarin-associated bleeding due to alterations in platelet function (Table 35–6). Other products have been reported to alter the prothrombin time (Table 35–7). In general, these are potential interactions based on the known or implied properties of the herbal

medicinals. Little is known about the actual risk of these compounds in patients taking warfarin.

Without reliable and substantive information about dietary supplements and potential interactions, and because of likely inconsistencies in product contents, it may be appropriate for patients taking warfarin to avoid using these agents altogether. However, to avoid potential adverse effects associated with interactions between dietary supplements and warfarin, vigilant and routine assessment of supplement use is necessary to avoid potential adverse effects associated with interactions between these products and warfarin.

Additional Web-based information regarding herbal and natural products can be found at The Natural Pharmacist (www.tnp.com), The Pharmacist's Letter (www.natural pharmacist.com), or the National Institutes of Health (http://dietary-supplements.info.nih.gov). Anticoagulation practi-

Table 35–6 Dietary Supplements That May Increase Bleeding Complications in Patients Taking Warfarin[52–56]

Product	Comments
agrimony	contains salicylates
aloe gel	reported to possess antiplatelet activity
aspen	reported to possess antiplatelet activity
black cohosh	reported to possess antiplatelet activity
black haw	reported to possess antiplatelet activity
bogbean	reported to possess antiplatelet activity
boldo	antiplatelet activity associated with inhibition of thromboxane A2 production
cassia	may inhibit platelet aggregation
clove	may inhibit platelet aggregation
dandelion	reported to possess antiplatelet activity
dihydroepiandrosterone (DHEA)	may enhance fibrinolysis by reducing levels of plasminogen activator inhibitor (PAI-1) and tissue plasminogen activator antigen (TPA antigen)
feverfew	may inhibit platelet aggregation
garlic	reduces platelet aggregation; reported to cause hemorrhage when used alone
german sarsaparilla	reported to possess antiplatelet activity
ginger	potent inhibitor of thromboxane synthetase resulting in inhibition of cyclooxygenase-dependent platelet aggregation
ginkgo*	potent inhibitor of platelet activating factor resulting in inhibition of cyclooxygenase-dependent platelet aggregation; reported to cause hemorrhage when used alone and in conjunction with warfarin
ginseng	reported to inhibit platelet aggregation and thromboxane A2 production
licorice	reported to possess antiplatelet activity
meadowsweet	contains salicylates
onion	reported to possess antiplatelet activity
policosanol	reported to possess antiplatelet activity
poplar	contains salicylates
senega	reported to possess antiplatelet activity
tamarind	reported to possess antiplatelet activity
willow	contains salicylates
wintergreen	reported to possess antiplatelet activity

*Interaction with warfarin substantiated by case reports.

tioners are encouraged to report suspected interactions through the FDA Medwatch program (www.fda.gov/medwatch) and to appropriate medical journals in the form of case reports, case series, or clinical investigations.

VARIABILITY

Many drug interactions involving warfarin have been characterized with respect to mean or typical response. However, significant variability among patients occurs with respect to their susceptibility to various interactions, the magnitude of response, the time of onset, and the duration of effect.[63] To a certain extent, even the methods by which drug interactions are reported influence the observed variability in patient response to drug interactions with warfarin.[64] Although reports of drug interaction investigations might adequately describe pharmacokinetic characteristics of warfarin in the presence of interacting drugs, the investigations frequently involve the use of normal volunteers, thus limiting the characterization of pharmacodynamic response. Case reports overcome this disadvantage through descriptions of patient-specific responses to drug interactions, but they are limited by underreporting and selective reporting, which can lead to overestimation of the frequency and magnitude of an interaction.

Table 35–7 Dietary Supplements That May Influence the Anticoagulant Effect of Warfarin[52–62]

Product	Comments
agrimony	reported to possess procoagulant properties
alfalfa	contains coumarin derivatives
aniseed	contains coumarin derivatives
arnica	contains coumarin derivatives
artemesia	contains coumarin derivatives
asa foetica	contains coumarin derivatives
bladder wrack	reported to contain anticoagulant properties
bogbean	contains coumarin derivatives
bromelains	reported to possess fibrinolytic properties
buchu	contains coumarin derivatives
capsicum	contains coumarin derivatives, and reported to possess fibrinolytic properties
cassia	contains coumarin derivatives
celery seed	contains coumarin derivatives
chamomile	contains coumarin derivatives
Chinese wolfberry*	(Lycium barbarum) may inhibit CYP2C9; reported to increase INR in patients taking warfarin
coenzyme Q10	contains a vitamin K derivative (ubidecareonone); reported to decrease INR in patients taking warfarin
dan-shen*	(Salvia miltiorrhiza) contains coumarin derivatives; reported to increase INR in patients taking warfarin
dong quai*	(danggui; Angelica sinensis) contains coumarin derivatives; reported to increase INR in patients taking warfarin
dandelion	contains coumarin derivatives
fenugreek*	contains coumarin derivatives; reported to increase INR in patients taking warfarin
garlic	may enhance fibrinolysis; reported to cause hemorrhage when used alone
ginseng*	may possess fibrinolytic properties; reported to reduce INR in patients taking warfarin; however, a clinical trial reported no influence in INR when fixed doses of ginseng were added to stable warfarin therapy
goldenseal	reported to possess procoagulant properties
grapefruit juice*	inhibits CYP1A2 and CYP3A4; reported to increase INR in patients taking warfarin; however, a clinical trial reported no influence in INR when consistent quantities of grapefruit juice were added to stable warfarin therapy
horse chestnut	contains coumarin derivatives
horseradish	contains coumarin derivatives
inositol nicotinate	reported to possess fibrinolytic properties
licorice	contains coumarin derivatives
meadowsweet	contains coumarin derivatives
melilot	contains coumarin derivatives
mistletoe	reported to possess procoagulant properties
nettle	contains coumarin derivatives
onion	reported to possess fibrinolytic properties
papain*	reported to increase INR in patients taking warfarin
parsley	contains coumarin derivatives
passion flower	contains coumarin derivatives
pau d'arco	reported to possess anticoagulant properties
prickly ash	contains coumarin derivatives
quassia	contains coumarin derivatives
red clover	contains coumarin derivatives
St. John's Wort*	induction of CYP3A4
sweet clover	contains coumarin derivatives
sweet woodruff	contains coumarin derivatives
tonka beans	contains coumarin derivatives
wild carrot	contains coumarin derivatives
wild lettuce	contains coumarin derivatives
yarrow	reported to possess procoagulant properties

*Interaction with warfarin substantiated by case reports

Individual patient variables also influence susceptibility, magnitude, onset, and duration of drug interactions.[65] Comorbid diseases, concurrent use of other medications, patient age, and current diet are among the factors that influence clotting factor synthesis and degradation and the absorption, metabolism, and elimination of the interacting drug, as well as the pharmacokinetic and pharmacodynamic characteristics of warfarin (Figure 35–1). In addition, recent advances in the understanding of the stereochemical characteristics of warfarin metabolism serve to describe further the difficulty in predicting patient response to warfarin drug interactions.

Warfarin is available for clinical use as a racemic mixture of (R) and (S) enantiomers that differ with respect to both pharmacodynamic and pharmacokinetic properties, including sites and extent of oxidative metabolism.[66] Genetic variations in metabolizing enzyme availability and/or activity can also influence the pharmacokinetic characteristics of warfarin, the pharmacokinetic characteristics of the interacting drug, and/or other variables known to affect patient responses to drugs.[67,68]

Given the significant variability in patient response to drug interactions, prevention of adverse clinical outcomes associated with drug interactions is dependent on careful management of anticoagulated patients. Practitioners who care for patients treated with warfarin must

- recognize situations that increase the risk of clinically significant drug interactions
- educate patients regarding drug interaction prevention
- continuously monitor prescription and nonprescription drug use
- monitor and adjust warfarin therapy to prevent adverse outcomes

RISK FACTORS FOR DRUG INTERACTIONS

The clinical significance of warfarin drug interactions is dependent on the physiologic response of individual patients to changes in the hypoprothrombinemic effect of warfarin. Drug interactions can cause elevations or reductions in PT or result in hemorrhagic complications or thromboembolic recurrence. Despite the possibility of adverse outcomes, however, concurrent use of warfarin and interacting drugs is not an absolute contraindication.[63]

Clinically significant drug interactions can occur when an interacting drug is added during warfarin therapy, when an interacting drug is discontinued during warfarin therapy, or when an interacting drug is used intermittently during warfarin therapy. These therapeutic situations represent significant risk factors for drug interactions and require intervention in order to avoid adverse outcomes. By anticipating patient response to the addition, discontinuation, or intermittent use of the interacting drug and by planning appropriate monitoring frequency and dosage alterations to avoid changes in PT response, clinically significant drug interactions can be prevented.

PATIENT EDUCATION

The prevention of adverse clinical outcomes associated with drug interactions is also dependent on effective, ongoing education of patients treated with warfarin.[69] Stressing the following three points during patient education will help patients to avoid warfarin drug interactions:

1. Patients must notify all health care providers of their status as anticoagulation patients.
2. Patients must obtain assistance in selecting nonprescription medications, including vitamins, minerals, nutritional supplements, herbal remedies, homeopathic and naturopathic compounds, and home remedies.
3. Patients must report to their health care providers any changes in prescription and nonprescription drug use, including initiation, discontinuation, and intermittent use, and any changes in dosage of their current medications.

Patients must be instructed to report their status as anticoagulation patients to all health care providers from whom they receive care, including physicians, physician assistants, nurse-practitioners, dentists, and pharmacists. With this knowledge, health care providers can participate in preventing hemorrhagic or thromboembolic complications in their patients by helping them to avoid the use of interacting drugs.

Also, patients must be instructed to obtain assistance in the selection of over-the-counter medications for minor medical

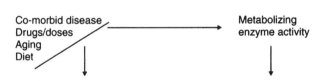

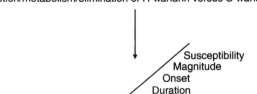

Co-morbid disease
Drugs/doses
Aging
Diet

Metabolizing enzyme activity

- Clotting factor synthesis/degradation
- Absorption/metabolism/elimination of interacting drug
- Absorption/metabolism/elimination of R-warfarin versus S-warfarin

Susceptibility
Magnitude
Onset
Duration

Figure 35–1 Factors influencing variability of warfarin drug interactions

problems so that interacting drugs can be avoided. This point is of particular importance because of the increasing availability, on a nonprescription basis, of many medications that interact with warfarin and that were previously available only by prescription.

Finally, patients must be counseled to report immediately to the clinicians who provide their anticoagulation monitoring all information pertaining to the initiation, discontinuation, and intermittent use of prescription and nonprescription drugs, regardless of the indication, duration, or frequency of their use of these medications. When clinicians are alerted to changes in medication use, appropriate monitoring and dosage adjustments can be initiated in order to avoid adverse outcomes.

MONITORING OF MEDICATION USE

Routine assessment of prescription and nonprescription drug use is an essential component of managing anticoagulation patients and plays a significant role in the prevention of adverse clinical outcomes associated with drug interactions. Patient management protocols should include guidelines for assessing medication use on an ongoing basis as a component of routine evaluation of warfarin therapy.

Current prescription drug use can be evaluated by using a series of open to closed questions in order to determine name, dosage form, dose, frequency, indication, compliance, and prescriber of each agent. Compliance assessment includes the following determinations:

- whether and why doses are missed or duplicated
- how medications are used in cases of changes in symptoms for which they were prescribed
- whether the patient receives assistance with medication administration from another individual
- whether the patient takes medications that were previously prescribed, does not take medications that are currently prescribed, and/or uses medications prescribed for others

Nonprescription drug use can be most efficiently evaluated with the use of a "by indication" or "by system" approach. Questioning should include an assessment of herbal remedies; homeopathic and naturopathic compounds; vitamins, minerals, and nutritional supplements; and home remedies used for various indications. Frequency and duration of use, as well as most recent use, should be evaluated.[70]

It might be necessary to evaluate visually all medications to gain a more complete understanding of current medication use. Patients can be asked to bring to the anticoagulation clinic all prescription and over-the-counter medications that are available to them at home, regardless of current or past use, as well as vitamins; minerals; nutritional supplements; and herbal, homeopathic, and naturopathic products. Labels should be compared with actual use, and administration devices and other reminder techniques also should be evaluated.[71]

PREVENTION OF ADVERSE EVENTS

In many instances, the initiation or discontinuation of agents that interact with warfarin is reported prospectively or concurrently to the clinician responsible for warfarin management. Patient management then involves anticipating response, planning appropriate dosing alterations, and/or monitoring frequency in order to prevent adverse clinical outcomes. In other circumstances, drug interactions are detected as a component of routine patient evaluation. Given the significant variability in individual patient response to drug interactions, clinicians are faced with the inability to predict susceptibility, magnitude, onset, and duration of drug interactions in selected patients and must adjust patient monitoring accordingly. Frequency of monitoring is directed by the following[19]:

- the pharmacokinetic and pharmacodynamic characteristics of warfarin and of the interacting drug
- consideration of the influence of dosage, route of administration, and drug metabolites
- an assessment of the characteristics of the interaction in a group of similar patients
- consideration of the time course associated with the mechanism of the interaction

The prevention of adverse clinical outcomes associated with drug interactions can be ensured by avoiding therapy with interacting drugs. When noninteracting alternatives are not available or are unacceptable, however, complications associated with drug interactions can be prevented by diligent PT monitoring, routine physical assessment of patient response, and appropriate warfarin dosage alterations.

REFERENCES

1. Jankel CA, McMillan JA, Martin BC. Effect of drug interactions on outcomes of patients receiving warfarin or theophylline. *Am J Hosp Pharm.* 1994;51:661–666.

2. Crussell-Porter LL, Rindone JP, Ford MA, Jaskar DW. Low-dose fluconazole therapy potentiates the hypoprothrombinemic response of warfarin sodium. *Arch Intern Med.* 1993;153:102–104.

3. Ahmad S. Lovastatin: warfarin interaction. *Arch Intern Med.* 1990; 150:2407.

4. Gaw A, Wosornu D. Simvastatin during warfarin therapy in hyperlipoproteinaemia. *Lancet.* 1992;340:979–980. Letter.

5. Souto JC, Oliver A, Montserrat I, Mateo J, Sureda A, Fontcuberta J. Lack of effect of influenza vaccine on anticoagulation by acenocoumarol. *Ann Pharmacother.* 1993;27:365–368.

6. Mieszczak C, Winther K. Lack of interaction of ketoprofen with warfarin. *Eur J Clin Pharmacol.* 1993;44:205–206.

7. Ermer JC, Hicks DR, Wheeler SC, Kraml M, Jusko WJ. Concomitant etodolac affects neither the unbound clearance nor the pharmacologic effect of warfarin. *Clin Pharmacol Ther.* 1994;55:305–316.

8. Unge P, Svedberg L-E, Blom NH, Andersson T, Lagerstrom PO, Idstrom JP. A study of the interaction of omeprazole and warfarin in anticoagulated patients. *Br J Clin Pharmacol.* 1992;34:509–512.

9. Scarfe MA, Israel MK. Possible drug interactions between warfarin and combination of levamisole and fluorouracil. *Ann Pharmacother.* 1994;28:464–467.

10. Wajima T, Mukhopadhyay P. Possible interactions between warfarin and 5–fluorouracil. *Am J Hematol.* 1992;40:238–243. Letter.

11. Quinn DI, Day RO. Drug interactions of clinical importance. *Drug Saf.* 1995;12:393–452.

12. Freedman MD, Olatidoye AG. Clinically significant drug interactions with the oral anticoagulants. *Drug Saf.* 1994;10:381–394.

13. Wehbe TW, Warth JA. A case of bleeding requiring hospitalization that was likely caused by an interaction between warfarin and levamisole. *Clin Pharmacol Ther.* 1996;59:360–362.

14. Stoysich AM, Lucas BD, Mohinddin SM, Hilleman DE. Further elucidation of pharmacokinetics interaction between diltiazem and warfarin. *Int J Clin Pharmacol Ther.* 1996;34:56–60.

15. Adachi Y, Yokoyama Y, Nanno T, Yamamoto T. Potentiation of warfarin by interferon. *Br Med J.* 1995;311:292. Letter.

16. Cheung B, Lam FM, Kumana CR. Insidiously evolving, occult drug interaction involving warfarin and amiodarone. *Br Med J.* 1996;312: 107–108.

17. Sellers EM, Koch-Weser J. Potentiation of warfarin-induced hypoprothrombinemia by chloral hydrate. *New Engl J Med.* 1970;283: 827.

18. Guthrie SK, Stoysich AM, Bader G, Hilleman DE. Hypothesized interaction between valproic acid and warfarin. *J Clin Psychopharmacol.* 1995;15:138–139. Letter.

19. Hansten PD, Horn JR. *Drug Interactions Analysis and Management Facts and Comparisons.* St. Louis, MO, 2002.

20. Sanoski CA, Bauman JL. Clinical observations with the amiodarone/warfarin interaction. *Chest.* 2002;121:19–23.

21. Kolesar JM, Johnson CL, Freeberg BL, Berlin JD, Schiller JH. Warfarin-5-FU interaction—a consecutive case series. *Pharmacotherapy.* 1999;19:1445–1449.

22. Aldridge MA, Ito MK. Fenofibrate and warfarin interaction. *Pharmacotherapy.* 2001;21:886–889.

23. Bair JD, Oppelt TF. Warfarin and ropinirole interaction. *Ann Pharmacother.* 2001;35:1202–1204.

24. Jahnchen E. Enhanced elimination of warfarin during treatment with cholestyramine. *Br J Clin Pharmacol.* 1978;5:437.

25. Parrish RH, Waller B, Gondalia BG. Sucralfate-warfarin interaction. *Ann Pharmacother.* 1992;26:1015–1016. Letter.

26. Orme M. Enantiomers of warfarin and phenobarbital. *N Engl J Med.* 1976;295:1482.

27. Heimark LD. The mechanism of the warfarin-rifampin drug interaction in humans. *Clin Pharmacol Ther.* 1987;42:388.

28. Lee CR, Thrasher KA. Difficulties with anticoagulation management during coadministration of warfarin and rifampin. *Pharmacotherapy.* 2001;21:1240–1246.

29. Abemethy DR, Kaminsky LS, Dickinson TH. Selective inhibition of warfarin metabolism by diltiazem in humans. *J Pharmacol Exp Ther.* 1991;257:411–415.

30. Grind M, Murphy M, Warrington S, Aberg J. Method for studying drug-warfarin interactions. *Clin Pharmacol Ther.* 1993;54:381–387.

31. Beckey NP, Parra D, Colon A. Retrospective evaluation of a potential interaction between azithromycin and warfarin in patients stabilized on warfarin. *Pharmacotherapy.* 2000;20:1055–1059.

32. Robertson P, Hellriegel ET, Arora S, Nelson M. Effect of modafinil at steady state on the single-dose pharmacokinetic profile of warfarin in healthy volunteers. *J Clin Pharmacol.* 2002;42:205–214.

33. Gidal BE, Sorkness CA, McGill KA, Larson R, Levine RR. Evaluation of a potential enantioselective interaction between ticlopidine and warfarin in chronically anticoagulated patients. *Ther Drug Monit.* 1995;17:33–38.

34. Levy RH, Bajpai M. Phenytoin. Interactions with other drugs: mechanistic aspects. In: Levy RH, Mattson RH, Meldrum BS, eds. *Antiepileptic Drugs.* 4th ed. New York: Raven Press, 1995.

35. Slaughter RL, Edwards DJ. Recent advances: the cytochrome P450 enzymes. *Ann Pharmacother.* 1995;29:619–624.

36. Hermans JJR, Thijssen HHW. Human liver microsomal metabolism of the enantiomers of warfarin and acenocoumarol: p450 isozyme diversity determines the differences in their pharmacokinetics. *Br J Pharmacol.* 1993;110:482–490.

37. Chan TYK. Adverse interactions between warfarin and nonsteroidal antiinflammatory drugs: mechanisms, clinical significance, and avoidance. *Ann Pharmacother.* 1995;29:1274–1283.

38. Alderman CP, Moritz CK, Ben-Tovim D. Abnormal platelet aggregation associated with fluoxetine therapy. *Ann Pharmacother.* 1992;26: 1517–1519.

39. Hanger HC, Thomas F. Fluoxetine and warfarin interactions. *NZ Med J.* 1995;108:157. Letter.

40. Fiske WD, Connell JM, Benedek IH. Lack of pharmacokinetic interaction between aspirin and warfarin. *Am J Ther.* 1995;2:407–413.

41. Frazee LA, Reed MD. Warfarin and nonsteroidal antiinflammatory drugs: why not? *Ann Pharmacother.* 1995;29:1289–1291. Editorial.

42. Turpie AGG, Gent M, Laupacis A, et al. A comparison of aspirin with placebo in patients treated with warfarin after heart-valve replacement. *N Engl J Med.* 1993;329:524–529.

43. Stading JA, Skrabal MZ, Faulkner MA. Seven cases of interaction between warfarin and cyclooxygenase-2 inhibitors. *Am J Health-Syst Pharm.* 2001;58:2076–2080.

44. O'Donnell DC, Hooper JS. Increased international normalized ratio in a patient taking warfarin and celecoxib. *J Pharm Technol.* 2001;17:3–5.

45. Linder JD, Monkemuller KE, Davis JV, Wilcox CM. Cyclooxygenase-2 inhibitor celecoxib: a possible cause of gastropathy and hypoprothrombinemia. *South Med J.* 2000;93:930–932.

46. Karim A, Tolbert D, Piergies A, et al. Celecoxib does not significantly alter the pharmacokinetics or hypoprothrombinemic effect of warfarin in healthy subjects. *J Clin Pharmacol.* 2000;40:655–663.

47. Schwartz JI, Bugianesi KJ, Ebel DL, et al. The effect of rofecoxib on the pharmacodynamics and pharmacokinetics of warfarin. *Clin Pharmacol Ther.* 2000;68:626–636.

48. Rosenbaum MD, Blendon RJ, Benson J, et al. Survey of Americans and dietary supplements. National Public Radio/Henry J Kaiser Family Foundation/Harvard University Kennedy School of Government, 1999.

49. Eisenberg DM, Davis RB, Ettner SL, et al. Trends in alternative medicine use in the United States 1990–1997: results of a follow-up national survey. *JAMA.* 1998;280:1569–1575.

50. Kurtzweil P. An FDA guide to dietary supplements. *FDA Consumer.* US Food and Drug Administration Publication no. 99-2323, January 1999.

51. Boullata JI, Nace AM. Safety issues with herbal medicine. *Pharmacotherapy.* 2000;20:257–269.

52. Newell CA, Anderson LA, Philipson JD. *Herbal Medicinals: A Guide for Health Care Professionals.* London: The Pharmaceutical Press; 1996.

53. Miller LG. Herbal medicinals. Selected clinical considerations focusing on known or potential drug-herb interactions. *Arch Intern Med.* 1998;158:2200–2211.

54. Heck AM, DeWitt BA, Lukes AL. Potential interactions between alternative therapies and warfarin. *Am J Health Syst Pharm.* 1999;56:125–138.

55. Vaes LPJ, Chyka PA. Interactions of warfarin with garlic, ginger, ginkgo or ginseng: nature of the evidence. *Ann Pharmacotherapy.* 2000;34:1478–1482.

56. Wittkowsky AK. Drug interactions update: drugs, herbs and oral anticoagulation. *J Thrombosis Thrombolysis.* 2001;12:67–71.

57. Hoult JR, Paya M. Pharmacological and biochemical actions of simple coumarins: natural products with therapeutic potential. *Gen Pharmacol.* 1996;27:713–722.

58. Sullivan DM, Ford MA, Boyden TW. Grapefruit juice and the response to warfarin. *Am J Health Syst Pharm.* 1998;55:1581–1583.

59. Bartle WR. Grapefruit juice might still be a factor in warfarin response. *Am J Health Syst Pharm.* 1999;56:676.

60. Chan TYK. Interaction between warfarin and danshen (salvia miltiorrhiza). *Ann Pharmacotherapy.* 2001;35:501–504.

61. Lam AY, Elmer GW, Mohutsky MA. Possible interaction between warfarin and lycium barbarum L. *Ann Pharmacother.* 2001;335:1199–1201.

62. Lambert JP, Cormier J. Potential interaction between warfarin and boldo-fenugreek. *Pharmacotherapy.* 2001;21:509–512.

63. Hansten PD, Horn JR. Principals of oral anticoagulant drug interactions. In: Hansten PD, Horn JR, eds. *Drug Interactions and Updates Quarterly.* Vancouver, WA: Applied Therapeutics, Inc; 1993:57–61.

64. Hansten PD, Horn JR. Pitfalls in the evaluation of drug interaction literature. In: Hansten PD, Horn JR, eds. *Drug Interactions and Updates Quarterly.* Vancouver, WA: Applied Therapeutics, Inc; 1993:31–34.

65. Wells PS, Holbrook AM, Crowther NR, Hirsh J. Interactions of warfarin with drugs and food. *Ann Intern Med.* 1994;121:676–683.

66. Rettie AK, Wienkers LC, Gonzalez FJ, Trager WF, Korzekwa KR. Impaired (S)-warfarin metabolism catalyzed by the R144C allelic variant of CYP2C9. *Pharmacogenetics.* 1994;4:39–42.

67. Chan E, McLachlan A, O'Reilly R, Rowland M. Stereochemical aspects of warfarin drug interactions: use of a combined pharmacokinetic-pharmacodynamic model. *Clin Pharmacol Ther.* 1994;56:286–294.

68. Aithal GP, Day CP, Kesteven PJ, Daly AK. Association of polymorphisms in the cytochrome P450 CYP2C9 with warfarin dosing requirement and risk of bleeding complications. *Lancet.* 1999;353:717–719.

69. Wyness MA. Evaluation of an educational programme for patients taking warfarin. *J Adv Nurs.* 1990;15:1052–1063.

70. Segall A. A community survey of self-medication activities. *Med Care.* 1990;28:301–310.

71. Stoller EP. Prescribed and over-the-counter medicine use by the ambulatory elderly. *Med Care.* 1988;26:1149–1157.

Chapter 36

Dietary Considerations

Janet Hiatt Dailey

INTRODUCTION

The medical literature contains a number of case reports that suggest significant changes in the intensity of anticoagulation in previously stable patients as a result of changes in dietary consumption of vitamin K. Although a host of potential factors can cause radical changes in the International Normalized Ratio (INR), diet can be an important factor to consider in the management of an anticoagulated patient. Thus, investigating variations in vitamin K intake is an essential component of managing patients who take warfarin.

VITAMIN K DIFFERENTIATION

The term *vitamin K* refers to a group of fat-soluble vitamins that are derivatives of 2-methyl-l,4-naphthioquinone. Two forms of vitamin K are available to humans. Vitamin K_1, or phylloquinone, is the main form of vitamin K in foods, whereas vitamin K_2, or menaquinone, although present in fermented foods such as cheeses, natto, and animal liver, is primarily synthesized by gram-positive bacteria that normally reside in the small intestine.[1,2] In addition to vitamin K_1, dihydrovitamin K_1 has been recently recognized during the hydrogenation process of vitamin K_1–rich vegetable oils.[3]

Physiologic Role of Vitamin K

Vitamin K plays an important role in the biosynthesis of clotting factors II, VII, IX, and X (see Chapter 16). In addition to the hemostatic function of vitamin K, other vitamin K proteins that are not structurally related to clotting factors are involved in bone and cartilage metabolism.[2,4–6]

Daily Recommended Dietary Allowance

The daily adult recommended dietary allowance (RDA) of phylloquinone is 80 μg/day and 65 μg/day for men and women, respectively.[7] To estimate the average consumption of vitamin K in a typical American diet, researchers measured the phylloquinone content of various foods in the US Food and Drug Administration Total Diet Study. This study analyzed more than 250 different foods consumed by 3,600 participants of various ages who had completed three days of dietary data. The food, purchased four times per year from retail markets from different geographic regions within the United States, was analyzed in triplicate using high-performance liquid chromatography. Of interest, when comparing the dietary intake of vitamin K to the established RDA recommendations, Booth and colleagues[7] determined that vitamin K consumption was inadequate in some age groups within the United States and excessive in others. Approximately 9.2% (59 μg/day) and 17.5% (66 μg/day) less vitamin K than recommended by the current RDA was consumed by women and men, respectively, in the 25–30-year-old group. In contrast, infants up to age six months consumed seven times the amount of vitamin K of the established RDA of 10 μg/day. The higher level was the result of the high vitamin K content found in many infant formula products.[8] In addition, children age 2 to 10 years were found to have a higher vitamin K intake than the respective RDA recommendations.[7] Their consumption of vitamin K did not increase as they became older, perhaps because of their reluctance to eat vegetables and/or a decrease in supervision of their eating habits. An assessment of dietary phylloquinone intake of 362 postmenopausal women in New England based on three consecutive days of recording estimated that the mean intake of vitamin K was 156 ± 147 (mean ± standard deviation) µg per day.[9]

The discovery of dihydrovitamin K_1 might result in a change in the current RDA for vitamin K. Vitamin K_1 and dihydrovitamin K_1 can be measured in plasma. Total vitamin K intake, therefore, would include the sum of dihydrovitamin K_1

and vitamin K_1, which is not reflected in the current RDA. Using analytic methodology described above, researchers[3] determined that the combined amount of dihydrovitamin K_1 and vitamin K_1 exceeded the RDA recommendation for vitamin K in the 25–35-year-old group. The impact of dihydrovitamin K_1 levels on the nutritional status of patients is unknown; however, if the summation of dihydrovitamin K_1 and vitamin K_1 is deemed clinically important, foods that are low in vitamin K_1 but abundant in dihydrovitamin K_1 will need to be included when counseling anticoagulation patients on dietary concerns. Foods containing greater than 10 µg/100 g of vitamin K_1 or dihydrovitamin K_1 content based on analysis by Booth et al[3,4] are depicted in Table 36–1.

Table 36–1 Phylloquinone (Vitamin K_1) and Dihydrophylloquinone Content of Core Foods in the US Food and Drug Administration Total Diet Study

Food Name	Average Serving Size (g)	Mean Vitamin K Content (µg/100g)	Estimated Portion Size (equivalent to 100 g)	Vitamin K per Serving (µg)	Dihydro-Vitamin K (µg/100g)	Dihydro-Vitamin K per Serving (µg)
Eggs:						
Scrambled	64	12.0	2 (large)	7.5	NA	NA
Meat, poultry, and fish:						
Chicken, fried, fast-food	85	1.3	1 piece	1.1	19.0	20.0
Tuna, canned in oil, drained	56	24.0	3.5 oz	14.0	NA	NA
Legumes and nuts:						
Mixed nuts, no peanuts, dry roasted	28	13.0	3.5 oz	3.6	NA	NA
Grain products:						
Blueberry muffin, commercial	57	25.0	2½ muffins	14.0	3.9	2.2
Biscuit, refrigerated dough, baked	70	4.6	3½ biscuits	3.2	30.0	21.0
Butter-type crackers	30	13.1	28 crackers	3.9	59.0	18.0
Graham crackers	28	8.9	14 crackers	0.5	21.0	6.0
Saltine crackers	30	3.6	33 crackers	1.1	21.0	6.4
Fruits:						
Avocado, raw	30	14.0	1 small	4.3	NA	NA
Vegetables:						
Asparagus, fresh/frozen, boiled	90	80.0	7 spears	72.0	NA	NA
Broccoli, fresh/frozen, boiled	78	113.0	½ cup	88.0	NA	NA
Brussels sprouts, fresh/frozen, boiled	78	289.0	5 sprouts	225.0	NA	NA
Cabbage, fresh, boiled	75	98.0	⅔ cup	73.0	NA	NA
Carrot, fresh, boiled	78	15.0	⅔ cup	12.0	NA	NA
Cauliflower, fresh/frozen, boiled	62	20.0	½ cup, pieces	12.0	NA	NA
Celery, raw	55	32.0	2.5 stalks	17.0	NA	NA
Coleslaw with dressing, homemade	120	100.0	¾ cup	119.0	12.0	14.0
Collards, fresh/frozen, boiled	85	440.0	½ cup	374.0	NA	NA
French fries, fast-food	68	4.4	20 pieces	3.0	36.0	25.0
Green beans, fresh/frozen, boiled	62	16.0	¾ cup	9.7	NA	NA
Sauerkraut, canned	118	13.0	½ cup	15.0	NA	NA
Spinach, fresh/frozen, boiled	90	360.0	½ cup	324.0	NA	NA
Iceberg lettuce, raw	89	31.0	5 leaves	28.0	NA	NA
Green peas, fresh/frozen, boiled	80	24.0	½ cup	19.0	NA	NA
Okra, fresh/frozen, boiled	80	40.0	½ cup, slices	32.0	NA	NA
Mixed vegetables, frozen, boiled	82	19.0	½ cup	15.0	NA	NA

continues

Table 36–1 continued

Food Name	Average Serving Size (g)	Mean Vitamin K Content (µg/100g)	Estimated Portion Size (equivalent to 100 g)	Vitamin K per Serving (µg)	Dihydro-Vitamin K (µg/100g)	Dihydro-Vitamin K per Serving (µg)
Mixed dishes and meals:						
Beef chow mein, from Chinese carryout	250	31.0	⅓ cup	78.0	NA	NA
Fish sandwich on bun, fast-food	158	17.0	⅔ sandwich	26.0	4.8	7.6
Meat loaf, homemade	85	12.0	3.5 oz	10.0	NA	NA
Taco/tostada, from Mexican carryout	171	16.0	½ taco/tostada	28.0	4.7	8.0
Tuna noodle casserole, homemade	240	20.0	3.5 oz.	48.0	3.4	8.2
Desserts:						
Apple pie, fresh/frozen, commercial	125	11.0	⅛ pie	14.0	22.0	27.0
Brownies, commercial	57	14.0	5 brownies (3" × 1" × ⅞")	8.0	16.0	8.9
Cake doughnuts with icing, any flavor	47	9.8	3 doughnuts	4.6	31.0	15.0
Chocolate cake with chocolate icing, commercial	64	13.0	2 pieces	8.4	15.0	9.8
Chocolate chip cookies, commercial	30	10.0	8 cookies	3.0	45	14
Pumpkin pie, fresh/frozen, commercial	125	10.0	⅛ pie	11.0	18.0	16.0
Sandwich cookies with cream filling, commercial	30	8.7	10 cookies	2.6	38.0	11.0
Sugar cookies, commercial	30	11.0	6 cookies	3.4	49.0	15.0
Sweet roll/danish, commercial	65	11.0	2 rolls	7.3	25.0	17.0
Snacks:						
Popcorn, popped in oil	22	20.0	9 cups	4.4	NA	NA
Potato chips	28	15.0	3.5 oz	4.1	NA	NA
Condiments and sweeteners:						
Dill cucumber pickles	28	13.0	1 ½ large (3¾ long, 1¼" diameter)	3.7	NA	NA
Jelly, any flavor	19	12.0	5 Tbsp	2.3	NA	NA
Sweet cucumber pickles	28	23.0	3 large (3" long. ¾" diameter)	6.3	NA	NA
Fats and dressings:						
French salad dressing, regular	29	51.0	7 Tbsp	15.0	NA	NA
Margarine, stick, regular	14	33.0	7 Tbsp	4.6	57.0	8.0
Mayonnaise, regular, bottled	14	41.0	7 Tbsp	5.7	42.0	5.9
Infant and junior foods:						
Creamed spinach, strained/junior	113	292.0	3.5 oz.	330.0	NA	NA
Green beans, strained/junior	113	26.0	3.5 oz.	29.0	NA	NA
Milk-based infant formula, high iron, ready to feed	30	12.0	3.5 fl oz.	3.5	NA	NA
Milk-based infant formula, low iron, ready to feed	30	13.0	3.5 fl oz.	4.0	NA	NA
Peas, strained/junior	113	17.0	3.5 oz	19.0	NA	NA
Soy-based infant formula, ready to feed	30	16.0	3.5 fl oz.	4.7	NA	NA

Source: Data from SL Booth, JA Pennington, and JA Sadowski, Dihydro-Vitamin K 1: Primary Food Source and Estimated Dietary Intakes in the American Diet, *Lipids* 1996;31:715–720.

DETERMINATION OF VITAMIN K CONTENT IN FOOD

Several analytic methods, including chick bioassay, thin-layer chromatography, and gas chromatography, have been used to determine the vitamin K content in foods. Until recently, the reported vitamin K content of foods was unreliable because a variety of analytic methods were used.[8] New developments in analytic techniques, however, have improved the quantitation of vitamin K with the use of high-performance liquid chromatography.[10]

Vegetables

Historically, green leafy vegetables have been considered foods with a high content of vitamin K. Ferland and Sadowski[2] investigated whether climate, geographical location of growth, or soil conditions influence the vitamin K content of vegetables. Specifically, the researchers evaluated cabbage, Swiss chard, leaf lettuce, spinach, and kale grown simultaneously between the months of June and August in Boston and Montreal. The dark green and leafy plants (kale, spinach, Swiss chard, leaf lettuce) had the highest level of vitamin K. The plants with the greatest amount of vitamin K_1 content at maturation were the spinach and kale, grown in Boston and Montreal, respectively. The concentration of vitamin K_1 in most of the vegetables differed, depending on the maturation of the plant. The more mature the plant, the higher was the concentration of vitamin K_1. In addition, the researchers discovered that the outer leaves of the cabbage contained more vitamin K_1, compared with the inner leaves, regardless of the geographical area. Interestingly, all of the vegetables grown in Montreal had levels of vitamin K_1 that were 1.5–3.3 times higher than the vitamin K_1 levels of those grown in Boston, which suggests that perhaps differences in climate or soil influence vitamin K_1 content. Post-trial soil analyses indicated that Montreal's soil was richer in minerals and cation exchange capacity than Boston's soil.

Oils

A variety of oils derived from peanuts, corns, almonds, sunflowers, safflowers, walnuts, sesame seeds, olives, rapeseed, and soybeans contain high levels of vitamin K. The vitamin K content of these oils is listed in Table 36–2. Ferland and Sadowski[5] report that soybean, rapeseed, and olive oils are rich sources of phylloquinone, whereas peanut and corn oils are not. Foods not typically recognized as containing high amounts of vitamin K need to be considered as potential sources of vitamin K when oils high in vitamin K are used in their preparation. For example, processed bakery items can

Table 36–2 Vitamin K Content of Various Oils

Type	No. of Brands	Average Vitamin K* (μg/100 g [mean $\pm$ SEM])
Peanut	3	0.65 $\pm$ 0.27
Corn	2	2.91 $\pm$ 1.28
Almond	1	6.70
Sunflower	2	9.03 $\pm$ 0.17
Safflower	2	9.13 $\pm$ 2.64
Walnut	1	15.00
Sesame	2	15.50 $\pm$ 3.30
Olive	6	55.50 $\pm$ 6.30
Rapeseed	4	141.00 $\pm$ 17.0
Soybean	5	193.00 $\pm$ 28

*Average values obtained by triplicate per brand.

Key: SEM, standard error of the mean.

Source: Adapted with permission from G Ferland and JA Sadowski, Vitamin K1 (Phylloquinone) Content of Edible Oils: Effects of Heating and Light Exposure, *Journal of Agricultural and Food Chemistry*, Vol 40, p 1870, © 1992, American Chemical Society.

contain high levels of vitamin K if they are made with vitamin K–rich oils.

Food Preparation

Not only the type of oil but the various processing conditions in which oils are incorporated can influence the content of vitamin K. Ferland and Sadowski[5] determined the vitamin K_1 content via reversed-phase high-performance liquid chromatography of 10 commercially available oils under various processing conditions. For example, vitamin K_1 content was evaluated in oils, with the exception of almond, walnut, and sesame, under heating conditions. A small amount of vitamin K_1 (7% and 11%) was lost after 20 minutes and 40 minutes, respectively, of heating to temperatures of 185°–190° C. The researchers report that the oils with the highest percentage of lost vitamin K_1 were peanut, corn, and olive. In addition, the stability of vitamin K_1 in oils is altered when they are exposed to various light sources. For example, Ferland and Sadowski[5] also note that when oils (specifically safflower and rapeseed) were exposed to fluorescent light and sunlight for 22 days, their vitamin K content decreased. In addition, the method of storing oils appears to have an effect on the stability of vitamin K_1.

It is suggested that oils stored in amber bottles versus clear bottles will have a higher content of vitamin K_1. Interaction between warfarin and foods containing oils can be minimized by selecting an oil with a lower vitamin K content (peanut, corn, safflower, sunflower), purchasing oils in clear glass containers and exposing them to sunlight, and becoming familiar with the sources of oil added to processed foods.[4,5]

Nutritional Supplements

A number of case reports document significant interactions between enteral nutrition products and warfarin. Since the earliest of these reports, many manufacturers have reduced the amount of vitamin K in their products. Some liquid nutrition preparations, however, are hidden sources of vitamin K and can hinder the effectiveness of warfarin therapy. Enteral preparations containing vitamin K are listed in Table 36–3.

Prescribed and over-the-counter vitamins also might be sources of vitamin K. Vitamins containing vitamin K that are readily accessible to consumers are listed in Table 36–4.

CASE REPORTS OF INTERACTIONS

Case reports documenting interactions between diet and warfarin are listed in Table 36–5. In a review of published cases documenting food interactions with warfarin. Wells and colleagues[11] categorize each report by using a strict criterion as to whether the case represents a clinically important interaction. Of the cases reported, the authors conclude that sufficient evidence was present to rate the consumption of large amounts of avocado and broccoli as "highly probable" and "probable," respectively, for causing an interaction with warfarin.

Table 36–3 Vitamin K Content in Nutrition Therapy per Liter

Enteral Nutritional Therapy/Manufacturer	Vitamin K (µg/L)	Enteral Nutritional Therapy/Manufacturer	Vitamin K (µg/L)
Milk-based formulas:		Nutren 1.0 Liquid (Clintec Nutrition)	50
Compleat Regular Formula Lilquid (Novartis Nutrition)	67	Osmolite Liquid (Ross)	43
		Osmolite HN Liquid (Ross)	61
Meritene Powder (Novartis Nutrition)	77	Portagen Powder (Mead Johnson Nutritionals)	106
Lactose free products:		Renal Liquid (Mead Johnson Nutritionals)	118
Compleat Modified Formula Liquid (Novartis Nutrition)	67	Replete-Oral Liquid (Clintec Nutrition)	50
		Resource Plus Liquid (Sandoz Nutrition)	55
Comply Liquid (Mead Johnson Nutritionals)	144	Resource Liquid (Sandoz Nutrition)	38
Criticare HN Liquid (Mead Johnson Nutritionals)	131	Sustacal Liquid (Mead Johnson Nutritionals)	240
Deliver 2.0 (Mead Johnson Nutritionals)	250	Tolerex Powder (Sandoz Nutrition)	37
Ensure with Fiber Liquid (Ross)	58	Travasorb MCT Powder (Clintec Nutrition)	75
Ensure Plus Liquid (Ross)	57	Travasorb HN Powder (Clintec Nutrition)	75
Ensure HN Liquid (Ross)	85	Travasorb STD Powder (Clintec Nutrition)	75
Ensure Liquid and Powder (Ross)	43	TwoCal HN Liquid (Ross)	85
Ensure Plus HN Liquid (Ross)	85	Ultracal Liquid (Mead Johnson Nutritionals)	68
Impact Liquid (Novartis Nutrition)	67	Vital High Nitrogen Powder (Ross)	54
Introlite Liquid (Ross)	61	Vivonex T.E.N. Powder (Novartis Nutrition)	22
Isocal Liquid (Mead Johnson Nutritionals)	132		
Isocal HN Liquid (Mead Johnson Nutritionals)	106	*Specialized formulas:*	
Isosource Liquid (Novartis Nutrition)	62	Glucerna Liquid (Ross)	56.3
Isosource HN Liquid (Novartis Nutrition)	62	Nutrihep Liquid (Clintec Nutrition)	120
Isotein HN Powder (Novartis Nutrition)	56	Pulmocare Liquid (Ross)	85
Jevity Liquid (Ross)	61	Suplena Liquid (Ross)	84
Nutren 1.5 Liquid (Clintec Nutrition)	75	Traumacal Liquid (Mead Johnson Nutritionals)	127
Nutren 2.0 Liquid (Clintec Nutrition)	100		

Table 36–4 Vitamins Containing Vitamin K

Vitamin K Products/Manufacturer	Vitamin K (μg Content per Tablet)
ABC to Z (Nature's Bounty)	25
Centrum, Jr Plus Iron (Lederle)	10
Centrum, Jr Plus Extra C (Lederle)	10
Centrum, Jr Plus Extra Calcium (Lederle)	10
Centrum Silver (Lederle)	10
Children's SunKist Multivitamins Plus Iron (Ciba)	5
Complete (L Perrigo)	25
Decagen (Goldline)	25
Geritol Extend (SmithKline-Beecham)	80
Myadec (Parke-Davis)	25
Ondrox (Unimed)	25/6 tablets
Sigtab-M (Roberts)	25
Sunkist Multivitamins Plus Extra C (Ciba)	5
Total Formula (Vitaline)	70

PATIENT EDUCATION

Practitioner's Role

The magnitude of the interaction between diet and warfarin is difficult to quantitate for a variety of reasons. The variability of vitamin K content in foods prepared differently; the effects of seasonal variation and geographic region; physiologic factors, such as plasma triglyceride levels; and individual variability in vitamin K consumption all contribute to the problems encountered in predicting the impact of diet variations on the intensity of anticoagulation therapy.[12] For example, a high intake of vitamin K–rich vegetables can interfere with oral anticoagulant therapy, as documented by case reports, and changes in dietary vitamin K consumption contribute to alterations in intensity of anticoagulation. In order to prevent adverse events associated with dietary intake of vitamin K, clinicians first must obtain accurate diet histories from patients so that any potential sources of vitamin K can be stabilized, minimized, or eliminated and then make dietary recommendations during patient counseling.

Table 36–5 Case Reports of Food and Warfarin Interaction

Author/Date	Number of Patients	Duration of Interaction	Food	Amount of Vitamin K (μg) Reported	Response
Blickstein et al, 1991[13]	1 AC	NA	Avocado, 100 g/day	8	INR ↓ 2.5 to 1.7 and returned to 2.5 after avocado was stopped
	1 AC	2 days	Avocado, 200 g/day	16	INR ↓ from 2.7 to 1.6
Kalra et al, 1988[14]	1 AC	2 months	Animal liver, 75 gm/week	NA	20% ↑ in nicoumalone dose
	1 AC	4 months	Stopped liver	NA	PT >300; TT <3%
Karlson et al, 1986[15]	10 AC	1 time	250 g broccoli	300–800	Slight rise of TT value; remained therapeutic
			250 g spinach	160–500	Slight rise of TT value; remained therapeutic
			41 g wine		No effect
	11 AC	1 week	250 g spinach	300–800	More marked ↑ in TT than broccoli
			250 g broccoli	160–500	TT value exceeded therapeutic limit by day 3
Kempin, 1983[16]	1 AC	NA	1 lb broccoli (0.45 kg/daily)	NA	PT was never therapeutic after discharge from hospital

continues

Table 36–5 continued

Author/Date	Number of Patients	Duration of Interaction	Food	Amount of Vitamin K (μg) Reported	Response
	1 AC	NA	Broccoli (soup and raw) (230 g–340 g/day)	NA	PT could not be maintained in therapeutic range
Lader et al, 1980[17]	1 AC	1 week	Osmolite	1,200	↑ Daily doses of warfarin from 5 mg to 15 mg; PT ↓ to control levels
O'Reilly, 1979[18]	8 AC	21 days	Wine, 10 oz. and 20 oz.	None	No significant change in one-stage prothrombin activity
O'Reilly and Rytand, 1980[19]	1 AC	2 weeks	Ensure	480	Prothrombin activity ↑ from 20%–30% to 70%
Parr et al, 1982[20]	1 AC	NA	Osmolite	NA	↑ warfarin from 7.5 mg/day to 10 mg/day
	1 AC	approx. 10 days	Osmolite	NA	PT ↑ to 3.5 × control after enteral feeding was stopped
Pedersen et al, 1991[21]	13 AC	7 days	Vitamin K–rich vegetables	Mean 1,100	9/13 above therapeutic range
	5 AC	1 day	Vitamin K–rich vegetables	Mean 1,000	2/5 above therapeutic range
	7 AC	2 days	Vitamin K–rich vegetables	Mean 1,000	3.7 above therapeutic range
	7 AC	6 days	Vitamin K–poor vegetables	Mean 135	No change in plasma coagulant activity
Qureshi et al, 1981[22]	1 AC	6 weeks	High vitamin K diet	1,277	PT 16.2–18.7 seconds (mean 17.6) on warfarin 20 mg
	1 AC	6 weeks	Low vitamin K diet	360	PT 22.1–24.5 seconds (mean 23.5) on warfarin 20 mg
Udall 1965[1]	10 NAC	3 weeks	Diet devoid of vitamin K	None	PT ↑ from 14.8 seconds to 16.0 seconds

Key: AC, anticoagulated; approx., approximately; INR, International Normalized Ratio; NA, not available; NAC, not anticoagulated; PT, prothrombin time; TT, thrombotest.

Diet History

The purpose of obtaining a diet history from a patient on warfarin is to assess the individual's typical dietary vitamin K intake. When unexplained fluctuations in intensity of anticoagulation occur, dietary information can be evaluated to assess possible changes in vitamin K intake as a source of warfarin instability. Thus, dietary assessment is an ongoing process and part of the routine evaluation of the patient.

Interviewing a patient for a diet history is far more complex than simply asking "What did you have for dinner this past week?" In fact, it might require a nutritional assessment of several weeks of diet recall in order to obtain sufficient and detailed information regarding food preferences. For instance, more information is conveyed when a diet history assesses specific items, such as collard greens versus the general description of "green vegetables." By evaluating specific food selection, an accurate account of the consumption of vitamin K can be obtained. In fact, a minimum of five days of dietary recording is thought to be necessary to estimate an individual's typical vitamin K intake.[9] A variety of tools, including a seven-day food diary and a food frequency questionnaire, can be implemented to ascertain a patient's usual and current intake of vitamin K.

In addition to assessing typical diets of individual patients, the process of diet recall also can be used to identify regional or cultural dietary habits. For instance, the diets of patients residing on tropical islands of the United States would be expected to differ significantly from the diets of patients living in the Northern Plains states. Some foods commonly consumed in the United States (see Table 36–1) might not be familiar to everyone on anticoagulation therapy. Likewise, patients from various ethnic backgrounds might consume foods common to native homelands. Because of the influences of customs and cultures, clinicians must be aware that unusual foods with a high vitamin K content might be consumed by some patients. Table 36–6 lists the names of various foods not typically found on many grocery lists that are abundant in vitamin K.

Thorough diet histories also need to include an assessment of nutritional supplements, homeopathic and naturopathic products, and vitamin preparations that might be sources of

Table 36–6 Phylloquinone Content in Unusual Foods

Food Name	Mean Vitamin K Content (μ/100 g)	Estimated Portion Size (Equivalent to 100 g)	Food Name	Mean Vitamin K Content (μ/100 g)	Estimated Portion Size (Equivalent to 100 g)
Fruits:			Kaiwaredaikon, raw leaf	80	NA
Kiwi fruit	25	1¼ medium	Kale, raw leaf	817	NA
Pumpkin, canned	16	½ cup	Komatsuna, raw leaf	280	NA
Legumes and nuts:			Leek, raw	14	1 cup chopped
Pecan, dry	10	3.5 oz	Lettuce, red leaf	210	NA
Pistachio	70	3.5 oz	Malabar gourd, raw leaf	22	NA
Meat, poultry, and fish:			Onion, green scallion, raw	207	⅔ cup chopped
Abalone	23	3.5 oz	Osh, raw leaf	310	NA
Vegetables:			Parsley—raw leaf	540	1½ cups chopped
Algae—purple laver	1,385	3.5 oz	cooked leaf	900	1½ cups chopped
Konbu	66	NA	Perilla, raw leaf	650	NA
Hijiki	327	NA	Purslane, raw	381	NA
Amaranth, raw leaf	1,140	NA	Roctish—raw leaf	290	NA
Artichoke, globe	14	⅓ medium	cooked leaf	420	NA
Asatsuki, leaf	190	NA	Samat—raw leaf	350	NA
Ashitaba, leaf	590	NA	cooked leaf	960	NA
Basella, raw leaf	160	NA	Squash, summer, peel only	80	NA
Bell tree dahli—raw leaf	630	NA	Toumyao (Chinese)	380	NA
cooked leaf	1,110	NA	Tziton, raw leaf	250	NA
Chard, Swiss, raw leaf	830	NA	Watercress, raw	250	3 cups
Chive, raw	190	33 Tbsp chopped	*Fats and dressings:*		
Chrysanthemum, garland boiled	350	1 cup pieces	oils—canola (rapeseed)	141	7 Tbsp
Coleslaw with dressing, homemade	100	¾ cup	sesame	10	7 Tbsp
			soybean	193	7 Tbsp
Collards, fresh/frozen, boiled	440	½ cup	walnut	15	7 Tbsp
Coriander—raw leaf	310	6¼ cups	*Beverages:*		
cooked leaf	1,510	NA	Tea—black, leaves (dry)	262	NA
Endive, raw	231	2 cups chopped	green, leaves (dry)	1,428	NA

vitamin K. Clinicians should encourage patients to bring in bottles of all such products that they use and review the ingredients on the labels.

Dietary Recommendations

A significant reduction in the serum phylloquinone concentration occurs when foods with high vitamin K content are eliminated from the diet.[23] A low vitamin K diet has been developed,[24] but because of the diversity of "typical" diets and the large variation in vitamin K consumption among patients, it can be difficult to adhere to such a diet. Rather, it is important that patients maintain a consistent dietary vitamin K intake. In fact, a diet containing a consistent amount of vitamin K was effective in increasing the number of INRs within the therapeutic range in patients with poor anticoagulant stability.[25]

In some cases, minimization or elimination of an inconsistently consumed source of excessive vitamin K is necessary. For example, it might be appropriate to ask certain patients to avoid green tea available in Asian restaurants if the intake of this source of excessive vitamin K is infrequent. For other patients, avoidance of more routinely consumed vitamin K–containing products might be necessary, particularly if routine consumption interferes with the ability to reach a therapeutic level of anticoagulation despite escalating doses of warfarin. The following four points represent the foundation of patient education regarding dietary intake of vitamin K:

1. Recognize foods and food products containing high quantities of vitamin K.
2. Maintain a consistent intake of vitamin K–containing foods and food products.
3. Avoid drastic changes in diet.
4. Inform health care providers of any changes in intake of vitamin K–containing foods and food products.

These points should be components of ongoing education provided to patients taking warfarin. It is important, however, to recognize that, despite detailed counseling, some patients might initially interpret these dietary considerations as meaning that all vitamin K–containing foods should be eliminated from the diet. This misinterpretation can be avoided by careful ongoing education and by consistent and thorough dietary assessments.

CONCLUSION

Dietary alterations in which excessive vitamin K sources are added or eliminated can lead to changes in intensity of anticoagulation or increase the risk of thromboembolic and hemorrhagic complications of warfarin, respectively. These interactions can be avoided by maintaining a consistent intake of vitamin K–containing foods and food products. When dietary changes occur, adverse clinical outcomes can be prevented by adjusting warfarin doses to limit the impact of changes in vitamin K intake. An ongoing dialogue between the patient and the provider, which includes thorough assessments of vitamin K intake, is an essential component of patient management.

REFERENCES

1. Udall JA. Human sources and absorption of vitamin K in relation to anticoagulation stability. *JAMA*. 1965;194:127–129.

2. Ferland G, Sadowski JA. The vitamin K_1 (phylloquinone) content of green vegetables: effects of plant maturation and geographical growth location. *J Agric Food Chem*. 1992;40:1874–1877.

3. Booth SL, Pennington JAT, Sadowski JA. Dihydrovitamin K_1: primary food sources and estimated dietary intakes in the American diet. *Lipids*. 1996;31:715–720.

4. Booth SL, Sadowski JA, Pennington JAT. Phylloquinone (Vitamin K1) content of foods in the U.S. Food and Drug Administration's Total Diet Study. *J Agric Food Chem*. 1995;43:1574–1579.

5. Ferland G, Sadowski JA. Vitamin K_1 (phylloquinone) content of edible oils: effects of heating and light exposure. *J Agric Food Chem*. 1992;40:1869–1873.

6. Shearer MJ. Vitamin K. *Lancet*. 1995;345:229–234.

7. Booth SL, Pennington JAT, Sadowski JA. Food sources and dietary intakes of vitamin K_1 (phylloquinone) in the American diet: data from the PDA total dietary study. *J Am Diet Assoc*. 1996;96:149–154.

8. Schneider DL, Fluckiger HB, Manes JD. Vitamin K_1 content of infant formula products. *Pediatrics*. 1974;53:273–275.

9. Booth SL, Sokoll LJ, O'Brien ME, et al. Assessment of dietary phylloquinone intake and vitamin K status in postmenopausal women. *Eur J Clin Nutr*. 1995;49:832–841.

10. Mummah-Schendel LL, Suttie JW. Serum phylloquinone concentrations in a normal adult population. *Am J Clin Nutr*. 1986;44:686–689.

11. Wells PS, Holbrook AM, Crowther NR, Hirsh J. Interactions of warfarin with drugs and food. *Ann Intern Med*. 1994;121:676–683.

12. Sadowski JA, Hood SH, Dallal GE, Garry PJ. Phylloquinone in plasma from elderly and young adults: factors influencing its concentration. *Am J Clin Nutr*. 1989;50:100–108.

13. Blickstein D, Shaklai M, Inbal A. Warfarin antagonism by avocado. *Lancet*. 1991;337:914–915.

14. Kalra PA, Cooklin M, Wood G, et al. Dietary modification as cause of anticoagulation instability. *Lancet*. 1988;2:803.

15. Karlson B, Leijd B, Hellstrom K. On the influence of vitamin K–rich vegetables and wine on the effectiveness of warfarin treatment. *Acta Med Scand*. 1986;220:347–350.

16. Kempin SJ. Warfarin resistance caused by broccoli. *N Engl J Med*. 1983;308:1229–1330.

17. Lader E, Yang L, Clarke A. Warfarin dosage and vitamin K in Osmolite. *Ann Intern Med.* 1980;93:373–374.

18. O'Reilly RA. Lack of effect of mealtime wine on the hypoprothrombinemia of oral anticoagulant. *Am J Med Sci.* 1979;277:189–194.

19. O'Reilly RA, Rytand DA. Resistance to warfarin due to unrecognized vitamin K supplementation. *N Engl J Med.* 1980;303:160–161.

20. Parr MD, Record KE, Griffith GL, et al. Effect of enteral nutrition on warfarin therapy. *Clin Pharm.* 1982;1:274–276.

21. Pedersen FM, Hamberg O, Hess K, Ovesen L. The effect of dietary vitamin K on warfarin-induced anticoagulation. *J Intern Med.* 1991;229:517–520.

22. Qureshi G, Reinders TP, Swint JJ, Slate MB. Acquired warfarin resistance and weight-reducing diet. *Arch Intern Med.* 1981;141:507–509.

23. Suttie JW, Mummah-Schendel LL, Shah DV, Lyle BJ, Greger JL. Vitamin K deficiency from dietary vitamin K restriction in humans. *Am J Clin Nutr.* 1988,47:475–480.

24. Ferland G, Macdonald DL, Sadowski JA. Development of a diet low in vitamin K_1 (phylloquinone). *J Am Diet Assoc.* 1992;92:593–597.

25. Sorano GG, Biodni G, Conti M, et al. Controlled vitamin K content diet for improving the management of poorly controlled anticoagulated patients: a clinical practice proposal. *Haemostasia.* 1993;23:77–82.

Chapter 37

Managing Anticoagulation during Surgery and Other Invasive Procedures

Clive Kearon

INTRODUCTION

Long-term anticoagulation presents a problem when the need for surgery arises because anticoagulation is associated with bleeding from the operative site, patients have an increased risk of thromboembolism when therapy is interrupted, and warfarin's antithrombotic effects take days to recede after it is stopped and a similar length of time to reestablish after it is restarted. There is uncertainty about the optimal perioperative management of anticoagulation for patients who have been receiving oral anticoagulant therapy. Rational decisions can only be made if one can quantify the risks of thrombosis and bleeding that are associated with different approaches to management (Exhibit 37–1). The risk of thromboembolism and associated morbidity depends largely on (1) the indication for anticoagulation (ie, prevention of venous or arterial thrombosis), (2) the prevalence of risk factors for thromboembolism in individual patients, and (3) whether or not surgery increases the risk of postoperative thromboembolism.[1] The risk of anticoagulant-induced bleeding is generally low preoperatively but high during and shortly after major surgery.

Based on an individual assessment of risk factors for arterial or venous thrombosis and the risk of postoperative bleeding, this chapter outlines an approach to the perioperative management of anticoagulation that is designed to optimize patient safety and efficient health care delivery. The risks of venous and arterial thromboembolism associated with different conditions and the relative risk reduction for thromboembolism achieved by anticoagulation are summarized in Table 37–1.[1] Derivation of these estimates and an analysis of the risks and benefits of using supplementary intravenous unfractionated heparin (UFH) as "bridging therapy" while oral anticoagulation is subtherapeutic before and after surgery have been detailed elsewhere.[1] As the risk of thromboembolism and bleeding are often influenced by the surgical procedure, it is helpful to consider anticoagulant management separately for the preoperative and postoperative periods. However, before proposing how patients with different indications for long-term anticoagulant therapy should be managed before surgery, approaches to the delivery of preoperative "bridging therapy" will be described. The term *bridging therapy* refers to the use of therapeutic-dose UFH or low–molecular-weight heparin (LMWH) and does not include lower doses of UFH and LMWH that are used to prevent venous thromboembolism.[2]

PREOPERATIVE "BRIDGING THERAPY"

Although the practice has not been evaluated by randomized trials, it is generally recommended that patients with the highest risk of arterial or venous embolism who require interruption of oral anticoagulant therapy for surgery should receive therapeutic-dose heparin therapy (UFH or LMWH) during much of the interval when the International Normalized Ratio (INR) is subtherapeutic.[3,4] Because the INR does not start to fall until ~29 hours after a dose of warfarin and then decreases with a half-life of ~22 hours, if "bridging therapy" is used preoperatively, it is reasonable before surgery to start it ~60 hours after the last dose of warfarin (eg,

Exhibit 37–1
FACTORS INFLUENCING PERIOPERATIVE ANTICOAGULANT MANAGEMENT

- Risk of thromboembolism without anticoagulation
  - during the preoperative period
  - during the postoperative period
- Risk reduction for thromboembolism with anticoagulation
- Risk of bleeding with anticoagulation
  - during the preoperative period
  - during the postoperative period
- Consequences of thromboembolism (venous or arterial)
- Consequences of bleeding
- Fear of thromboembolism or bleeding
- Cost of supplemental perioperative anticoagulation

Table 37–1 Rates of Thromboembolism Associated with Different Indications for Oral Anticoagulation and Risk Reduction with Anticoagulation

Indication	Control Rate	Risk Reduction
Venous thromboembolism		
Acute venous thromboembolism		
0–1 month	40%/month*	80%
1–3 months	10%/2 months*	80%
Recurrent venous thromboembolism‡	15%/year*	90%
Arterial thromboembolism		
NVAF	4.5%/year	66%
NVAF and previous embolism	12%/year	66%
Mechanical heart valve	8%/year	75%
Acute arterial embolism		
0–1 month	15%/month	66%

*An increase in the risk of venous thromboembolism associated with surgery (estimated to be 100-fold) is not included in these rates.
‡Last episode of venous thromboembolism more than three months previously but require long-term anticoagulation because of high risk of recurrence.
NVAF = nonvalvular atrial fibrillation.

Source: Reproduced, with minor modifications, from Kearon and Hirsh.[1]

third morning after last evening dose).[5,6] In the past, this generally necessitated admission to the hospital to receive intravenous UFH, which was stopped ~6 hours before surgery.[1]

A popular alternative to intravenous UFH is to use LMWH, administered subcutaneously as an outpatient, for bridging therapy.[3,4,7,8] With this approach, doses of LMWH that are recommended for treatment of venous thromboembolism are administered once[6] or twice[7,8] daily, generally for two (preceding INR 2.0 to 3.0) or three (preceding INR 3.0 to 4.0) days before surgery. In order to avoid persistence of heparin during surgery, it is suggested that the last dose of LMWH should be given no less than 18 hours preoperatively with a twice-daily regimen (eg, ~100 U/kg of LMWH) or 30 hours preoperatively with a once-daily regimen (eg, ~150–200 U/kg of LMWH), and that an additional 6-hour interval between the last dose of LMWH and surgery may be appropriate if neuraxial anesthesia is planned. Use of bridging therapy after surgery is discussed under Postoperative Management of Anticoagulation.

PREOPERATIVE MANAGEMENT OF ANTICOAGULATION

In order to assess the risks associated with temporarily stopping anticoagulants, the consequences as well as the absolute risk of thromboembolic events need to be considered. Arterial thromboembolism often results in death (about 40% of events) or major disability (about 20% of events),[9–12] whereas recurrent venous thromboembolism rarely presents as sudden death (about 6% of cases),[13] and major permanent disability due to venous thromboembolism is also unusual (estimated at less than 5% of events) in treated patients. It is therefore logical to consider patients whose indication for long-term anticoagulation is the prevention of arterial thromboembolism separately from those whose indication is the prevention of venous thrombosis (Figure 37–1).

Arterial Thromboembolism

Prophylaxis of arterial thromboembolism is most commonly undertaken inpatients with atrial fibrillation and/or valvular heart disease (native or prosthetic). Patients with nonvalvular atrial fibrillation have an average risk of systemic embolism of about 4.5% per year in the absence of antithrombotic therapy.[9] In individual patients, this risk varies from about 1% to 20%, depending on the prevalence of risk factors (ie, previous embolism, hypertension, age $\geq$75 years, left ventricular dysfunction, diabetes, mitral stenosis).[9,14–16] The average rate of major thromboembolism in nonanticoagulated patients with mechanical heart valves is estimated to be 8%, with the risk in individuals also varying widely according to the prevalence of risk factors (ie, caged ball or disk valves,

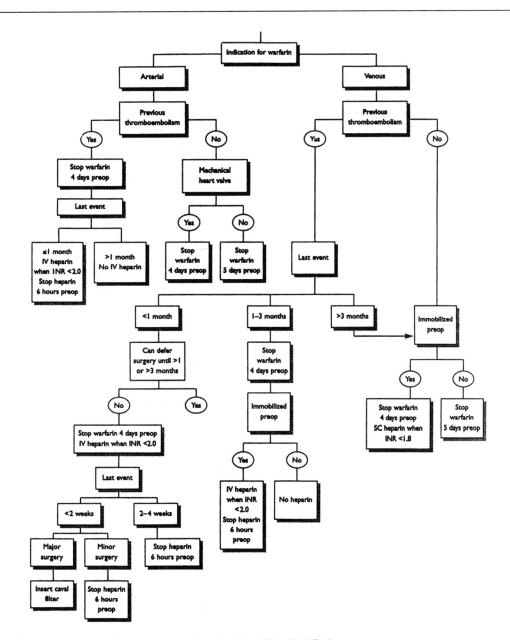

Preop, preoperatively; IV, intravenous; SC, subcutaneous; INR, International Normalized Ratio.
IV heparin denotes use of bridging therapy in the above algorithm; in most circumstances subcutaneous LMWH can be used for this purpose (see text).

Figure 37–1 Algorithm outlining an approach to the management of anticoagulation before elective surgery. Source: Reprinted with permission from C. Kearon, Perioperative Management of Angicoagulants, In *Critical Decisions in Thrombosis and Haemostasis*, J.S. Ginsberg, C. Kearon, and J. Hirsh, eds., © 1998.

mitral position, atrial fibrillation, previous embolism, age ≥70 years).[17–20]

Previous thromboembolism is the single most important risk factor for stroke in patients with atrial fibrillation,[9,10,15,16] and it is also an important risk factor in patients with prosthetic heart valves. Consequently, the period of subtherapeutic oral anticoagulation should be kept to a minimum in patients with previous embolism and in others with multiple risk factors (Figure 37–1). In patients whose INR is 2.0–3.0, it takes about four days for the INR to spontaneously fall to 1.5 or less,[5,6] an intensity of anticoagulation that is not expected to be associated with a increase in intraoperative bleeding.[5,21–25] If the INR is 3.0 to 4.0, this is expected to take five days. Therefore, in patients with a higher than average risk of embolism, such as those with a previous episode, four (INR 2.0 to 3.0) or five (INR 3.1 to 4.0) daily doses of warfarin should be withheld preoperatively, and the INR should be measured the day before surgery to determine if it has decreased adequately. If the INR is more than 1.7 the day before surgery, 1 mg of vitamin K can be given orally to accelerate the reversal of anticoagulation and INR can be repeated the day of surgery.[26] If necessary, plasma can then be given prior to surgery if the INR is still not acceptable to the surgeon (ie, INR 1.3–1.7, one unit; INR 1.7–2.0, two units); however, administration of blood products should be avoided for elective surgery. Checking the INR the morning of the day before surgery may also provide a convenient opportunity to administer a single therapeutic dose of LMWH if the INR is 1.8 or less, without embarking on the more complex task of providing two or three days of outpatient bridging therapy.

There is evidence that the risk of recurrent arterial thromboembolism in patients with atrial fibrillation is highest within a month of an acute event (about 0.5% per day),[27–29] and this is also likely to be true for patients with mechanical heart valves. To minimize the possibility of preoperative embolism, bridging therapy (see above) is recommended when the INR drops to less than 2.0 in such patients (Figure 37–1). Many physicians use such bridging therapy in a broader spectrum of patients that are at risk of cardioembolism, particularly those with mechanical heart valves.[3,4,30,31]

Venous Thromboembolism

Venous indications for long-term anticoagulation are usually the prevention of recurrent venous thromboembolism, a risk that declines rapidly during the three months after an acute episode.[32,33] It is estimated that stopping anticoagulation within one month of an acute event is associated with a very high risk of recurrent venous thromboembolism (ie, 40% over a one-month period) (Table 37–1) and that this risk is intermediate if anticoagulants are stopped during the second and third months of treatment (ie, 10% over a two-month period).[1]

If feasible, surgery should be deferred following an acute episode of venous thromboembolism until patients have received at least one month, and preferably three months, of anticoagulation (Figure 37–1). If this is not feasible and surgery is performed within one month of an acute event, bridging therapy should be used while the INR is less than 2.0. If it is necessary to perform surgery within two weeks of an acute episode of venous thromboembolism, the risk of pulmonary embolism is probably acceptable if bridging therapy is withheld for 18 hours or less (eg, with intravenous UFH, 6 hours preoperatively and 12 hours postoperatively) and the duration of surgery is short. Consequently, patients undergoing less extensive surgery who do not have a high risk of postoperative bleeding can be managed with bridging therapy. However, within two weeks of an acute episode of proximal deep vein thrombosis or pulmonary embolism, patients undergoing major surgery should have a vena caval filter inserted preoperatively or intraoperatively.[1]

If the most recent episode of venous thromboembolism was between one and three months previously, warfarin should be withheld for only four doses to minimize the period of thrombotic risk; however, unless patients are immobilized (ie, already hospitalized) bridging therapy or use of prophylactic doses of UFH or LMWH (in this case, including prophylactic doses) are not necessarily preoperatively. As previously described, the INR of outpatients can be checked the day before surgery and, depending on its value, a single dose of oral vitamin K or subcutaneous LMWH can be considered at that time.

Anticoagulation for more than three or six months is usually reserved for patients with multiple episodes of venous thromboembolism or a single episode of thrombosis that was not provoked by a temporary risk factor such as recent surgery. The latter group of patients may have had idiopathic venous thromboembolism or may have a chronic risk factor such as active malignancy or an underlying hereditary hypercoaguable state. Interruption of warfarin therapy during this phase of treatment is estimated to be associated with a much lower risk of thromboembolism than if it is stopped during the first three months of therapy (ie, 15% per year). Consequently, it is reasonable to withhold five doses of warfarin prior to surgery in patients who have already been treated with three or more months of anticoagulation. Additional preoperative prophylaxis needs to be provided only to patients with an INR of less than 1.8 if they are immobilized in the hospital.

POSTOPERATIVE MANAGEMENT OF ANTICOAGULATION

In relation to the management of anticoagulation, two factors distinguish the postoperative from the preoperative period. First, major surgery is associated with a marked increase in the risk of venous thromboembolism; in the short term, this is estimated to be a 100-fold increase in risk.[1] However, unlike venous thromboembolism, there is no convincing clinical evidence that surgery increases the risk of arterial embolism. Second, recent surgery is a major risk factor for anticoagulant-induced bleeding.[34–41] Whereas bleeding is uncommon when warfarin is started after major surgery,[2,25,42,43] bleeding is expected to be substantial if therapeutic doses of UFH or LMWH are administered within days of operation.[35,37,40,44] For example, when both are started within 24 hours of major orthopaedic surgery, prophylactic doses of LMWH (ie, less than half the dose used for bridging therapy) are associated with more bleeding than is warfarin.[2,42,43] Although the consequences of an episode of major bleeding in the postoperative period (eg, case fatality estimated at 3%)[34,45] are generally less severe than those of an episode of thromboembolism, because the absolute risk of thromboembolism prior to reestablishing oral anticoagulation is often extremely low, administration of bridging therapy has the potential to do more harm than good during this interval.[1] A number of recent small studies suggest that, with appropriate patient selection, major episodes of bleeding are uncommon (~1%) when LMWH is used for bridging therapy pre- and postoperatively.[6–8]

As there is a delay of about 12–24 hours after warfarin administration before the prothrombin time begins to increase, warfarin should be restarted as soon as possible after surgery unless patients have additional invasive procedures planned or are actively bleeding (Figure 37–2). In patients who are undergoing procedures that are associated with a low risk of bleeding, warfarin can even be restarted shortly before surgery.

Arterial Thromboembolism

In patients who have surgery performed within a month of an episode of arterial thromboembolism, the risk of recurrence is sufficiently high that postoperative intravenous UFH is probably warranted until the INR reaches 2.0, provided that the risk of bleeding is not very high (Figure 37–2).

If intravenous UFH is being used for postoperative bridging therapy, it should be started with a loading dose approximately 12 hours after surgery, at a rate of no more than 18 units per kilogram per hour.[46] In the absence of a loading dose, the first activated partial thromboplastin time measurement should be deferred for 12 hours in order for a stable anticoagulant response to have been attained. Compared with therapeutic-dose subcutaneous LMWH, intravenous UFH has the advantage of being rapidly eliminated and effectively reversed for protamine sulphate if bleeding occurs.[47]

If therapeutic-dose subcutaneous LMWH is being used, it should probably not be started until ~24 hours after surgery and only after hemostasis has been achieved. Twice-daily dosing may be preferable to once-daily dosing in the early postoperative period as lower peaks of anticoagulant effect are induced, and the smaller twice-daily dose is expected to be eliminated sooner if bleeding occurs close to the time of injection; however, this is speculative and both once[6] and twice[7,8] daily regimens have been used postoperatively.

Bridging therapy is not recommended for patients who have undergone major surgery who are at high risk for bleeding even if there has been an episode of arterial embolism within a month of surgery.[1] Instead, subcutaneous UFH or LMWH, in doses recommended for thromboembolism prophylaxis of high-risk patients, should be given until the INR reaches 1.8.[2]

Venous Thromboembolism

As surgery is a major risk factor for venous thromboembolism, the need for antithrombotic prophylaxis is much greater postoperatively than it is preoperatively. Patients who have had an episode of venous thromboembolism within three months of surgery have a very high risk of recurrence postoperatively. Consequently, bridging therapy is recommended in this setting until the INR is 2.0 or greater, provided the surgeon does not feel that the patient is a high risk for bleeding.[1] Although patients who have a vena caval filter remain at high risk of recurrent venous thrombosis, they are at least partially protected from pulmonary embolism[48] and, consequently, bridging therapy can be avoided in these patients in the early postoperative period.

Provided there have been no previous episodes of thromboembolism within three months prior to surgery, postoperative bridging therapy is not indicated. Subcutaneous heparin is recommended in doses used for venous thromboembolism prophylaxis of high-risk patients. If patients are discharged before their INR has reached 1.8 and it is feasible for them to receive subcutaneous heparin at home, this is recommended. As there is a concern that restarting warfarin may induce a transient hypercoagulable state in patients with protein C or protein S deficiency,[49] patients with these conditions should restart warfarin at no more than the expected maintenance dose and should receive heparin until the INR is 2.0 or greater for at least two consecutive days.

QUALIFYING REMARKS

The recommendations outlined above are strongly influenced by a number of assumptions. It is proposed that, for most patients, warfarin be withheld preoperatively long enough for the INR to spontaneously fall to a value of 1.5 or lower before surgery without the need for bridging therapy. As the INR will be prolonged to some extent for much of this time, it is estimated that this interruption of warfarin will

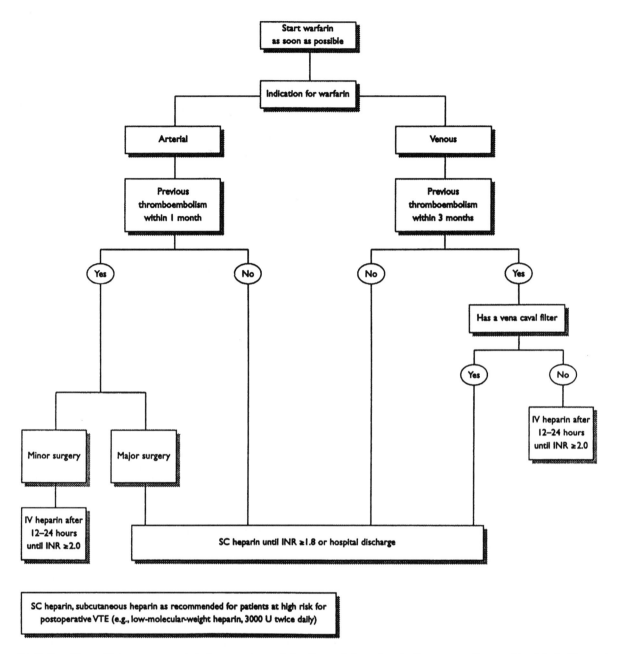

Figure 37–2 Algorithm outlining an approach to the management of anticoagulation after elective surgery. Source: Reprinted with permission from C. Kearon, Perioperative Management of Angicoagulants, In *Critical Decisions in Thrombosis and Haemostasis*, J.S. Ginsberg, C. Kearon, and J. Hirsh, eds., © 1998.

expose patients to a small risk of thromboembolism preoperatively (ie, equivalent to the thromboembolic risk associated with one day of no anticoagulation).[50–52] For the same reason, where warfarin is restarted the day of surgery, it is estimated that patients are exposed to a similar small risk of thromboembolism postoperatively while oral anticoagulant therapy is being reestablished. It has also been assumed that the risk of thromboembolism associated with a day without anticoagulation is one 365th part of the risk associated with a year without therapy. Hence, a 10% per year risk of throm-

boembolism translates to a daily risk of ~0.03%, or a one in 3,650 probability of an event. If stopping oral anticoagulation induces a transient "rebound" hypercoagulable state,[53–58] or restarting anticoagulation induces a transient "paradoxical" hypercoaguable state,[49] the daily risk of thromboembolism may be underestimated. However, there is no convincing clinical evidence to support either of these phenomena.[58] As patients with inherited protein S and protein C deficiency are believed to have a higher than average risk for warfarin-induced thrombosis, it is recommended that oral anticoagulation be reintroduced slowly, under the cover of concomitant heparin therapy (prophylactic or therapeutic doses), in such patients.

Another approach to management in this setting is to shorten the interval when the INR is subtherapeutic by withholding fewer doses of warfarin preoperatively while giving a small dose of oral vitamin K (eg, 1 mg) to accelerate reversal of anticoagulation. The safety of this approach is not known, and though it appears reasonable for most patients if surgery needs to be performed before the INR can spontaneously decrease to an acceptable level, unless accompanied by bridging therapy, this practice is discouraged for patients with mechanical heart valves.[59,60]

There is also uncertainty about the need to reverse anticoagulation before some different surgical procedures. It does not appear to be necessary for dental extractions[3,61] or for extracapsular cataract removal under local anesthetic.[62] Similarly, the American Society for Gastrointestinal Endoscopy recommends that, because of a low associated risk of bleeding, diagnostic upper endoscopy, flexible colonoscopy with or without biopsy, diagnostic endoscopic retrograde cholangiopancreatography, and biliary stent implantation can be performed with an INR of up to 2.5.[63] In general, it is more acceptable to perform surgical procedures while on anticoagulant therapy if the site of potential bleeding is accessible (eg, mouth or skin) rather than remote (eg, percutaneous biopsy of internal organs).

The assumption that underlies the use of bridging therapy is that it is effective at preventing thromboembolism. While there is good evidence that UFH and LMWH are effective at preventing venous thromboembolism,[2,64] there is less certainty for the prevention of cardioembolism, particularly with the use of LMWH. Compared to aspirin, LMWH (dalteparin 100 IU/kg, twice daily) did not reduce the frequency of early recurrent stroke in patients with atrial fibrillation (odds ratio = 1.1, 95% confidence interval, 0.6 to 2.2),[29] a finding that is consistent with subgroup analyses of other studies that have evaluated LMWH in acute ischemic stroke.[65,66] However, in the International Stroke Trial, UFH (5,000 or 12,500 IU twice daily) was more effective than aspirin at preventing early recurrent stroke (42% risk reduction).[28] There are fewer data, and none from randomized trials, about the efficacy of UFH and LMWH for the prevention of embolism in patients with mechanical heart valves.

Indirect comparisons suggest that subcutaneous UFH is substantially less effective than oral anticoagulants at preventing thromboembolic complications in pregnant women with mechanical heart valves; however, less than currently recommended therapeutic doses of UFH were often used in these patients.[67,68] A number of cases of fatal mechanical valve thromboses have been documented in pregnant women who were being treated with therapeutic-dose LMWH (~100 IU/kg, twice daily), including 2 of 8 women in a prospective study (Lovenox® [enoxaparin] product monograph). At least partly arising from these reports, the product monograph for this LMWH preparation states that it is not recommended for thromboprophylaxis in patients with prosthetic heart valves; this does not preclude that LMWH reduces the risk of thromboembolism in patients with mechanical heart valves when oral anticoagulation is interrupted.[69] In the absence of treatment with thrombolytic therapy and aspirin (but not with such therapy), therapeutic or near-therapeutic doses of UFH approximately halve the frequency of stroke associated with acute myocardial infarction, supporting the hypothesis that UFH can reduce cardioembolism.[70] Taken together, the above data suggest that UFH, and particularly LMWH, is less effective than warfarin at preventing cardioembolism. Doses of UFH and LMWH that are greater than those used to treat venous thromboembolism might be more effective at preventing cardioembolism; however, such doses are more likely to cause bleeding, particularly following recent surgery.

It is concluded that, provided the number of days without warfarin is kept to a minimum, most patients on oral anticoagulant therapy can have elective surgery performed without the need for bridging therapy. Further, except for those patients who have the highest risk of postoperative thromboembolism, bridging therapy should be avoided within two days of major surgery because of the associated risk of bleeding.

Finally, perioperative management of anticoagulation can cause anxiety for patients, surgeons, anesthetists, and anticoagulant clinic personnel. Good communication among all of these parties is essential to ensure that an optimal management strategy is identified, that this strategy is then successfully executed, and that the potential for recrimination is minimized in the unlikely event of a serious thrombotic or hemorrhagic complication.

REFERENCES

1. Kearon C, Hirsh J. Managing anticoagulation before and after surgery in patients who require oral anticoagulants. *N Engl J Med*. 1997; 336(21):1506–1511.

2. Geerts WH, Heit JA, Clagett GP, Pineo GF, Colwell CW, Anderson FA, Jr, et al. Prevention of venous thromboembolism. *Chest*. 2001;119: 132S–175S.

3. Ansell J, Hirsh J, Dalen J, Bussey H, Anderson D, Poller L, et al. Managing oral anticoagulant therapy. *Chest*. 2001;119:22S–38S.

4. Heit JA. Perioperative management of the chronically anticoagulated patient. *J Thromb Thrombolys*. 2002;12:81–87.

5. White RH, McKittrick T, Hutchinson R, Twitchell J. Temporary discontinuation of warfarin therapy: changes in the International Normalized Ratio. *Ann Intern Med*. 1995;122:40–42.

6. Tinmouth AH, Morrow BH, Cruickshank MK, Moore PM, Kovacs MJ. Dalteparin as perioperative anticoagulation for patients on warfarin and at high risk of thrombosis. *Ann Pharmacother*. 2001;35:669–674.

7. Spandorfer JM, Lynch S, Weitz HH, Fertel S, Merli GJ. Use of enoxaparin for the chronically anticoagulated patient before and after procedures. *Am J Cardiol*. 1999;84:478–480, A10.

8. Turpie AGG, Johnson J. Temporary discontinuation of oral anticoagulants: role of low molecular weight heparin (Dalteparin). *Circulation*. 2002;102:II-826 (abstract 3983).

9. Atrial Fibrillation Investigators. Risk factors for stroke and efficacy of antithrombotic therapy in atrial fibrillation. Analysis of pooled data from five randomized trials. *Arch Intern Med*. 1994;154: 1449–1457.

10. European Atrial Fibrillation Trial Study Group. Secondary prevention in non-rheumatic atrial fibrillation after transient ischaemic attack or minor stroke. *Lancet*. 1993;342:1255–1262.

11. Caplan LR, Hier DB, D'Cruz I. Cerebral embolism in the Michael Reese Stroke Registry. *Stroke*. 1983;14:530–536.

12. Anderson CS, Jamrozik KD, Broadhurst RJ, Stewart-Wynne EG. Predicting survival of 1 year among different subtypes of stroke. *Stroke*. 1994;25:1935–1944.

13. Douketis JD, Kearon C, Bates S, Duku EK, Ginsberg JS. Risk of fatal pulmonary embolism in patients with treated venous thrombo-embolism. *JAMA*. 1998;279:458–462.

14. Atrial Fibrillation Investigators. Echocardiographic predictors of stroke in patients with atrial fibrillation. *Arch Intern Med*. 1998; 158:1316–1320.

15. Hart RG, Halperin JL. Atrial fibrillation and thromboembolism: a decade of progress in stroke prevention. *Ann Intern Med*. 1999;131: 688–695.

16. Albers GW, Dalen JE, Laupacis A, Manning WJ, Petersen P, Singer DE. Antithrombotic therapy in atrial fibrillation. *Chest*. 2001;119: 194S–206S.

17. Mok CK, Boey J, Wang R, Chan TK, Cheung KL, Lee PK, et al. Warfarin versus dipyridamole-aspirin and pentoxifylline-aspirin for the prevention of prosthetic heart valve thromboembolism: a prospective randomized clinical trial. *Circulation*. 1985;72:1059–1063.

18. Cannegieter SC, Rosendaal FR, Briet E. Thrombembolic and bleeding complications in patients with mechanical heart valve prostheses. *Circulation*. 1994;89(2):635–641.

19. Horstkotte D, Scharf RE, Schultheiss HP. Intracardiac thrombosis: patient-related and device-related factors. *J Heart Valve Dis*. 1995;4: 114–120.

20. Stein PD, Alpert JS, Bussey HI, Dalen JE, Turpie AG. Antithrombotic therapy in patients with mechanical and biological prosthetic heart valves. *Chest*. 2001;119:220S–227S.

21. Tinker JH, Tarhan S. Discontinuing anticoagulant therapy in surgical patients with cardiac valve prostheses. Observations in 180 operations. *JAMA*. 1978;239;738–739.

22. Francis CW, Marder VJ, Evarts CM, Yaukoolbodi S. Two-step warfarin therapy. Prevention of postoperative venous thrombosis without excessive bleeding. *JAMA*. 1983;249:374–378.

23. Taberner DA, Poller L, Burslem RW, Jones JB. Oral anticoagulants controlled by the British comparative thromboplastin versus low-dose heparin in prophylaxis of deep vein thrombosis. *Br Med J*. 1978;1:272–274.

24. Rustard H, Myhre E. Surgery during anticoagulant treatment. The risk of increased bleeding in patients on oral anticoagulant treatment. *Acta Med Scand*. 1963;173:115–119.

25. Francis CW, Pellegrini VD, Jr, Leibert KM, Totterman S, Azodo MV, Harris CM, et al. Comparison of two warfarin regimens in the prevention of venous thrombosis following total knee replacement. *Thromb Haemost*. 1996;75:706–711.

26. Crowther MA, Julian J, McCarty D, Douketis J, Kovacs M, Biagoni L, et al. Treatment of warfarin-associated coagulopathy with oral vitamin K: a randomised controlled trial. *Lancet*. 2000;356: 1551–1553.

27. Cerebral Embolism Task Force. Cardiogenic brain embolism. *Arch Neurol*. 1986;43:71–84.

28. International Stroke Trial Collaborative Group. The International Stroke Trial (IST): a randomized trial of aspirin, subcutaneous heparin, both or neither among 19,435 patients with acute ischaemic stroke. *Lancet*. 1997;349:1569–1581.

29. Berge E, Abdelnoor M, Nakstad PH, Sandset PM. Low molecular-weight heparin versus aspirin in patients with acute ischaemic stroke and atrial fibrillation: a double-blind randomised study. HAEST Study Group. Heparin in Acute Embolic Stroke Trial. *Lancet*. 2000;355:1205–1210.

30. Douketis JD, Crowther MA, Cherian SS. Perioperative anticoagulation in patients with chronic atrial fibrillation who are undergoing elective surgery: results of a physician survey. *Can J Cardiol*. 2000;16: 326–330.

31. Douketis JD, Crowther MA, Cherian SS, Kearson CB. Physician preferences for perioperative anticoagulation in patients with a mechanical heart valve who are undergoing elective noncardiac surgery. *Chest*. 1999;116:1240–1246.

32. Coon WW, Willis PW. Recurrence of venous thromboembolism. *Surgery*. 1973;73:823–827.

33. Heit JA, Mohr DN, Silverstein MD, Petterson TM, O'Fallon WM, Melton LJ, III. Predictors of recurrence after deep vein thrombosis and pulmonary embolism: a population-based cohort study. *Arch Intern Med*. 2000;160:761–768.

34. Collins R, Scrimgeour A, Yusuf S, Peto R. Reduction in fatal pulmonary embolism and venous thrombosis by perioperative administration of subcutaneous heparin. *N Engl J Med*. 1988;318:1162–1173.

35. Levine MN, Hirsh J, Gent M. Prevention of deep vein thrombosis after elective hip surgery: a randomized trial comparing low molecular weight heparin with standard unfractionated heparin. *Ann Intern Med*. 1991;114:545–551.

36. Coon WW, Willis PW. Hemorrhagic complications of anticoagulant therapy. *Arch Intern Med*. 1974;133:386–392.

37. Green RM, DeWeese JA, Rob CG. Arterial embolectomy before and after the Fogarty catheter. *Surgery*. 1975;77:24–33.

38. Treiman RL, Cossman DV, Foran RF, Levin PM, Cohen JL, Wagner WH. The influence of neutralizing heparin after carotid endarterectomy on postoperative stroke and wound hematoma. *J Vasc Surg*. 1990;12:440–446.

39. Wilson JR, Lampman J. Heparin therapy: a randomized prospective study. *Am Heart J*. 1979;97:155–158.

40. Nieuwenhuis HK, Albada J, Banga JD, Sixma JJ. Identification of risk factors for bleeding during treatment of acute venous thromboembolism with heparin or low molecular weight heparin. *Blood*. 1991;78(9): 2337–2343.

41. Basu D, Gallus AS, Hirsh J, Cade J. A prospective study of the value of monitoring heparin treatment with the activated partial thromboplastin time. *N Engl J Med*. 1972;287(7):324–327.

42. Hull R, Raskob G, Pineo G, Rosenbloom D, Evans W, Malloy T, et al. A comparison of subcutaneous low–molecular-weight heparin with warfarin sodium for prophylaxis against deep-vein thrombosis after hip or knee implantation. *N Engl J Med*. 1993;329:1370–1376.

43. Colwell CW Jr, Collis DK, Paulson R, McCutchen JW, Bigler GT, Lutz S, et al. Comparison of enoxaparin and warfarin for the prevention of venous thromboembolic disease after total hip arthroplasty. *J Bone J Surg*. 1999;81-A:932–940.

44. Hull RD, Raskob GE, Rosenbloom D, Panju AA, Brill-Edwards P, Ginsberg JS, et al. Heparin for 5 days as compared with 10 days in the initial treatment of proximal venous thrombosis. *N Engl J Med*. 1990;322:1260–1264.

45. Kakkar VV, Cohen AT, Edmonson RA, Phillips MJ, Cooper DJ, Das SK, et al. Low molecular weight versus standard heparin for prevention of venous thromboembolism after major abdominal surgery. *Lancet*. 1993;341:259–265.

46. Raschke RA, Reilly BM, Guidry JR, Fontana JR, Srinivas S. The weight-based heparin dosing nomogram compared with a "standard care" nomogram. *Ann Intern Med*. 1993;119:874–881.

47. Hirsh J, Warkentin TE, Shaughnessy SG, Anand SS, Halperin JL, Raschke R, et al. Heparin and low–molecular-weight heparin: mechanisms of action, pharmacokinetics, dosing, monitoring, efficacy, and safety. *Chest*. 2001;119:64S–94S.

48. Decousus H, Leizorovicz A, Parent F, Page Y, Tardy B, Girard P, et al. A clinical trial of vena caval filters in the prevention of pulmonary embolism in patients with proximal deep-vein thrombosis. *N Engl J Med*. 1998;338:409–415.

49. Harrison L, Johnston M. Massicotte MP, Crowther M, Moffat K, Hirsh J. Comparison of 5-mg and 10-mg loading doses in initiation of warfarin therapy. *Ann Intern Med*. 1997;126:133–136.

50. Bern MM, Lokich JJ, Wallach SR, Bothe A, Jr, Benotti PN, Arkin CF, et al. Very low doses of warfarin can prevent thrombosis in central venous catheters. *Ann Intern Med*. 1990;112(6):423–428.

51. Levine M, Hirsh J, Gent M, Arnold A, Warr D, Falanga A, et al. Double-blind randomised trial of very–low-dose warfarin for prevention of thromboembolism in stage IV breast cancer. *Lancet*. 1994;343:886–889.

52. Blackshear JL, Baker VS, Rubino F, Safford R, Lane G, Flipse T, et al. Adjusted-dose warfarin versus low-intensity, fixed-dose warfarin plus aspirin for high-risk patients with atrial fibrillation: stroke prevention in atrial fibrillation III randomised clinical trial. *Lancet*. 1996;348:633–638.

53. Grip L, Blomback M. Schulman S. Hypercoagulable state and thromboembolism following warfarin withdrawal in post-myocardial-infarction patients. *Eur Heart J*. 1991;12:1225–1233.

54. Palareti G, Legnani C, Guazzalocac G, Frascaro M, Grauso F, De Rosa F, et al. Activation of blood coagulation after abrupt or stepwise withdrawal of oral anticoagulants—a prospective study. *Thromb Haemost*. 1994;72:222–226.

55. Valles J, Aznar J, Santos T, Villa P, Fernandez A. Platelet function in patients with chronic coronary heart disease on long-term anticoagulant therapy: effect of anticoagulant stopping. *Haemostasis*. 1993;23:212–218.

56. Raskob GE, Durica SS, Morrisey JH, Owen WL, Comp PC. Effect of treatment with low-dose warfarin-aspirin on activated factor VII. *Blood*. 1995;85(11):3034–3039.

57. Genewein U, Haeberli A, Straub PW, Beer JH. Rebound after cessation of oral anticoagulant therapy: the biochemical evidence. *Br J Haematol*. 1996;92:479–485.

58. Palareti G, Legnani C. Warfarin withdrawal—pharmacokinetic-pharmacodynamic considerations. *Clin Pharmacokinet*. 1996;30:300–313.

59. Shields RC, McBane RD, Kuiper JD, Li H, Heit JA. Efficacy and safety of intravenous phytonadione (vitamin K_1) in patients on long-term oral anticoagulant therapy. *Mayo Clin Proc*. 2001;76:260–266.

60. Bonow RO, Carabello B, de LA, Jr, Edmunds LH, Jr, Fedderly BJ, Freed MD, et al. Guidelines for the management of patients with valvular heart disease: executive summary. A report of the American College of Cardiology/American Heart Association Task Force on Practice Guidelines (Committee on Management of Patients with Valvular Heart Disease). *Circulation*. 1998;98:1949–1984.

61. Wahl MJ. Dental surgery in anticoagulated patients. *Arch Intern Med*. 1998;158:1610–1616.

62. McCormack P, Simcock PR, Tullo AB. Management of the anti-coagulated patient for ophthalmic surgery. *Eye*. 1993;7(Pt 6):749–750.

63. American Society for Gastrointestinal Endoscopy. Guideline on the management of anticoagulation and antiplatelet therapy for endoscopic procedures. *Gastrointest Endosc*. 1998;48:672–675.

64. Hyers TM, Agnelli G, Hull RD, Morris TA, Samama M, Tapson V, et al. Antithrombotic therapy for venous thromboembolic disease. *Chest*. 2001;119:176S–193S.

65. Bath PM, Lindenstrom E, Boysen G, De Deyn P, Friis P, Leys D, et al. Tinzaparin in acute ischemic stroke (TAIST): a randomised aspirin-controlled trial. *Lancet*. 2001;358:702–710.

66. Bath PM, Iddenden R, Bath FJ. Low–molecular-weight heparins and heparinoids in acute ischemic stroke: a meta-analysis of randomized controlled trials. *Stroke*. 2000;31:1770–1778.

67. Chan WS, Anand S, Ginsberg JS. Anticoagulation of pregnant women with mechanical heart valves: a systematic review of the literature. *Arch Intern Med*. 2000;160:191–196.

68. Salazar E, Izaguirre R, Verdejo J, Mutchinick O. Failure of adjusted doses of subcutaneous heparin to prevent thromboembolic phenomena in pregnant patients with mechanical cardiac valve prostheses. *J Am Coll Cardiol*. 1996;27:1698–1703.

69. Montalescot G, Polle V, Collet JP, Leprince P, Bellanger A, Gandjbakhch I, et al. Low molecular weight heparin after mechanical heart valve replacement. *Circulation*. 2000;101:1083–1086.

70. Collins R, Peto R, Baigent C, Sleight P. Aspirin, heparin, and fibrinolytic therapy in suspected acute myocardial infarction. *N Engl J Med*. 1997;336:847–860.

Chapter 38

Managing the Patient with Cancer

Robert D. Bona, Amy D. Hickey, and Donna M. Wallace

INTRODUCTION

Patients with cancer and thromboembolic disease represent a therapeutic challenge. The association between cancer and thrombosis, first reported by Armand Trousseau in the 1800s, has been verified recently in a prospective study of 250 patients with deep vein thrombosis (DVT) where a statistically and clinically significant association between idiopathic DVT and the subsequent development of overt cancer was established.[1] This risk was even greater in patients who had recurrent venous thrombosis during the two-year follow-up period. Hemostatic complications represent the second most common cause of mortality in patients with cancer.[2] Further, patients with cancer and venous thrombosis (VT) have a higher mortality than those without VT.[3]

The principal causes of thrombosis described in Virchow's triad are particularly applicable to the patient with cancer. Damage to vascular endothelium caused by vascular access devices or invasion by cancer can alter the usual fibrinolytic and anticoagulant activity of the endothelium. Venous stasis resulting from prolonged periods of bed rest, necessitated by a deteriorating clinical status or surgery, or tumors that cause pressure on a major vessel (eg, renal cell, adrenocortical, and testicular cancers) can heighten the risk of VT. Some malignant diseases can cause hyperviscosity (eg, polycythemia vera, Waldenstom's macroglobulinemia) and interfere with blood flow. Finally, coagulation abnormalities resulting in hypercoagulable states can heighten the risk of thrombosis. Coagulation abnormalities identified in this population in- clude increased levels of fibrin degradation products, increased fibrinopeptide A, thrombocytosis, hyperfib- rinogenemia, increased production of procoagulants by cancer cells, and decreased levels of antithrombin and protein C. Table 38–1 lists some of the clinical thrombotic syndromes seen in patients with cancer. The many co-morbid conditions, treatment complications, and treatment itself make anticoagulation of this population a unique and difficult challenge. Abnormal results on routine coagulation tests have been described in up to 90% of patients with cancer.[4] The use of anticoagulant therapy must be undertaken with a careful risk/benefit consideration. Although the safety of anticoagulation in patients with cancer has been questioned, results from the authors' service and other services have shown that warfarin can be administered relatively safely.[5,6] However, two large studies have shown an increased risk of bleeding with warfarin therapy in this population. The first, a retrospective study published by Hutten et al[7] and the second published in preliminary form by Prandoni et al,[8] have indeed shown an increase in the risk of bleeding in this population while treated with warfarin. The latter two studies were quite large by comparison (260 and 181 with cancer, respectively), and the reliability of the estimated risk of bleeding may be more accurate than the earlier smaller studies. It also appears true that the risk of recurrent thrombosis is higher in cancer patients receiving warfarin as secondary prophylaxis for VT compared with patients without cancer.[7,8] It is more difficult, however, to maintain a therapeutic International Normalized Ratio (INR) in these

Table 38–1 Clinical Thrombotic Syndromes Seen in Patients

Embolic Clinical Events	Associated Malignancies and Comments
Deep vein thrombosis, upper extremity	Occurring in all malignancies
Deep vein thrombosis, lower extremity most common	Vascular devices—arterial and/or venous
Pulmonary embolism	Diagnosis complicated by lung cancer or pulmonary metastasis
Disseminated intravascular coagulation, chronic or acute Superior vena cava syndrome	Adenocarcinoma, gastrointestinal cancer, and certain leukemias Lung cancer and lymphoma
Migratory superficial thrombophlebitis usually involving upper extremities (Trousseau's syndrome)	Gastrointestinal and pancreatic cancers
Hepatic vein thrombosis (Bud-Chiari syndrome), portal vein thrombosis	Myeloproliferative disease (e.g., polycythemia vera), essential thrombocytopenia
Nonbacterial thrombotic endocarditis	Adenocarcinoma
Digital and cerebral microvascular thrombosis	Myeloproliferative disease (eg, polycythemia vera), essential thrombocytothemia
Intestinal infarction	Has been described in renal cell cancer

patients, and they need more frequent monitoring to avoid complications.[5,6] Patients with cancer might have nontherapeutic INR values for a greater proportion of the time because of associated problems of metastatic liver disease, malnutrition, chemotherapy, noncompliance, or other, unidentified factors.

PROPHYLAXIS

Preventive nursing and medical measures should be employed in the standards of care for all patients with cancer. Additionally, prophylaxis of venous thrombosis should be a concern in their care, especially for hospitalized patients at bed rest or undergoing surgery or for those for whom long periods of immobility are anticipated. This could take the form of low-dose or adjusted-dose subcutaneous heparin, low–molecular-weight heparin (LMWH), warfarin, pneumatic compression devices, and gradient thromboembolism deterrent or pulsatile stockings. Prompt evaluation of any symptoms suggesting arterial or venous thromboembolism is warranted in these high-risk patients. A 1990 study demonstrated that prophylaxis with warfarin at 1 mg/day reduced thrombosis associated with indwelling catheters in patients receiving cancer chemotherapy[9] as does a single daily dose of an LMWH.[10] Low-dose warfarin (target INR, 1.5–2.0) also has been shown to decrease thromboembolic events in women with metastatic breast cancer.[11]

TREATMENT

General Approach

The patient with cancer who develops a VT can present a challenging clinical problem. It may be appropriate to withhold therapy in patients with advanced metastatic disease; however, the symptoms of VT (leg pain, leg swelling, breathlessness, chest pain) can often be palliated with judiciously used anticoagulant drugs. In individuals with less advanced disease, therapy is aimed at preventing fatal pulmonary embolism, preventing recurrent pulmonary embolism, decreasing symptoms in the involved limb, and reducing morbidity because of postphlebitic syndrome as much as possible.

Standard Therapy

The patient who develops a venous thrombosis should be treated initially with heparin to maintain the activated partial thromboplastin time 1.5 to 2.5 times the mean normal value (assuming that this range represents a heparin concentration of 0.4 to 0.8 units/mL as determined by an in vitro heparin anti-Xa titration curve). The single published study[12] that evaluated the safety of intravenous heparin in cancer patients compared with patients without cancer demonstrated that this approach was safe. An alternative to standard unfractionated heparin is LMWH. A number of studies have been published that demonstrate, at the very least, equal efficacy and safety of LMWH when compared with standard heparin for the initial treatment of venous thrombosis.[13] Some emerging data would, in fact, support the superiority of LMWH over unfractionated heparin for the initial treatment of VT. A recent preliminary publication analyzed a subset of patients enrolled in the CORTES trial. Patients with cancer who had VT and were treated with an LMWH compared with unfractionated heparin had improved phlebographic responses measured 21 days after initiation of treatment and had fewer recurrences in the follow-up period. Two studies[14,15] demonstrated that patients with VT can be safely treated at home with LMWH. Although neither of these studies exclusively evaluated patients with cancer, such patients were not excluded from the studies and frequently comprised a significant number of the study sample. It would seem rea-sonable then to assume that LMWH would be as safe and effi-cacious as standard heparin for the initial treatment of venous thrombosis in patients with cancer. Studies evaluating the safety and efficacy of home therapy are currently being conducted.

The long-term secondary prophylaxis of venous thrombosis in these patients presents a clinical challenge. Warfarin has been used in this setting, and two prospective, cohort studies[16,17] demonstrated that the hemorrhagic risk is not significantly greater in cancer patients when compared with patients without cancer receiving warfarin. The targeted INR was 2 to 3 in both of these studies. However, two larger studies (one retrospective and one prospective) have shown an increased risk of bleeding with warfarin in this population. The risk of recurrent thrombosis appears to be approximately threefold greater in cancer patients when compared with patients without cancer who receive warfarin for secondary prophylaxis of venous thrombosis.[7,8] If warfarin is used, it should be started on the first day of heparin therapy. The heparin should be continued for at least five days and until the INR is therapeutic for two consecutive days.

The duration of anticoagulation with warfarin is usually 3 to 6 months in individuals without ongoing risk factors. However, in individuals with ongoing risk factors, the rate of recurrent thrombosis is high after warfarin is discontinued.[7] Patients with cancer frequently have a persistent hypercoagulable state due either to the disease itself or treatment with chemotherapy or hormonal therapy.[18] It has been the authors' practice, therefore, to continue warfarin anticoagulation until the risk factors have resolved (eg, chemotherapy, persistent cancer, and so forth).

Alternate Approach

Secondary prophylaxis also can be achieved with dose-adjusted subcutaneous unfractionated heparin or LMWH.

Although studies involving large numbers of patients with cancer have not been performed, it is likely that this treatment regimen would be effective. A preliminary report[19] of a small sample of patients supports this belief.

Patients at high risk of serious hemorrhage with anticoagulation (ongoing significant blood loss, pericardial metastases) can be treated with the insertion of an inferior vena caval filter in order to prevent life-threatening pulmonary embolism. This approach, however, is associated with a high rate of recurrent VT and/or filter thrombosisis.[20] Further, pulmonary embolism is not completely prevented, especially after the filter has been in place for longer than one year. Nonetheless, this procedure can be life saving and should be considered in patients who have a major contraindication to anticoagulation.

Treatment of the Patient Who Develops Recurrent Disease While on Warfarin

Patients who develop recurrent VT while on warfarin and who have consistently had a therapeutic INR should be considered warfarin failures. The approach to this group of patients has not been standardized and represents a difficult and potentially serious clinical situation. It has been the authors' practice to treat these patients initially with heparin or LMWH for 5 to 7 days. Secondary prophylaxis can be attempted with warfarin and a higher targeted INR (3–4) or subcutaneous adjusted-dose heparin (or LMWH). The former approach may be efficacious, but it will likely be associated with a higher bleeding risk.[21] The latter approach (LMWH) has been studied in small groups of patients by several investigators[19,22,23] and appears to be reasonably effective. Two studies[22,23] report on a total of five patients who had recurrent VT while maintained on warfarin. Therapy with LMWH was effective in preventing recurrent VT in all five patients. In another, preliminary report, Blinder et al[19] treated eight patients with recurrent VT despite therapeutic warfarin. Treatment appeared to be efficacious and safe in these patients. The insertion of an inferior vena caval filter can be considered, but it is the authors' opinion that in the absence of ongoing anticoagulation, there will be a high risk of filter thrombosis.

ASSESSMENT DURING CHRONIC ANTICOAGULATION

Meaningful communication among all members of the health care team, including the patient, family members, and caregivers, is essential when caring for patients with cancer.

Extra time might be needed to educate the patient and caregivers about anticoagulant therapy. A thorough patient history is vital. It should include a record of all concomitant medications and complete information regarding any chemotherapy that the patient is receiving. There should be an awareness of the chemotherapy cycle, any changes in the chemotherapy itself, the expected blood count during its nadir, and any possible cumulative drug effect. Frequent communication with the patient's hematologist-oncologist is advised.

The routine care of this population should include frequent laboratory testing, with particular focus on a drop in the hematocrit and hemoglobin levels, which could indicate a possible bleeding event, as well as thrombocytopenia to a level that could put a patient on warfarin at risk for bleeding.

Liver function tests are used routinely to assess liver toxicity or disease. Abnormalities in liver function will interfere with the metabolism of warfarin and necessitate a change in dosing. Some patients with liver metastasis actually have prolonged prothrombin times (PTs) and INRs when on very low doses of warfarin or none at all.

Malnutrition, biliary tract disease, and certain classes of antibiotics can cause vitamin K deficiency and lead to an increased sensitivity to warfarin. In the patient with cancer, the effects of multiple medications, chemotherapy, and the disease process itself can cause nausea, vomiting, diarrhea, anorexia, and mouth, gum, and throat sores or ulcerations. The short-term decrease in oral intake of vitamin K or intestinal malabsorption can potentiate the effect of warfarin therapy and result in a prolonged PT/INR.

The patient's medications should be reviewed at each visit, with particular attention given to those known to interact with warfarin.

Patients with cancer may utilize complementary and alternative medicine in combination with or instead of conventional therapies. One anti-cancer diet urges individuals to choose "good" fats, for example, the omega-3 fatty acids or the monounsaturated fats in olive oil. However, it is possible that many of these compounds can have effects on platelet function and coagulation proteins.[24-27] Dietary supplements may also contain unknown amounts of vitamin K.

The use of alternative therapies can affect the INR response to warfarin, and health care providers should be alert to unexplained difficulties in establishing a therapeutic INR. Patients should be asked specifically about alternative therapies, including vitamin therapy and other dietary supplements, as they may not recognize their potential impact on the effect of anticoagulation drugs.

Pain management is essential in helping the patient to attain the best possible quality of life. Many combinations of drugs, including nonsteroidal anti-inflammatory drugs, opiates, corticosteroids and other adjuvant analgesics, antihistamines, and tricyclic antidepressants and other central nervous system drugs are utilized. Problems can arise when pain medications cause confusion, forgetfulness, or central nervous system disturbances that lead to unintentional noncompliance with instructions for taking anticoagulants. These side effects can also result in trauma or injury that causes thrombosis or bleeding. Just as important is any potential interaction of the prescribed pain medication and warfarin.

Depression, denial, and other psychosocial factors can also lead to noncompliance regarding anticoagulation.

CONCLUSION

The standard principles and practices that are implemented in caring for all patients on anticoagulant therapy are also applied when caring for the patient with cancer. This patient, however, presents additional challenges, and appropriate dose adjustment is required more frequently because of the patient's often complicated and changing clinical status. Nonetheless, it might be more difficult to maintain a stable or therapeutic INR. Keeping these principles in mind, the clinician can manage anticoagulation therapy for the patient with cancer safely and effectively.

REFERENCES

1. Prandoni P, Lensing AW, Büller HR, et al. Deep vein thrombosis and the incidence of subsequent symptomatic cancer. *N Engl J Med.* 1992; 327:1128–1133.

2. Luzzatto G, Schafer AI. The prethrombotic state in cancer. *Semin Oncol.* 1990;17:147–159.

3. Sorensen HT, Mellemkjaer L, Olsen JH, Baron JA. Prognosis of Cancer Associated with Venous Thromboembolism. *New Engl J Med.* 2000;343:1846–1850.

4. Edwards RL, Rickles FR, Moritz TE, et al. Abnormalities of blood coagulation tests in patients with cancer. *Am J Clin Pathol.* 1987;88:596–602.

5. Bona RD, Hickey AD, Wallace DM. Warfarin is safe as secondary prophylaxis in patients with cancer and a previous episode of venous thrombosis. *Am J Clin Oncol.* 2000;23:71–73.

6. Krauth D, Holden A, Knapic N, Liepman M, Ansell J. Long-term anticoagulation in patients with cancer. *Cancer.* 1987;59:983–985.

7. Hutten BA, Prins MH, Gent M, et al. The incidence of recurrent thromboembolic and bleeding complications among patients with venous thromboembolism in relation to both malignancy and achieved International Normalized Ratio. *J Clin Oncol.* 2000;18:3078–3083.

8. Prandoni P, Lensing AWA, Piccioli A, Noventa P, Bagatella P, Bernardi E, Girolami B, Marchiori P, Sabbion P, Simioni P, Prins MH,

Girolami A. Recurrent venous thromboembolism and bleeding complications during anticoagulant treatment in patients with cancer and venous thrombosis. *Thromb Haemost*. 2001, Supplement, abstract OC901.

9. Bern MM, Lokich JJ, Wallach SR, et al. Very low doses of warfarin can prevent thrombosis in central venous catheters. *Ann Intern Med*. 1990;112:423–428.

10. Monreal M, Alastrue A, Rull M, et al. Upper extremity deep venous thrombosis in cancer patients with venous access devices—prophylaxis with a low molecular weight heparin (Fragmin). *Thromb Haemost*. 1996;75:21–23.

11. Levine M, Hirsh J, Gent M, et al. Double-blind randomized trial of very–low-dose warfarin for the prevention of thromboembolism in stage IV breast cancer. *Lancet*. 1994;343:886–889.

12. Wester JPJ, de Valk HW, Nieuwenhuis HK, et al. Risk factors for bleeding during treatment of acute venous thromboembolism. *Thromb Haemost*. 1996;76:682–688.

13. Siragusa S, Cosmi B, Piovella F, Hirsh J, Ginsberg J. Low molecular weight heparins and unfractionated heparin in the treatment of patients with acute venous thromboembolism: results of meta-analysis. *Am J Med*. 1996;100:269–277.

14. Koopman MMW, Prandoni P, Piovella F, et al. Treatment of venous thrombosis with intravenous unfractionated heparin administered in the hospital as compared with subcutaneous low molecular weight heparin administered at home. *N Engl J Med*. 1996;334:682–687.

15. Levine M, Gent M, Hirsh J, et al. A comparison of low molecular weight heparin administered primarily at home with unfractionated heparin administered in the hospital for proximal deep vein thrombosis. *N Engl J Med*. 1996;334:677–681.

16. Prandoni P. Antithrombotic strategies in patients with cancer. *Thromb Haemost*. 1997;78:141–144.

17. Bona RD, Hickey AD, Wallace DM. Efficacy and safety of oral anticoagulation in patients with cancer. *Thromb Haemost*. 1997;78:137–140.

18. Agnelli G. Venous thromboembolism and cancer: a two-way clinical association. *Thromb Haemost*. 1997;78:117–120.

19. Blinder MA, Govindan R, Beeki V, Clark RC. Exonaparin for the treatment of venous thromboembolism in patients with malignancy: a pilot study. *Blood*. 1996;88(suppl 1):180.

20. Decousus H, Leizorovicz A, Parent F, et al. A clinical trial of vena caval filters in the prevention of pulmonary embolism in patients with proximal deep vein thrombosis. *N Engl J Med*. 1998;338:409–415.

21. Levine M, Raskob GE, Landefeld S, Hirsh J. Hemorrhagic complications of anticoagulant therapy. *Chest*. 1985;I08:291S–301S.

22. Walsh-McMonagle D, Green D. Low molecular weight heparin in management of Trousseau's syndrome. *Cancer*. 1997;80:649–655.

23. Zuger M, Demarmels Biasiutti F, Wuillemin WA, Furlan M, Lammle B. Subcutaneous low molecular weight heparin for treatment of Trousseau's syndrome. *Ann Hematol*. 1997;75:165–167.

24. Chan T. Interaction between warfarin and dashan (salvia miltiorrhiza). *Ann Pharmacotherapy*. 2001;35:501–503.

25. Heck A, Dewitt B, Lukes A. Potential interactions between alternative therapies and warfarin. *Am J Health-Systems Pharm*. 2000;57:1221–1227.

26. Junker R. Effects of diets containing olive oil, sunflower oil or rapeseed oil on the hemostatic system. *Thromb Haemost*. 2001;85:280–286.

27. Vaes L, Chyka P. Interactions of warfarin with garlic, ginger, ginko, or ginseng: nature of the evidence. *Ann Pharmacol*. 2000;34:178–182.

Chapter 39

The Challenges and Opportunities
of Anticoagulation Compliance

Cheryl Nadeau and Barbara Delmore

INTRODUCTION

One of the many challenges faced by health care professionals is the issue of patient compliance with treatments. Lack of compliance interferes with patient safety,[1-4] full recovery, healing, and adequate disease management.[3] Noncompliance with drug therapies not only limits their effectiveness, but in some instances is associated with grave clinical consequences, repeated hospitalizations, and substantial economic burden.[5] Hospital readmission rates due to medication noncompliance have been estimated to be between 5% and 40%.[3]

The costs of managing the consequences of poor medication compliance have been estimated to be greater than $100 billion annually in the United States alone.[3,6] In addition, there are direct and indirect costs to the patient. Direct costs include additional prescriptions, avoidable emergency department visits, hospitalizations, and additional physician visits. Indirect costs are related to lost productivity as a result of morbidity and mortality.[7,8]

At least 38% of patients fail to follow short-term treatment plans, and at least 43% do not adhere to recommendations for long-term treatment. More than 75% of patients are unwilling or unable to follow recommended lifestyle changes.[9] Despite its frequency, health professionals often do not detect patient noncompliance, even physicians with considerable clinical experience. This chapter addresses the concerns and challenges caused by poor compliance with anticoagulation therapy and presents opportunities that can help reduce noncompliance.

COMPLIANCE BACKGROUND

Patient compliance is an age-old problem that dates back to the time of Hippocrates, who stated "the physician must not only be prepared to do what is right himself, but also to make the patient . . . cooperate."[10] Historically, numerous terms have been coined to describe patients who deviate from instructions. During early efforts at tuberculosis control, such patients were called "ignorant," "vicious," "recalcitrant," or "defaulters." Later came terms such as *faithless, untrustworthy,* and *unreliable.*[11] The currently used terms are *compliance, adherence,* and *concordance.* The term *compliance* has been defined in various ways to characterize the extent to which a person's behavior coincides with medical or health advice.[4] The term *adherence* then became the preferred term because it encompasses the total collaborative patient-clinician process and avoids negative connotations.[4,7,12] Concordance is described as a "state of agreement," which can be achieved by a therapeutic alliance reached through negotiation. The term encompasses the patient's fears, expectations, health beliefs, and ideas.[4] The distinction between the terms *compliance, adherence,* and *concordance* is meaningless from the patient's perspective.[2,12] None of these terms accurately represents patients' motivations for choosing to take their medications a certain way. "Patients do not judge outcomes by percentage of medicine taken, but how that medicine affects their lives."[12]

COMPLIANCE CHALLENGES

Medication compliance is defined as using "the right drug in the correct dose at the right interval"[13] as well as the correspondence between the patient's dose history and prescribed regimen.[14] Compliance can be total, partial, nil, or erratic[15] and may be intentional or unintentional.[16] The most common medication compliance problems are delayed doses and/or missing doses. Toxicity and adverse effects may result when patients miss doses for extended periods and then resume taking the drug at full dose.[14] Multiple patterns of poor adherence are often seen within the same individual. Failure to persist with chronic therapy is particularly prevalent with asymptomatic diseases.[5]

Noncompliance with medication taking is not only important to the individual patient but can impact results of clinical research trials. Noncompliant patients included in randomized trials may increase costs because of the inability of the researchers to detect treatment effects, thus increasing sample sizes.[5,17] Therefore, many trials eliminate noncompliant patients during the earlier trial phases to increase their internal validity. Such methods may lead to results that generalize poorly to everyday patient care in that practice and research do not match. As explained by Hughes et al,[5] randominized clinical trials remain the "gold standard" for comparing alternative treatments, yet the high internal validity required to demonstrate efficacy comes at the expense of external validity.[18] To that end, research still remains important in determining compliance characteristics and opportunities. Currently, the difficulty lies in the methodological limitations and variances, which make comparison of studies and compliance methods difficult. Similar themes arise continuously and are discussed within this chapter.

COMPLIANCE FROM THE CLINICIAN'S PERSPECTIVE

It is not surprising that patients who comply with treatment regimens have better health outcomes than noncompliant patients. It has been suggested that certain predispositions, such as genetics, personal history, and personality influence compliance behaviors.[17] Other determinants identified as affecting compliance include a person's subjective norms, health beliefs, attitudes, and coping style. A person's beliefs about what others want him or her to do may affect intention or commitment to carry out a specific behavior.[19] Exhibit 39–1 identifies other factors affecting compliance.

Whether practitioner or patient, we are all affected by culture, which brings its own set of personal biases. In addition, practitioners develop professional biases that they

Exhibit 39–1
OTHER FACTORS IDENTIFIED AS AFFECTING COMPLIANCE[1,4,7,9,12–14,19–23]

- Noninvolvement of patient in designing the treatment plan
- Trust in the clinician–patient relationship
- Multiple drug prescribers
- Cost of medications
- Duration of drug therapy
- Language barriers
- Personal values
- Complex drug regimens
- Lack of knowledge
- Adverse side effects of drugs
- Degree of behavior change required
- Cultural background
- Poor morale, perceptions of poor health or poor quality of life

impart to the patient and need to be aware of how these biases may affect a patient and, ultimately, compliance.[23]

COMPLIANCE FROM THE PATIENT'S PERSPECTIVE

The majority of compliance research by the health care profession has focused on the extent, methods of measurement, and potential determinants of noncompliance. Some authors propose one particular option to solve noncompliance; others suggest a combination of strategies.[6,14] Regardless, all the aforementioned become meaningless when compromised by an incomplete understanding of the importance of the medicine to the patient. Simply, patients may not have the same expectation in mind as practitioners. The patient may view compliance as a false measure developed for the health practitioner's convenience, yet with little value to the patient.[24]

Patients are more concerned with human functioning than medically defined physiologic function. Health care providers dedicated to improving compliance must first recognize outcomes that are valued by patients and the motivations for their behavior. A person's interpretation of the cause of an illness and his or her perceived control regarding a chronic condition may affect the decision to seek medical care, take preventive actions toward an illness, and adhere to medical advice.[7] To truly gain an understanding of medication-taking behavior, one must consider the patient's perspective. Exhibit 39–2 illustrates some common rationales for noncompliance.

Patients use a variety of criteria to determine the value of medication. They may place equal or greater value on per-

Exhibit 39–2
COMMON RATIONALES FOR PATIENT NONCOMPLIANCE

- Lack of timely continuity in diagnosis/treatment due to scheduling tests and appointments
- Lack of immediate results
- Despondency caused by bureaucracy of health care system (referrals, etc.)
- Failure to complete medication schedule due to improved systems
- Cost of drug, co-pays, and transportation
- Lost work time
- Failure to recognize importance of treatment in asymptomatic diseases
- Influence of others, misinterpretation of news reports, Internet, etc.
- Side effects interfering with social function

sonal and often competing nonclinical outcomes. Morris and Schultz's[24] meta-analysis discovered this concept; medication value was essentially based upon the patient's desired outcomes. For some it was pain relief, for others it was returning to a normal life or resuming hobbies. From the patient's perspective, medication was ineffective if the desired outcomes were not reached, even if clinical indicators of improvement were present. Some patients realized therapeutic efficacy in this study after stopping and resuming the medicine when they felt bad without it. From a clinician's point of view, this behavior would be considered noncompliant. From the patient's perspective, this action was necessary to validate the treatment.[24]

Noncompliance from the patient's perspective may be intentional yet rational. It may result from practical difficulties such as taking time off from work for appointments or not being able to coordinate pill taking with their daily schedule. It may just be a result of the difficulties in navigating through the health care system. Barriers faced by patients today such as obtaining referrals and/or preauthorization requirements for physicians and tests can create significant time lapses between the patient reporting the symptoms and the diagnosis being made. The time elapsed can create two situations: worsening of symptoms and the loss of numerous work days to keep appointments.

Noncompliance may be a result of a patient's denial of a chronic illness that requires a change in daily routines. The "intrusion" may act as a daily reminder of the illness and "lack of wholeness" felt by the patient,[25] which is especially true in patients with asymptomatic diseases. Patients may be unwilling to endure physical responses such as medication side effects in order to decrease the risk of some future health problem, especially when the patient feels worse when following the prescribed regimen. In an attempt to improve their quality of life (QOL), patients may alter their medication regimen to avoid side effects. Drug side effects may be the reason why some patients are noncompliant with the regimen.[24] For example, many patients who need diuretics do not take them as prescribed because the increased urination interferes with sleep or social function.

Some patients may choose to disregard the clinician's recommendations completely and turn to alternative methods such as herbal products or dietary supplements. From the patients' perspective, they have not failed to comply; they have chosen to take another action. For them compliance is not an issue. They consider the clinician's instruction in light of other factors and eventually arrive at a decision about their treament.[6]

Patients tend to think very seriously before taking a new drug. They consider their subjective norms, health beliefs, attitudes, coping styles, and past behaviors. They do not usually arrive at a clinician's office meekly awaiting instructions. In general, they tend to hold sets of beliefs and theories about health and illness, and often about specific problems and treatments as well. Today's patients are demanding consumers. The majority want a great deal of information from their health professionals, and many want to take an active part in health decisions.[6] Although the patient may take into account the clinician's recommendations, they will often go to external sources as well, such as family, friends, neighbors, printed information, health-related programming/advertising on radio or television, or the Internet. Further impacting the patient's decision are media reports of medical controversies, contradictions, and even reversals regarding medical recommendations.[26] Therefore, the decision to comply may be reached after the patient synthesizes the information gathered from external sources with the clinician's recommendations and the patient's own beliefs. The majority who do not comply do not feel guilty at not following instructions; they will have reached a rational and sensible decision within the framework of their own lives and beliefs. Although their decision may appear irrational to others, it is not irrational to the individual.[6]

COMPLIANCE ISSUES IN THE ELDERLY

Elderly patients are at particular risk of noncompliance, often unintentionally, due to physical or cognitive barriers.[16] Persons over age 65 take approximately one-third of all prescription medications and about 40% of all nonprescription medications.[27] Elderly patients with multiple chronic conditions may take eight or more prescription drugs daily. Elderly individuals taking more than five medications simultaneously have a significantly greater risk for developing an adverse drug reaction and are at increased risk for hospitalization.[27] These patients tend to have complicated medication regimens, with medications often being prescribed by multiple health care providers. Further complicating the issue is the fact that patients often take over-the-counter (OTC) drugs without the prescribers' awareness, setting up the potential for serious drug interactions. Costs of medication, especially for the elderly living on a fixed income, can also impact compliance.[28] Exhibit 39–3 explains some causes for medication regimen noncompliance in the elderly.

It is not unusual for elderly persons to be unaware of the names of some or all of the medications they are taking, when the medication was prescribed, or for what purpose. On occasion an elderly person may be taking two doses of the same medication, one with a brand name and one with a generic name. Thrifty habits developed throughout a lifetime can also lead to polypharmacy issues. Many elderly do not discard old medications and may independently add a previously prescribed drug to a daily regimen. They may assume that because the drug was once ordered for a particular condition, it must be appropriate when a similar diagnosis is made.[27]

Social isolation can be a major contributor to nonadherence in the elderly due to lack of: (a) supervision in taking medications, (b) assistance in opening pill bottles, or (c) remembering to take medications.[1,12,13,16,19] Often overlooked by health care providers is the fact that many elderly patients are primary care providers for an ill spouse and frequently neglect their own medications and health care needs. Side effects of medication(s) such as urinary frequency, gastrointestinal disturbances, dry mouth, constipation, or dizziness may affect elderly patients' ability to perform their activities of daily living, which may also lead to noncompliance.

Cognitive and physical function can also play an important role in compliance. Forgetfulness, confusion, dementia, poor recall, or diminished hearing can all affect compliance.[16] Arthritic hands may cause inability to open pill bottles. Poor eyesight may create difficulty in distinguishing between pill bottles or reading labels, especially when the label becomes blurred with use.[1,12,13,29,30] The ability to remember specific doses and the time to take them, and then to take the medication as prescribed is a complex process. Cognition can be affected by multiple factors, including acute infection, change in environment, or the existence of one or more comorbidities.[30]

Elderly patients may have more difficulty with readiness to receive and process information following an acute hospital stay and/or follow-up office visit. Misunderstanding prescriptions and recommendations is also extremely common. Clinicians often use medical terms that patients do not understand, and patients are often too inhibited or inarticulate to frame their questions.[9,31]

COMPLIANCE AND ANTICOAGULATION

Anticoagulation therapy has been well proven to reduce the risk of mortality in cardiovascular events, prevent stroke, and reduce mortality in other disease processes.[1] Currently there are over two million people in the United States taking warfarin sodium.[32] Compliance is a significant concern with this drug because it has a narrow therapeutic index. The management of anticoagulation therapy involves the avoidance of two equally serious clinical failures: overanticoagulation and underanticoagulation. Both situations can be life threatening and both have been areas for medical malpractice and professional negligence litigation in the United States.[33]

Safe and efficacious anticoagulation therapy is dependent on maintaining the International Normalized Ratio (INR) level within the therapeutic range. Fluctuations in INR levels place the patient at risk of bleeding or thromboembolic complications.[34] The relationship between time in therapeutic range and episodes of bleeding and thromboembolism are exponential; small departures from target range are associated with small to moderate increases in bleeding and thromboembolism, while large departures are associated with large increases in bleeding and thromboembolism.[30,35,36] Numerous factors can affect the INR level, including changes in diet or medication, onset of a new illness, travel or interruption of warfarin therapy. In addition, adherence to one medication does not imply adherence with another. Because the efficacy of warfarin is affected by the patient's adherence to concurrent medications, examining adherence to warfarin therapy as an isolated entity is not as useful as examining total adherence for all the patient's medications.[37] Additionally, some patients who require anticoagulation therapy for clinical reasons lack the personal and social resources to safely comply with their prescribed anticoagulation therapy regimen.[35] Safe and effective anticoagulation therapy is in large part dependent on a cooperative and compliant patient.

Lack of patient compliance in anticoagulation management not only poses the obvious dangers of over- or underanti-

---

Exhibit 39–3
CAUSES FOR NONCOMPLIANCE IN THE ELDERLY

- Complicated medication regimens
- Polypharmacy
- Side effects
- Multiple prescribers
- Misunderstanding instructions
- Economic impact
- Social isolation
- Cognitive function
- Sensory impairment
- Physical function

coagulation to the individual; there is also the wider issue of how poor compliance may affect the perceived efficacy of treatment. Subtherapeutic INR levels might result in prescribed increases in dosage or discontinuation of the drug because it is believed to be ineffective. The conclusion is often based on the assumption that the patient has taken the medication as prescribed when noncompliance may be the cause for the lack of efficacy.[3] The higher the adherence rate with prescribed warfarin therapy, the lower the percentage of INRs outside the therapeutic range. Changes in warfarin dosage are more commonly made in nonadherent patients.[37–39]

Issues related to compliance with anticoagulation therapy are the same as those with other disease processes except for fear of bleeding. Lancaster et al[40] found the experience of bleeding during anticoagulant therapy was associated with a significant decrease in health perceptions even when those bleeding episodes were clinically minor. Fear of bleeding was not a substantial anxiety for anticoagulant-treated patients until they actually experienced bleeding. The study also looked at the impact of long-term warfarin therapy on QOL and found that when carefully managed, warfarin therapy was well tolerated and did not significantly impinge on a patient's QOL. It also found that, on average, elderly patients with atrial fibrillation who were taking warfarin did not perceive themselves to be any less healthy than a comparable group who were treated without anticoagulation. Once aware of the heightened risk of stroke, many patients reported that they felt safer with warfarin therapy.

Arsten et al[1] performed a case-control study to identify determinants of noncompliance with anticoagulation therapy. Results of this study demonstrated that patients who were noncompliant with warfarin therapy shared distinctive clinical characteristics. Notably, younger male patients who have not experienced a thromboembolic event were more likely to forgo INR testing or to stop anticoagulation therapy completely. Noncompliant patients were found to be less likely to know why warfarin had been prescribed. These patients tended not to have a primary physician. Additionally, the study found that noncompliant patients perceived markedly different benefits and barriers to anticoagulation than compliant patients. Noncompliant patients considered regular blood tests to be a big problem; they felt that their life was adversely affected by taking warfarin and failed to perceive health benefit from anticoagulation therapy.

Formal anticoagulation settings, besides maintaining INR levels within therapeutic ranges, can reduce thromboembolic events and hemorrhagic complications.[34] Clinics, hospital-based or other, have been recommended as a method of delivery for anticoagulant care. Physicians and patients equate these settings with safe care because of the primary anticoagulation focus and the education and follow-up involved.[34,41–43] (See Chapter 1, The Value of an Anticoagulation Management Service.)

METHODS OF MEASURING COMPLIANCE

Unfortunately there is no completely accurate method of measuring compliance in taking medication, but numerous methods of measuring compliance have been reported, including direct observation of a patient taking medication, biochemical validation, patient self-report, prescription refills, pill counts, and electronic medication monitoring. Direct observation of a patient taking medication is invalidated if the patient "cheeks" the medicine.[12] Biochemical validation is flawed in many ways because assays are not available for many compounds. Blood and urine tests for therapeutic drug monitoring are influenced by variable drug absorption, metabolism, and clearance, and may give an inaccurate impression of overall compliance. Levels of short-acting drugs reflect recent dosing but provide no information on drug-taking behavior several days before the test. If a patient is more compliant just prior to a clinic visit, the blood or urine drug assay may overestimate compliance.[15]

Patient self-reports (eg, history taking, diaries, questionnaires, self-report scales) may be flawed because patients tend to respond in a socially desirable manner.[19] It may also be erroneous not because patients consciously falsify dosing reports, but because they may have forgotten about doses take or missed.[44]

Prescription refills are questionable for assessment of dosing compliance because they provide no information on timing or intake quantity. Many patients request refills regularly when reminded even if they have not run out of the drug, whereas others stockpile medications or have quantities of medications in several areas of convenience. Pill counts are also unreliable measures of adherence, particularly if patients fail to bring their medication with them at the time of the clinic visit. In addition, some patients may empty their pill bottles just before the clinic visit to deceive the clinician. Electronic medication monitoring devices record the opening of a box or bottle to remove tablets or capsules. Although these devices provide more accurate information, they do not document that the medication was actually taken by the patient, only that it was removed from the container.[15]

OPPORTUNITIES TO IMPROVE COMPLIANCE

Enhancing patient compliance in taking medication requires personalized intervention focusing on the unique meaning that health and illness have for each individual. The most effective strategy is to use a comprehensive approach encompassing patients' readiness to adhere; their sense of medication self-efficacy; their personal biases related to adherence; as well as their physical, economic, psychological, functional, social, and QOL characteristics.[12,45] Exhibits 39–4 through 39–10 identify opportunities to improve compliance.

Exhibit 39–4
STRATEGIES TO ENHANCE THE
CLINICIAN–PATIENT RELATIONSHIP[9,12,14,15,46]

- Establish a clinician-patient relationship that encourages trust and communication.
- Consult the patient regarding his or her ability to comply with the necessary drug regimen.
- Use written agreements outlining behavioral expectations.
- Describe treatment plans, goals, and rationale using simple unambiguous language.
- Explore physical, emotional, and financial factors related to treatment and develop a mutual plan that will help overcome identified barriers.

Exhibit 39–5
IMPORTANT INFORMATION FOR PATIENTS
ON WARFARIN

- Importance of getting INR monitored regularly
- Drug interactions with warfarin (prescription, OTC, herbal/dietary supplements)
- Risks of over- and undercoagulation
- Signs of unusual bleeding
- Interaction of warfarin with dietary intake of vitamin K
- When to seek treatment if bleeding occurs

Clinician-Patient Relationship

Patients are more likely to adhere to a regimen when the relationship with their clinician allows them to express their concerns about a condition or treatment.[14] Patients and their significant others need to be viewed as partners in the treatment plan to identify strategies to help strengthen patient compliance. Misunderstanding and misinformation are avoided if proper assessment of the patient's knowledge, beliefs, and expectations about treatment are discussed.[23] Compliance success is more likely if patients are involved in treatment decisions and are aware of the potential risks that may affect their future QOL.[9] (See Exhibit 39–4.)

Medication Regimens

Simplicity in medication regimen is tantamount to compliance and is achieved by minimizing the frequency of dosing, the number of prescribed drugs, and the duration of treatment.[14,15,29] Another strategy is to prescribe medications in concert with the patient's daily activities. Care should be taken when prescribing medications that come in multiple

Exhibit 39–6
STRATEGIES TO ENHANCE PATIENT
UNDERSTANDING AND INFORMATION
RETENTION[12,14,35,46,47]

- State the most important information first.
- Keep information simple and without medical jargon.
- Have patients repeat the treatment plan in their own words to validate understanding.
- Reinforce oral with printed information.
- Ensure that patients can read, the information is on the appropriate reading level, print size can be clearly seen, and language appropriate.
- Have patients write down the instructions and repeat back to the practitioner if dosage instructions are provided by telephone.
- Instruct patients that if they experience adverse effects, miss a dose(s), or make a mistake with the dosage schedule, to call the clinician (patients should not take it upon themselves to adjust their warfarin dosage without professional guidance).
- Review information at each patient encounter.

dosages. For example, warfarin comes in nine different doses; patients with multiple warfarin dosages can easily take the wrong one. Safety and compliance strategies for warfarin therapy may include either prescribing fewer different dosages or prescribing just one strength and having the patient break pills in half or take more than one pill of the same dosage.[47] (See Exhibit 39–5.) Successful medication regimen compliance includes educating the patient on the purpose and action of therapy.

Patient Instructions

Patient instructions should be written and reviewed with the patient before they leave the office/clinic. Exhibit 39–6 suggests strategies to include in instructions, especially when patients are given large amounts of information and may have retention problems.

Memory Strategies

Exhibit 39–7 suggests strategies to use if the patient expresses difficulty remembering a medication regimen.

Follow-Up

At all follow-up visits, monitor compliance with the treatment plan as well as the efficacy and side effects of the prescribed medicine. Exhibits 39–8 and 39–9 propose techniques for enhancing compliance.

Exhibit 39–7
REMINDER STRATEGIES[12,48]

- Keep medication next to familiar objects, such as a toothbrush or coffeepot.
- Have appointed family members or friends place reminder calls.
- Use a medication chart that can be checked off after each dose is taken.
- Use pill containers that can be prefilled with medication for a week at a time.
- Place reminders on household appliances or personal items.
- Use alarm devices that remind patients of dosing times.

Exhibit 39–8
TECHNIQUES TO ENHANCE COMPLIANCE AT FOLLOW-UP VISITS[15,27,47]

- Assess carefully for any changes in patients' medication, including OTC drugs and dietary supplements.
- Have patients bring their warfarin on each visit to ensure they are taking the correct dosage.
- Probe in a nonjudgmental and nonthreatening manner about compliance before making any dosage changes. If the patient has not been taking the medication, increasing the dosage will not solve the problem.
- Ask patients if they have seen any health care providers since their last visit. This question may be a reminder that a new medication was added or that warfarin therapy has been or will be interrupted for an invasive procedure.
- Instruct patients that one designated health care provider should manage their warfarin therapy. Multiple clinicians may prescribe different dosages, creating confusion and the potential for adverse effects.

Exhibit 39–9
STRATEGIES FOR ENHANCING COMPLIANCE WITH FOLLOW-UP APPOINTMENTS[14]

- Telephone or postcard appointment reminders prior to the appointment may be helpful.
- If unable to reach patients by telephone, missed appointment letters may be necessary. Patients who stop receiving care are unlikely to take their medication.
- Have a system in place to follow up missing appointments.
- Calling patients when they miss an appointment demonstrates concern for their well-being and may enhance the patients' trust in the clinician.

Compliance in the Elderly

Compliance in the elderly population can be especially challenging because of complex issues related to multiple co-morbidities, complex drug regimens, physical and cognitive challenges associated with aging, and social and financial issues. Although many of the compliance strategies previously discussed are equally effective with the elderly population, Exhibit 39–10 shows some compliance strategies that may be particularly helpful for this age group.

Exhibit 39–10
COMPLIANCE STRATEGIES FOR THE ELDERLY[12,16,27,29,30,48,49]

- Coordinate medication prescribing among all the patient's health care providers to prevent duplication of drugs and drug interactions.
- Review the patient's medication regimen at each visit, including inquiring about OTC, herbals, and dietary supplements.
- Include adult children or significant other(s) in medication education and encourage their participation in administering, reminding, or validating that medications are taken.
- Assess the patient's ability to purchase medication. Prescribe the least expensive drug that will achieve the desired therapeutic effect.
- Start medication education for hospitalized patients well before discharge day so that the patient does not feel overwhelmed. Have a family member or significant other present for teaching.
- Consider having a visiting nurse perform a home assessment.
- Prescribe the least amount of drugs at the lowest possible dose that will achieve the desired therapeutic effect.
- Provide the patient an accurate medication schedule, written in large print, to take home, which includes name of drug, purpose, dosage, time to take, and side effects.
- Counteract forgetfulness by considering reminder devices such as watch alarms, pill boxes, microelectronic monitoring devices, or check-off charts.
- Perform a functional assessment of the patient's ability to perform activities of daily living (ADLs) (eg, eating, toileting, bathing) and instrumental ADLs (eg, shopping, food preparation, managing finances) and a cognitive assessment to detect memory impairment. These assessments may be indicative of the patient's ability to manage medication.
- Instruct the patient to bring appropriate aids, such as eyeglasses or hearing aid, to each visit.
- Suspect the most recently prescribed medication or a combination of medications at onset of newly observed confusion or disorientation.

SUMMARY

Noncompliance exasperates health professionals, many of whom assume that in all cases the locus of the problem is the patient.[50] Morris and Schultz refer their readers to Trostle, who so aptly described noncompliance as an "unvoidable byproduct of collisions between the clinical world and other competing worlds of work, play, friendship and family life."[24] People who take medicine live in these worlds continuously; they are patients intermittently. Opportunities for health care professionals to help patients achieve their highest level of wellness will be limited by the degree that they recognize and accept these worlds as vital components of the patient's perspective.[24]

The success of any treatment regimen is dependent on the patient's willingness to follow it. No study has been able to offer a universally acceptable and effective solution to the noncompliance problem. Understanding compliance is as complex as understanding human nature. Patients will make reasoned decisions about accepting a clinician's advice, taking medications, or changing aspects of lifestyle based on their own beliefs and personal circumstances regardless of how illogical or unreasonable that decision may seem to others.

Health professionals can best serve patients not by encouraging and cajoling them into taking prescribed medications, but by taking a supportive role in learning how they can contribute to the decisions patients make about their health care. Focusing on details misses the real crux of noncompliance. Understanding an individual's health-related behavior and the many interrelated factors involved is essential. Forming a treatment plan that falls within the framework of the patient's circumstances and beliefs, as well as helping the patient identify barriers and strategies to overcome them, is the real opportunity to help a patient achieve his or her highest level of wellness. Shared decision making provides an opportunity for health professionals to understand the context within which patients reach their decisions and for the patient's decision-making abilities to be acknowledged and accepted.[6]

REFERENCES

1. Arsten JH, Gelfand JM, Singer DE. Determinants of compliance with anticoagulation: a case-control study. *American Journal of Medicine*. 1997;103(1):11–17.

2. Coons SJ. Medication compliance: the search for answers continues (ed). *Clin Ther*. 2001;8:1294–1295.

3. Dunbar-Jacob J, Mortimer-Stephens MK. Treatment adherence in chronic disease. *J Clin Epidemiol*. 2001;54:S57–S60.

4. Falk M. Compliance with treatment and the art of medicine (ed). *Am J Cardiol*. 2001;88(6):668–669.

5. Hughes DA, Bagust A, Haycox A, Walley T. The impact of non-compliance on the cost-effectiveness of pharmaceuticals: a review of the literature. *Health Econ*. 2001;10:601–615.

6. Donovan JL. Patient decision making: the missing ingredient in compliance research. *International J Tech Assess Health Care*. 1995; 11(3):443–455.

7. Patel RP, Taylor SD. Factors affecting medication adherence in hypertensive patients. *Ann Pharmacother*. 2002;36:40–44.

8. Johnson JA, Bootman LJ. Drug-related morbidity and mortality: a cost-of-illness model. *Arch Intern Med*. 1995;155(18):1949–1956.

9. DiMatteo MR. Enhancing patient adherence to medical recommendations. *JAMA*. 1994;271(1):79.

10. Turner BJ, Hecht FM. Improving on a coin toss to predict patient adherence to medications. *Ann Intern Med*. 2001;134:1004–1006.

11. Steiner JF, Earnest MA. The language of medication-taking. *Ann Intern Med*. 2000;132(11):926–930.

12. Huss K, Travis P, Huss R. Adherence issues in clinical practice. *Lippincott's Primary Care Pract*. 1997;1(2):199–206.

13. Barat I, Andreasen F, Damsgaard E. Drug therapy in the elderly: what doctors believe and patients actually do. *Br J Clin Pharmacol*. 2001; 51(6):615–625.

14. Schaffer SD, Yoon SL. Evidence-based methods to enhance medication adherence. *Nurse Pract*. 2001;26(12):50–54.

15. Tashkin DP. Multiple dose regimens impact on compliance. *Chest*. 1995;107(suppl 5):176S–182S.

16. Raynor DK, Nicolson M, Nunney J, et al. The development and evaluation of an extended adherence support programme by community pharmacists for elderly patients at home. *Int Pharm Pract*. 2000; September:157–164.

17. Horwitz RI, Horwitz SM. Adherence to treatment and health outcomes. *Arch Intern Med*. 1993;153:1863–1868.

18. Pedhazur EJ, Schmelkin LP. *Measurement, Design, and Analysis: An Integrated Approach*. Hillsdale, NJ: Lawrence Erlbaum Associates, Publishers; 1991.

19. Sherbourne CD, Hays RD, Ordway L, et al. Antecedents of adherence to medical recommendations: results from the medical outcomes study. *J Behav Med*. 1992;15(5):447–465.

20. Svensson S, Kjellgren KI, Ahlner J, et al. Reasons for adherence with antihypertensive medication. *Int J Cardiol*. 2000;76:157–163.

21. Hudson S. Medication management in the community: some considerations about compliance. *Home Care Provider*. 2001;August: 114–115.

22. Mitchell J, Mathews HF, Hunt LM, et al. Misunderstanding prescription medications among rural elders: the effects of socioeconomic status, health status, and medication profile indicators. *Gerontologist*. 2001; 41(3):348–356.

23. Charonko CV. Cultural influences in "noncompliant" behavior and decision making. *Holistic Nurs Pract*. 1992;6(3):73–78.

24. Morris LS, Schulz RM. Medication compliance: the patient's perspective. *Clin Ther*. 1993;15(3):593–605.

25. Alvarez CA. Noncompliance or human nature? *Clin Nurse Specialist*. 2001;15(2):51.

26. Kravitz RL, Hays RD, Sherbourne CD, et al. Recall of recommendations and adherence to advice among patients with chronic medical conditions. *Arch Intern Med*. 1993;153:1869–1878.

27. Schafer SL. Prescribing for seniors: it's a balancing act. *J Am Acad Nurse Pract.* 2001;13(3):108–112.

28. Wolfe SC, Schirm V. Medication counseling for the elderly: effects on knowledge and compliance after hospital discharge. *Geriatr Nurs.* 1992;May/June:134–138.

29. Cramer JA. Enhancing patient compliance in the elderly. Role of packaging aids and monitoring. *Drugs & Aging.* 1988;12(1):7–15.

30. Conn V, Taylor S, Miller R. Cognitive impairment and medication adherence. *J Gerontol Nurs.* 1994;July:42–47.

31. Balkrishnan R. Predictors of medication adherence in the elderly. *Clin Ther.* 1998;20(4):764–770.

32. Fihn S. Aiming for safe anticoagulation. *New Engl J Med.* 1995;333(1):54–55.

33. McCormick WP. Medical-legal implications of anticoagulation. *J Thromb Thrombolysis.* 2001;12(1):95–97.

34. Lafata JE, Martin SA, Kaatz S, et al. The cost-effectiveness of different management strategies for patients on chronic warfarin therapy. *J Gen Intern Med.* 2000;15:31–37.

35. Ansell JE, Buttaro ML, Thomas OV, et al. Consensus guidelines for coordinated outpatient oral anticoagulation therapy management. *Ann Pharmacother.* 1997;31:604–613.

36. Ansell JE, Hirsh J, Dalen J, et al. Managing oral anticoagulant therapy. *Chest.* 2001;119(suppl 1):22S–35S.

37. Mason BJ. Anticoagulant clinic warfarin adherence rates and assessment. *J Pharm Technol.* 1996;12:97–101.

38. Kumar S, Haigh JRM, Rhodes LE, et al. Poor compliance is a major factor in unstable outpatient control of anticoagulant therapy. *Thromb Haemostasis.* 1989;62(2):729–732.

39. Hixon-Wallace JA, Dotson JB, Blakey SA. Effect of regimen complexity on patient satisfaction and compliance with warfarin therapy. *Clin Appl Thromb/Hemost.* 2001;7(1):33–37.

40. Lancaster TR, Singer DE, Sheehan MA, et al. The impact of long-term warfarin therapy on quality of life. *Arch Intern Med.* 1991;151:1944–1948.

41. Baglin T. Decentralised anticoagulant care (ed). *J Clin Pathol.* 1998;51(2):89–90.

42. Chiquette E, Amato MG, Bussey HI. Comparison of an anticoagulation clinic with usual medical care. *Arch Intern Med.* 1998;158:1641–1647.

43. Pubentz MJ, Calcagno D, Teeters JL. Improving warfarin anticoagulation therapy in a community health system. *Pharm Prac Manage Q.* 1998;October:1–16.

44. Claxton AJ, Cramer J, Pierce C. A systematic review of the associations between dose regimens and medication compliance. *Clin Ther.* 2001;23(8):1296–1304.

45. Konkle-Parker DJ. A motivational intervention to improve adherence to treatment of chronic disease. *J Acad Nurse Pract.* 2001;13(2):61–68.

46. Roter DL, Hall JA. Strategies for enhancing patient adherence to medical recommendations. *JAMA.* 1994;271(1):80.

47. Nadeau C, Alpert B, Costantino T, et al. The challenges of oral anticoagulation. *Patient Care.* 2000;December 15:33–49.

48. Raynor DK, Booth TG, Blenkinsopp A. Effects of computer-generated reminder charts on patients' compliance with drug regimens. *Br Med J.* 1993;May 1:1158–1161.

49. Esposito L. The effects of medication education on adherence to medication regimens in an elderly population. *J Adv Nurs.* 1995;21(5):935–943.

50. Moore KN. Compliance or collaboration? The meaning for the patient. *Nurs Ethics.* 1995;2(1):71–76.

Chapter 40

Quality of Life Issues

Nichola Davis, Daniel E. Singer, and Julia H. Arnsten

INTRODUCTION

The number of patients for whom long-term anticoagulation is indicated has increased dramatically during the past 10 years.[1–10] This increase is largely due to randomized trials demonstrating that anticoagulants prevent strokes in patients with nonrheumatic atrial fibrillation.[1–6] Anticoagulants have also been shown to reduce the risk of mortality and cardiovascular morbidity after acute myocardial infarction.[7,8]

In real world practice, as opposed to clinical trials, anticoagulation is a demanding therapy for both patients and physicians. Patients are generally prescribed warfarin for asymptomatic conditions, yet they are required to make significant lifestyle changes in order to obtain long-term benefit. These changes include frequent office visits and laboratory tests, avoidance of physical trauma and contact sports, abstention from alcohol, and careful monitoring of diet and concurrent medications. In addition, patients on warfarin are susceptible to both minor and major bleeding events, ranging from epistaxis to intracranial hemorrhage. Therefore, warfarin therapy can substantially diminish patients' quality of life. In fact, many physicians have cited impairment of quality of life and inconvenience of blood test monitoring as reasons for not prescribing warfarin in certain situations.[11–13]

Despite evidence from randomized trials that demonstrates warfarin's efficacy in preventing strokes and cardiovascular morbidity and mortality, patients are likely to vary with respect to the risk they are willing to accept from a potentially dangerous treatment in order to avoid a relatively unlikely adverse outcome. In addition, patients might be willing to accept only minimal lifestyle burdens in order to avoid events that may occur in the distant future. This point is well-illustrated in the clinical trials of warfarin for atrial fibrillation, in which 8% to 26% of patients were withdrawn because of noncompliance or general refusal to continue.[1–5]

Evaluating the impact of chronic anticoagulation therapy on quality of life is important because the success of warfarin therapy depends on a favorable balance between the perceived benefits of treatment and the associated inconveniences. Several studies have addressed this topic. These studies can be classified into two types: (1) health status surveys of patients for whom chronic anticoagulation is indicated and (2) decision analyses estimating the adjustment in quality of life generated by chronic anticoagulation therapy. This chapter reviews the available literature on the impact of anticoagulation on quality of life and defines important questions for future research.

MEASURING QUALITY OF LIFE

Quality of life and health status are useful criteria for evaluating medical outcomes and making treatment decisions. Assessment of quality of life has become an increasingly important component of clinical and epidemiological research and is also used in clinical practice, policy analysis, and population monitoring. Because quality of life is influenced by social, environmental, economic, and occupational factors, the more specific term *health-related quality of life* is often used to refer to the physical, mental, functional, and social domains affected by health. In studying health-related quality of life, each domain is individually assessed, using specific questions pertaining to its most important components. For example, physical functioning may be assessed by asking about limitations in performing activities such as climbing stairs, while social functioning may be assessed by asking about limitations in usual activities with family or friends.[14] Health-related quality of life is usually measured using multi-item scales that meet basic standards of reliability, validity, sensitivity, practicality, and interpretability.[15,16] Many such generic and disease-specific scales are commonly available and have been extensively reviewed.[17]

ESTIMATING THE IMPACT OF ANTICOAGULATION THERAPY ON QUALITY OF LIFE

Patients' perceptions of the impact of long-term warfarin therapy on health-related quality of life have been examined in three studies, including two in the United States and one in Europe.[18–20] The earliest of these was a survey of perceived health status among patients participating in a randomized trial of warfarin to prevent stroke in atrial fibrillation in the United States.[18] Quality of life was measured using a combination of generic and disease-specific scales. Generic measures included assessments of physical and social functioning, emotional well-being, bodily pain, general health perceptions, and health distress and concern. A six-item disease-specific scale (see Table 40–1) was developed to assess problems with taking warfarin. The items in this scale were chosen with the help of the patients and staff of a large anticoagulation therapy unit.

The survey was conducted during an unblinded, randomized, controlled trial, and the generic scale was assessed on both warfarin-treated and control patients. Any differences in health status attributable to warfarin therapy could therefore be easily identified. In fact, this study found no difference between warfarin-treated and control patients on any of the generic measures. Warfarin-treated patients who had experienced a bleeding episode, however, reported more health distress and concern, and significantly worse general health perceptions than did warfarin-treated patients who had no bleeding complications.

The disease-specific scale used to assess attitudes toward warfarin therapy was administered to warfarin-treated patients only. As shown in Table 40–1, most patients did not feel that warfarin affected or restricted their lifestyle. Though only 37% felt that taking warfarin benefited their health, and only 39% felt that warfarin protected their future health, more than 50% of the patients responded "not sure" to these last two questions. This distribution of responses is consistent with the fact that these patients were participating in a randomized controlled trial, and the benefits of warfarin for stroke prevention in atrial fibrillation were not yet known.

The impact of warfarin therapy on quality of life was further examined in a case-control study of the determinants of noncompliance with anticoagulation that was also conducted in the United States.[19] Cases in this study were patients who had self-discontinued warfarin therapy, and controls were patients who were still taking warfarin. Both cases and controls could have any indication for anticoagulation. Surveys assessed a variety of health status perceptions, including the disease-specific items detailed in Table 40–1. Attitudes among the control patients toward taking warfarin are described in the table. As shown, control patients in this study reported greater negative and positive impact of warfarin therapy on quality of life than patients in the randomized trial. As would be expected, noncompliant cases reported even greater negative impact of warfarin therapy than control patients (data not shown).

Table 40–1 Perceived Benefits and Barriers to Anticoagulation

Statements about Taking Warfarin	Patients Agreeing with Statement (%)	
	Randomized Trial (n=177)	Case-Control Study (n=89)
Taking warfarin restricts my physical activity.	2	15
Taking warfarin affects my lifestyle.	7	31
I worry about bleeding while taking warfarin.	13	30
Regular blood tests are a problem.	22	34
Taking warfarin benefits my health.	37	80
Taking warfarin protects my future health.	39	85

Source: Reprinted with permission from Lancaster, Singer, and Sheehan et al, The Impact of Long-Term Warfarin Therapy on Quality of Life: Evidence from a Randomized Trial, *Archives of Internal Medicine*, Vol 151, pp 1944–1949, © 1991, American Medical Association.

The marked difference in perceptions of warfarin's impact on quality of life between the patients in the randomized trial and the control patients in the case-control study is not explained by differences in age or length of time on warfarin. The case-control study, however, was conducted four years after the randomized trial, during which time several studies confirming warfarin's efficacy and safety were published. The dissemination of these results into clinical practice may explain the increase in positive perceptions of warfarin therapy, as later patients may have felt more certain that taking warfarin protected their health because their physicians and nurses were more certain of warfarin's effects. The higher prevalence of negative perceptions of warfarin in the case-control study may be explained by the fact that the respondents in the first study were participants in a randomized trial, and therefore may not be representative of general patient populations.

The third published study of quality of life among chronically anticoagulated patients was conducted in Europe and was a cross-sectional survey of patients in two anticoagulation clinics.[20] The indications for long-term anticoagulation among this population were diverse and included atrial fibrillation, mechanical heart valves, recurrent deep venous thrombosis, and antiphospholipid antibody syndrome. Most respondents to this survey (89%) reported that warfarin therapy added little or no limitation to their everyday life. However, 38% stated that they were worried about bleeding during therapy, and 21% reported restrictions in their leisure activity due to warfarin. These negative perceptions of warfarin's impact on quality of life are consistent with the results of the U.S. case-control study shown in Table 40–1. Difficulty getting to the clinic was also a source of concern for many of the patients (47%) in this study. Positive perceptions of warfarin were less common than in the U.S. study, with 52% of respondents reporting that warfarin therapy improved their health. When respondents were stratified by age, gender, and education level, there were notable differences in beliefs regarding warfarin therapy. Older respondents (above age 65) found it less difficult to maintain a stable level of anticoagulation, which may reflect a higher level of compliance in this age group.[19]

CLINICAL DECISION ANALYSIS

In addition to multi-item scales, another common method of evaluating quality of life is formal utility assessment, a component of clinical decision analysis. In a decision analysis, all available choices and the potential outcomes of each are explicitly identified, and a model of the decision is constructed in the form of a decision tree. Branches of the tree represent the possible therapeutic options and the potential outcomes of each available option. Each outcome has a specified likelihood, derived from the clinical literature, and

a relative value. The relative value of the outcome is generally described numerically on a scale ranging from 0.0 to 1.0, where perfect health is assigned the value of 1.0 and death is assigned a value of 0.0. Utility assessment differs from health status surveys by allowing each subject to express his or her values for common health states on a 0 to 1 scale.

Various techniques are used to generate these health state values, or "utilities."[21,22] Formally, the most valid utilities are derived from patient experience using two available methods: the standard gamble and the time trade-off. In the standard gamble, or lottery technique, the patient is presented with a series of scenarios and asked to choose between successive pairs of alternatives until the patient is indifferent between the alternatives offered. For example, a patient with atrial fibrillation might be asked to choose between living with the disability resulting from a stroke and a gamble between immediate death and a stroke-free state of health. The patient is first given a 10% chance of immediate death and a 90% chance of stroke-free survival. In this scenario, most patients will choose the gamble over the certain stroke. If the probabilities are reversed, such that the chance of immediate death is 90% and the chance of stroke-free survival is 10%, most patients will choose not to take the gamble but rather to live in a post-stroke disabled state. The probabilities are varied until the point is reached at which the patient is ambivalent between the disabled post-stroke state and the gamble. If this occurs when the chance of stroke-free survival is 25% and the chance of death is 75%, then the utility of stroke is considered to be 0.25, or the probability of the best outcome at the point of indifference.

The time trade-off is another common technique for estimating health-state utilities. In this technique, the patient is asked to consider two health states that differ in duration. For example, a patient with atrial fibrillation might be asked, "would you rather live for 10 years after a stroke or for 9 years without complications?" In this scenario, most patients will choose to give up one year of life to avoid a stroke. The duration of life without complications is reduced in a series of questions until the point is reached at which the patient is indifferent between longevity, albeit with the disability from a stroke, and a shortened, but stroke-free, life-span. If the patient is willing to accept just 4 years of health in order to avoid 10 years of life after stroke, then the utility of stroke is 0.4. The time trade-off approach may avoid the problem of risk aversion that can arise with the stark choices posed by the standard gamble method.

During the past 15 years, several studies have included estimates of the impact of anticoagulation therapy on quality of life generated by using decision analytic techniques.[23–32] In these studies, utility values were calculated for several health states, including systemic and intracranial hemorrhage, short-term and disabling stroke, and taking warfarin per se. For this review, the estimates of the utility of taking warfarin per se are of primary interest.

Many of the earlier studies utilized physician proxies rather than patient-derived utilities in constructing decision analyses. Utility of taking warfarin in these studies ranged from 0.99 to 1.0, assuming little or no disutility in taking warfarin.[23–27] In several of these studies sensitivity analyses were performed in which the utility of taking warfarin was varied to determine how different values would affect the final decision. The inconvenience of taking warfarin was shown to be an extremely important variable. In one study,[24] when the utility of taking warfarin was 0.96 rather than 1.0, warfarin and no treatment were equally valued for the treatment of chronic atrial fibrillation. Another study[27] found that this threshold was 0.91–0.93, depending on the patient's age. Interpreting these values as a time trade-off, a utility of 0.96 means that if a patient is willing to give up 4% or more of his or her life to avoid the inconvenience and worry of taking warfarin, then that patient should not take warfarin. The difficulty in interpreting these values lies in the fact that it is entirely unknown how many patients would in fact choose a utility of 1.0 and how many would choose a lower utility.

More recent decision analyses have used patient-generated utilities for taking warfarin.[30–32] In one study, designed to assess the cost-effectiveness of anticoagulation in patients with nonvalvular atrial fibrillation, quality-of-life estimates were obtained from 57 patients using the time trade-off method.[30] Each patient was asked to estimate the utility of daily therapy with warfarin, including blood tests every four weeks and the requirement to avoid contact sports and excessive intake of alcoholic beverages. Patients were also asked to estimate the utilities of daily therapy with aspirin, of mild and moderate-to-severe strokes (either ischemic or hemorrhagic), of recurrent neurological events, and of nonintracranial hemorrhage. The well state was assigned a utility of 1.0 and death was assigned a utility of 0.0.

The mean utilities for each health state are listed in Table 40–2. Patients assigned daily warfarin a mean utility of 0.988, indicating that they would give up no more than 1.2% of their remaining life in order to avoid taking warfarin. In contrast, moderate-to-severe neurologic defect was assigned a utility of 0.39, indicating that patients would be willing to give up 61% of their life to avoid this state. While these utility values are consistent with and lend credibility to the physician-derived estimates in the earlier decision analyses, they are more believable because they are based on patient interviews. The estimate of 0.988 for warfarin's utility suggests that the vast majority of patients are willing to accept the inconveniences of warfarin therapy in order to avoid future adverse outcomes. There is, however, a subgroup of patients who consider the necessary lifestyle changes too burdensome and would not opt for warfarin therapy. Moreover, patients may not act according to the rational standards of decision analysis. They might assign taking warfarin a near-perfect utility value, yet quit taking it because of inconvenience.

Table 40–2 Quality of Life Utility Estimates for Atrial Fibrillation Patients

Therapy	No therapy	1.0
	Aspirin	0.998
	Warfarin	0.988
Neurologic event (ischemic or hemorrhagic with residual)	Mild	0.75
	Moderate-to-severe	0.39
	Recurrent	0.12
Other states	Non-intracranial hemorrhage	0.76
	Death	0.0

Source: Adapted from Gage BF, Cardinalli AB, Albers GW, Owens DK. Cost-effectiveness of warfarin and aspirin for prophylaxis of stroke in patients with nonvalvular atrial fibrillation. *Journal of the American Medical Association* 274 (1995):1839–1845.

The patient-derived utilities in Table 40–2 were corroborated by a second decision analysis, in which subjects with atrial fibrillation were interviewed using a computer-based utility assessment program.[31] The median utility assigned to taking warfarin was 0.997 and did not differ significantly between subjects who were and were not taking warfarin. However, 16% of patients assigned a utility to taking warfarin of less than 0.975, indicating that they were willing to give up 2.5% of their life to avoid the inconvenience of this therapy. A wide variation in patient utilities for stroke was observed among the 70 patients interviewed for this study. The median utility assigned for mild stroke was 0.94, for moderate stroke was 0.07, and for major stroke was 0.0. For some patients, quality of life with a moderate or major stroke was considered worse than death.

Another recent decision analysis assessed utilities for taking warfarin among 97 elderly participants (ages 70–85) with chronic atrial fibrillation using the time trade-off method.[32] This analysis was unique in that each participant's risk for both thromboembolic events and adverse effects from warfarin, based on age and co-morbidity, was used to create an individual decision tree. Participants were then able to incorporate this information when defining their utility for treatment with warfarin. In this study, only 61% of participants preferred anticoagulation with warfarin to no treatment, which is considerably fewer than the proportion who would be recommended for treatment according to current consensus guidelines. Of 38 participants in this study whose decision tree indicated that they would prefer no warfarin, 45% had been prescribed warfarin. Conversely, of 28 patients who indicated that they would prefer warfarin, 47% had not been prescribed this therapy. This study highlights the importance of incorporating patient preferences in deciding whether to prescribe warfarin, as it has a variable impact on individual quality of life.[32]

CONCLUSIONS

Despite proven efficacy in the prevention of cerebrovascular and cardiovascular morbidity and mortality, warfarin therapy may lead to lifestyle changes and side effects that significantly impair quality of life. For a few patients, the inconveniences and anxieties that chronic anticoagulation impose are substantial and may outweigh its benefits. However, the vast majority of patients taking anticoagulants report little impairment of quality of life or are willing to tolerate the burdens of anticoagulation in order to avoid future adverse outcomes.

Devices allowing self-testing of prothrombin times represents a new technical advance that may improve patients' quality of life on anticoagulants. Patients using home prothrombin time monitors in controlled trials have reported high levels of satisfaction and have almost universally wanted to continue to use the devices after the studies ended.[33–36] In a randomized trial comparing self-management with home prothrombin monitoring to usual care, treatment-related quality-of-life measures were significantly higher in the intervention group than in the control group. These measures included general treatment satisfaction, daily hassles, self-efficacy, and distress.[36] Patients using home monitors have also reported a greater sense of control and involvement in the management of their illness and have found the monitors more convenient and less painful than frequent laboratory tests.[34]

The most important practical impact of anticoagulation's effect on quality of life is on patient adherence. Adherence to both medication dosing and blood test monitoring is necessary to safely realize the benefits of anticoagulation. In order to maximize patient adherence, the impact of anticoagulation therapy on quality of life must be fully understood, and interventions must be tailored to reduce this impact. The research reviewed in this chapter provides a foundation for understanding the impact of warfarin therapy on quality of life, but it is limited by its cross-sectional nature. Further prospective studies are needed to provide a richer sense of anticoagulation's effect on quality of life and to suggest interventions to improve this important outcome of anticoagulation.

REFERENCES

1. The Boston Area Anticoagulation Trial for Atrial Fibrillation Investigators. The effect of low-dose warfarin on the risk of stroke in patients with nonrheumatic atrial fibrillation. *N Engl J Med.* 1990;323: 1505–1511.

2. Petersen P, Godtfredsen J, Boysen G, Andersen ED, Andersen B. Placebo-controlled, randomised trial of warfarin and aspirin for prevention of thromboembolic complications in chronic atrial fibrillation: the Copenhagen AFASAK study. *Lancet.* 1989;1:175–179.

3. Stroke Prevention in Atrial Fibrillation Investigators. Stroke prevention in atrial fibrillation study: final results. *Circulation.* 1991;84:527–539.

4. Connolly SJ, Laupacis A, Gent M, Roberts RS, Cairns JA, Joyner C. Canadian atrial fibrillation anticoagulation (CAFA) study. *J Am Coll Cardiol.* 1991;18:349–355.

5. Ezekowitz MD, Bridgers SL, James KE, et al. Warfarin in the prevention of stroke associated with nonrheumatic atrial fibrillation. *N Engl J Med.* 1992;327:1406–1412.

6. EAFT (European Atrial Fibrillation Trial) Study Group. Secondary prevention in nonrheumatic atrial fibrillation after transient ischaemic attack or minor stroke. *Lancet.* 1993;342:1256–1262.

7. Smith P, Arnesen H, Holme I. The effect of warfarin on mortality and reinfarction after myocardial infarction. *N Engl J Med.* 1990;323:147–152.

8. Anticoagulants in the Secondary Prevention of Events in Coronary Thrombosis (ASPECT) Research Group. Effect of long-term anticoagulant treatment on mortality and cardiovascular morbidity after myocardial infarction. *Lancet.* 1994;343:499–503.

9. Turpie AG, Gunstensen J, Hirsh J, Nelson H, Gent M. Randomized comparison of two intensities of oral anticoagulant therapy after tissue heart valve replacement. *Lancet.* 1988;1:1242–1245.

10. Saour JN, Sieck JO, Mamo LA, Gallus AS. Trial of different intensities of anticoagulation in patients with prosthetic heart valves. *N Engl J Med.* 1990;322:428–432.

11. Kutner M, Nixon G, Silverstone F. Physicians' attitudes toward oral anticoagulants and antiplatelet agents for stroke prevention in elderly patients with atrial fibrillation. *Arch Intern Med.* 1991;51:1950–1953.

12. Chang HJ, Bell JR, Deroo DB, Kirk JW, Wasson JH, Dartmouth Primary Care Coop Project. Physician variation in anticoagulating patients with atrial fibrillation. *Arch Intern Med.* 1980;150:81–84.

13. McCrory DC, Matchar DB, Samsa G, Sanders LL, Pritchett EL. Physician attitudes about anticoagulation for nonvalvular atrial fibrillation in the elderly. *Arch Intern Med.* 1995;155:277–281.

14. Stewart AL, Ware JE, eds. *Measuring Functioning and Well-Being: The Medical Outcomes Study Approach.* Durham, NC: Duke University Press; 1992.

15. Stewart AL. Psychometric considerations in functional status instruments. In: *Functional Status Measurement in Primary Care*, WONCA Classification Committee. New York, NY: Springer-Verlag; 1990:3–26.

16. Testa MA, Simonson DC. Current concepts: assessment of quality-of-life outcomes. *N Engl J Med.* 1996;334:835–840.

17. Wilkin D, Hallam L, Doggett M. *Measures of Need and Outcome for Primary Care.* New York, NY: Oxford University Press; 1992.

18. Lancaster TR, Singer DE, Sheehan MA, et al. The impact of long-term warfarin therapy on quality of life: evidence from a randomized trial. *Arch Intern Med.* 1991;151:1944–1949.

19. Arnsten JH, Gelfand JM, Singer DE. Determinants of compliance with anticoagulation: a case-control study. *Am J Med.* 1997;103:11–17.

20. Barcellona D, Contu P, Sorano G, et al. The management of oral anticoagulant therapy: the patient's point of view. *Thromb Haemost.* 2000;83:49–53.

21. Weinstein MC, Fineburg HV. *Clinical Decision Analysis*. Philadelphia, PA: WB Saunders; 1980.

22. Pauker SG, Kassirer JP. Decision analysis. *N Engl J Med*. 1987;116:250–258.

23. Caro JJ, Groome PA, Flegel KM. Atrial fibrillation and anticoagulation: from randomised trials to practice. *Lancet*. 1993;341:1381–1384.

24. Disch DL, Greenberg ML, Holzberger PT, Malenka DJ. Managing chronic atrial fibrillation: a Markov decision analysis comparing warfarin, quinidine, and low dose amiodarone. *Ann Intern Med*. 1994;120:449–457.

25. Flegel KM, Hutchinson TA, Groome PA, Tousignant P. Factors relevant to preventing embolic stroke in patients with non-rheumatic atrial fibrillation. *J Clin Epidemiol*. 1991;44:551–560.

26. Gustafsson C, Asplund K, Britton M, Norrving B, Olsson B, Marke L. Cost effectiveness of primary stroke prevention in atrial fibrillation: Swedish national perspective. *BMJ*. 1992;305:1457–1460.

27. Tsevat J, Eckman MH, McNutt RA, Pauker SG. Warfarin for dilated cardiomyopathy: a bloody tough pill to swallow? *Med Decis Making*. 1989;9:162–169.

28. Naglie IG, Detsky AS. Treatment of chronic nonvalvular atrial fibrillation in the elderly. *Med Decis Making*. 1992;12:239–249.

29. Beck JR, Pauker SG. Anticoagulation and atrial fibrillation in the brady-cardia-tachycardia syndrome. *Med Decis Making*. 1981;1285–301.

30. Gage BF, Cardinalli AB, Albers GW, Owens DK. Cost-effectiveness of warfarin and aspirin for prophylaxis of stroke in patients with nonvalvular atrial fibrillation. *JAMA*. 1995;274:1839–1845.

31. Gage B, Cardinalli A, Owens D. The effect of stroke and stroke prophylaxis with aspirin or warfarin on quality of life. *Arch Int Med*. 1996;156:1829–1836.

32. Protheroe J, Fahey T, Montgomery A. Effects of patients' preferences on the treatment of atrial fibrillation: observational study of patient-based decision analysis. *West Jour Med*. 2001;174:311–315.

33. White RH, McCurdy SA, von Marensdorff H, Woodruff DE, Leftgoff L. Home prothrombin time monitoring after the initiation of warfarin therapy. *Ann Int Med*. 1989;111:730–737.

34. Ansell JE, Patel N, Ostrovsky D, Nozzolillo E, Peterson AM, Fish L. Long-term patient self-management of oral anticoagulation. *Arch Int Med*. 1995;155:2185–2189.

35. Anderson DR, Harrison L, Hirsh J. Evaluation of a portable prothrombin time monitor for home use by patients who require long-term oral anticoagulant therapy. *Arch Int Med*. 1993;153:1441–1447.

36. Sawicki P. A structured teaching and self-management program for patients receiving oral anticoagulation. *JAMA*. 1999;281:145–150.

Chapter 41

Frequency of Testing and Therapeutic Effectiveness

David B. Matchar and Gregory P. Samsa

INTRODUCTION

Anticoagulation with warfarin has been shown to reduce the risk of thromboembolism in a variety of applications. Anticoagulation is effective for prophylaxis of venous thrombosis in high-risk surgery; treatment of venous thrombosis and pulmonary embolism; and prevention of systemic embolism in patients with acute myocardial infarction, valvular heart disease, atrial fibrillation, and both tissue and mechanical heart valves. Recent research[1] also suggests a potentially major role in secondary prevention of myocardial infarction.

While anticoagulation decreases the risk of thromboembolism, it engenders other significant risks, particularly the risk of major bleeding. Thus, the objective of high-quality anticoagulation care is to minimize the risk of both thromboembolism and bleeding. How can this be done? Abundant evidence suggests that AC provided by a knowledgeable provider in an organized system of follow-up with reliable prothrombin time (PT) monitoring and good patient communication and education will achieve the best results. Within this context of care, an important question is how frequently the International Normalized Ratio (INR) should be monitored. This question is particularly relevant, as very frequent testing (ie, once a week or more often) would require new strategies such as patient self-testing (PST) or patient self-management (PSM). The following text describes the strength of evidence pertaining to the relationship between frequency of testing and patient outcomes, focusing on very frequent testing.

EVENT RATES VERSUS TIME IN TARGET RANGE: A SURROGATE MEASURE OF QUALITY

If the objective of high-quality anticoagulation care is to minimize the risk of thromboembolism and bleeding, then the obvious measure of anticoagulation quality is clinical event rates per person-year of follow-up. For statistical reasons, however, it is difficult to evaluate quality based on this measure. For example, to demonstrate statistically that a new anticoagulation strategy reduces bleeding risk by 40% (ie, from 5% to 3%) would require a randomized trial with over 3,000 patient-years of follow-up. Because this approach is not practical to answer each question about each detail of anticoagulation care, it is important to select a satisfactory alternative or surrogate measure. The widely accepted alternative is time in therapeutic range (TTR).

A strong relationship between TTR and bleeding or thrombosis rates has been observed in a number of studies with different patient populations, different target ranges, and different scales for measuring intensity of anticoagulation (ie, PT, PT ratio, and INR).[2–12] In a large, representative study by Cannegieter et al,[2] the relationship between TTR and major bleeds was approximately exponential (ie, small departures from the target range were associated with small to moderate increases in bleeding rates, while large departures from the target range were associated with large increases in bleeding rates). A similar relationship holds for TTR and thromboembolism rates; when bleeding and thromboembolism are considered simultaneously, the overall relationship is U-shaped (Figure 41–1).

Data from clinical trials on success in achieving TTR are difficult to compare across studies because different methods are used to measure TTR. The most common method expresses the proportion of INR values within therapeutic range as the number of INRs within range divided by the number of PT tests. This method is likely to underestimate the TTR because the result is affected by the tendency of physicians to perform repeated tests soon after obtaining an out-of-range INR (ie, to verify the initial INR or assess the effect of a dosage adjustment).

Another approach is the "cross section of the files" method, where a given date is selected and the proportion of INRs within therapeutic range using the most recent INR value is calculated for each patient. The cross section of the files method is inefficient in that it fails to utilize test results between the assessment dates.

Two other methods try to overcome these problems and assess actual days spent in or out of range. The equidivision method[12] assumes that the change between two consecutive INR measurements occurs halfway between the two tests. It has been shown to be reproducible, but not valid.[13] The second, the linear interpolation method of Rosendaal et al,[14] is based on calculating the actual time in target range by first linearly interpolating between observed test values and then defining the TTR as the number of patient-days of follow-up that were within target range divided by the total number of patient-days included in the follow-up period.

The results of all these methods depend on the choice of target INR range; therefore, results are more favorable if the target range is expanded, even in the absence of any actual improvements in quality of anticoagulation management. Another deficiency is that the various methods of assessment treat small departures from target range as identical to large departures, even though the former would have much less impact on clinical outcomes than the latter. These differences must be taken into account when comparing results across multiple studies. The data in Table 41–1 indicate the various methodologies used for determining TTR and arrange results based on the model of anticoagulation management.

There is further difficulty in comparing results across trials because of the different models of anticoagulation management employed in trials. Thus, the knowledge of the provider will vary, as will the system of follow-up, the quality of PT monitoring, and the quality of patient communication and education. Correlating the model of care with adverse event rates (but not with TTR) is also complicated by the fact that the older literature based results on a PT ratio, whereas therapy based on an INR with low- and high-intensity levels of treatment is of relatively recent onset. Nevertheless, where data are available (Table 41–1), results indicate a wide range of success in achieving TTR. A usual care model appears to yield the worst results with a TTR between 33% and 64%. Even in randomized controlled trials where patient care is often highly structured, TTR varies between 48% and 83%. Achieved TTR appears to be best in either an anticoagulation

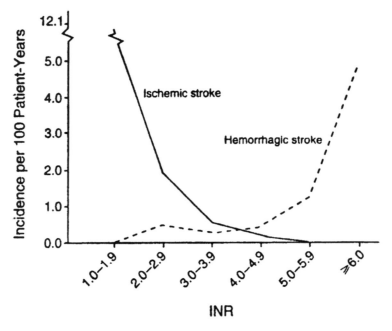

Figure 41–1 U-Shaped curve indicating incidence of ischemic and hemorrhagic stroke according to International Normalized Ratio category. Source: Reprinted with permission from Cannegieter et al, Optimal Oral Anticoagulant Therapy in Patients with Mechanical Heart Valves, *The New England Journal of Medicine*, Vol 333, pp 11–17, Copyright © 1995, Massachusetts Medical Society. All rights reserved.

Table 41-1 Time in Therapeutic Range (A Surrogate Measure for Quality) Achieved under Different Models of Anticoagulation Management and with Different Testing Frequencies

Study	Predominant Model of Management	PTR v INR	% TTR*	% Above Range	% Below Range	Frequency of Monitoring	Method of Determining TTR‡	Major Diagnosis
Garabedian-Ruffalo et al, 1985[18]	UC	PTR	64	—	—		% in range	Mixed
Gottlieb/Salem-Schatz, 1994[19]	UC	PTR	50	30	20	every 25 days†	Days in range	Mixed
Holm et al, 1999[20]	UC	INR	63	8	29	—	% in range	Mixed
Beyth/Landefeld, 1997[21]	UC	INR	33	16	51	—	—	Mixed
Horstkotte et al, 1996[17]	UC	INR	59	16	50	19 days†	% in range	Valves
Sawicki, 1999[22]	UC	INR	34	16	50	—	% in range	AF/Valves
Palareti et al, 1996[23]	AMS	INR	68	6	26	15 days†	Days in range	Mixed
Cannegieter et al, 1995[2]	AMS	INR	61	8	31	18.9 days†	Days in range	Valves
Lundstrom et al, 1989[24]	AMS	TT	92	—	—	—	% in range	AF
Garabedian-Ruffalo et al, 1985[18]	AMS	PTR	86	—	—	—	% in range	Mixed
White et al, 1989[25]	AMS	PTR	75	—	—	—	Days in range	Mixed
Ansell et al, 1995[26]	AMS	PTR	68	10	22	16 days†	% in range	Mixed
Conte et al, 1986[27]	AMS	PTR	59	12	29	—	—	Mixed
Seabrook et al, 1990[28]	AMS	PTR	66	7	7	Once monthly	% in range	Mixed
White et al, 1989[25]	PST	PTR	93	—	—	—	Days in range	Mixed
Beyth/Landefeld, 1997[21]	PST	INR	56	14	30	—	—	Mixed
Ansell et al, 1995[26]	PSM	PTR	89	5	6	13.8 days†	% in range	Mixed
Horstkotte et al, 1996[17]	PSM	INR	92	—	—	4 days†	% in range	Valves
Sawicki, 1999[22]	PSM	INR	57	10	33	—	% in range	AF/Valves
AFASAK, 1989[11]	RCT	INR	73	0.6	26	—	—	AF
BAATAF, 1990[9]	RCT	PTR	83	9	8	Every 3 weeks	Days in range	AF
SPAF I, 1991[29]	RCT	PTR	71	5	23	At least once per month	% in range	AF
SPAF II, 1994[30]	RCT	PTR/INR	74	5	21	At least once per month	% in range	AF
SPAF III, 1996[31]	RCT	INR	61	14	25	At least once per month	% in range	AF
SPINAF, 1992[8]	RCT	PTR	56	15	29	Monthly	% in range	AF
CAFA, 1991[10]	RCT	INR	44	16	40	Every 3 weeks	Days in range	AF
AFASAK 2, 1999[32]	RCT	INR	73	9	18	Not more than every 4 weeks	Days in range	AF
EAFT, 1995[3]	RCT	INR	59	9	32	Every 5 weeks	% in range	AF
Hellemons et al, 1999[33]	RCT	INR	48	24	28	Every 2–6 weeks	% in range	AF
Hutten et al, 1999[13]	RCT	INR	61	—	—	—	Days in range	DVT/PE

AF = atrial fibrillation; AMS = anticoagulation management service; INR = International Normalized Ratio; Mixed = mixed indications for anticoagulation; PSM = patient self-management; PST = patient self-testing; PTR = prothrombin time ratio; RCT = randomized controlled trial; TT = thrombotest; TTR = time in therapeutic range; UC = usual care; valves = cardiac prosthetic valve.

*Time in range represents mean or median percent of prothrombin times or days in range.

†Those studies that documented the achieved frequency of monitoring as opposed to the stated goal for monitoring interval.

‡% in range = the proportion of PT tests in range divided by the total number of tests; days in range = the estimated days or time in range as determined by various methodologies.

management service model or with PST/PSM (approximately 60% to 90%).

STRENGTH OF THE RELATIONSHIP BETWEEN FREQUENCY OF TESTING AND OUTCOMES

Some investigators have attempted to develop predictive models with the goal of reducing the frequency of testing without sacrificing quality.[15] A few recent clinical trials, however, suggest that TTR, and presumably fewer adverse events, can be maximized by more frequent testing.[16,17] This is particularly true in studies utilizing PST where access to testing is virtually unlimited.

In order to focus on frequency of testing alone, Horstkotte et al[16] performed a repeated measures experiment on 200 patients following placement of a mechanical heart valve. In chronological order, patients were followed by their private physician using their usual testing intervals (usual care), or by their private physician with a planned testing interval of 2 weeks. Other patients performed their own PT test and managed their own therapy (PSM) with a planned testing interval of 8 days, 4 days, and 2 days. Actual mean intervals were 24, 17, 7, 4, and 2 days, respectively, and the percentages of INR measurements within target range were 48%, 64%, 76%, 89%, and 90%, respectively. Comparing usual care with a 24-day interval with usual care with a 17-day interval (ie, 48% versus 64% TTR) illustrates the benefit of more frequent testing within the context of usual care. Comparing PSM with an 8-day interval with PSM and a 4-day interval (ie, 76% versus 89% TTR) illustrates the benefit of more frequent testing within the context of PSM. The lack of a difference in TTR between 4- and 2-day intervals (ie, 89% versus 90%) illustrates that a threshold exists beyond which more frequent testing is not beneficial. The comparison between usual care and PSM reflects the effects of not only test frequency but also patient knowledge, empowerment, compliance, and other potential factors that can influence TTR. Although not definitive (ie, all patients proceeded from long to short time intervals, and the generalizability of the patient population is uncertain), Horstkotte et al's experiment provides perhaps the most direct evidence available in support of the benefits of increased frequency of testing.

CONCLUSIONS

While these studies supporting a relationship between frequency of testing and TTR are neither definitive nor entirely generalizable, they do consistently support the hypothesis that frequency of testing improves outcomes. This information can serve to provide part of the rationale for identifying practical, efficient strategies for increasing INR test frequency and for performing randomized controlled trials to determine the effectiveness of these strategies in real-world settings.

REFERENCES

1. Hirsh J, Dalen JE, Anderson D, et al. Oral anticoagulants: mechanism of action, clinical effectiveness, and optimal therapeutic range. *Chest.* 1998;114:445S–469S.

2. Cannegieter SC, Rosendaal FR, Wintzen AR, van der Meer FJM, Vandenbroucke JP. The optimal intensity of oral anticoagulant therapy in patients with mechanical heart valve prostheses: the Leiden artificial valve and anticoagulation study. *N Engl J Med.* 1995;333:11–17.

3. European Atrial Fibrillation Trial Study Group. Optimal oral anticoagulant therapy in patients with nonrheumatic atrial fibrillation and recent cerebral ischemia. *N Engl J Med.* 1995;333:5–10.

4. van der Meer FJM, Rosendaal FR, vandenbroucke JP, Briet E. Bleeding complications in oral anticoagulant therapy: an analysis of risk factors. *Arch Intern Med.* 1993;153:1557–1562.

5. Forfar JC. Prediction of hemorrhage during long-term oral coumadin anticoagulation by excessive prothrombin ratio. *Am Heart J.* 1982;103:445–446.

6. Charney R, Leddomado E, Rose DN, Fuster V. Anticoagulation clinics and the monitoring of anticoagulant therapy. *Int J Cardiol.* 1988;18:197–206.

7. Wilson DB, Dunn MI, Hassanein K. Low intensity anticoagulation in mechanical cardiac prosthetic valves. *Chest.* 1991;100:1553–1557.

8. Ezekowitz MD, Bridgers SL, James KE, et al. Warfarin in the prevention of stroke associated with nonrheumatic atrial fibrillation. *N Engl J Med.* 1992;327:1406–1412.

9. Boston Area Anticoagulation Trial for Atrial Fibrillation Investigators. The effect of low dose warfarin on the risk of stroke in patients with nonrheumatic atrial fibrillation. *N Engl J Med.* 1990;323:1505–1511.

10. Connolly SJ, Laupacis A, Gent M, et al. Canadian atrial fibrillation anticoagulation (CAFA) study. *J Am Coll Cardiol.* 1991;18:349–355.

11. Petersen P, Boysan G, Godtfredsen J, et al. Placebo-controlled, randomized trial of warfarin and aspirin for prevention of thromboembolic complications in chronic atrial fibrillation: the Copenhagen AFASAK Study. *Lancet.* 1989;1:175–179.

12. Duxbury BmcD. Therapeutic control of anticoagulant treatment. *Br Med J.* 1982;284:702–704.

13. Hutten BA, Prins MH, Redekop WK, Tljssen JGP, Heisterkamp SH, Buller HR. Comparison of three methods to assess therapeutic quality control of treatment with vitamin K antagonists. *Thromb Haemost.* 1999;82:1260–1263.

14. Rosendaal FR, Cannegieter SC, van der Meer FJM, Briet E. A method to determine the optimal intensity of oral anticoagulant therapy. *Thromb Haemost.* 1993;39:236–239.

15. Kent DL, Domokos V, McDonell M, Henikoff J, Fihn SD. A model for planning optimal follow-up for outpatients on warfarin anticoagulation. *Med Decis Making.* 1992;12:132–141.

16. Horstkotte D, Piper C, Wiemer M. Optimal frequency of patient monitoring and intensity of oral anticoagulation therapy in valvular heart disease. *J Thromb Thrombolysis.* 1998;5:S19–S24.

17. Horstkotte D, Piper C, Wiemer M, et al. Improvement of prognosis by home prothrombin estimation in patients with life-long anticoagulant therapy. *Eur Heart J.* 1996;17(suppl):230. Abstract.

18. Garabedian-Ruffalo SM, Gray DR, Sax MJ, et al. Retrospective evaluation of a pharmacist-managed warfarin anticoagulation clinic. *Am J Hosp Pharm.* 1985;42:304–308.

19. Gottlieb LK, Salem-Schatz S. Anticoagulation in atrial fibrillation: does efficacy in clinical trials translate into effectiveness in practice? *Arch Intern Med.* 1994;154:1945–1953.

20. Holm T, Lassen JF, Husted SE, Heickendorff L. Identification and surveillance of patient on oral anticoagulant therapy in a large geographic area—use of laboratory information systems. *Thromb Haemost.* 1999;82(suppl):858–859.

21. Beyth RJ, Landefeld CS. Prevention of major bleeding in older patients treated with warfarin: results of a randomized trial. *J Gen Intern Med.* 1997;12:66. Abstract.

22. Sawicki PT, Working Group for the Study of Patient Self-Management of Oral Anticoagulation. A structured teaching and self-management program for patients receiving oral anticoagulation. A randomized controlled trial. *JAMA.* 1999;281:145–150.

23. Palareti G, Leali N, Coccheri S, et al. Bleeding complications of oral anticoagulant treatment: an inception-cohort, prospective collaborative study (ISCOAT). *Lancet.* 1996;348:423–428.

24. Lundstrom T, Ryden L. Haemorrhagic and thromboembolic complications in patients with atrial fibrillation on anticoagulant prophylaxis. *J Intern Med.* 1989;225:137–142.

25. White RH, McCurdy A, Marensdorff H, et al. Home prothrombin time monitoring after the initiation of warfarin therapy: a randomized, prospective study. *Ann Intern Med.* 1989;111:730–737.

26. Ansell J, Patel N, Ostrovsky D, et al. Long-term patient self-management of oral anticoagulation. *Arch Intern Med.* 1995;155:2185–2189.

27. Conte RR, Kehoe WA, Nielson N, Lodhia H. Nine-year experience with a pharmacist-managed anticoagulation clinic. *Am J Hosp Pharm.* 1986;43:2460–2464.

28. Seabrook GR, Karp D, Schmitt DD, Bandyk DF. An outpatient anticoagulation protocol managed by a vascular nurse-clinician. *Am J Surg.* 1990;160:501–504.

29. Stroke Prevention in Atrial Fibrillation Investigators. Stroke prevention in atrial fibrillation study: final results. *Circulation.* 1991;84:527–539.

30. Stroke Prevention in Atrial Fibrillation Investigators. Warfarin versus aspirin for prevention of thromboembolism in atrial fibrillation: stroke prevention in atrial fibrillation II study. *Lancet.* 1994;343:687–691.

31. Stroke Prevention in Atrial Fibrillation Investigators. Adjusted-dose warfarin versus low-intensity, fixed-dose warfarin plus aspirin for high-risk patients with atrial fibrillation: stroke prevention in atrial fibrillation III randomized clinical trial. *Lancet.* 1996;348:633–638.

32. Gullov AL, Koefoed BG, Petersen P. Bleeding during warfarin and aspirin therapy in patients treated with atrial fibrillation. The AFASAK 2 study. *Arch Intern Med.* 1999;159:1322–1328.

33. Hellemons BSP, Langenberg M, Lodder J, et al. Primary prevention of arterial thromboembolism in non-rheumatic atrial fibrillation in primary care: randomized controlled trial comparing two intensities of Coumadin with aspirin. *Br Med J.* 1999;319:958–964.

Chapter 42

Duration of Anticoagulation Therapy in Venous Thromboembolic Disease

David R. Anderson

Few issues in the management of patients with deep vein thrombosis and pulmonary embolism (venous thromboembolism) remain as contentious as the optimal duration of oral anticoagulant therapy. An extensive number of clinical trials in the past decade have refined the initial treatment of venous thromboembolism very clearly. A parenteral heparin agent, administered for a minimum of five days, followed by oral anticoagulation with a vitamin K antagonist whose dose is adjusted to maintain the International Normalized Ratio between 2.0 and 3.0 for a minimum three-month period is very effective therapy for acute venous thromboembolism.[1] Only about 4% to 8% of patients treated with this regimen will develop recurrent venous thromboembolism in the initial three months following diagnosis.[1]

The combination of a heparin preparation followed by oral anticoagulation is an effective "one-two punch" for the treatment of acute venous thromboembolism. Heparin, the more potent of the two anticoagulants, dampens the prothrombotic potency of the acute thrombosis. Then oral anticoagulants serve primarily to prevent the secondary recurrence of the thrombotic process. The decision to initiate anticoagulation to treat acute deep vein thrombosis or pulmonary embolism is usually straightforward. The more difficult management decision is determining when a sufficient amount of oral anticoagulant therapy has been administered and the treatment may be safely discontinued. This chapter reviews the available data from clinical trials that can be used in judging the appropriate duration of oral anticoagulant therapy

for acute venous thromboembolism. However, for individual patients, there are no absolute answers. Physicians, other health care providers, and patients must keep the following points in mind when considering the decision regarding the optimal duration of oral anticoagulant therapy:

- Oral anticoagulants are very effective therapy for the secondary prevention of venous thromboembolism. It is very unusual for patients to develop recurrent venous thromboembolism while receiving oral anticoagulants, particularly after they have received therapy for three months.[1,2]
- There is an ongoing risk of major hemorrhage while patients are receiving oral anticoagulants, which increases with patient age.[3,4]
- Oral anticoagulants are inconvenient to use for patients and physicians and there is a cost associated with their administration. For women of child-bearing age there is also a risk of fetal malformation during pregnancy with oral anticoagulant use.[5]

In any individual patient, careful consideration of the benefits of continuing oral anticoagulant therapy must be carefully weighed against its risks, cost, and inconvenience. Patient preferences should play an important role in management decisions regarding the long-term use of oral anticoagulants, particularly when there is clinical equipoise in considering the need for continuing the medication.

RISK OF RECURRENT VENOUS THROMBOEMBOLISM

Until recently, the standard therapy for all patients developing an acute episode of venous thromboembolism was heparin followed by three to six months of oral anticoagulation, and the rate of recurrent venous thromboembolism following this treatment course was perceived to be low. However, over the past decade patients with acute venous thromboembolism who were treated with oral anticoagulants for a 3- to 6-month period were followed by several long-term prospective studies for 5 to 8 years after the completion of anticoagulation.[6,7] The rates of recurrent venous thromboembolism over this time period were found to be surprisingly high and varied from 20% to 30% (Table 42–1). The rate of recurrence was greatest in the first 6 to 12 months following the discontinuation of anticoagulant therapy, and this risk declined somewhat over time.[6,7]

These long-term cohort studies have identified clinical risk factors that increase a patient's likelihood of recurrent venous thromboembolism.[6–8] Patients with proximal deep vein thrombosis, cancer, and previous venous thromboembolism are at significantly increased risks of recurrent venous thromboembolism (Table 42–1). On the other hand, episodes of venous thromboembolism that occur in association with a recent surgical procedure carry a significantly lower risk of recurrence (Table 42–1).

RANDOMIZED TRIALS OF OPTIMAL DURATION OF ORAL ANTICOAGULATION

In the 1990s three randomized controlled trials compared short (4 to 6 weeks) with longer (3 to 6 months) courses of oral anticoagulation following parenteral heparin for the treatment of acute venous thromboembolism.[9–11] Each of these studies demonstrated a statistically significant benefit for the longer courses of anticoagulation (Table 42–2). These studies also identified similar risk factors for recurrent venous thromboembolism as those seen in the cohort studies. That is, recurrence rates were lower and the benefit of lower courses of anticoagulation were less apparent in patients who developed deep vein thrombosis following a transient risk factor such as surgery. However, patients with cancer had higher rates of recurrence and did particularly poorly with the shorter courses of anticoagulation.[9–11]

More recently the DOTAVK study compared the use of 3 versus 6 months of oral anticoagulation for the first episode of proximal deep vein thrombosis or pulmonary embolism.[12] The rates of recurrent venous thromboembolism and major bleeding were not different in the two groups. However, the DOTAVK study confirmed the previously described low risk of recurrence in patients with a transient risk factor and the higher risk of recurrence for patients with permanent risk factors.

The findings of these clinical trials have demonstrated that acute venous thromboembolism is a heterogenous disease and its natural history varies depending upon the risk factors that resulted in the development of the disorder in the first place. This has implications regarding the optimal duration of oral anticoagulant therapy. Although surgery is a very common risk factor for venous thromboembolism and extensive and even fatal thromboembolic events may occur postoperatively, once patients have been treated successfully with parenteral heparin and 3 months of anticoagulation, the risk of recurrent venous thromboembolism is small even after anticoagulants are discontinued.

On the other hand when patients develop venous thromboembolism in association with a permanent risk factor such as metastatic cancer, the rate of recurrent venous thromboembolism is substantive and ongoing. In this setting clini-

Table 42–1 Risk Factors for Recurrent Venous Thromboembolism

Study	Design	N	Follow-Up	Recurrence Rate	Risk Factors HR (95% CI)
Hasson (2000)[7]	Prospective cohort	738	5 years	21.5%	Proximal DVT 2.4 (1.5–3.9) Cancer 2.0 (1.2–3.2) Previous VTE 1.7 (1.2–2.5) Recent Surgery 0.3 (0.1–0.6)
Prandoni et al (1996)[6]	Prospective cohort	355	8 years	29.1%	Cancer 1.7 (1.3–2.3) Thrombophilia 1.4 (1.0–2.0) Recent Surgery 0.4 (0.2–0.6)

N = number; HR - hazard ratio; CI = confidential interval.

Table 42-2 Optimal Duration of Anticoagulation Studies

	Short Course (%)	Longer Course (%)	P
BTS (1992)[9]			
N	358	354	
Duration	4 weeks	12 weeks	
Recurrent VTE	28 (7.8)	11 (3.1)	0.04
Major bleeding	5 (1.4)	4 (1.1)	NS
Deaths	26 (7.3)	28 (7.9)	NS
Levine et al (1995)[11]			
N	105	109	
Duration	4 weeks	12 weeks	
Recurrent VTE	9 (8.6)	9 (0.9)	<0.01
Major bleeding	0 (0)	1 (0.9)	NS
Deaths	9 (8.6)	9 (8.3)	NS
Schulman et al (1995)[10]			
N	443	454	
Duration	6 weeks	6 months	
Recurrent VTE	90 (20.3)	49 (10.8)	<.001
Major bleeding	1 (0.2)	5 (1.1)	0.23
Deaths	22 (5.0)	17 (3.7)	NS
DOTAVK (2001)[12]			
N	270	269	
Duration	3 months	6 months	
Recurrent VTE	21 (8.1)	23 (8.7)	NS
Major bleeding	5 (1.9)	7 (2.6)	NS
Deaths	NA	NA	

N = number; VTE = venous thromboembolism; NS = not significant.

cians may opt to continue oral anticoagulants indefinitely given the high risk of recurrent venous thromboembolism following the discontinuation of oral anticoagulants.

IDIOPATHIC VENOUS THROMBOEMBOLISM

Patients who develop venous thromboembolism in the absence of an identifiable risk factor are labeled as having idiopathic disease. The risk of recurrent venous thromboembolism in these patients following the discontinuation of oral anticoagulant therapy falls between those of patients having transient (eg, surgery) or permanent (eg, metastatic cancer) risk factors. Determining the optimal duration of oral anticoagulation in patients with idiopathic venous thromboembolism was the subject of two recent clinical trials.[13,14]

In the LAFIT study, Kearon and associates performed a randomized controlled trial that demonstrated 3 months of oral anticoagulation were less effective than 2 years of therapy for the treatment of a first episode of idiopathic venous thromboembolism.[13] Only 1.3% of the patients per year re-ceiving prolonged oral anticoagulants developed recurrent venous thromboembolism compared to 27.4% of patients per year in the 3-month arm (P < 0.001). About 4% of patients in the 2-year oral anticoagulant arm had a major bleeding complication compared to 0% in the 3-month arm (P = 0.08). The LAFIT study was stopped prematurely because an interim analysis demonstrated the substantive benefit of prolonged oral anticoagulation. As a result, this study did not address whether patients who continued oral anticoagulant for 2 years had a lower rate of recurrent venous thromboembolism after discontinuing oral anticoagulants than patients receiving the shorter course of therapy.[13]

This latter point is of particular interest because of the results of the recent WODIT study.[14] This randomized controlled trial compared the rates of recurrent venous thromboembolism in patients with idiopathic deep vein thrombosis or pulmonary embolism who received either 3 months or 12 months of oral anticoagulation. Similar to LAFIT, the WODIT study reported that the rates of recurrent venous thromboembolism were higher in the 3-month than the 12-month arm during the first year of follow-up. However, there was an apparent rebound of venous thromboembolic events in both groups after anticoagulants were discontinued, and over the

2-year follow-up period, overall rates of recurrent venous thromboembolism in the two groups were similar.[14]

Given the results of the LAFIT and WODIT studies, the optimal duration of oral anticoagulant therapy for patients with idiopathic venous thromboembolism remains uncertain. Based on the LAFIT study, 3 months of therapy seem insufficient. However, considering the WODIT results, even with one year of therapy there is a substantive recurrence rate once anticoagulants are discontinued. Until results from additional clinical trials are available, decisions regarding the duration of anticoagulant therapy in this patient group should give strong consideration to an individual patient's risk factors for bleeding and preferences regarding therapy.[3]

HEREDITARY AND ACQUIRED HYPERCOAGULABLE STATES

In recent years a number of hereditary and acquired thrombophilic blood factors have been described that increase an individual's risk for developing venous thromboembolism. There has been much interest in determining whether the presence of a hereditary or acquired thrombophilic anomaly increases the risk of recurrent venous thromboembolism beyond that of individuals experiencing a single episode who lack one of these factors. The only thrombophilic factor consistently associated with an increased risk of recurrent venous thromboembolism is the presence of the lupus anticoagulant or anticardiolipin antibodies.[13,15] Not only are these patients at high risk of recurrent venous thromboembolism, but uncontrolled studies would support that once they experience a thrombembolic event, they should receive higher intensity anticoagulation, maintaining the target INR between 2.5 and 3.5, and remain on therapy indefinitely.[3,15]

The most common hereditary factors associated with an increased risk of venous thromboembolism are heterozygous factor V Leiden (resistance to activated protein C) and the prothrombin gene mutation. Although these are risk factors for a venous thromboembolism, there is not clear evidence that they are associated with an increased risk of recurrent disease compared to other patients with a previous history of venous thromboembolism who lack these anomalies.[13,16-18]

Previous studies have reported the presence of antithrombin or protein C or protein S deficiency carries a small but significant increased risk of recurrent venous thromboembolism.[17] However, a more recent, albeit smaller, study did not confirm this association.[13] It must be considered that the measurements of these intrinsic anticoagulants may vary with time and that the results may be lowered by the presence of oral anticoagulation (protein C and protein S) and heparin (antithrombin). Ideally, abnormal antithrombin, protein C, or protein S assay results should be confirmed on at least one occasion while patients are not receiving the confounding anticoagulant before a patient is labeled as having a deficiency of one of these factors.

The risk of venous thromboembolism for patients who have combined deficiencies of one or more hereditary or acquired thrombophilic abnormalities or who are homozygous for factor V Leidan is increased beyond the simple additive effects of a single defect.[19] Based on uncontrolled studies, it would be recommended that extended duration or indefinite treatment with oral anticoagulants be considered for patients with idiopathic and/or recurrent venous thromboembolism.

SECOND EPISODE OF ANTICOAGULATION

If a patient has a second documented episode of venous thromboembolism, how long should oral anticoagulants be continued? This was the subject of a randomized controlled trial by Schulman and colleagues[20] who compared 6 months of oral anticoagulation with indefinite therapy for such patients. They determined there was a substantive reduction in the risk of recurrent venous thromboembolism by extending anticoagulation indefinitely, 2.6%, versus 20.7% in patients who received the shorter course of oral anticoagulant treatment.[20] Predictably there was a trade-off with increased major bleeding in the extended oral anticoagulant arm compared to the group who received oral anticoagulation for 6 months (8.6% versus 2.7%; P = 0.084). The findings of this study would suggest indefinite anticoagulation be advised in patients with recurrent venous thromboembolism unless there is a major risk for bleeding.

OTHER FACTORS THAT MAY INFLUENCE ANTICOAGULATION DURATION DECISIONS

Presence of Inferior Veno-Caval (IVC) Filter

Patients with acute venous thromboembolism usually have IVC filters inserted either because of an acute contraindication to anticoagulation (eg, massive trauma) or because of failure of anticoagulation (eg, recurrent pulmonary embolism despite therapeutic levels of anticoagulation). The question is whether once the IVC filter is inserted patients require long-term oral anticoagulation to prevent thrombosis of the filter itself.[21] This concern has been reinforced by the results of a randomized controlled trial evaluating the use of IVC filters to reduce the risk of pulmonary embolism in patients with acute proximal deep vein thrombosis. This study demonstrated that despite use of anticoagulation, there was a substantive increased risk of recurrent deep vein thrombosis, including some IVC clots, in patients with filters (20.8%

versus 11.6%; P = 0.02) compared to controls.[22] However, there have been no randomized trials to specifically address the value of oral anticoagulants for preventing the thrombosis of IVC filters. Although uncontrolled studies have not supported the routine need for long-term anticoagulation in patients who have IVC filters, clinicians must be aware of the potential for recurrent thromboembolism, particularly in patients with idiopathic venous thromboembolism or those with cancer.[21]

Post-Phlebitic Syndrome

The major risk factor for the development of the post-phlebitic syndrome is recurrent deep vein thrombosis in the ipsilateral limb.[6] For some patients who have developed chronic swelling and leg discomfort after an initial episode of deep vein thrombosis, consideration may be given to extending the duration of oral anticoagulation to minimize the likelihood of a second episode.

Massive Pulmonary Embolism

Some patients may prevent with massive, life-threatening pulmonary embolism as their initial manifestation of idiopathic venous thromboembolism. In this setting consideration should be given to extending the duration of anticoagulation indefinitely if there are no major contraindications. After a patient has suffered from one life-threatening episode of pulmonary embolism, avoiding a second such episode is highly desirable.

CONSIDERATIONS FOR DISCONTINUING ORAL ANTICOAGULANT THERAPY

Whenever a decision is made to discontinue oral anticoagulant therapy, particularly in the setting of idiopathic venous thromboembolism, patients need to be aware that they become at increased risk of recurrent disease. They should be reminded of the symptoms of deep vein thrombosis and pulmonary embolism and be instructed to present to medical attention should any of these develop. Patients should also be reminded about high-risk settings for recurrent venous thromboembolism (eg, future surgery, pregnancy) and be told of the importance of relaying historical information to physicians involved in their subsequent care.

Patients should be cautioned to avoid settings that might result in prolonged venous stasis. If traveling, they should mobilize their legs on a regular basis. Patients should consider delaying travel for several months after stopping anti-coagulants to minimize the risk of developing recurrent symptoms when away from home.

Finally, physicians should consider repeating diagnostic imaging testing at the time of completion of oral anticoagulant treatment. This is particularly useful for patients with deep vein thrombosis that was diagnosed using venous ultrasound imaging.[23] The extent of deep vein thrombosis usually decreases but does not resolve completely over the course of anticoagulant therapy. Making a diagnosis of recurrent deep vein thrombosis with ultrasonography is problematic because of the difficulty in distinguishing acute from chronic disease. The availability of this baseline scan to be compared with a new study at the time of recurrent symptoms will greatly aid the radiologist in interpreting the ultrasonographic findings.

SUMMARY

Recent clinical trials have helped clarify that venous thromboembolism is a heterogenous disease and the duration of oral anticoagulant therapy requires consideration of the risk factors surrounding the development of each patient's condition. Table 42–3 summarizes some general recommendations and guidelines regarding the optimal duration of anticoagulant therapy for acute venous thromboembolism. Health care professionals need to be aware that considerable controversy still surrounds the issue of optimal oral anticoagulation duration.

Table 42–3 Guidelines for Optimal Duration of Anticoagulant Treatment for Venous Thromboembolism

Risk Factor	Duration of Therapy
First episode	
• Transient reversible factor (eg, surgery)	3 months
• Cancer (metastatic)	Indefinite
• Antiphospholipid antibody syndrome	Indefinite
• Idiopathic, including heterozygous factor V Leiden	Minimum 6 months
• Complex combinations of thrombophilia	Consider indefinite
Recurrent episode	
• Transient reversible factor	3 months
• Other setting	Indefinite

REFERENCES

1. Hyers M, Agnelli G, Hull R, et al. Antithrombotic therapy for venous thromboembolic disease. *Chest*. 1998;114:561S–578S.

2. Douketis JD, Kearon C, Bates S, et al. Risk of fatal pulmonary embolism in patients with treated venous thromboembolism. *JAMA*. 1998;279(6):458–462.

3. Van der Meer FJM, Rosendaal FR, Vandenbroucke JP, et al. Bleeding complications in oral anticoagulant therapy. An analysis of risk factors. *Arch Intern Med*. 1993;153:1557–1562.

4. Levine M, Baskob G, Landefeld S, Kearon C. Hemorrhagic complications of anticoagulation treatment. *Chest*. 1998;114:511S–523S.

5. Ginsberg J, Hirsh J. Use of antithrombotic agents during pregnancy. *Chest*. 1998;114:524S–530S.

6. Prandoni P, Lensing A, Cogo A, et al. The long-term clinical course of acute deep vein thrombosis. *Ann Intern Med*. 1996;125:1–7.

7. Hasson P, Sorbo J, Erikson H. Recurrent venous thromboembolism after deep vein thrombosis. *Arch Intern Med*. 2000;160:769–774.

8. Heit J, Mohr D, Silverstein M, et al. Predictors of recurrence after deep vein thrombosis and pulmonary embolism. *Arch Intern Med*. 2000; 160:761–768.

9. Sudlow M, Campbell I, Angel J, et al. Optimum duration of anticoagulation for deep-vein thrombosis and pulmonary embolism. *Lancet*. 1992;340:873–876.

10. Schulman S, Rhedin A, Lindmarker P, et al. A comparison of six weeks with six months of oral anticoagulant therapy after a first episode of venous thromboembolism. *N Engl J Med*. 1995;332:1661–1665.

11. Levine M, Hirsh J, Gent M, et al. Optimal duration of oral anticoagulation therapy: a randomized trial comparing four weeks with three months of warfarin in patients with proximal deep vein thrombosis. *Thromb Haemost*. 1995;74:606–611.

12. Pinede L, Ninet J, Duhaut P, et al. Comparison of 3 and 6 months of oral anticoagulant therapy after a first episode of proximal deep vein thrombosis or pulmonary embolism and comparison of 6 and 12 weeks of therapy after isolated calf deep vein thrombosis. *Circulation*. 2001;103:2453–2460.

13. Kearon C, Gent M, Hirsh J, et al. A comparison of three months of anticoagulation with extended anticoagulation for a first episode of idiopathic venous thromboembolism. *N Engl J Med*. 1999;340:901–907.

14. Angelli G, Prandoni P, Santamaria MG, et al. Three months versus one year of oral anticoagulant therapy for idiopathic deep vein thrombosis. *New Engl J Med*. 2001;345:165–169.

15. Schulman S, Svengusson E, Granqvist S, et al. Anticardiolipin antibodies predict early recurrence of thromboembolism and death among patients with venous thromboembolism following anticoagulation therapy. *Am J Med*. 1998;104:332–338.

16. Eichinger S, Pabinger I, Stumpflen A, et al. The risk of recurrent venous thromboembolism in patients with and without factor V Leiden. *Thromb Haemost*. 1997;77:624–628.

17. Simioni P, Prandoni P, Lensing A, et al. The risk of recurrent venous thromboembolism in patients with an Arg506 → Gln mutation in the gene for factor V (factor V Leiden). *N Engl J Med*. 1997;336:399–403.

18. Lindmarker P, Schulman S, Sten-Linder M, et al. The risk of recurrent venous thromboembolism in carriers and non-carriers of the G1691A allele in the coagulation factor V gene and the G20210A allele in the prothrombin gene. *Thromb Haemost*. 1999;81:684–689.

19. De Stefano V, Martinellli I, Mannucci P, et al. The risk of recurrent deep venous thrombosis among heterozygous carriers of both factor V Leiden and the G20210A prothrombin mutation. *N Engl J Med*. 1999;341:801–806.

20. Schulman S, Granqvist S, Holmstrom M, et al. The duration of oral anticoagulant therapy after a second episode of venous thromboembolism. *N Engl J Med*. 1997;336:393–398.

21. Streiff M. Vena caval filters: a comprehensive review. *Blood*. 2000;95:3669–3677.

22. Decousus H, Leizorovicz A, Parent F, et al. A clinical trial of vena caval filters in the prevention of pulmonary embolism in patients with proximal deep vein thrombosis. *N Engl J Med*. 1998;338:409–415.

23. Fraser J, Anderson DR. Deep vein thrombosis: recent advances and optimal investigation with ultrasonography. *Radiology*. 1999;211:9–16.

Chapter 43

Questions, Answers, and Pearls from Anticoagulation Health Care Providers on Common Issues Related to Anticoagulation Therapy

Lynn B. Oertel

This chapter is a compilation of frequently asked questions posed by clinicians primarily working in anticoagulation clinics in various settings across the country. The questions were accumulated over time, and once assembled, patterns began to emerge in their content. These patterns illustrated common areas of concern relative to patient management issues such as drug interactions, warfarin dosing regimens, or perplexing patient cases. As a result, it is possible to conclude that all anticoagulation providers, despite disparities in their clinic size, patient populations, work settings, or clinical experience, face similar challenges.

Many of the following questions originate from clinicians who were participants in an Internet-based continuing education course on anticoagulation management, and others were acquired from various educational settings. Of note, the participants in the Internet-based continuing education course submitted questions electronically to a list-server, an electronic mail bulletin board. Participants on the list-server, including past and present course students, university faculty, and a designated panel of expert clinicians, were free to contribute responses. All list-server participants were able to benefit from reading the questions and posted responses.

This chapter is organized according to content areas representative of the frequently asked questions. Questions with similar themes are combined and edited. Likewise, excerpts from several responses to questions are edited to illustrate alternate points of view. These responses frequently reflect an expert's opinion, but not in all cases. Varied clinical experiences and practice variations from region to region may explain differences of opinion and respective recommendations. As such, the author cannot take responsibility for the accuracy of all responses, as they are not necessarily reflective of a uniform standard. Nevertheless, this type of exchange provides a rich, multidisciplinary learning environment in which clinicians can participate.

INTERACTIONS WITH WARFARIN

Frequently recurring questions are about potential interactions with warfarin. Most relate to drug-drug interactions, but a number of questions pertain to herbal and other supplemental preparations. The list-server was particularly effective in promoting a discussion among clinicians relative to their own patient care experiences. Ultimately, the overall effect was one of collegial support and encouragement for health care providers as they face challenging, easily frustrating, and often unpredictable situations related to patient care.

In their responses, clinicians often warned that a patient's response to medication changes or herbal supplements is often unpredictable and that diligent patient observation is warranted. Timely communication, patient education, compliance, and attentive monitoring mechanisms to assess such interactions was repeatedly emphasized.

It is difficult to keep abreast of all the new pharmacologic and herbal agents. Thus, a current pharmacology reference or online source to keep informed of potential interactions is recommended. For an excellent overview on warfarin interactions see Chapter 35, Warfarin Drug Interactions.

Some of the more interesting questions follow. A compilation of responses from various clinicians is included to illustrate the complexity of the situations.

Q: Is there an interaction with warfarin and grapefruit juice?

Flavenoids (found in grapefruit juice) are known to inhibit hepatic cytochrome P450 enzymes CYP1A2 and CYP3A4. These enzymes are responsible for oxidation of R-warfarin, which undergoes roughly 60% oxidation (and 40% reduction). Comparatively, S-warfarin is about 90% oxidized, but primarily by CPY2C9 (with a minimal contribution by CPY3A4). Since the S isomer is more potent than the R isomer, the potential interaction between grapefruit juice and warfarin can be expected to be of minor significance and variable among individuals.

Q: Can anyone tell me if flaxseed or flaxseed oil affects warfarin?

Flaxseed oil contains omega-3 fatty acids and inhibits platelet aggregation, so while it may not affect warfarin, it could presumably increase the bleeding risk by affecting platelets.

Another response: I have three patients who insisted on taking flaxseed oil. It has increased their INRs (International Normalized Ratios) dramatically.

Q: Are artichokes high, medium, or low in vitamin K content?

One clinician responded with the following information obtained from the Natural Medicines Comprehensive Database: "No interactions are known to occur, and there is no known reason to expect a clinically significant interaction with artichoke." For more information on botanical medicine, visit the Natural Medicines Comprehensive Database at http://www.naturaldatabase.com.

An alternate opinion suggested that the vitamin K_1 content of an artichoke is low based on another reference. See Table 36–6 in Chapter 36, Dietary Considerations.

Q: Is there any interaction between alcohol and warfarin?

Alcohol affects liver function, and clinicians described the difficulties in maintaining therapeutic INRs and lack of compliance in patients with chronic alcohol abuse. Indulgence in alcohol puts the patient at risk for falls or injury. Patients are reminded that a slight stumble or fall in an average person may be insignificant, but with anticoagulation, a significant risk for injury is present.

Q: Does anyone know of any interaction with Viagra and warfarin?

Clinicians responded by indicating that there does not seem to be an effect on the INR. No known interactions

specific to warfarin are listed in the *Physician's Desk Reference.* (Entry on-line via Micromedix Inc.)

PATIENT MONITORING

Q: I am in the process of putting together an anticoagulation management service at my hospital. What patient management systems are used?

A number of computerized programs are available to assist with patient management in terms of patient tracking and quality assurance. Several of these software programs also include a computerized dosing application. Each program has its strengths and weaknesses depending upon the purpose for which it will be used. There are numerous factors to consider when making a choice, and it may require input not only from clinicians who will use the system but also from local technical support services for potential integration into an existing network. There are also financial costs to consider as licensing fees vary greatly. For a more detailed discussion, see Chapter 9, Software Applications in Anticoagulation Management.

If you are not in a position to implement a computerized management program, a number of aids have been developed by clinicians to assist in day-to-day patient tracking and data management. If your intended clinic size is relatively small, use of such forms will assist with your clinic organization and create a consistent approach to patient care. See Appendix 8B, INR Flowsheet Tools and Appendix 8A, Data Collection Tools.

Q: Are there clinics that manage home-based patients who may never physically appear at the anticoagulation clinic for follow-up visits?

A number of patient follow-up scenarios exist for patient management. Although most clinicians would agree that face-to-face visits are ideal for patient assessment, education, and management, this is often not possible due to a host of reasons. Therefore, an alternative approach is telephone management and, to a lesser extent, a mail system using a postcard or letter to inform stable patients of stable results, warfarin dose, and date of next INR. Telephone-managed patients still benefit from the coordinated approach provided by the anticoagulation clinic when face-to-face visits are impossible to arrange. Of note, there are no reimbursement opportunities for telephone-managed patients. In addition, most clinics require at least one face-to-face visit at the onset of management in order to make an initial assessment and begin education.

Q: How do most clinics handle the phenomenon of "winter snowbirds" (patients who live in the northern states and head south for the winter months)?

Most clinics manage these patients by telephone during their prolonged stay in warmer climates. They cite continuity of care and patient preference as the main reasons to continue despite the long distance. Ideally, arrangements are made for a standing INR order at the patient's laboratory of choice (provided the international sensitivity index of the reagent is reasonable) and the results are faxed to the home clinic. Not everyone agrees, however, and some report added problems such as difficulty in reaching patients at the phone numbers provided, obtaining lab results in a timely fashion, and lack of appropriate medical follow-up in patients with changing medical conditions. In addition, patients who temporarily relocate to locales with different time zones place additional burdens on clinic staff to obtain INR results and contact patients. Patients who spend extended periods away from home should strongly consider establishing a relationship with a primary care physician in their locale.

In such cases, the patient should be asked to decide whether he or she would like to transfer anticoagulation management as well. If the home clinic continues management, this needs to be clearly communicated to all parties to avoid potential errors.

Clinics should evaluate the type of impact these snowbirds place on their services and weigh the benefits against the inconveniences. Once a decision is made, it should become the policy of the clinic and be communicated to all patients and referring physicians. The Anticoagulation Forum (see Web site: www.acforum.org) maintains a list of anticoagulation clinics across the country and may provide a useful reference to locate a clinic for transfer of patient care.

Q: Are there any recommendations for monitoring complete blood counts (CBCs), urinalysis (UA), and stool for occult blood for patients receiving long-term warfarin therapy?

Although there are no standards specific to this question, many clinics adopt local standards of practice that address the specific needs of their patient population and policies of the work setting. For example, a Veterans Affairs anticoagulation clinic obtains a UA, CBC, creatinine, and albumin every 6 months and a stool specimen for occult blood every 12 months. The justification was that they have a traditionally older patient population, many of whom take numerous medications and have concurrent medical problems. Other clinics may request this type of information through the patient's referring or primary care physician. Other clinics clearly state in their scope of practice policy that routine screening diagnostic testing is the responsibility of the patient's primary care provider.

PATIENT MANAGEMENT—WARFARIN DOSING AND PROTOCOLS

Q: What is the history and track record of published algorithms and protocols for warfarin dose management? I realize many factors come into play when making dosing adjustments, but are there any basic guidelines to go by?

Warfarin dosing protocols and algorithms are appearing with more frequency in the literature. Some have a strong history of clinical use, but the degree to which each has been studied in a systematic, controlled fashion is variable. These protocols provide a systematic, organized methodology with which to evaluate a patient's response to warfarin and make appropriate dose adjustments. However, they should be used merely as guidelines. No protocol can account for all of the confounding factors that may exist when a patient shows up for a prothrombin time test. Nothing replaces good clinical judgment in most situations. See examples of dosing protocols in Appendix 31A, Management Tools for the Clinician.

Q: I am preparing to set up a new anticoagulation clinic in our large cardiology practice. Could you please provide some input on how other clinics dose warfarin?

Most clinicians use a single strength tablet and use multiples or halves of it to individualize patient dose requirements. This strategy limits patient confusion when compared to strategies using multiple tablet strengths. A wide range of weekly mg totals is achieved using multiples or halves of the same strength tablet. For example, a patient uses a 5 mg size tablet and requires a weekly total of 30 mg to maintain a therapeutic INR. Dose instructions for this patient based on the number of tablets per day are as follows: take 1 tablet Sunday, Tuesday, Wednesday, Friday, and Saturday; and ½ tablet on Monday and Thursday. This scheme provides a total weekly dose of 30 mg/week. Clinics that use a similar strategy have reported good results, approaching 80% of patients in therapeutic range. To avoid dose errors, patients are provided with a written dose calendar based on the number of tablets per day, along with a reminder on the mg strength (and color) of tablet used.

Access to multiple strength tablets may increase the possibility of dose errors and add unnecessary patient costs. Many experts agree that there is no pharmacological benefit to prescribing the same number of mg per day given the relatively long half-life of warfarin and variable effect on the INR.

Q: What is the best approach to managing brief interruptions of therapy? How long should I hold warfarin prior to a diagnostic procedure?

This is a frequently cited concern and many issues must be taken into account. Experts agree that communication between the patient's physician and the anticoagulation provider is key to avoiding prolonged and sometimes unnecessary interruptions in warfarin therapy. A careful review of the patient's risk of bleeding with anticoagulation needs to be weighed against the risks of recurrent thromboembolism without anticoagulation. Some high-risk patients will need coverage with heparin while their INR is subtherapeutic in order to proceed safely with surgery or an invasive procedure. Each patient needs a careful evaluation of these risks followed by a management plan specific to his or her needs.

Many procedures involving the gums, teeth, and cataracts can be safely performed without interruption of warfarin therapy, provided the INR is at the low end of the therapeutic range.

Responses from other clinicians suggest the use of tranexamic acid mouthwash to minimize oral bleeding without interrupting warfarin therapy.

Patient response to withholding warfarin is variable. In general, withholding warfarin for three to five days will likely cause a drop in the INR to subtherapeutic or normal levels. (see White et al. *Ann Intern Med* 1995;122:40–42 and Chapter 37, Managing Anticoagulation during Surgery and Other Invasive Procedures).

Q: Does anyone have any comments or suggestions regarding INR monitoring and warfarin dose changes when patients are prescribed a course of antibiotics?

Most clinicians agree that more frequent INR monitoring is needed during such times. Some clinics have policies to decrease the warfarin dose and check INRs every three to four days after patients begin trimethoprim-sulfamethoxazole (Bactrim) or metronidazole (Flagyl), since the INR change is usually significant. Others disagree and do not make dose adjustments until indicated by rising INR values.

Checking the INR three to five days after the initiation of an antibiotic seems prudent. Future dose adjustments may be necessary, and close monitoring of the INR is advised. In most circumstances, patients (not the prescribing physician) inform the clinic when such medications are added, and this is not always done in a timely manner. Despite best efforts with patient education and communication, clinic staff often find out about these changes after the fact.

Q: The orthopaedic surgeons in our community maintain patients status post knee and hip surgeries at an INR goal range of 1.5 to 2.0 for short-term therapy. We have not found documentation in the literature to support this INR goal. Does anyone have experience managing this population of patients?

This is a common example of differing opinions on the optimal therapeutic INR range for a specific population. Continuing research will help define subsets of patients, along with risk-stratification models, that will provide clinicians with improved standards with which to base practice. The American College of Chest Physicians publishes a consensus conference on antithrombotic therapy as a supplement to the *Chest* journal. This reference should be viewed as a definitive source for setting standards of care in clinical practices. All anticoagulation providers should be familiar with its content and develop policies and procedures accordingly.

There is evidence in the literature documenting an INR intensity range of 2.0 to 3.0 as most effective. Several clinicians described their positive experiences with changing physician practice after having presented data on the target INR range of 2.0 to 3.0. Physician groups were willing to change the INR intensity range or, in some cases, to develop a compromise INR range of 2.0 to 2.5. Patients stand to benefit the most from this type of collaboration to improve patient care.

BRIDGE THERAPY USING LMWH

Q: Are there any recommendations or protocols for substitution of low–molecular-weight heparins (LMWHs) for warfarin in patients who require surgery or invasive procedures?

To date, a few abstracts have been published of small groups of patients successfully using LMWH as "bridging" therapy around the time of an invasive procedure. Despite the lack of extensive scientific data, this method of bridging anticoagulation before and after invasive procedures using LMWH is done frequently. It is probably appropriate to use "treatment" doses of any LMWH for this purpose. It also may be appropriate to limit the length of the preprocedure period by using minidose vitamin K to reverse the effects of warfarin, rather than relying on a long period of time to allow the INR to drift below the lower limit of the therapeutic range.

Guidelines at one university center are based on (1) whether the anticoagulation needs to be reduced or reversed for the procedure and (2) the patient-specific relative risk of thromboembolism during periods of reduced or reversed anticoagulation. For example, if surgery needs to be performed in a patient with a high risk for recurrence of thromboembolic disease, then

- Hold warfarin for three to five days preoperatively, *or* hold warfarin for two to three days preoperatively and administer vitamin K_1, 1 mg IV or 2.5 mg PO two days preoperatively (may repeat on day −1).
- Initiate unfractionated heparin (UFH) SQ/IV or LMWH when INR falls below lower limit of therapeutic range.
- Stop IV UFH 6 hours preoperatively or stop SQ UFH/LMWH 12 hours preoperatively.
- Resume UFH/LMHW 12 to 24 hours postoperatively and continue until INR lower limit of therapeutic range.
- Resume warfarin 12 to 24 hours postoperatively.

METHODS FOR DETERMINING INR VALUES (POINT-OF-CARE TESTING DEVICES)

Q: We are considering performing fingersticks (point-of-care testing) to increase our patient compliance. What has been your experience with patient preference and costs?

In terms of direct cost—possibly more expensive. In terms of time and quality of health care—priceless. Many older patients are difficult venous draws, and most patients prefer the fingerstick method. We schedule patients every 15 minutes and 45 minutes are allotted for an educational visit.

Patients appreciate the appointment schedule because they no longer wait for a turn in the laboratory.

The fingerstick method allows the clinic to run more efficiently in terms of nursing time since the INR result is known and patients are instructed about their dose while at the office.

Q: When using a point-of-care device, what INR value is considered "critical" to require a venous draw to verify accuracy of the result? How accurate are these devices? Is it necessary to carry out a correlation study at my institution before I purchase such a device?

Several point-of-care devices are available today and are Food and Drug Administration (FDA) approved for professional office use as well as patient home use. The results of correlation studies performed to achieve FDA approval are available for review. In general, the correlation between central laboratory INRs and point-of-care devices is not as strong at either end of the spectrum, particularly at the higher end, as they are toward the therapeutic spectrum.

Individual clinics must determine a threshold for "critical" INR values and develop a plan for follow-up. A description of the procedure should be part of the clinic's policy and procedure manual. At the present time, regional differences in practice are evident. For example, one clinic reported using 6.0 or higher as the threshold to require a venous INR sample. Other clinics simply repeat the INR on the same device and if the repeat value is close, accept it, and do not require plasma INRs on elevated fingerstick results.

Despite the above controversies, many experts agree that when one obtains an elevated INR (either from point-of-care device or plasma sample from a central laboratory), attention should be focused on patient assessment, that is, on how the patient is doing clinically. In most circumstances, the clinical decision for patient management and education will be the same for an INR value of 6.1 obtained via finger-stick or 7.3 obtained via plasma sample. The appropriate action to follow when such circumstances present themselves should be documented in the organization's policy and procedure manual.

Q: Can point-of-care devices be used safely during the initiation phase of anticoagulation therapy?

Most experts agree that point-of-care testing devices are safe and reliable during all phases of warfarin therapy. See Chapter 28, Capillary Whole Blood Prothrombin Time Monitoring: Instrumentation and Methodologies.

Q: Does anyone have experience with patients who are post-dialysis and having problems with obtaining accurate INR values with a point-of-care device? Is there something in the dialysis process that affects the point-of-care system?

During dialysis treatment, patients are heparinized with 2,000 to 10,000 units of heparin. Heparin alters the results of the INR on these devices and may explain erroneous results.

INR PERFORMANCE AND BENCHMARKING

Q: Does anyone have any pointers for determining "time in therapeutic range"? What's a realistic goal? What are national averages?

The literature suggests that an anticoagulation management service should aim to achieve 60%–80% of INRs in therapeutic range. This should be achieved whether patient management is performed manually or aided by computerized software programs. Of course, computerization of the patient INR data is preferred, as this will facilitate calculation of INR performance measures.

The literature describes three major methods for evaluating INR performance. The first is a frequency measure or percentage of INR tests in range. It is a straightforward calculation of the fraction of tests in range with no time considerations. Secondly, a time-weighted INR distribution (more commonly referred to as percentage of time in range) uses a linear interpolation between sequential INR tests to assign a portion of time at a given INR level. Last, the cross section of the files method is performed by selecting a random date and identifying the closest INR value for each patient in order to determine the percentage in range. In reports where these methods are used and the accumulated INR data are significant, the percentage of time in range value and cross section of the files values have been similar to the percentage of INR tests in range. Although more validation studies are needed, the cross section of the files approach may provide clinicians with an accurate and relatively easy method to assess time in range. (For a more detailed discussion on time in range, see Rosendaal FR, Cannegieter SC, van der Meer FJM, Briet E. A method to determine the optimal intensity of oral anticoagulant therapy. *Thromb Haemost.* 1993;69:236–239.)

Q: I've heard about an accepted "fudge factor" to use when calculating time in range. Please comment.

Many clinicians express frustrations over the apparent discrepancies in methods used for calculating time in range or percentage of INR tests in range. For example, some clinics exclude patients from the analysis during their initiation phase, that is, the first four to six weeks of therapy. Some clinics allow +/– 0.1 –0.3 INR units outside the stated INR range as "allowed" values and count these values as "in range." (The rationale here is that a single INR value just slightly out of range would not necessarily mandate a dose change.) Some clinics exclude the time period around a temporary interruption in warfarin therapy from the analysis.

In addition, clinics that primarily manage unstable, medically complex patients may never achieve as high a percentage in range as do clinics with stable, healthier patients. When INR statistics are reported, one should evaluate the method used to determine results and then draw one's own conclusions until such time as a universal consensus is reached on this statistic.

CLINIC ADMINISTRATIVE ISSUES

Q: Are there any recommendations for anticoagulation clinic staff related to clinic population size?

Generally speaking, one full-time professional (RN or pharmacist) is able to manage a clinic composed of approximately 300 patients. Of course the scope and responsibilities of the anticoagulation management service will impact this professional staff to patient ratio. Factors such as clinic operations, local organizational issues, and method(s) used to determine INR values are just a few of the factors that will affect this ratio. Perhaps the more-sensitive figure to consider when evaluating staffing requirements is an estimate of the number of INR tests and/or patient appointments scheduled per day. Although four weeks is generally accepted as the maximum length of time between INR tests, the average mean time between INR tests is often two to three weeks. This figure, along with an evaluation of the characteristics of the clinic's patient population, may help predict staffing needs. Once the clinic population expands beyond 300, the addition of a part-time clerical person will be necessary to assist with the phone calls, patient tracking, and related paperwork. See Chapter 4, Personnel Needs and Division of Labor and Appendix 4A, Policies and Procedures Examples.

CLINIC REIMBURSEMENT

Q: What can my institution expect to receive in reimbursement for services under evaluation and management (E/M) codes 99211 (office visit) and 85610 (laboratory)?

The Ambulatory Prospective Payment schedule is published by the Centers for Medicare and Medicaid. The amount reimbursed by Medicare and private insurers will vary according to fee schedules established for different regions. The business or finance departments within your institution can assist you to determine the dollar amount you are eligible for based on services provided and methodologies you employ. The rules and regulations for Medicare reimbursement are available at cms.hhs.gov. (See Chapter 12, Reimbursement Basics for Anticoagulation Services.)

Q: We work in an ambulatory clinic and manage warfarin therapy for patients who reside in long-term care facilities. We use a point-of-care device for some of our patients to determine the INR, and for others we receive a faxed INR report from an outside laboratory service. Can we bill using the E/M code 99211 in these situations?

For nonphysician providers to bill services using the E/M code 99211, a number of "incident to" rules must be fulfilled. For example, the service must be part of the physician's treatment plan, the physician must supervise the nonphysician provider, and the physician must be physically on site. Also, the nonphysician provider who performs the service must be an employee of the physician group. Evaluation and management criteria must meet the requirements for each level of service. In general, nonphysician providers are only eligible to bill level 1 visits for established patients, and thus the E/M code 99211 must be used. Nurse practitioners and physician assistants may bill for services using their own provider number and may bill at higher levels of service, if warranted, but the reimbursement rate is generally 15% lower than the physician's fee schedule.

Check with your financial advisors/auditors in your institution to see if you meet the requirements for submitting reimbursement for services using the 99211 code. If your clinic is part of a hospital and not a private physician's office, then you probably are not eligible for reimbursement under this provision code.

In cases where INR results are faxed to your clinic and patients are not seen in person, insurers do not provide reimbursement for telephone consultation.

Q: Are there any references to help me support the cost justification needed to develop an anticoagulation management service?

There is a growing body of evidence in the literature to justify the cost to establish an anticoagulation management service. Often, the approach to justifying the costs is to present data addressing the cost savings due to reduced utilization of expensive hospital resources (emergency department visits, hospitalizations). Helpful references can be found in the 1998 issue of the *Chest* supplement in the chapters titled "Oral Anticoagulants: Mechanisms of Action, Clinical Effectiveness, and Optimal Therapeutic Range" and "Making Decisions about Antithrombotic Therapy in Heart Disease: Decision Analytic and Cost-Effectiveness Issues."

CHALLENGING PATIENT SITUATIONS

Q: We have a patient who had an allergic reaction to warfarin in the past and now needs a valve replacement. Does anyone have any information on Miradon?

Miradon (anisindione), a product of Schering Laboratories, is an oral anticoagulant. The indications for use are prophylaxis and treatment of deep vein thrombosis, treatment of atrial fibrillation with embolization, prophylaxis and treatment of pulmonary embolism, and as an adjunct in the treatment of coronary occlusion. It is similar to warfarin but has a longer half-life and time to peak levels. It works by interfering with the hepatic synthesis of vitamin K–dependent clotting factors. (Source: *Clinical Pharmacology 2000*, Gold Standard Multimedia.)

Q: I have a 37-year-old male patient who takes warfarin for atrial fibrillation and stroke prevention. He also has a pacemaker. He wants to have a tattoo. Is there a contraindication to this?

Tattooing is a very personal decision and ultimately up to the patient. If the INR is within therapeutic limits, let the patient make the decision after counseling on the increased risk of bleeding and infection. Tattoo artists may refuse to work with clients who take anticoagulants.

Another response focused on the fact that this patient has a pacemaker. Getting a tattoo poses an increased risk of endocarditis if sterile technique is broken. Advice to this patient would be to not do it.

Chapter 44

Point-of-Care Testing: Patient Self-Testing and Patient Self-Management

Jack E. Ansell

INTRODUCTION

Point-of-care testing, also known as near-patient testing, on-site monitoring, and decentralized testing (see Chapter 28), describes an analytic process that does not take place in a centralized clinical laboratory but rather where the patient receives care (eg, at the bedside, in an office, or at home). In the mid-1980s, a new generation of instruments for prothrombin time (PT) measurement was introduced that allowed for true point-of-care testing as an option for PT monitoring of oral anticoagulation.[1] Although microsample technology and point-of-care instrumentation for PT measurement already existed in a rudimentary form,[2] it was cumbersome and not conducive to patient self-testing. The new technology allowed for fingerstick sampling of capillary whole blood with instrumentation that was lightweight, portable, simple to use, accurate, and precise. Chapter 28 discusses the types of instruments and their accuracy and precision, whereas this chapter focuses on clinical studies that assess the value of these instruments for patient self-testing at home and for patient self-management of warfarin therapy.

PATIENT SELF-TESTING

Given the simplicity and portability of these capillary whole blood PT monitors, it is not surprising that studies have been conducted to determine the suitability of patient self-testing and home monitoring with an eye toward improving clinical outcomes (safety and efficacy) and patient satisfaction. Evaluations of self-testing generally have been concerned with the answers to two questions:

1. Can patients perform their own PTs accurately?
2. Does self-testing produce a level of care that is at least as good as standard testing?

A number of studies have addressed the potential of patient self-testing or self-monitoring. Many studies have had too few patients to show differences in outcomes such as hemorrhage or thrombosis and thus have used the surrogate marker of time in therapeutic range as an end-point for effectiveness and safety.

With regard to the first question, Belsey et al[3] showed that a point-of-care instrument can be used by individuals with little laboratory experience. The portable monitor was subject to few operational problems, and trained technologists and nontechnically trained staff achieved comparable results with it. Although the study was designed to evaluate decentralized PT testing for office management, the conclusion that individuals with little or no laboratory training can accurately perform the test suggests the potential for patient self-testing.

In a multi-institutional trial,[4] simultaneous capillary whole blood and venous samples from 201 warfarin-treated patients and 52 control patients were compared with standard laboratory methodology at each institution, as well as with a reference laboratory. The study analyzed the ability and accuracy of patients to perform their own measurements in comparison with the ability and accuracy of health care providers. The monitor International Normalized Ratio (INR) significantly correlated to the INR of the reference laboratory for both the health care provider (venous sample, r = 0.93) and the patient (capillary sample, r = 0.93). Monitor PT results for fingersticks performed by both the patient and the health care provider were also equivalent and correlated highly (r = 0.91). A follow-up report from the same group of investigators[5] indicates that, after standardized training (approximately one hour), 83% of patients were able to obtain accurate PTs on the first attempt and an additional 10% were successful after the second try. Although 85% of the patients graded the monitor easy to use, with only 7.5% finding its use difficult, 92% of the patients preferred the fingerstick sampling methodology. The correlation of fingerstick sample to each hospital site (five sites) ranged from r = 0.89 to r = 0.93.

More recently, Andrew et al[6] reported on the ability and accuracy of 93 patients (82 adults and 11 children) who performed weekly fingerstick PTs at home during a six-week period, compared with venous samples collected within three hours at a study site and tested both on the instrument and in a reference laboratory. The patients' home monitor results were highly correlated with the study site venous results (r = 0.92, n = 535). Again, the patients favored the fingerstick sampling (95%), and 85% of the patients graded the monitor easy to use at home.

Further studies have specifically evaluated patient self-monitoring at home in therapeutic trials and have found advantages over traditional laboratory management. It is important to take note of what type of control group is used in randomized studies since this will influence the degree of difference in outcomes. Most studies have used a routine medical care model of anticoagulation management as the control group, while others have compared patient self-testing to the outcomes achieved by an anticoagulation management service. The former is likely to yield a higher rate of adverse events compared to the latter. White et al[7] report on a model of care in which patients were given portable PT monitors at the time of hospital discharge, instructed in their use, and asked to perform their own PT tests at home. The patients then reported their results to an anticoagulation management service (AMS) that adjusted the warfarin dose. Self-testing patients (n = 23), compared with the AMS control group (n = 23), had a greater percentage of INR results within therapeutic range (93% versus 75%; p = 0.003) and were significantly less likely to be outside of therapeutic range during the follow-up period (6.3% versus 23%; p < 0.0001).

Anderson et al[8] confirm the feasibility and accuracy of patient self-testing at home in their study of a cohort of 40 individuals who monitored their own therapy during a period of 6-24 months. The patients monitored their own PTs every two weeks and periodically had venous samples drawn within four hours of self-testing for reference plasma PTs. Based on either a narrow or expanded target therapeutic range, the authors observed a mean level of agreement per patient, with reference plasma PTs of 83% by narrow criteria and 96% by expanded criteria. All but one patient, or 97.5% of the total patients, preferred home testing to standard management.

In a large prospectively randomized study, Beyth et al[9] reported on 325 newly treated older patients with a variety of indications for anticoagulation. Of these patients, 163 performed patient self-testing and had their doses managed by a single investigator, and 162 of the patients were managed by their private physicians (routine medical care or RMC) based on venous sampling. During the initial 6-month period, the patient self-testing group experienced a 5.6% incidence of major hemorrhage compared to a 12% incidence in the personal physician–managed group (p = 0.049). Recurrent venous thromboembolism occurred at a rate of 8.6% in the self-testing group compared to 13% of the physician managed group, but the difference was not significant.

In another study, Kaatz et al[10] compared anticoagulation management using a point-of-care instrument in the clinic with patient self-testing at home, but with the dose managed by clinic personnel. There was no significant difference in time in therapeutic range between the home testing group and the clinic group (63.4% vs 64.7%, respectively). These studies are summarized in Table 44–1.

PATIENT SELF-MANAGEMENT

In 1974, well before the studies discussed above, Erdman et al[11] published the first study of the potential role that patients could play in facilitating the management of anticoagulants by adjusting their own doses. Each of 200 patients with prosthetic heart valves managed his or her own therapy based on a personalized guidance table that indicated the correct dose to achieve a particular PT result. PTs were obtained by standard methods at centralized laboratories, and patients were given their results for dose adjustments. Investigators found that 71% of patients managed before the introduction of this study were satisfactorily anticoagulated at any given time, whereas 98% of patients participating in the study were satisfactorily anticoagulated.

Schachner et al[12] continued and updated the study of Erdman et al.[11] Comparison of 59 patients in a self-managed group and 60 patients in a physician-managed group demonstrated that those in the former group were more likely to have therapeutic PTs (0.53 PT per patient out of range) versus those in the latter group (2.9 PTs per patient out of range). Self-managed patients also experienced fewer embolic episodes than physician-managed patients (1.1% per patient year versus 4.7% per patient year; p < 0.0005) and fewer bleeding episodes (5.7% per patient year versus 7.5% per patient year; p < 0.05).

The advent of capillary whole blood PT point-of-care testing enabled Ansell et al[13,14] to assess the ability of patients

Table 44-1 Studies of Patient Self-Testing and Patient Self-Management of Oral Anticoagulation Stratified by Whether the Comparator Group Is Routine Medical Care or an Anticoagulation Management Service Model of Care

Study	Study Groups	Time in Range	Adverse Events
Beyth et al. (2000)[9] (RCT)	PST* vs RMC	56% vs 32%	14% vs 25%
Horstkotte et al. (1996)[17] (RCT)	PSM vs RMC	92% vs 59%	5.4% vs 4.5%
Hasenkam et al. (1997)[16] (cohort)	PSM vs RMC	77% vs 59%	no AEs
Sawicki (1999)[18] (RCT)	PSM vs RMC	57% vs 34%	3 vs 1
Kortke & Korfer (2001)[19] (RCT)	PSM vs RMC	78% vs 61%	2.9% vs 4.7%
White et al. (1989)[7] (RCT)	PST* vs AMS	87% vs 68%	no AEs
Kaatz et al. (2001)[10] (RCT)	PST* vs AMS	63% vs 65%	NA
Ansell et al. (1995)[14] (cohort)	PSM vs AMS	88% vs 66%	no AEs
Watzke et al. (2000)[20] (RCT)	PSM vs AMS	86% vs 80%	2 vs 0
Cromheecke et al. (2000)[21] (crossover)	PSM vs AMS	55% vs 49%	no AEs

*Dose management for PST group performed by an anticoagulation management service.

RCT = randomized control trial; PST = patient self-testing; PSM = patient self-management; RMC = routine medical care; AMS = anticoagulation management service; AE = adverse event; NA = not available

to measure their own PTs and adjust their own warfarin doses. The investigators recently analyzed the results of such care delivered over a 7-year span to 20 patients, ranging in age from 3 years to 87 years, with diverse indications for anticoagulation.[14] These patients performed their own PT tests at home and adjusted their own warfarin doses, based on physician guidelines. The results, summarized in Table 44–2, prove this mode of therapy to be at least as safe and effective, if not more so, as care provided to a control group managed by an anticoagulation clinic. Self-managed patients were found to be in therapeutic range for 88.6% of PT determina-

tions versus 68% of PT determinations in the controls (p<0.001). Also, fewer dose changes were required by study patients (10.7%) than by controls (28.2%; p<0.001). Complication rates did not differ between the groups. Patient satisfaction was extremely high with this mode of therapy, which empowered patients by allowing them to manage their own care and possibly improved their understanding of and compliance with therapy.

Bernardo[15] has even more experience with this mode of therapy in Germany, where patient self-management is becoming widespread. Investigators initially used a KC 1A

Table 44-2 Long-Term Patient Self-Management of Oral Anticoagulation

Clinical Outcomes	Self-Managed Patients	Control Patients	p Value
Number of patients	20	20	
Weekly warfarin dose	37.5 mg	34.8 mg	>.10
Mean duration in study (Month) (Range)	44.7 (3–87)	42.5 (3–86)	>.10
Number of PTs (mean/patient)	2,153 (107.7)	1,608 (80.4)	>.05
Mean interval between PTs (days)	13.8	16.0	>.10
PTs above range	5.2%	10.3%	<.001
PTs below range	6.3%	21.8%	<.001
PTs in range	88.6%	68.0%	<.001
Dose changes	10.7%	28.2%	<.001
Incorrect dose changes	3.1%	—	

Note: 20 patients followed over a period of 7 years measured their own PTs and adjusted their own warfarin doses based on guidelines provided by study investigators. Patient outcomes are compared with 20 matched controls.

Source: Reprinted with permission from JE Ansell et al, *Archives of Internal Medicine*, Vol 155, p 2185, © 1995, American Medical Association.

coagulometer and subsequently the CoaguChek instrument to measure PT. A report on 216 self-monitored and self-managed patients between 1986 and 1992 indicates that 83.1% of the PT results were within target therapeutic range and no serious adverse events occurred. In a randomly selected subgroup of 92 self-managed patients compared retrospectively with a group of 317 patients managed by traditional means (118 patient years versus 374 patient years), the investigators found fewer hemorrhagic events (3.38% versus 4.38%) and fewer embolic events (0 versus 8 episodes) in the self-management group than in the traditionally managed group. Hasenkam et al[16] confirmed the effectiveness of self-management in 20 patients with prosthetic valves, reporting that these patients were in the therapeutic range 77% of the time compared to 53% of the time for 20 retrospectively matched control patients.

In the first prospective randomized trial of this model of care, Horstkotte et al[17] report the outcomes from a study of 150 patients with prosthetic heart valves who managed their own therapy (n = 75) compared with a control group who were managed by their personal physicians (n = 75). The self-managed patients tested themselves approximately every 4 days and achieved a 92% degree of satisfactory anticoagulation as determined by the INR. The physician-managed patients were tested approximately every 19 days and only 59% of the INRs were in therapeutic range. The self-managed individuals experienced a 4.5% per year incidence of any type of bleeding and a 0.9% per year rate of thromboembolism, compared to 10.9% and 3.6% rates respectively in the physician-managed group (p = 0.038 between the two groups).

Sawicki et al[18] reported on patients randomized between patient self-management (PSM) (n = 90) and management by their personal physicians (n = 89). As an outcome measure, they compared the distribution of INRs from the midpoint of each patient's therapeutic range at 3 months and 6 months (cross section of the files method) compared to baseline. Patients in the self-managed group were significantly closer to their target INR and had a greater percentage of values within therapeutic range at three months (57% vs 34% within range), while the differences were not significant at six months. Based on a survey of patient preferences, general treatment satisfaction and daily hassle scores improved in the self-management group and remained unchanged in the routine care group. Using a similar control group, Kortke and Korfer[19] reported preliminary results from a large randomized controlled German study (Early Self-Controlled Anticoagulation Study or ESCAT). Three hundred five PSM patients achieved a greater frequency of INRs in range (78.3%) vs 295 RMC patients (60.5%). There was a significant difference in major adverse events between groups as well (4.7% in the RMC group vs 2.9% in the PSM group; p = 0.042).

Using anticoagulation clinic care as the control group, Watzke et al[20] compared weekly INR patient self-manage-

ment in 49 patients with management by an anticoagulation management service in 53 patients. The self-management group was within therapeutic range a greater percentage of the time and had a significantly smaller mean deviation from the target INR. Lastly, Cromheecke et al[21] conducted a randomized crossover study with 50 patients managed by an AMS or by self-management. Although the differences did not achieve statistical significance, there was a trend toward greater time in therapeutic range in the self-management group (55% vs 49%).

These studies are summarized in Table 44–2. Results indicate that when PST or PSM are compared against a routine medical care model of management, the outcomes of time in therapeutic range or adverse events are considerably better than when an AMS is the comparator group.

Based on the foregoing, portable PT monitors offer the potential to lower the risk/benefit ratio of anticoagulant therapy; to improve patient satisfaction and possibly patient compliance; and, by reducing the labor intensity of physician management, to encourage the more widespread use of warfarin for proven indications. Although these results need further confirmation by large randomized prospective trials, they suggest that future management of anticoagulation should include patient self-monitoring and patient self-management of therapy.

PATIENT EDUCATION

Certain guidelines that have been developed for educating and training patients apply to all patient education situations. Because of the high risk/benefit ratio of warfarin and the potentially serious consequences of nontherapeutic levels of anticoagulation, however, special considerations are warranted in patient education for anticoagulation therapy. Also, the majority of patients taking oral anticoagulants are older, and a number of special guidelines for teaching older patients apply.

Patient education in the use of capillary whole blood monitors should begin with the identification of good candidates. Certainly, not all patients will be able or willing to perform the test and keep the necessary records to ensure safe and accurate monitoring.

The important consideration in the identification of a good candidate is incentive. Patients cannot be expected to comply unless they have a specific incentive to do so. Incentives differ among patients and often depend on their individual circumstances. Less frequent clinic visits, particularly for patients who have difficulty reaching the clinic, might be sufficient incentive to learn the information. Patients who have an aversion to phlebotomy or who have poor venous access might appreciate the ease in obtaining results from a fingerstick. Some patients will be grateful for the opportunity to learn about their conditions and to take an active role in their treatments. Patients at increased risk for hemorrhage, or individuals whose PT seems to fluctuate widely for a variety of reasons, might welcome the opportunity for more frequent (and less invasive) monitoring and the potential to increase the amount of time spent within the desired therapeutic range. For some patients, the recommendation of self-testing by a trusted physician will suffice. Most important, the trainer, along with the patient, must identify a willingness and an ongoing incentive to perform the test as required.

Other important considerations in the identification of good candidates are:

- adequate motor skills to perform the test
- sufficient mentation and memory
- sufficient reading and writing capabilities
- adequate eyesight, with or without glasses, to see the screen

For some patients who lack these abilities, related caregivers might be willing to take the responsibility for monitoring.

Patient education is twofold. Patients must be educated about anticoagulation so that they understand what they are being asked to do and why (see Chapter 10), and they must be trained in the use of the monitor. Ensuring that patients have the skills and information required for correct use of the PT monitor involves a different yet complementary approach than that required for teaching about anticoagulation. The challenge for the health care provider is to convey the necessary information to the patient and train the patient in the use of the monitor without conveying excessive or superfluous information. Seley[22] offers 10 strategies for successful patient teaching:

1. assessment of the patient's needs
2. determination of the patient's readiness to learn
3. establishment of measurable goals
4. division of information into manageable bits
5. demonstration and practice
6. written instructions
7. feedback and review
8. lifestyle modifications
9. reinforcement
10. follow-up and referrals

Trainers should simplify the process as much as possible and provide backup written instructions to which patients can refer during training and later at home. Instructions for performing the actual test should be written in short, clear sentences or phrases. The text print should be large and clear; small, poor-quality photocopies are unacceptable. The tasks that the patient must perform at home should be clearly listed in simple, straightforward, and consistent terms and be located in an easily accessible place, such as the first page of a booklet. The trainer should refer to the list throughout the training sessions. Technical language is to be avoided whenever possible.

When instructing patients in the actual use of the instrument, the trainer must remember that the majority of patients probably cannot program a VCR or coffee machine and perhaps are uncomfortable with computers. Consequently, they might be intimidated by the apparent complexity of the monitoring device and accompanying materials. The transition from clinic to home testing can be facilitated if patients have been monitored in a clinic that uses the capillary whole blood monitor. The trainer should remember that older patients like and need consistency, and their routine should be disrupted as little as possible. For a patient who is accustomed to having blood drawn in a laboratory and then receiving a telephone call about dosage changes, learning about the machine and its use can be overwhelming. All efforts should be made to facilitate this transition and to inspire self-confidence in the patient.

Once patients have performed the test, they must record their results. Large, clearly marked spaces should be provided for writing the results. Often, a printed calendar to use both as a testing schedule and a place for recording results is helpful. The trainer must discuss the following points with each patient and verify that the patient understands the instructions before leaving the clinic:

- the days the patient will perform the test
- where the patient writes down the results, preferably in an easily accessible place for the patient to refer to again (eg, on the calendar)
- time of day when it is most convenient for the patient to perform the test
- what the patient must do to plan the test at that time and how the trainer can help with the plan
- where in the house it will be most convenient to perform the test
- how the patient pictures the process running smoothly in the home and how the trainer can help in clarifying the picture

The trainer should try to anticipate any problems that a specific patient might have and make a plan with the patient to solve them (eg, some patients need to keep a spare pair of reading glasses in the case with the machine).

Follow-up visits should be scheduled and recorded on the calendar. More than one visit might be necessary to train a patient in all aspects of home testing. The trainer should not assume that patients remember everything they were taught, even though they seemed to understand the instructions during the training session. Patients should know whom to call when they have problems and the individual's telephone number. Ideally, this would be the same person to call for a medical problem, such as bruising, or to make appointments.

Finally, the trainer must give patients the opportunity to express concerns and ask questions. Many patients look forward to interacting with a health care provider, especially one whom they know, and they should be assured that the trainer will be available for them. It is also important for the trainer to reinforce the incentive identified by each patient and the trainer at the beginning of the session.

REFERENCES

1. Lucas FV, Duncan A, Jay R, et al. A novel whole blood capillary technique for measuring the prothrombin time. *Am J Clin Pathol.* 1987;88:442–446.

2. Shoshikes M, Grunwald E. A capillary test tube technique for the determination of capillary whole blood prothrombin time. *J Lab Clin Med.* 1959;53:617–621.

3. Belsey RE, Fischer PM, Baer DM. An evaluation of a whole blood prothrombin analyzer designed for use by individuals without formal laboratory training. *J Fam Pract.* 1991;33:266–271.

4. Ansell J, Becker D, Andrew M, et al. Accurate and precise prothrombin time measurement in a multicenter anticoagulation trial employing patient self-testing. *Blood.* 1995;86(suppl 1):864a.

5. Becker R, Becker D, Andrew M, et al. Anticoagulation monitoring: accurate results with patient self-testing in a multicenter clinical trial. *J Am Coll Cardiol.* 1996;27(suppl A):317A.

6. Andrew M, Ansell J, Becker D, Becker R, Triplett D, Shepherd A. Multicenter trial of accurate home self-testing in oral anticoagulant patients with a novel whole blood system. *Blood.* 1996:88(suppl 1):179a.

7. White RH, McCurdy SA, von Marensdorff H, Woodruff DE, Leftgoff L. Home prothrombin time monitoring after initiation of warfarin therapy. *Ann Intern Med.* 1989;111:730–737.

8. Anderson DR, Harrison L, Hirsh J. Evaluation of a portable prothrombin time monitor for home use by patients who require long-term oral anticoagulant therapy. *Arch Intern Med.* 1993;153:1441–1447.

9. Beyth RJ, Quinn L, Landefeld C. A multicomponent intervention to prevent major bleeding complications in older patients receiving warfarin. *Ann Intern Med.* 2000;133:687–695.

10. Kaatz S, Elston-Lafata J, Gooldy S. Anticoagulation therapy home and office monitoring evaluation study. *J Thromb Thrombolys.* 2001;12;111.

11. Erdman S, Vidne B, Levy MJ. A self-control method for long-term anticoagulation therapy. *J Cardiovasc Surg.* 1974;15:454–457.

12. Schachner A, Deviri E, Shabat S. Patient-regulated anticoagulation. In: Butchart EG, Bodnar E, eds. *Thrombosis Embolism and Bleeding.* London: ICR Publishers; 1992;318–324.

13. Ansell J, Holden A, Knapic N. Patient self-management of oral anticoagulation guided by capillary (fingerstick) whole blood prothrombin times. *Arch Intern Med.* 1989;149:2509–2511.

14. Ansell JE, Patel N, Ostrovsky D, Nozzolillo E, Peterson AM, Fish L. Long-term patient self-management of oral anticoagulation. *Arch Intern Med.* 1995;155:2185–2189.

15. Bernardo A. Experience with patient self-management of oral anticoagulation. *J Thromb Thrombolysis.* 1996;2:321–325.

16. Hasenkam JM, Kimose II, Knudsen L, et al. Self-management of oral anticoagulant therapy after heart valve replacement. *Eur J Cardiothorac Surg.* 1997;11:935–942.

17. Horstkotte D, Piper C, Wiemer M, et al. Improvement of prognosis by home prothrombin estimation in patients with life-long anticoagulant therapy. *Eur Heart J.* 1996;17(suppl):230.

18. Sawicki PT, Working Group for the Study of Patient Self-Management of Oral Anticoagulation. A structured teaching and self-management program for patient receiving oral anticoagulation. A randomized controlled trial. *JAMA.* 1999;281:145–150.

19. Kortke H, Korfer R. International Normalized Ratio self-management after mechanical heart valve replacement: is an early start advantageous? *Ann Thorac Surg.* 2001;72:44–48.

20. Watzke HH, Forberg E, Svolba G, Jimenez-Boj E, Krinniger B. A prospective controlled trial comparing weekly self-testing and self-dosing with the standard management of patients on stable oral anticoagulation. *Thromb Haemost.* 2000;83:661–665.

21. Cromheecke ME, Levi M, Colly LP, et al. Oral anticoagulation self-management and management by a specialist anticoagulation clinic: a randomized cross-over comparison. *Lancet.* 2000;556:97–101.

22. Seley JJ. Ten strategies for successful patient teaching. *Am J Nurs.* 1994;94:63–65.

Chapter 45

Patient Selection and Training for Patient Self-Testing and Patient Self-Management of Oral Anticoagulation

Alan K. Jacobson

BACKGROUND

One of the major advances in the management of anticoagulation over the past decade has been the recognition that the method of management plays a critical role in the safety and efficacy of therapy. Systematic management of anticoagulant therapy has been shown to provide a significant reduction in both thromboembolic and hemorrhagic events.[1,2] Routine management or "usual care" tends to be a passive approach where a monitoring episode is initiated by a patient reporting to a laboratory for prothrombin time (PT) testing, and the result then being transmitted to the health care professional for interpretation and action. Under this approach, no test—no action. While many criteria have been suggested as critical components of a systematic management approach,[3] the essence of such an approach is direct, active management by a qualified health care provider ensuring: reliable patient scheduling and tracking; accessible, accurate, and frequent PT testing; patient specific decision support and interaction; and ongoing patient education and quality control (QC) (Figure 45–1, Exhibit 45–1).

The ability to provide highly accurate testing combined with sophisticated interpretive and dosage adjustment guidelines is of no use if the patient never has the test performed and the management system has no way of detecting that the test was never performed.

STRUCTURAL MODELS FOR ANTICOAGULATION MANAGEMENT

Testing has been performed traditionally in a central laboratory with the results being interpreted by a health care provider who then contacts the patient with any changes in treatment regimen. An alternative approach became available in the mid-1980s with the introduction of portable point-of-care PT (POC-PT) devices for use in the clinic setting. This provided the ability of having the patient and the result in the same place at the same time, offering potential improvements in efficiency and communication. However, even though centralized POC-PT testing offered the patient a single consolidated visit for both testing and interpretation, it still required the patient to come to the provider's office for each monitoring episode.

In the mid- to late-1980s, POC-PT testing began in Germany and the United States, but was developed with particular enthusiasm in Germany. Within a short time, formalized training programs had been developed within Germany to provide this model of management to patients. The initial German training programs were primarily for inpatients and provided extensive training, not only in patient self-testing (PST) but also in patient self-management (PSM) with the patient being trained to be responsible for management of anticoagulant dosage adjustments.[4]

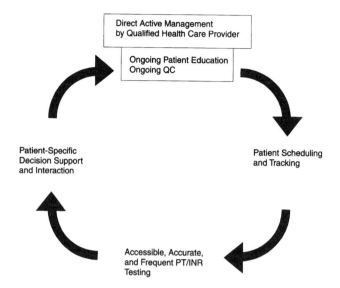

Figure 45–1 Systematic anticoagulation management. Source: Data from Premier Innovation Institute.

By 1990, an official association had developed, the Association for Self Anticoagulation (ASA), which has a formal link with the German Heart Association. The ASA has developed guidelines for the development of patient training programs with over 150 certified training centers currently throughout Germany and over 42,000 patients performing PST/PSM.

In the United States, the Food and Drug Administration (FDA) approved two devices for patient home use in 1997, and three additional manufacturers have devices under development. Extensive evaluations of the accuracy of these portable devices have been performed and results are essentially the same as would be expected from a central laboratory.[5–8] Several studies have been performed to evaluate the use of these devices by the patient in the home environment, in the setting of both PST and PSM.[9–12]

The availability of POC-PT testing allows for a spectrum of structural models for the management of anticoagulant therapy[13] (Exhibit 45–2). However, none of these models inherently provides systematic, active management. It is the combination of an active management system with the structural model of management most appropriate for a given patient that will result in optimal management for that patient.

RATIONALE FOR PATIENT SELF-TESTING

There are several aspects of PST that are theoretically appealing. First, PST provides the ability for testing with a frequency that is not practical in centralized models. There are preliminary data to suggest that optimal patient outcomes, at least in terms of time in therapeutic range, can be obtained with a frequency of testing of once or twice a week.[14] This provides the ability to detect any drift in International Normalized Ratio (INR) stability prior to the drift resulting in a clinically significant event. Second, PST enhances patients' involvement in their own care. PST allows the patient to evaluate how lifestyle events affect INR stability. The timely feedback may then allow the patient to modify lifestyle elements and thereby improve INR stability. Finally, PST provides for a level of consistency in instrumentation and reagents that is often not achieved in a usual care or even systematic care model.

PATIENT SELECTION

Patient selection is a critical consideration in all aspects of anticoagulation, both in determining whether a patient is even an appropriate candidate for anticoagulant therapy as well as in determining which method of management is most appropriate for that patient. The most concise criteria for patient selection are to assess whether the patient is willing, able, and reliable to perform self-testing. While the specific criteria will vary depending on the specific management option, these three general criteria are the essence of patient selection. Patients who have the potential to benefit the most from PST include those who have limited access to testing due to distance or disability, and those who require increased testing frequency (ie, those patients with heart failure, cirrhosis, or marked variation in their PT values) (Exhibit 45–3).

In the case of PST, the testing and management is not necessarily restricted to the patient but may be provided by a qualified provider. For pediatric patients and for patients

Exhibit 45–1
CHARACTERISTICS OF SYSTEMATIC ANTICOAGULATION MANAGEMENT

1. Management by Qualified Health Care Provider
   - Patient care comes under the management of a single individual. Responsibilities include
     – ensuring that patient education is adequate and maintained
     – ensuring that there is ongoing QC of patient outcomes and management procedures
     – ensuring direct and active oversight of anticoagulation management

2. Patient Scheduling and Tracking
   - *Reliable, predictable scheduling method:* The planning of patient visits should be recorded using a calendar format whether it be a paper system or a more automated process.
   - *Tracking of missed visits and recording of test results:* In addition to a scheduling methodology, there must be a feedback system to identify when patients have missed their visits. The system also should maintain a continuous record of lab test results.
   - *Feedback, contact, and action on missed appointments and capture of outside results:* Integral to the "direct and active" management process would be the process of contacting patients who have missed their appointments or have out-of-range INR results captured at another location.
   - *Enabling technologies/approaches:*
     – standard operating procedures
     – patient database, preferably computerized
     – scheduling tools
     – feedback mechanism (ie, automated queries of patient database)

3. Accessible, Accurate, and Frequent PT/INR Testing
   - *Access to testing:* Patients must have ready access to the testing modality, be it a central laboratory or point-of-care device.
   - *Reliable PT testing:* Effective control of pre-analytical, analytical, and postanalytical variables is necessary to ensure reliability of results.
   - *Results reported in INR:* Whether obtained at a central laboratory or using a POC testing device, the results should be reported using the INR metric.
   - *Enabling technology/approach:* Point-of-care testing (professional or patient).

4. Patient-Specific Decision Support and Interaction
   - *Patient assessment by qualified health care provider:* Optimally, this person would be a nurse, pharmacist, PA, or other licensed care provider. The care provider should have some form of anticoagulation management training.
   - *Integration and correlation of INR results with patient-specific considerations:* Test results, patient assessment, and dosage decision making are integrated during the evaluation.
   - *Dosing recommendations, education, and follow-up plan:* Patient-specific education is correlated with clinical issues and medication adjustment; follow-up interval is individualized but guideline based.
   - *Enabling technologies/approaches:*
     – anticoagulation training courses/preceptorships
     – protocols and operating procedures
     – dosing algorithms

with disabilities that would preclude their being able to competently perform their own testing, the availability of a parent, spouse, or qualified care provider allows these patients to be considered for PST.

TRAINING THE PATIENT FOR PST/PSM

Patient training needs to cover three broad categories of information—anticoagulation therapy, POC-PT testing, and management of test results. All patients receiving long-term anticoagulant therapy should be provided with general background training relating to the basic aspects of anticoagula-

tion theory. In an ideal setting, training would be provided by a multidisciplinary team including nursing, pharmacy, laboratory, and dietary staff. Topics to be covered would include: (1) mechanism of anticoagulant action; (2) narrow therapeutic dosing window; (3) interpretation of test results (PT/INR); (4) factors that affect the PT—diet, drugs, liver function; (5) bleeding risks and monitoring; (6) testing frequency; and (7) indication and duration of therapy (Exhibit 45–4).

Those patients being considered for PST then will require additional training in the actual performance of PST-PT. Training approaches have not been evaluated in controlled settings and it is unclear as to what constitutes the absolute minimum training required for competent performance of

Exhibit 45–2
STRUCTURAL MODELS FOR ANTICOAGULATION MANAGEMENT

1. Laboratory Testing with Professional Management of Results
   - testing performed in a central facility on a venipuncture specimen
   - result reporting and management occur at a later time
2. Point-of-Care Testing by a Professional with Professional Management of Results
   - testing performed in a central facility on a fingerstick specimen
   - consolidated visit includes testing, interpretation, and management
3. Point-of-Care Testing by a Patient with Patient or Professional Management
   - testing performed at patient location on fingerstick specimen
   - patient reports result to professional provider for management (PST)
   - patient interprets results and provides management (PSM)

Any of the above may be provided in a passive (no effective mechanism to ensure and track patient testing—respond to results when and if obtained) or active (specific mechanisms to actively ensure monitoring is occurring on a timely basis) manner.

Exhibit 45–3
CATEGORIES OF PATIENTS LIKELY TO ACHIEVE GREATEST BENEFIT FROM PST

1. Patients who have difficulty with access to testing due to
   - distance
   - disability
   - scheduling conflicts
2. Patients who require increased frequency of testing, due to
   - liver disease
   - congestive heart failure
   - highly variable INR results

Exhibit 45–4
CATEGORIES OF PATIENT EDUCATION

1. Basic Anticoagulation Theory: Provided to all patients receiving warfarin.
   - indication, duration, and desired therapeutic range for anticoagulation
   - basic mechanism of anticoagulant effect of warfarin
   - rationale for monitoring
   - impact of diet, drugs, and liver function on INR
2. Technique of Fingerstick INR Testing: Provided to those patients who will be performing their own testing (PST).
   - storage and handling of supplies, care of testing device
   - fingerstick technique
   - reporting of results
3. Management of INR Results: Provided to those patients who will interpret their own INR results and manage their own warfarin dosage adjustments (PSM).

erations that should be taken into account when initiating a training program.

Most patients are able to demonstrate competent performance of PST-PT following a single training session of about two hours' duration. The most efficient format is a group training session with one instructor for two or three patients. This session includes theory, demonstration, and hands-on patient experience. Indications for and approaches to quality control performance also need to be covered.

PST Theory

Desirable topics to cover in the theory section include

- basics of PT testing methodology
- interpretation of the INR and its limitations
- mechanics of fingerstick testing
- storage and handling of supplies

This can be accomplished through a combination of videotape materials, slide-based lectures, handouts, or oral presentation with informal illustration on overhead transparencies or a chalkboard.

PST Demonstration

Once patients understand the basic theory, it is appropriate to demonstrate the mechanics of testing on the particular brand of instrument that they will be using. Demonstration should include

- instrument setup
- layout of supplies
- testing technique

PST-PT. Initial European programs required very rigorous training that often required a minimum of six hours. However, much of this time was spent on dosing adjustment instruction and was performed in an inpatient setting. The majority of patients in the United States have anticoagulation initiated on an outpatient basis and this must be considered in the design of the training program. What follows are consid-

Hands-On Experience with PST

The final component is for the patient to gain competence with actual hands-on experience using the device. This can be accomplished in either a stepwise process by having the patient utilize liquid control solutions (to gain comfort with use of the device prior to applying an actual fingerstick whole blood sample), or by proceeding directly to the use of patient fingerstick samples.

To ensure ongoing patient competence, it is appropriate to recommend a transitional period prior to complete reliance on PST-PT results as the basis for dosing adjustments. During this transition period, typically two to four weeks, patients are instructed to perform PST-PT determinations once or twice a week. This transition period helps the patient become comfortable with the performance of fingersticks and with the operation of his or her monitor. At the end of the transition period, the patient is seen back in the clinic and performs a test on their device in the clinic, with a comparison test also being performed by the clinic staff. This provides the opportunity to document patient versus professional equivalence of results, verify proper functioning of the patient device, review patient technique, and answer patient questions. The patient then is asked to perform once a week PST-PT with clinic follow-up after eight weeks. The second clinic visit follows the same format as the first, and if patient performance is felt to be clinically acceptable, he or she is then placed on a maintenance surveillance schedule of weekly PST-PT determinations supplemented by clinic visits approximately every 6–12 months. At the interval clinic visits, patient versus professional equivalence in INR determinations and device integrity are reassessed.

QUALITY CONTROL

We have had experience with multiple approaches to quality control (QC) with POC-PT devices. Some devices incorporate the QC checks onto the test strips (on-board QC) and others rely on external methods (liquid or electronic). Unfortunately, there is little literature or data to guide the appropriate frequency of QC testing. It is clear that QC protocols that may be appropriate for high-volume testing equipment in the central laboratory may not be appropriate for single-use supplies such as utilized in PST-PT programs. Having had experience with multiple approaches, it appears that using a single therapeutic intensity liquid control solution once a month and once with each new box of test strips is reasonable. The routine use of multiple intensity QC solutions or the routine use of higher frequency QC testing is of unclear additional value. The routine use of electronic QC alternatives is under evaluation and holds significant promise. Aside from the baseline QC outlined above, it appears that the availability of external QC primarily serves a reassur-

ance function that provides the patient with a mechanism to ensure the integrity of test strips and device functioning should a question arise.

MANAGEMENT OF PST-PT RESULTS

In many European countries, programs have been set up to train patients in comprehensive management of PST-PT results, including dosage adjustment. Two approaches are used. The most comprehensive approach is to train the patients in dosing theory and allow them to exercise independent judgment in deciding how to adjust the dose.[15] The second approach is to provide the patient with a dosing algorithm.[16] Obviously the first approach requires training that is more comprehensive than for the algorithm approach.

In the United States, there is currently no FDA approval for patients to be involved in dosing adjustment (although it is unlikely that PDA approval is needed). We utilize patient self-testing, not patient self-management. However, due to the increased frequency of testing, most physicians and anticoagulation clinics would be overwhelmed if they had to receive and respond to every test result. Therefore, most providers simply provide the patient with a desired therapeutic range, and unless the test results are outside of that range, the physician is not notified. All patients should be provided with a diary or patient log in which they record the date and INR result of each test, the lot number of the test strips utilized, any QC results, and any appropriate clinical comments. The accuracy of the patient diary can be assessed at the time of the interval clinic visits by downloading the POC-PT device memory and comparing the device log with the patient diary.

One prototype system has been developed to provide automated ongoing results collection from PST patients. This system allows the patient to call the clinic computer utilizing a regular touch pad telephone and, by responding to voice prompts, verify anticoagulant dose, report current INR measurement, and notify changes in clinical status. This provides the capability to maintain a comprehensive database of patient results and enhance the ability to verify ongoing timeliness of patient testing with a minimal use of personnel resources.

SUMMARY

We have a variety of management options for patients receiving oral anticoagulant therapy. Some patients are managed entirely by professional testing and result interpretation, others perform their own testing but rely on professional guidance for dosage adjustment, while in some settings patients are fully responsible for both testing and dosage management.[17] As one moves across this spectrum, there is an increasing need for the patient to be willing, able, and reliable to participate in his or her own care. Similarly, there is an increasing need for additional training to allow the patients more control over their own management. Optimal patient results are obtained when the particular method of management chosen is provided within an active, systematic management system to ensure that patient scheduling, testing, and decision support are provided in a consistent, reliable, and timely manner.

REFERENCES

1. Ansell JE. Anticoagulation management as a risk factor for adverse events: grounds for improvement. *J Thromb Thromboly.* 1998;5:S13–S18.

2. Bussey HI, Chiquette E, Amato MG. Anticoagulation clinic care versus routine medical care: a review and interim report. *J Thromb Thromboly.* 1996;2:315–319.

3. Ansell JE, Buttaro ML, Thomas OV, Knowlton CH. Consensus guidelines for coordinated outpatient oral anticoagulation therapy management. Anticoagulation Guidelines Task Force. *Ann Pharmacother.* May 1997;31(5):604–615.

4. Bernardo A. Experience with patient self-management of oral anticoagulation. *J Thromb Thromboly.* 1996;2:321–325.

5. Kaatz SS, White RH, Hill J, et al. Accuracy of laboratory and portable monitor International Normalized Ratio determinations: comparison with a criterion standard. *Arch Inter Med.* 1995;155:1861–1867.

6. van den Besselaar AM, Breddin K, Lutze G, Parker-Williams J, Taborski U, Vogel G, Tritschler W, Zerback R, Leinberger R. Multicenter evaluation of a new capillary blood prothrombin time monitoring system. *Blood Coagul Fibrinolysis.* December 1995;6(8):726–732.

7. McCurdy SA, White RH. Accuracy and precision of a portable anticoagulation monitor in a clinical setting. *Arch Intern Med.* 1992;152:589–592.

8. Anderson DR, Harrison L, Hirsh J. Evaluation of a portable prothrombin time monitor for home use by patients who require long-term oral anticoagulant therapy. *Arch Intern Med.* 1993;153:1441–1447.

9. Bernardo A, et al. Long-term experience with patient self-management of oral anticoagulation. *Ann Hematol.* 1996;72 (Supp. I):A62.

10. Hasenkam JM, Knudsen L, Kimose HH, et al. Practicability of patient self-testing of oral anticoagulant therapy by the International Normalized Ratio (INR) using a portable whole blood monitor: a pilot investigation. *Thrombos Res.* 1997;85:77–82.

11. White RH, McCurdy SA, von Marensdorff H, Woodruff DE, Leftgoff L. Home prothrombin time monitoring after the initiation of warfarin therapy: a randomized, prospective study. *Ann Intern Med.* 1989;111:730–737.

12. Zerback R, Horstkotte D. Patient self-monitoring in follow-up of long-term anticoagulant therapy. *Z Kardiol.* 1998;87 Suppl 4:68–74.

13. Ansell JE, Hughes R. Evolving models of warfarin management: Anticoagulation clinics, patient self-monitoring, and patient self-management. *Am Heart J.* 1996;132:1095–1100.

14. Horstkotte D, Piper C, Wiemer M. Optimal frequency of patient monitoring and intensity of oral anticoagulation therapy in valvular heart disease. *J Thromb Thromboly.* 1998;5:S19–S24.

15. Sawicki PT. A structured teaching and self-management program for patients receiving oral anticoagulation: a randomized controlled trial. Working Group for the Study of Patient Self-Management of Oral Anticoagulation. *JAMA.* 1999;281:145–150.

16. Ansell JE, Patel N, Ostrovsky D, Nozzolillo E, Peterson AM, Fish L. Long-term patient self-management of oral anticoagulation. *Arch Intern Med.* 1995;155:2185–2189.

17. Ansell JE. Empowering patients to monitor and manage oral anticoagulation therapy. *JAMA.* 1999;281:182–183.

Chapter 46

Managing Oral Anticoagulation Therapy in the Netherlands

W.G. Mimi Breukink-Engbers

INTRODUCTION

The Netherlands is a small country in Western Europe with a surface area of 34,000 km² and 16 million inhabitants. (See Figures 46–1 and 46–2.) It has a tradition of over 50 years of managing oral anticoagulation therapy in outpatients by specialized centers, the *trombosediensten* (thrombosis centers). Even within some hospitals the management of some inpatients is delegated to such a service. The centers are recognized by the Ministry of Public Health, Welfare, and Sports and must satisfy certain standards and requirements. The following section describes the history and features of the organization of these centers in the Dutch health care system.

HISTORY

The Dutch anticoagulation centers have a history of over 50 years. In 1949, Professor Jordan, an internist, established the first Dutch post-thrombosis-care-center in the Academic Hospital in Utrecht. His aim was to create a center to provide optimal oral anticoagulant therapy in outpatients by concentrating knowledge about anticoagulant treatment. The reasons for doing so were medical, social, and financial. Until that time, patients with deep venous thrombosis treated with oral anticoagulants had to stay in a hospital for several weeks, since anticoagulation monitoring was only available in the hospital. By bringing together knowledge of monitoring anticoagulation therapy in a specialized center and being able

to send out specially educated staff (nurses) to visit the patients at their home, he raised the quality of medical treatment as well as the quality of life for the patient, avoiding the costs of hospitalization.

The knowledge and skills developed in his center consisted of

- knowledge of the pharmacology of oral anticoagulants
- knowledge of the interaction of oral anticoagulants with other drugs and various diseases
- knowledge of dosage
- knowledge of laboratory techniques
- personal patient guidance

In 1952 a second center was established in The Hague under the auspices of the local division of the Dutch Red Cross. It was called a *trombosedienst* (thrombosis center). A rapid expansion of the number of thrombosis centers followed, initiated by the intensive involvement of the Dutch Red Cross. In 1957, by negotiations with the authorities, a fixed system of financing was set up. In 1971, the centers (more than 30 in number at that time) founded the Federatie van Nederlandse Trombosediensten (FNT, Federation of Dutch Thrombosis Centers).

The Federation of Dutch Thrombosis Centers

Members of the FNT can be anticoagulation centers that have a lead physician, are able to visit patients at their home

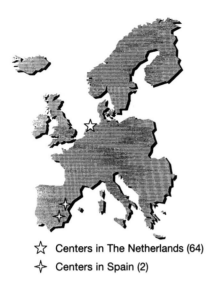

☆ Centers in The Netherlands (64)
✧ Centers in Spain (2)

Figure 46–1 Dutch anticoagulation centers in Europe

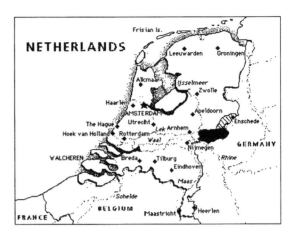

■ Ascon Region East—Gelderland
▨ Ascon Region Enschede

Figure 46–2 The Netherlands and the East Netherland Anticoagulation Center ASCON

when needed, and can perform prothrombin time measurements either within the center or within an associated medical laboratory. The laboratory has to meet the quality standards of the FNT: The laboratory results must be standardized as International Normalized Ratio (INR) values, and both internal and external quality controls are required (see below).[1,2]

As of April 2002, there are 63 Dutch anticoagulation centers throughout The Netherlands and two in Spain for patients staying there for holidays or spending the winter (Figure 46–1). The members of the FNT serve approximately 300,000 patients annually. That means more than 4 million blood samples collected for prothrombin time measurements. Some centers are associated with a hospital, a medical laboratory, or a medical diagnostic center, but most are independent corporations.

The aim of the FNT is to monitor and improve the quality and to preserve the interests of the member centers. This includes the following goals:

- providing guidelines for monitoring anticoagulant therapy
- providing recommendations and educational material for patients
- organizing refresher courses for staff and physicians of the centers
- stimulating scientific research in the field of thrombosis and coagulation
- negotiating with the health and financial authorities

Communication between the members of the FNT takes place at meetings of the delegates from each center at least three times a year and through a Web site (www.fnt.nl). The board consists of nine delegates from different member centers. There are permanent committees for different issues, like the Thrombosis Center Accreditation Policy committee for quality assessment and certification and the complaints committee to manage patient complaints. Ad hoc committees are formed for other issues such as educational programs for physicians and staff involved in advising patients and prescribing the dose of oral anticoagulants. In cooperation with pharmacists, a standardized procedure has evolved to handle the prescription of interacting medications,[3] and a basic guide on oral anticoagulation has been published for physicians.[4]

In 1974 the FNT founded the Trombosestichting (Thrombosis Foundation) to stimulate research in the field of thrombosis and hemostasis and to raise funds for that purpose. To improve the quality of laboratory determinations, the RELAC (Reference Laboratory for Anticoagulation) foundation was set up (see below).

ORGANIZATION OF A DUTCH ANTICOAGULATION CENTER

An anticoagulation center consists of a central site and peripheral locations in a defined region. The management and administrative activities occur at the central site. Most of the centers have their own laboratory for prothrombin time determinations. The satellite locations are visited at least once a week by staff of the center who collect blood samples, obtain relevant information on patients, and give advice. After determination of the prothrombin time and reviewing the actual history of the patient, a physician or specially trained dose advisor estimates the dose of the anticoagulant and the date of the next checkup. The dose advice is sent by post and received by the patient on the next day. When more information or an urgent alteration of the dose or intake of vitamin K is needed, the staff phone the patient as well as the patient's pharmacist. If an INR is >8, the family physician is informed. When needed, a phone consultation between the physician of the center and the family physician or treating medical specialist takes place.

Every center has a lead physician who is responsible for all dose adjustments. The physicians are experienced in anticoagulation therapy and have attended a special course set up by the FNT. Almost all centers use a computerized system for dosing anticoagulation and storing the medical records. The existing systems are able to dose automatically in about 35% of cases.

A treating medical specialist or general practitioner is responsible for establishing the diagnosis and the indication for anticoagulation and usually starts the patient with one of the oral anticoagulants before the patient is referred to the center. In The Netherlands two coumarin derivates are available, the short-acting acenocoumarol 1 mg (Sintrom Mitis®) and the longer acting phenprocoumon (Marcoumar®). These coumarins differ from warfarin not only in half-life, but also in the mean dose needed to achieve a therapeutic INR (Table 46–1).[5] It mostly depends upon the experience of the treating physician as to which of the coumarin derivates is started. The physician of the center takes over the anticoagulation management when he or she accepts the indication and target range. If the physician of the center does not agree with the indication or target range, there will be a consultation between the two physicians.

At the first visit a short medical history is taken by the staff, and information is given about the anticoagulation therapy and the organization of the center. Most centers use the written educational material of the FNT supplied with leaflets and a checklist for this purpose. The nurses instruct the patients to phone the center when there are changes in medication, illnesses, or when they have any bleeding. They also invite patients to phone the center when invasive procedures or holidays are planned. For holidays there is the possibility to provide the patient with a letter in one of six different languages (Dutch, English, French, German, Italian, Spanish) with information about the indication for anticoagulation and the data of the most recent checks for use in case of emergency. If there is doubt about compliance to therapy or when special risk is suspected, the physician of the center contacts the referring physician or general practitioner to discuss whether the therapy should be changed.

The centers use guidelines and recommendations of the FNT for target ranges and duration of therapy. Two different INR ranges are used, depending on the indication for the anticoagulation therapy:

- Target range 2.5–3.5 INR, acceptable range 2.0–3.5 INR, for primary and secondary prevention of venous thrombosis and pulmonary embolism, atrial fibrillation, and cerebrovascular insufficiency
- Target range 3.0–4.0 INR, acceptable range 2.5–4.0 INR, for primary and secondary prevention of arterial thromboembolism, artificial heart valve prosthesis, venous thrombosis in patients with antiphospholipids, and recurrence of venous thromboembolism in patients treated with target range 2.5–3.5 INR

The lower level of target ranges is 0.5 INR higher than that of the acceptable ranges to prevent an insufficient intensity of the anticoagulation by dietary and other changes in lifestyle.

MANAGEMENT OF ANTICOAGULATION IN VENOUS THROMBOSIS

Since the publication of the TASMAN study,[6] patients with venous thrombosis are more frequently treated as outpatients. The general practitioner sends them to a diagnostic center or medical specialist for diagnosis and afterward they are sent home with low–molecular-weight heparin (LMWH) and an oral anticoagulant. A district nurse or a nurse of the anticoagulant center provides instruction about the injections. If patients are not able to inject themselves, the daily LMWH injections are given by the nurse. The physician of the center takes care of the management of the oral anticoagulation and the termination of the use of LMWH when oral anticoagulation is at a sufficient level. All is done in cooperation with the family physician or the treating medical specialist.

QUALITY ASSESSMENT

Improving the quality of monitoring of the centers is a main goal of the FNT. The most important methods are laboratory quality control, annual reports of the centers, and audits and certification of centers. A system of external quality control for the prothrombin time test has been set up

Table 46–1 The Coumarins Used in The Netherlands in Comparison to Warfarin

Coumarin	Mean Dose in Milligrams	Half-Life
Acenocoumarol 1 mg	2.4–2.5	8–10 hours
Phenprocoumon 3 mg	2.1–2.4	4–9 days
Warfarin	4–5	10–45 hours

by the FNT in collaboration with the RELAC laboratory. Ten times per year five blood samples are sent to every center to determine a prothrombin time. The samples are made from pooled plasma of patients on oral anticoagulants. Two of the samples are identical. A score based on the deviation of the result with respect to the national mean and standard deviation is given for each determination, not only for the prothrombin time itself, but also for the calculated INR value. Once a year a summary of the scores is reported to the centers, including a certificate when the center fulfills the standards of the FNT (at least 75% good scores). Since this quality control program was set up in 1974, the coefficient of variation between laboratories decreased from 10% to 6%.

All centers have to report annually several data to the FNT. These contain basic data, such as number of patients, indications for anticoagulation, number of controls, and some financial data, but also include the achieved intensity of anticoagulation, bleeding complications, and cerebral hemorrhages.

The acquired intensity of anticoagulation is reported as percentage in the intended range on two arbitrarily chosen days with at least a six-month interval using a "cross section of the files" method. In patients who are already treated for six months or longer, at least 70% of the results should be in the intended range. Centers that do not reach that standard are visited by a delegation of the FNT who explore what might be the reason and give support in improving the quality. In a joint medical report of the FNT, the data of the centers are summarized anonymously both for comparing by the centers and for the authorities to get an overview of the overall quality of anticoagulation therapy on a nationwide basis.

In 1992, the FNT set up a quality assessment committee that developed a quality manual for anticoagulation centers and a certification system based on audits by specially trained auditors. The auditors are physicians and other staff of member centers who have attended special training for that purpose. They make their observations during a one-day visit. The report of that visit is sent to the national quality assessment coordinator who decides if the center fulfills the standards for a certificate of quality. At present, 23 of the centers have obtained this certificate. As a result of this process of auditing, several more specified and new standards have been developed and are included in the second edition of the quality manual. A third edition is in preparation.

SELF-MANAGEMENT OF ANTICOAGULATION

Because of the network of anticoagulation centers spread over the country of The Netherlands, the need for self-management of anticoagulation was not felt to the same extent as elsewhere in the world. Both authorities and patients had to be convinced that it is as safe as the management by the Dutch anticoagulation centers. Two studies (one of them not yet published)[7] compared the management of Dutch anticoagulant centers with patient self-management and showed that it is safe and may even give better results in some cases. These conclusions and the efforts of FNT and patient associations caused the authorities to accept training and support for patient self-management as a regular service of anticoagulation centers since January 1, 2002.

Trainers for self-management must attend a basic train-the-trainer course of the FNT. A center with trained trainers can bill the health insurance companies for the training and counseling of patients. If, after the training, a patient is successful in managing his or her anticoagulation, then the center is responsible for delivering the instrument and materials for that purpose. Every three months the patient has a checkup in the anticoagulation center. If the results of self-management are insufficient, the physician of the center can decide to return to regular management, and the patient has to return the instrument. All agreements between patient and center are laid down in a contract signed by the patient and the responsible physician of the center. As this system has just started, data from experiences and results are not yet available.

SOME DATA OF THE DUTCH CENTERS

In the year 2000 the FNT had 66 member centers with 64 within The Netherlands and 2 in Spain. Data of 61 of the members in The Netherlands are used in the following summary.

The centers treated 301,420 patients and did 4,041,536 INRs. In total about 2% of the Dutch population was treated with oral anticoagulants. The overall frequency of INRs was 19 per patient per year. On average the monitoring of oral anticoagulant therapy costs 163 € per year of treatment. In long-term treated patients (over 6 months) the mean time between checks was 25 days, in short-term treated patients (2–6 months) it was 19 days, and in patients started in the last 2 months it was 12 days on average. Thirty-seven percent of the checks were done at the patient's home. About 50% of the patients started therapy in that year, and the same percentage discontinued therapy. The other 50% were on long-term treatment. Seventy-seven percent of the patients used acenocoumarol 1 mg, and 23% used phenoprocoumon 3 mg.

Indications for treatment were prevention of venous thrombosis and pulmonary embolism in 89,886 cases (30%) and valvular prosthesis, atrial fibrillation, or prevention of arterial thromboembolism in 210,971 cases (70%). In recent years, there was a clear increase in the number of patients with atrial fibrillation, while the number of patients with myocardial infarction and prevention of arterial thromboembolism decreased.

Table 46–2 Indications for Oral Anticoagulation Therapy in Patients Monitored in the Year 2000 by the East-Gelderland Anticoagulation Center

	Number	%
Atrial fibrillation	1442	29.8
Primary prevention of venous thrombosis in orthopaedic patients	896	18.5
Peripheral atherosclerosis and vascular surgery	415	8.6
Heart valve prosthesis	386	8.0
Deep venous thrombosis	378	7.8
Myocardial infarction	348	7.2
Cerebrovascular insufficiency and cerebral thromboembolism	339	7.0
Pulmonary embolism	199	4.1
Coronary surgery	197	4.1
Other	246	5.1
Total	4846	100

The acquired intensity of anticoagulation reported as the percentage in acceptable range (mean of "cross section of the files" on 2 arbitrary days with at least a 6-month interval) varied from 56% on average in just-started patients (<2 month) in the higher intensity group to 77% on average in the long-term treated (>6 month) patients in the lower intensity group. Some centers even reported results up to 91% in range. In long-term treated patients, the acquired intensity on phenoprocoumon is about 5–10% better than that for patients on acenocoumarol.

Major bleeding (leading to hospitalization, blood transfusion, or death, as well as all cerebral, joint, and muscular bleeding) was reported in 1.2% (range 0.2%–2.7%) of patients per year of treatment and 18% of the patients died from the bleeding episode. Minor bleeding occurred on average in 9.2% (range 0.3%–20.6%) of patients per year. Intracerebral bleeding was reported in 0.23% (range 0.00%–0.82%) of patients per year. Eighty-eight percent of those patients died. There is no standardized report of thromboembolic events.

PERFORMANCE OF A SINGLE CENTER

East Netherlands Anticoagulation Center (ASCON) consists of two outpatient clinics in the eastern part of The Netherlands (Figure 46–2). Both clinics have their own laboratory. Although one clinic, the former East Gelderland Anticoagulation Center TOG, is situated in a more rural area while the other, Enschede and surrounding area, serves a more urban region, the organization and results of the anticoagulation are comparable. There are about 50 peripheral sites for patient contacts and blood collection. Most peripheral sites are opened two times a week for approximately one hour. Many of the sites are located in nursing homes for the elderly. The clinics together are continuously treating approximately 7,000 persons, or annually about 10,000 different people. In total, 160,000 blood samples are collected per year, or an average of 250–450 samples daily per clinic.

Staff of the center consists of 6 physicians (of which one is the full-time managing and medical director and the others fill in together one full-time equivalent), 2 full-time coordinating nurses (one for each clinic), a quality assessment manager, 5 part-time laboratory employees (1 FTE), and 30 part-time nurses and nurse assistants (18 FTE) for contacting patients at the central site, going out to peripheral centers, making home visits, and taking blood samples. The physicians give most of the dosage advice, but the quality assessment manager and three of the other staff are also trained to give dosage advice. They use the computer system TRODIS (first version established in the 1970s at the Leiden University) for that purpose. The clinics have been linked to the same database since January 2002. Therefore it is possible for one physician to supervise both centers.

The East Gelderland clinic, started in 1976, covers a population of approximately 275,000 inhabitants. Prior to implementation, only 35% of patients had an INR in therapeutic range. Six months later, 70% of patients had achieved a therapeutic level. In 2000, the clinic treated 4,846 patients. Table 46–2 identifies the indications for treatment. Compared to 1998, the results for time-in-therapeutic range are slightly lower, but still within a good range (Table 46–3). Compared to 1998, the number of major hemorrhages were also greater in 2000 (2.2% vs. 2.7%, respectively).

Table 46–3 INR Values Obtained in Long-Term Treatment (Patients Monitored for at Least Six Months before the Day of Measurement) by the East-Gelderland Anticoagulation Center—Comparison of 1998 with 2000 Results

target group 2.0–3.5 INR	<2.0 INR (%)	2.0–3.5 INR (%)	>3.5 INR (%)	number of measurements
year 1998	4	83	13	2835
year 2000	5	79	16	3302
target group 2.5–4.0 INR	<2.5 INR (%)	2.5–4.0 INR (%)	>4.0 INR (%)	number of measurements
year 1998	8	80	12	2720
year 2000	8	78	14	2531

Cross section of the files at two different days in March and June.

CONCLUSION

The Dutch system of monitoring anticoagulation therapy by specialized centers provides a relatively inexpensive and safe method for treatment with anticoagulants. A system of quality assessment has been established to monitor and improve the quality of treatment. More efforts should be made to improve the recording of bleeding and standardized recording of thromboembolic events. Recently, the service of the Dutch anticoagulation centers has extended to counseling of patient self-management. Although it is more expensive, the possibility of patient self-management can be an important improvement, especially in patients' quality of life.

REFERENCES

1. *Standard for Quality Assurance. Part 4: Internal Quality Control in Haematology*. Eccls (1987). Vol. 4, no. 2. Berlin: Beuth Verlag.

2. *Standard for Quality Assurance, Part 5: External Quality Control in Haematology*. Eccls (1986). Vol. 3, no. 1. Berlin: Beuth Verlag.

3. Federatie van Nederlandse Trombosediensten. Geneemiddelinformatie van het Wetenschappelijk Instituut Nederlandse Apothekers en Stichting Health Base: Standaardafhandeling cumarin-interacties, August 1999, ISBN 90-705082-2-5.

4. Federatie van Nederlanse Trombosediensten. Vademecum voor poliklinische antistollingsbehandeling met cumarinederivaten, May 2000, ISBN 90-805082-1-7.

5. Keller C, Matzdorff AC, Kemkes-Mattes B. Pharmacology of warfarin and clinical implications. *Sem Thromb Hemost*. 1999;25:13–16.

6. Koopman MM, Prandoni P, Piovelli F, et al. Treatment of venous thrombosis with intravenous unfractionated heparin administered in the hospital as compared with subcutaneous low–molecular-weight heparin administered at home. The Tasman Study Group. *N Engl J Med*. 1996;334:682–687.

7. Comheecke ME, Levi M, Colly LP, et al. Oral anticoagulation self-management and management by a specialist anticoagulation clinic: a randomised cross-over comparison. *Lancet*. 2000;356:97–102.

Chapter 47

Managing Oral Anticoagulant Therapy: An Italian Perspective

Gualtiero Palareti and Armando Tripodi

Oral anticoagulation therapy (OAT) is becoming an increasingly important form of treatment for the care and prevention of thromboembolism and, more generally, vascular disease. As in most developed countries, a large number of patients are treated in Italy, and this number is constantly on the rise. According to our estimates, about 500,000 people, or just under 1% of the population, are currently receiving treatment in Italy.

OAT is effective in the clinical conditions it is indicated for. A factor that stands in the way of a more broad-based use of treatment, however, is the relatively high incidence of major hemorrhagic complications. The primary objective must be to enhance the safety of treatment. It is well known that periodic monitoring, both laboratory and clinical, is an indispensable condition for optimizing the therapeutic effectiveness of OAT. The quality of monitoring OAT is crucial for effective and safe treatment.

THE ITALIAN FEDERATION OF ANTICOAGULATION CLINICS

In 1989 the representatives of nine centers working in the field of OAT monitoring met in Parma (North Italy) and founded the Italian Federation of Anticoagulation Clinics (FCSA), whose overall aim is to improve the quality of OAT monitoring in our country (see Exhibit 47–1). The Federation seeks to set up new anticoagulation clinics (ACs) as an integral part of the network of services involved in the monitoring of anticoagulant patients. The guidelines for the setting up of ACs and the prerequisite conditions for recognition by the Federation are very simple (see Exhibit 47–2). Because of the increasing number of anticoagulant patients and the various initiatives of the Federation itself, the number of federated ACs over these years has grown steadily. Today they number over 250 and are spread out across the country (see Figure 47–1).

Despite the growth in the number of ACs in the FCSA, we estimate that only 25%–30% of anticoagulated patients are monitored by an AC. Of the rest, about 5% are followed by specialists, 1%–2% practice self-management, and the remaining 60%–70% are monitored by their general practitioners.

The basic activities of the FCSA include: (1) educational initiatives such as the drawing up of guidelines,[1] training courses for staff, an annual convention for members and anyone interested in the subject, and local conferences; (2) standardization of laboratory monitoring and quality control; and (3) collaborative studies.[2–7] These activities of the Federation address three distinct players: health authorities and institutions, both central (government) and local; the federated ACs and all health workers involved in AOT patient monitoring; and anticoagulant patients.

With regard to the National Health Service and local health authorities, our request is that all those who need this therapy should have the right to it, complete with all the safety that proper monitoring can provide. The federated ACs and all the operators (including general practitioners) are provided with training (via periodic courses), continuous education (through national and local conferences and the Internet), and invita-

Exhibit 47–1
MAIN GOALS OF THE ITALIAN FEDERATION
OF ANTICOAGULATION CLINICS

- Coordinate and support the activities of all those already involved nationally in the monitoring of anticoagulant patients.
- Promote the development of anticoagulation clinics (ACs) throughout Italy.
- Inform colleagues and national health authorities on the clinical and social importance of efficient and efficacious monitoring of anticoagulant patients.
- Draw up clinical and laboratory guidelines with proper indications.
- Encourage the standardization of laboratory methods, eg, adoption of an "external laboratory quality control scheme" and improvement of comparability of results and work methods among the federated ACs.
- Help in the training and continuous education of medical and paramedical staff involved.
- Promote collaborative studies between federated ACs.

Exhibit 47–2
WHAT IS REQUIRED OF AN
ANTICOAGULATION CLINIC FOR
FEDERATION TO THE ITALIAN FEDERATION

- Name a person in charge of the clinic, both for the laboratory and the clinical management of patients.
- Take part in at least one of the training courses regularly organized by the Federation.
- Take part in the external laboratory quality control scheme.
- Express prothrombin time result as International Normalized Ratio.
- Prescribe the daily dose of anticoagulant drug and set the date of the following control.
- Provide guidance in special clinical situations.

tions to take part in collaborative studies. Collaborative studies are important to the extent that they represent an opportunity to exchange valid diagnostic criteria and help standardize working procedures among the various ACs. For anticoagulant patients, our aim is to provide better information and health education, both prerequisites for good compliance. The Federation also promotes the creation at each center of voluntary associations of patients with a view to improving relations with the patients themselves and their organization. The main overall aim of all these activities is to improve the safety of anticoagulant therapy (Exhibit 47–3) and the patient's quality of life.

Exhibit 47–3
KEY FACTORS FOR THE EFFICACY AND
SAFETY OF TREATMENT

- Information and health education of patients
- Proper OAT indication, choice of therapeutic range, and duration of treatment
- Suitable laboratory diagnostics
- Correct prescription of daily dose of anticoagulant drug
- Use of specifically designed computerized systems
- Guidance in special clinical situations (eg, dental care, associated diseases, surgery, invasive procedures)
- Proper diagnosis and treatment of complications
- Analysis of the quality of results (both laboratory and clinical)

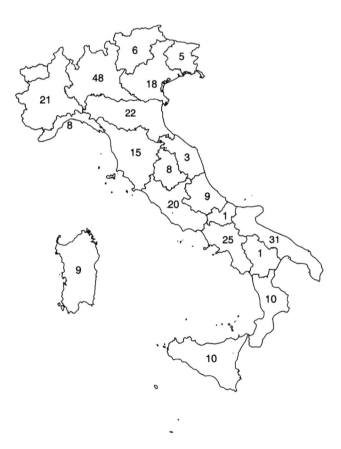

Figure 47–1 Regional distribution of the 270 anticoagulation clinics federated in the Italian Federation of Anticoagulation Clinics

OPERATIONAL RECOMMENDATIONS OF THE FCSA TO THE ANTICOAGULATION CLINICS

The Federation has drawn up a series of recommendations over recent years for its federated centers to standardize procedures and help provide proper monitoring.

Information and Health Education of Patients

Before beginning therapy, all OAT candidates must be given information and education necessary to understand the nature of treatment and achieve optimal results. Women must understand the side effects of OAT during pregnancy and what to do in case they become pregnant. Physicians must also be aware that a patient can refuse such treatment, especially if alternative therapies are available. Patients should be informed that OAT can reduce the risk of thrombotic events but that hemorrhagic risks may occur, especially if anticoagulation is poorly controlled, and that regular blood tests are required to be able to adjust daily drug doses. It is important that illustrative material containing all the necessary information on OAT be provided and be written in clear and understandable prose. The information should discuss the mechanism of action of the anticoagulant drug; interaction with diet, lifestyles, and associated drugs; the International Normalized Ratio (INR); and the importance of regular testing. Indications should be given on possible hemorrhagic complications and what to do in case of onset. It is important that there be a meeting with an expert (physician or nurse) to offer information on lifestyles and habits that might have an impact on the course of therapy and to explain any doubts that may have arisen. We recommend regular meetings with medical and nursing staff open to all anticoagulant patients so that problems and doubts can be discussed as a group.

All patients should receive initial medical visits to assess both their general conditions as well as the more specific conditions that led to OAT. The presence and extent of hemorrhagic or thrombotic risk factors should be taken into account. This will allow identification of the therapeutic target, expected duration of treatment, and need for regular specialized checkups.

All patients who opt to self-monitor OAT using a portable coagulometer should be given proper training in how to use the instrument, be provided with the necessary information and education prepared by professional staff, and be invited to follow a specially structured teaching program (see also those aspects regarding maintenance of the equipment and their quality control).

Regular Visits

Regular visits should be structured in such a way as to gather information on the history of the patient in the period since the previous INR, including compliance, new drugs, intervening diseases, changed lifestyle, and hemorrhage. These questions, which are written on the therapeutic prescription reports that the subjects receive at each INR and that are then presented at the following INR, are answered as simply as possible by the patients in writing. At the time of the blood test, the nurse collects the reports and checks the answers, asking further questions if necessary.

Once the INR value has been obtained, the daily dose needs to be provided for the forthcoming period and the date for the next appointment set. Determining the anticoagulant dose is not just a question of determining the INR; it should be seen as a medical assessment of the patient's overall clinical condition, complete with any possible changes in his or her recent history (eg, associated therapies, intervening diseases, onset of complications).

The patient's clinical computer records should be updated with the INR value, therapeutic prescription, and any eventual remarks on clinical condition.

Use of Computerized Systems and the Federation's Efforts To Standardize Them

The Federation encourages all ACs, specialists, and family practitioners, regardless of the number of patients followed, to adopt computerized systems specially designed to monitor anticoagulant patients. A wide range of such systems is today commercially available in our country. Some of these are essentially databases that can store all the information necessary and help manage patients; other, more sophisticated, systems can help the physician prescribe therapeutic doses. The software PARMA (Instrumentation Laboratory, Milan) is widely used in Italian ACs and offers algorithms for calculating the anticoagulant dose on the basis of patients' history, their anticoagulation target, and the INR value. A multicenter study recently performed by some Italian ACs showed that the use of this program helps increase the amount of time spent in the therapeutic range compared to exclusive management by AC physicians.[7]

The Federation lobbied the various companies that market software in our country dedicated to OAT monitoring. The aim was to allow a series of different programs to be used while at the same time standardizing the way the data are stored and allowing the transfer of results between one clinic and another. This was crucial for organizing collaborative studies between the federated ACs. With this in mind, a list of specific items was drawn up and passed to the manufacturers to allow the collection and centralization of data to the coordinating clinic of each study. (See Exhibit 47–4.)

Guidance in Special Situations

Anticoagulant patients, especially the elderly, frequently develop intercurrent diseases and often need invasive treatment (eg, dental surgery, general surgery, invasive diagnostic procedures). In these cases, the patient must be protected from excessive hemorrhagic or thrombotic risk following improper variations of the anticoagulant dose.

STANDARDIZATION OF LABORATORY MONITORING

The FCSA devoted much effort toward standardization of laboratory monitoring. This has been achieved in several ways.

Exhibit 47–4
FCSA RECOMMENDATIONS REGARDING COMPUTER FEATURES FOR MONITORING ANTICOAGULATED PATIENTS

- Software available on a series of computers
- Daily automatic backup
- A different code for each AC
- Facility to collect and centralize data from AC that may use different computerized systems
- Online database for patients under treatment
- Database not online for patients who have discontinued treatment
- Therapeutic range and target
- Date OAT is started, drug used, and date therapy is expected to finish (with alarm)
- Possibility of applying labels to groups of patients
- Clinical diary for each visit with relative data to be collected
- Recording of hemorrhagic, thrombotic, or other complications (standard list)
- Agenda
- Automatic search for those not presenting for regular visit
- Standard form for results/prescription of therapy
- Printout of results
- Possibility of searching every database field
- Programs for basic statistical elaboration and tests of laboratory quality control (% of INRs and % of time in the range, above or below)

Training Courses

On a regular basis (once a year), the Federation organizes training courses where the attendees learn how to measure the INR and how to standardize the parameters needed for its calculation (Exhibit 47–5). This proved to be most useful as it forms the basis for the adoption of similar procedures in different laboratories. During the last few years, the educational activity of the Federation was expanded by including lectures and training on thrombophilia testing (Exhibit 47–5). This proved useful as most of the anticoagulant clinics act also as thrombosis centers where thrombophilic patients are screened on a regular basis.

Support to Manufacturers

Manufacturers of thromboplastins are encouraged to provide the international sensitivity index (ISI) of their systems in accordance with World Health Organization guidelines.[8] Whenever requested, the Federation and its allied scientific committee through a limited number of laboratories are also available to help manufacturers in assigning specific ISI to thromboplastin house standards or working lots before they enter the market. This has helped to harmonize the system of reporting INRs across the country.

Quality Assessment

The External Quality Assessment Scheme has been operative since the beginning of the Federation. This is

---

Exhibit 47–5
MAIN TOPICS ADDRESSED DURING LABORATORY TRAINING COURSES ORGANIZED BY FCSA

INR determination

1. Principles of thromboplastin calibration
2. Variables influencing the INR calculation
- International sensitivity index (ISI) accuracy
- Preanalytical variability of prothrombin time measurement
- The choice of mean normal prothrombin time (MNPT)

Laboratory investigation of thrombophilic states

1. Why to test
2. When to test
3. How to test

provided three times per year free of charge to all federated anticoagulant clinics. Participation in the scheme is compulsory, and the performance achieved by individual participants will soon form the basis for accreditation of clinics. The scheme is focused mainly on the INR system. It consists of two types of exercises (Exhibit 47–6): basic exercises to assess performance and special exercises focused on problems of relevance for the standardization of the INR system.

In the basic exercises, lyophilized plasmas from anticoagulated patients covering the therapeutic range are sent to the participants. They are requested to measure the INR with their own systems and to report the results, together with information on the type of instrument/thromboplastin combination used for testing. Each individual result is compared to the consensus mean and the performance is expressed both as z-score (standardized difference from the consensus mean)

and percentage discrepancy (percentage difference from the consensus mean). The overall performance of the system is assessed by calculation of the standard deviation and coefficient of variation (CV). The overall CV value (ie, regardless of the systems used for testing), which had been greater than 20% when the Federation was founded, declined to 10%–20% subsequently.[9] Once the evaluation is completed, participants receive a full set of data, including data on individual performance based on the system used for testing and as a whole, Youden plots, and summary of performance achieved in the previous exercises. Comments and suggestions are also sent to participants whenever deemed useful.

Special exercises have been organized and carried out over the years to address some of the most important standardization issues. These include the investigation of the relationship between factor V and the INR,[10] the effect of instrumentation on the ISI-INR system,[11] and the usefulness of lyophilized plasmas with assigned prothrombin time in terms of international thromboplastin standards for local ISI calibration.[12]

SELF-TESTING AND SELF-MANAGEMENT

The Federation has recently started a program to guide the implementation of whole blood coagulation monitors in the laboratory control of oral anticoagulant therapy. This included the organization of studies aimed at assessing the comparability of results obtained with the monitors versus those obtained with conventional measurement[13] and the value of self-testing and self-management.[14] Further efforts include guidelines that describe the steps to be undertaken by all involved parties (ie, manufacturers, patients, and anticoagulant clinics) to ensure the reliability of results obtained with whole blood coagulation monitors. The guidelines include recommendations to manufacturers on how to calibrate their devices according to the state of the art[15]; requirements to train patients for self-testing and self-management; requirements to assess the accuracy of results obtained with whole blood coagulation monitors in comparison with conventional laboratory methods to measure the INR; and requirements for daily checks of the performance of whole blood coagulation monitors as well as the organization of external quality assessment schemes.

Exhibit 47–6
MAIN CHARACTERISTICS OF THE EXTERNAL QUALITY ASSESSMENT SCHEME ORGANIZED BY FCSA

Basic exercises

1. Aims: To assess the performance (three times a year) in determining the INR
2. Materials: Three lyophilized plasma samples from patients on oral anticoagulants at increasing levels of anticoagulation
3. Data analyses:
- Calculation of (consensus) mean, standard deviation, and coefficient of variation
- Calculation for each participant of the discrepancy (both as percentage deviation and z-score) from the mean
- Historical performance obtained in past exercises
- Suggestions and/or recommendations to participants as appropriate

Special exercises

1. Aims: To address, by means of field studies, issues that are relevant for the INR standardization
2. Materials and data analyses: As appropriate

REFERENCES

1. Palareti G, Dettori AG, Ciavarella N, et al. A guide to oral anticoagulant therapy. *Haemost.* 1998;28:1–46.

2. Palareti G, Leali N, Coccheri S, et al. Bleeding complications of oral anticoagulant treatment: an inception-cohort, prospective collaborative study (ISCOAT). Italian Study on Complications of Oral Anticoagulant Therapy. *Lancet.* 1996;348:423–428.

3. Palareti G, Manotti C, D'Angelo A, et al. Thrombotic events during oral anticoagulant treatment: results of the inception-cohort, prospective, collaborative ISCOAT study: ISCOAT study group (Italian Study on Complications of Oral Anticoagulant Therapy). *Thromb Haemost.* 1997;78:1438–1443.

4. Palareti G, Hirsh J, Legnani C, et al. Oral anticoagulation treat-ment in the elderly—a nested, prospective, case-control study. *Arch Intern Med.* 2000;160:470–478.

5. Palareti G, Legnani C, Lee A, et al. A comparison of the safety and efficacy of oral anticoagulation for the treatment of venous thromboembolic disease in patients with or without malignancy. *Thromb Haemost.* 2000;84:805–810.

6. Pengo V, Legnani C, Noventa F, Palareti G. Oral anticoagulant therapy in patients with nonrheumatic atrial fibrillation and risk of bleeding—a multicenter inception cohort study. *Thromb Haemost.* 2001;85:418–422.

7. Manotti C, Moia M, Palareti G, Pengo V, Ria L, Dettori AG. Effect of computer-aided management on the quality of treatment in anticoagulated patients: a prospective, randomized, multicenter trial of APROAT (Automated PRogram for Oral Anticoagulant Treatment). *Haematologica.* 2001;86:1060–1070.

8. WHO Expert Committee on Biological Standardization. Guidelines for thromboplastins and plasma used to control oral anticoagulant therapy. WHO Technical Report Series, N. 889, 1999.

9. Tripodi A, Chantarangkul V. Federazione dei Centri di Sorveglianza Anticoagulati (FCSA). Rapporto dei primi anni di attività del programma per la valutazione esterna di qualità (VEQ) dei centri federati. *Medicina di Laboratorio.* 2002. In press.

10. Tripodi A, Chantarangkul V, Akkawat B, Clerici M, Mannucci PM. A partial factor V deficiency in anticoagulated lyophilized plasmas was identified as a cause of the International Normalized Ratio discrepancy in External Quality Assessment Scheme. *Thromb Res.* 1995;78:283.

11. Chantarangkul V, Tripodi A, Mannucci PM. The effect of instru-mentation on the calibration of thromboplastin. *Thromb Haemost.* 1992;67:588.

12. Chantarangkul V, Tripodi A, Cesana BM, Mannucci PM. Calibration of local systems for International Normalized Ratio (INR) with lyophilized calibrant plasmas improves the interlaboratory variability of the INR in the Italian External Quality Assessment Scheme. *Thromb Haemost.* 1999;82:1621–1626.

13. Cosmi B, Palareti G, Moia M, et al. Accuracy of a portable pro-thrombin time monitor (Coagucheck) in patients on chronic oral anticoagulant therapy: a prospective multicenter study. *Thromb Res.* 2000;100:279–286.

14. Cosmi B, Palareti G, Moia M, et al. Assessment of patient capability to self adjust oral anticoagulant dose: a multicenter study on home use of portable prothrombin time monitor (Coagucheck). *Haemotologica.* 2000;85:826–831.

15. Tripodi A, Cosmi B, Pengo V, Poli D, Testa S. Controllo della terapia anticoagulante orale. Linee guida per l'utilizzo delti strumenti portatili. FCSA 2002.

Index